AF698745

Trace Metals and other Contaminants in the Environment 8

Hazardous Substances and Human Health

Exposure, Impact and External Cost Assessment at the European Scale

Trace Metals and other Contaminants in the Environment 8

Series Editor: Jerome O. Nriagu
Department of Environmental and Industrial Health
School of Public Health
University of Michigan
Ann Arbor, Michigan 48109-2029
USA

Other volumes in this series:

Volume 1: Heavy Metals in the Environment, edited by J.P. Vernet
Volume 2: Impact of Heavy Metals on the Environment, edited by J.-P. Vernet
Volume 3: Photocatalytic Purification and Treatment of Water and Air, edited by D.F. Ollis and H. Al-Ekabi
Volume 4: Trace Elements – Their Distribution and Effects in the Environment, edited by B. Markert and K. Friese
Volume 5: Metals, Metalloids and Radionuclides in the Baltic Sea Ecosystem, P. Szefer
Volume 6: Bioindicators and Biomonitors: Principles, Concepts and Applications, edited by B.A. Markert, A.M. Breure and H.G. Zechmeister
Volume 7: Long-term Performance of Permeable Reactive Barriers, edited by K.E. Roehl, T. Meggyes, F.-G. Simon and D.I. Stewart

Trace Metals and other Contaminants in the Environment 8

Hazardous Substances and Human Health

Exposure, Impact and External Cost Assessment at the European Scale

Till M. Bachmann

University of Stuttgart
Institute of Energy Economics and the Rational Use of Energy (IER)
Stuttgart, Germany

ELSEVIER

Amsterdam • Boston • Heidelberg • London • New York • Oxford
Paris • San Diego • San Francisco • Singapore • Sydney • Tokyo

Elsevier
Radarweg 29, PO Box 211, 1000 AE Amsterdam, The Netherlands
The Boulevard, Langford Lane, Kidlington, Oxford OX5 1GB, UK

First edition 2006

Copyright © 2006 Elsevier B.V. All rights reserved.

No part of this publication may be reproduced, stored in a retrieval system or transmitted in any form or by any means electronic, mechanical, photocopying, recording or otherwise without prior written permission of the publisher

Permissions may be sought directly from Elsevier's Science & Technology Rights Department in Oxford, UK: phone (+44) (0) 1865 843830; fax (+44) (0) 1865 853333; e-mail: permissions@elsevier.com. Alternatively you can submit your request online by visiting the Elsevier web site at http://www.elsevier.com/locate/permissions, and selecting *Obtaining permission to use Elsevier material*

Notice
No responsibility is assumed by the Publisher for any injury and/or damage to persons or property as a matter of products liability, negligence or otherwise, or from any use or operation of any methods, products, instructions or ideas contained in the material herein. Because of rapid advances in the medical sciences, in particular, independent verification of diagnoses and drug dosages should be made

Library of Congress Cataloging in Publication Data
A catalog record is available from the Library of Congress

British Library Cataloguing in Publication Data
A catalogue record is available from the British Library

ISBN-13: 978-0-444-52218-4
ISBN-10: 0-444-52218-2
D-93
Series ISSN: 0927-5215

For information on all book publications
visit our website at books.elsevier.com

Printed and bound in The Netherlands
06 07 08 09 10 10 9 8 7 6 5 4 3 2 1

Working together to grow
libraries in developing countries

www.elsevier.com | www.bookaid.org | www.sabre.org

ELSEVIER BOOK AID International Sabre Foundation

In memory of my beloved mother
who died from pancreas cancer in November 2004.

Preface

There is widespread public concern about hazardous chemicals that are contained in air, soil, water and food which is supported by scientific evidence, however, not as encompassing. Policy has therefore adopted a series of laws and regulations with regard to the emissions into and concentration levels in different media including food. As policy makers do not only have to consider the protection of the environment but also need to ensure a well-functioning economy at the same time, these limit or target values need to be set in a balanced way. The main problem, however, is to compare or rather optimize the different costs for achieving these targets with the benefits to society by having a smaller exposure to hazardous substances. According to neoclassical welfare economics theory, the optimal pollution level is found when the costs of the last implemented measure that just leads to the achievement of an environmental state (e.g., by implementing emission abatement techniques such as filters) are equal to the incremental increase in welfare (e.g., a better health status) valued in monetary terms. The assessment of the increases in welfare expressed in monetary values is associated with a rather high degree of uncertainty. This is due to the fact that not all aspects of environmental pollution can at present be valued (e.g., biodiversity loss) and due to the uncertainties in the employed model-based assessments involving information on emissions, description of the environmental fate of substances, behavioural patterns of people, effect models and their valuation approaches. As a result, current cost-benefit analyses are conducted in a way that they are complemented by qualitative aspects to a greater or lesser extent. It needs to be noted, however, that even in such cases in which the knowledge base is more reliable the target setting process in the end is primarily driven by political constraints and the outcome of complex international negotiations, rather than robust scientific evidence.

This book sets out to improve the reliability of cost-benefit analyses particularly of hazardous substances present in air, water, soil and food. It suggests that the human health risk assessment of chemicals is performed in a bottom-up analysis that is based on a spatially resolved multimedia modelling approach. In order to allow for cost-benefit analyses to be conducted, this approach is accompanied by monetary valuation of human health impacts.

Till M. Bachmann
University of Stuttgart
Institute of Energy Economics and the Rational Use of Energy
Stuttgart, Germany

September 2005

Acknowledgements

Any research conducted nowadays is marked by a high level of collaboration, even more so, when working in an interdisciplinary area of research. Hence, the work described in this book would have been impossible without the invaluable contributions, inspirations and comments of several colleagues. I would like to express my gratitude to the partners working in the EC-funded research project OMNIITOX for their excellent cooperation which has inspired me in developing the environmental fate, exposure and impact assessment model. In this respect, I especially feel grateful for fruitful discussions with Dr. David W. Pennington who also contributed to outlining Table 2-3.

In addition to that, I would like to thank my supervisors, Dr.-Ing. Rainer Friedrich and Dr. Olivier Jolliet, as the work described here would have not been possible without their fair comments and experience.

Special thanks go to my colleagues at the Institute of Energy Economics and the Rational Use of Energy, University of Stuttgart, Germany, for offering helpful comments and providing support especially with respect to database, Geographic Information System (GIS) and programming skills. I am particularly grateful for the implementation of trace elements into the software tool EcoSense and the provision of the respective deposition fields by my colleague Dr.-Ing. Bert Droste-Franke.

Furthermore, the developed approach relies on many data. I want to express my gratitude for all those data that are freely distributed especially when they have already been financed by the public (i.e., through taxes) as is regularly the case in the US. I also gratefully acknowledge the provision of global hydrological and lake data by the Center for Environmental Systems Research, University of Kassel, Germany.

The financial support of the European Commission through the "Energy, environment and sustainable development" programme given to the NewExt (New elements for the assessment of external costs from energy technologies, EC Project number: ENG1-2000-00129) and GREENSENSE projects (An applied integrated environmental impact assessment framework for the European union, EC Project number: EVG1-2000-00022) as well as through the "Sustainable and Competitive Growth" research programme given to the OMNIITOX-project (Operational Models aNd Information tools for Industrial applications of eco/TOXicological impact assessments, EC Project number: G1RD-CT-2001-00501) is also acknowledged. The realisation of this work would not have been accomplished without this external funding. In addition, I would like to thank the foundation *Stiftung Landesbank Baden-Württemberg: nature and the environment* for awarding a grant to this work.

And last but - for sure - not least, there is no way to adequately express my gratitude for the patient support of my wife, Martina Bachmann, who encouraged me to pursue my goals and, thus, has a considerable share in the realisation of this book. Also the birth of my two daughters, Lea and Mara, during the development of this work has been very inspiring and brought new perspectives and a so far unexperienced kind of happiness into my life.

Zusammenfassung

Die von der Europäischen Kommission geförderte Projektreihe 'ExternE' beschäftigt sich mit der Quantifizierung der durch Energiewandlungssysteme verursachten externen Kosten. Dabei wurden Expositionen und daraus folgende Schäden durch Schadstoffe, die in größeren Mengen in die Luft emittiert werden, abgeschätzt und bewertet. Es wird dem sogenannten Wirkungspfadansatz gefolgt, der durch die vorliegende Arbeit um Expositionen erweitert wurde, die über Boden und Wasser stattfinden. Diese Erweiterung wurde in Form eines Softwareprogramms mit Namen WATSON ('integrated WATer and SOil environmental fate, exposure and impact assessment model of Noxious substances') implementiert, das räumlich aufgelöst die Exposition gegenüber Schadstoffen durch Nahrungsaufnahme innerhalb Europas abschätzt.

Der Abschätzung der Exposition liegt eine Kopplung von Chemie-Transport-Modellen für Luft einerseits und Boden und Wasser andererseits zu Grunde. Dabei wurde für die Abschätzung im Bereich Luft auf das bestehende Softwareprogramm EcoSense zurückgegriffen (European Commission, 2003d), während das *environmental fate* im Boden und Wasser mit Hilfe eines neu entwickelten, räumlich aufgelösten Boxmodells abgeschätzt wird, das als Mackay-Modell level III/IV (Mackay, 1991) klassifiziert werden kann. Die beiden Chemie-Transport-Modelle unterscheiden sich nicht nur hinsichtlich der betrachteten Medien, sondern auch bezüglich der räumlichen Auflösung: das Luftmodell basiert auf einem regelmäßigen Gitter, das Boden-Wasser-Modell ist räumlich differenziert gemäß Einzugsgebietsinformationen. Beide *fate* Modelle verwenden Parameterwerte zur Beschreibung der Umwelt, die auf mehrjährigen Mittelwerten beruhen, und können somit als klimatologische Modelle bezeichnet werden. Das Chemie-Transport-Modell für Boden und Wasser weist weitere Besonderheiten auf. Dabei sind die räumliche Differenzierung von Kompartimenten, die pH-Abhängigkeit des Verteilungsverhaltens von Spurenelementen und verbesserte oder neue Prozesse wie bevorzugtes Fließen (*preferential flow*), Ernteentzug, Bodenerosion in Abhängigkeit von der Landnutzung und Unterscheidung von Flüssen und Seen zu nennen. Im Rahmen dieser Arbeit konnte gezeigt werden, dass diese Besonderheiten einen erheblichen Einfluss auf die menschliche Exposition haben.

Basierend auf den abgeschätzten Konzentrationen in der Umwelt erfolgt die Expositionsabschätzung, die für die Nahrungsaufnahme (Ingestion) komplexer ist als für die Exposition über die Atemwege (Inhalation). Dies ist darauf zurückzuführen, dass der Mensch eine Vielfalt an unterschiedlichen Lebensmitteln zu sich nimmt, deren landwirtschaftliche oder gewässerbezogene Produktion zudem räumlich verteilt ist. Die Expositionsabschätzung gegenüber Nahrungsmitteln basiert auf einem ortsabhängigen Ansatz zur Risikoabschätzung, der von der US-amerikanischen Umweltschutzbehörde für Sondermüllverbrennungsanlagen empfohlen wird (United States - Environmental Protection Agency, 1998), wobei versucht wird, keine Vorsorge-, sondern repräsentative Werte zu ermitteln. Die Expositionsabschätzung erfolgt auf der Ebene administrativer Einheiten, so dass der Verfügbarkeit von Nahrungs- und Bevölkerungsdaten Rechnung getragen wird. Handel wird als weiterer Bestandteil des *environmental fate* der Schadstoffe betrachtet. Es wird angenommen, dass er zu einer Vergleichmäßigung der Schadstoffkonzentrationen in den jeweiligen kommerziellen Nahrungs- und Futtermitteln innerhalb der geographischen Grenzen des Modells führt, bevor es zur Exposition von Mensch und Nutztier kommt. Als Maß für die aggregierte Exposition gegenüber Schadstoffen wird das Konzept des aufgenommenen Anteils der emittierten Menge einer Substanz genommen ('Intake Fraction', Bennett et al., 2002). Dadurch dass sehr unterschiedliche Zeiträume bei der Exposition über die Atemwege und über die Nahrung relevant sind, insbesondere wenn Pulsemissionsszenarien untersucht werden, wird die *Intake Fraction* getrennt nach Inhalation und Ingestion sowie für unterschiedliche Zeitspannen ausgewiesen. Eine weitere Neuerung besteht darin, dass die *Intake Fraction* nur die Schadstoffspezies berücksichtigt, die auch zur schädlichen Wirkung beitragen, weshalb von einer *effective Intake Fraction* gesprochen wird.

Zur vollständigen Verfolgung der Wirkungspfadanalyse mangelt es insbesondere an Informationen über Effekte durch die Nahrungsexposition, die anhand epidemiologischer Studien abgeleitet wurden. Daher erfolgt die Schadensabschätzung mit Hilfe des β_{ED10} *slope factor*-Ansatzes (Crettaz, 2000), der mit dem *Disability Adjusted Life Years* (DALYs)-Konzept kombiniert wird, das auch von der Weltgesundheitsorganisation (WHO) in Gesundheitsstatistiken verwendet wird. Da die DALYs Gesundheitsschäden durch Erkrankungen und vorzeitige Todesfälle in Äquivalenten von verlorenen Lebensjahren ('Years Of Life Lost', YOLLs) ausdrücken und aggregieren, kann eine monetäre Bewertung gemäß dem Standardansatz der ExternE-Projekte erfolgen. Als Schwachpunkt der publizierten und hier verwendeten DALY-Werte werden insbesondere die Gewichte für Gesundheitsbeeinträchtigungen gesehen, die Krankheitszeiten in Äquivalente an verlorenen Lebensjahren umwandeln.

Im Einklang mit der politischen Schwerpunktsetzung bezüglich Schadstoffüberwachung und -regulierung fokussiert sich die vorgestellte Analyse auf persistente Schadstoffe und insbesondere auf Schwermetalle. Im Einzelnen werden die Spurenelement Arsen, Cadmium, Chrom und Blei untersucht. Das entwickelte Modell ist momentan beschränkt bezüglich der potenziell zu analysierenden Schadstoffe. Entsprechend können nur Schadstoffe untersucht werden, die praktisch nicht volatil, d. h. aufgrund ihres Dampfdrucks nicht flüchtig sind. Zudem treten Schwermetalle (oder besser Spurenelemente) in verschiedenen Bindungsformen auf, die in unterschiedlichem Maße bioverfügbar und toxisch sind. Dem wird insofern Rechnung getragen, als das Verteilungsverhalten in Abhängigkeit vom pH-Wert modelliert und das Expositionsmaß effektiv ermittelt wird ('*effective Intake Fraction*', siehe oben). Ein Vergleich mit gemessenen Werten für Boden, Wasser und Nahrungsmittel hat ergeben, dass die in dieser Studie abgeschätzten Konzentrationen innerhalb der Erwartungswerte liegen.

Szenarioberechnungen wurden für Luft-Emissionen sowohl einzelner Kohlekraftwerke als auch auf gesamt-europäischer Ebene durchgeführt. In allen Fällen zeigte es sich, dass die menschliche Exposition über den Nahrungsweg gegenüber Ein-Jahres-Puls-Emissionen nicht nur langsam mit der Zeit ansteigt, sondern auch eine Verschiebung in der Bedeutung der Nahrungsmittel im Zeitverlauf stattfindet. Im Fall von Arsen war kurzfristig eine Mischung aus Getreide und Milchprodukten zu etwa 70 % für die Nahrungsmittelexposition verantwortlich, während langfristig die Milchprodukte allein 80 % ausmachten. Die Beitrag der Exposition über die Atemwege ist gegenüber der der Nahrungsaufnahme marginal und bestätigt Ergebnisse für Cadmium und Arsen (European Commission, 2000b). Der Vergleich der Kraftwerksstandorte ergab, dass die Variabilität der Exposition und der Schäden über den Nahrungspfad ähnlich groß ist wie über die Atemwege trotz des vergleichmäßigenden Effekts des Handels auf die Schadstoffkonzentrationen in den Nahrungsmitteln. Dieser Effekt des Handels lässt demnach die Standortunterschiede nicht in dem Maße verschwinden, wie es speziell von Spadaro und Rabl (2004) postuliert worden ist.

Die für die untersuchten Spurenelemente ermittelten Schadensfaktoren wurden mit denen für die klassischen Luftschadstoffe verglichen. Der Vergleich für Expositionen über die Atemwege ergab, dass die quantifizierbaren externen Kosten durch die gesamt-europäischen Emissionen der Spurenelemente in die Luft im Jahr 1990 vernachlässigbar klein gegenüber den durch SO_2, NO_x, NH_3, Primärpartikeln und NMVOCs verursachten Schäden sind. Der Unterschied beträgt vier Größenordnungen. Anders sieht es bei Expositionen gegenüber den Spurenelementen über die Nahrungswege aus. Diese können bis zu mehr als 10 % der durch die klassischen Luftschadstoffe verursachten gesamten quantifizierbaren externen Kosten ausmachen, wenn mit 0 % diskontiert wird. Diesbezüglich tragen vor allem die nicht-krebsbezogenen Effekte durch Blei bei, die zu einer Erhöhung des Blutdrucks führen. Allerdings hängt dieser Beitrag sehr stark von der Wahl der Diskontrate ab. Für den Fall, dass eine positive Diskontrate angenommen wird, werden die Schadensfaktoren für die Nahrungsaufnahme beträchtlich kleiner. Dies ist insbesondere auf die Persistenz der betrachteten Schadstoffe zurückzuführen (vgl. Hellweg, 2000; van den Bergh et al., 2000; Huijbregts et al., 2001; de Vries et al., 2004) gepaart mit ihrem vergleichsweise langsamen Ausbreitungsverhalten. Im Falle der Spurenelemente mit langsamer Dynamik, d. h. Arsen und Chrom, gelangen innerhalb der ersten 100 Jahre nach einer Ein-Jahres-Puls-Emission weniger als 2 % der potenziell zur Exposition beitragenden Menge über die Nahrung zum Menschen gemäß den hier vorgenommenen Abschätzungen. Somit sind die menschlichen Expositionen über Boden und Wasser generell dann besonders bedeutsam, wenn mittel- bis langfristige Zeiträume betrachtet werden. Diese Expositionen sind daher im besonderen Maße relevant bezüglich einer nachhaltigen Entwicklung und dabei insbesondere hinsichtlich der intergenerationellen Gerechtigkeit.

Der abgeschätzte geringe Beitrag der durch Spurenelemente verursachten quantifizierbaren externen Kosten zu den insgesamt quantifizierten externen Kosten durch die klassischen Luftschadstoffe konnte zuvor auch für Expositionen über die Nahrungsaufnahme von Dioxinen und Substanzen mit ähnlicher Wirkung (v. a. PCBs) für einzelne Länder gezeigt werden (Droste-Franke et al., 2003). Allerdings ist dabei zu berücksichtigen, dass die Anzahl der durch die vorliegende Arbeit zusätzlich bewertbaren Schadstoffe klein ist im Vergleich zu denen, die potenziell noch in Betracht zu ziehen sind. Ihr Beitrag zu den quantifizierbaren externen Kosten könnte erheblich sein. Dabei wird als hauptsächlich limitierender Faktor die Verfügbarkeit von Dosis-Wirkungsbeziehungen gesehen. Um zusätzlich noch solche Substanzen methodisch zu erfassen, für die Dosis-Wirkungsbeziehungen bekannt sind (wie etwa Quecksilber und Dioxine), bedarf es einer Weiterentwicklung des dargestellten methodischen Ansatzes. Zu nennen sind vor allem der betrachtete geographische Raum, der zumindest auf die Nordhemisphäre, wenn nicht sogar auf die ganze Erde erweitert werden müsste, und die vollständige Integration der Medien Luft, Boden und Wasser in einem Chemie-Transport-Modell.

Der verfolgte Ansatz stellt einen Mittelweg dar zwischen dem ambitionierten Ziel, Spurenelementkontaminationen räumlich aufgelöst auf europäischer Ebene zu erfassen, einerseits und der Modellierung dieser Substanzen gemäß dem aktuellen Kenntnisstand auf kleinerer Ebene andererseits. Die vorliegende Arbeit leistet einen wichtigen Beitrag zur Verbesserung der Wissensbasis hinsichtlich der Größenordnung der (durch den Menschen verursachten) Gesundheitsschäden und externen Kosten, da bisher insbesondere hinsichtlich der externen Kosten keine Informationen über andere Expositionspfade als die Inhalation vorhanden waren.

List of Figures

List of Tables

Abbreviations and acronyms

ADI	Acceptable Daily Intake
AQFD	Air Quality Framework Directive (EU)
AW	Ash Weight
BAT	Best Available Techniques
BMC	benchmark concentration
BMD	benchmark dose
CBA	Cost-Benefit Analysis
CLRTAP	Convention on Long-Range Transboundary Air Pollution
COD	Chemical Oxygen Demand
COI	Cost of illness
Corg	organic carbon
CORINAIR	Core Inventory of Air Emissions in Europe
CORINE	Coordinated Information on the Environment
CTD	Characteristic Travel Distance
DALY	Disability Adjusted Life Years
DNA	Deoxyribonucleic Acid
DW	Dry Weight
EC	European Commission
EEA	European Environment Agency
EMEP	Co-operative programme for monitoring and evaluation of long range transmission of air pollutants in Europe
ERICA	European rivers and catchments database
EU	European Union
EU15	the countries being member of the European Union as of 1995
EUROSTAT	Statistical Office of the European Communities
ExternE	Externalities of Energy
FAO	Food and Agriculture Organization of the United Nations
FBS	Food Balance Sheet
FW	Fresh Weight

GIS	Geographic Information System
GNP	Gross National Product
HELCOM	Baltic Marine Environment Protection Commission (Helsinki Commission)
HHRAP	Human Health Risk Assessment Protocol
HTP	Human Toxicity Potential
HYDRO1k	Family of hydrologically related GIS datasets based on a 1 km grid
IAEA	International Atomic Energy Agency
ICP	International Cooperative Programme on Effects of Air Pollution
ILSI	International Life Science Institute
IPPC	Integrated Pollution Prevention and Control (EU Directive)
ISC	Industrial Source Complex Model
ITP	Individual Time Preference
LAI	Leaf Area Index
LCA	Life Cycle Analysis
LCI	Life Cycle Inventory
LCIA	Life Cycle Impact Assessment
LOAEL	Lowest Observed Adverse Effect Level
MEI	Maximally Exposed Individual
MM	mineral matter
MOE	Margin Of Exposure
MOS	Margin Of Safety
n/a	not available or not applicable
NEW	Net Economic Welfare
NMVOC	Non-methane volatile organic compound
NOAEL	No Observed Adverse Effect Level
NUTS	Nomenclature des Unités Territoriales Statistiques (Nomenclature of Territorial Units for Statistics)
NUTS0	Administrative unit at the country level
NUTS1	Administrative unit at e.g. the federal state or canton level
NUTS2	Administrative unit between e.g. the federal state or canton and the municipal level
NUTS3	Administrative unit at the municipal level
OAT	one-factor-at-a-time (sensitivity screening approach)
OCC	Opportunity Cost of Capital
OCDD	Octachlorinated dibenzo-p-dioxin
ODE	ordinary differential equation
OM	organic matter
PAH	Polycyclic Aromatic Hydrocarbon (group of compounds)
PBT	Persistent, Bioaccumulative and Toxic chemicals

PCB	Polychlorinated biphenyl
PCDD	Polychlorinated dibenzo-p-dioxin
PCDF	Polychlorinated dibenzofuran
PEC	Predicted Environmental Concentration
PNEC	Predicted No Effect Concentration
POP	Persistent Organic Pollutant
PTO	person trade-off
QSAR	Quantitative Structure Activity Relationship
RA	Risk Assessment
RCF	Root Concentration Factor
RCR	Risk Characterisation Ratio
RfC	Reference Concentration
RfD	Reference Dose
RME	Reasonable Maximum Exposures
SCALE	Science, Children, Awareness, EU Legislation and Continuous Evaluation (initiative at the EU level)
SETAC	Society of Environmental Toxicology and Chemistry
SROM	Source Receptor Ozone Model
STP	Social Time Preference
t	tonnes (metric) , ,
TBT	tributyltin
TCDD	2,3,7,8-tetrachlorodibenzo(p)dioxin
TCDD	tetrachlorinated dibenzo-p-dioxin (usually the 2,3,7,8-substituted congener)
TD50	median Tumor Dose
TEF	Toxic Equivalency Factor
TEQ	Toxic Equivalent
TGD	Technical Guidance Documents
TRIM	Total Risk Integrated Methodology
TSCF	Transpiration Stream Concentration Factor
UK	United Kingdom
UN/ECE	United Nations Economic Commission for Europe
US	United States of America
US-EPA	United States - Environmental Protection Agency
US-EPA	United States Environmental Protection Agency
USLE	Universal Soil Loss Equation
USSR	Union of Soviet Socialist Republics
UWM	Uniform World Model
VLYL	Value of life years lost
VOC	Volatile Organic Compound

VOLY	Value of a life year
VOSL	Value of a statistical life
vPvB	Persistent and very Bioaccumulative chemicals
VSL	Value of a statistical life
WATSON	integrated WATer and SOil environmental fate, exposure and impact assessment model of Noxious substances
WFD	Water Framework Directive (EU)
WHO	World Health Organisation
WTA	Willingness to accept
WTM	Windrose Trajectory Model
WTP	Willingness to pay
YLD	Years of Life lived with a Disability
YOLL	Years of Life Lost
yr	year(s)

1 Introduction

The presently reached population together with the achieved degree of industrialisation can be considered the single most important driver for the usage and exploitation of natural resources although in many industrialised countries the perception to be overpopulated does not prevail. Not only the extraction of natural resources like minerals and fuels but also the release of sometimes hazardous substances to the environment need to be mentioned in this context. Although in many parts of the world policy has adopted respective laws in order to cut these emissions down to certain levels, the contaminants (still) released pose a potential threat to living organisms, be it humans, animals, plants or microorganisms in the affected regions. Economy which in principle takes care of the proper allocation of scarce resources comprising mineral resources, food, money, human capital amongst many others often fails when such side effects are not reflected in the prices of the respective goods being traded and finally consumed. These side effects are referred to as *externalities* or *external effects* and may in principle be positive or negative. In such *incomplete markets*, the market mechanism leads to allocation failures due to the lack of inclusion of external effects in the prices expressed in monetary terms. From a cost-benefit perspective, it is, therefore, necessary to convert these external effects into monetary units, especially in order to help in the policy decision-making process setting effort-effectiveness balanced regulatory standards. This in turn is done with the purpose to ensure societies to maintain or even increase their level of welfare.

Over the last decade in a series of projects funded by the European Commission, a methodology has been developed that assesses damages from pressures on the environment, most notably contaminant emissions to air due to energy conversion techniques (European Commission, 1995, 1999a; Friedrich and Bickel, 2001a). In a bottom-up analysis, this so-called *Impact Pathway Approach* follows the way of contaminants from their releases over their reactions and distributions in the environment (termed *environmental fate*) to the exposure and finally impacts on human health and other receptors such as building materials and crops.

In a second step, these impacts are then valued in order to yield damages in monetary terms. The monetised negative external effects are termed *external costs*. This approach is especially recognized in the area of externality valuation at the EU level (Rossetti di Valdalbero, 2004). Beside other criticisms, however, it lacks impact assessment schemes that take contaminations of the terrestrial and aquatic environments into account. Effects that were missing include: acidification and eutrophication, toxic impacts on non-human organisms potentially even leading to changes in biodiversity, and impacts on human health due to ingestion of food and drinking water. Damages to human health always by far (i.e., more than 90 %) dominate the external costs due to air pollution in the analyses undertaken so far (e.g., Friedrich and Bickel, 2001b; Droste-Franke and Friedrich, 2003). Additionally, the indirect exposure through food appears to be the dominant route of exposure to persistent substances (e.g., Finley and Paustenbach, 1994; Price et al., 1996) about which there exists public concern (Lindberg, 1989; Kabata-Pendias and Pendias, 1992; Council of the European Union, 1996a, 1996b; United Nations - Economic Commission for Europe, 1998; Parliament and Council of the European Union, 2000; European Commission, 2003f, 2003g; Barbante et al., 2004; Rat von Sachverständigen für Umweltfragen, 2004). Therefore, the framework for estimating external costs shall be extended particularly with respect to impacts on human health due to ingestion of contaminants.

Given that the existing Impact Pathway Analysis constitutes an approach to assess external costs from inhalation exposure, the purpose of the present work is to identify, provide and apply a methodological framework for the estimation of external costs due to ingestion exposures that is consistent with that for inhalation exposures. This means that the approach to be developed needs to fulfil the following requirements:

- providing assistance with respect to the evaluation of contaminants released by energy conversion techniques ending up in environmental media such as soil, water and foodstuff,
- providing the possibility to evaluate point sources like facilities as well as area sources such as economies across the whole of Europe in a spatially-resolved way,
- allowing for the assessment of impacts on human health at present as well as in the long run for example with respect to sustainability questions, and
- in contrast to risk assessments, striving for representative estimates rather than introducing a fair amount of conservatism.

Chapter 2 gives an introduction into human health and risk assessments in general and to the Impact Pahtway Approach in particular. It concludes with the formulation of the specific aims and requirements in terms of the modelling approach.

A general survey on existing environmental impact assessment frameworks will be given in Chapter 3. The realm of hazardous substances is rather large. Different substance groups, however, have different requirements as to the formulation of their environmental fate and exposure assessment. As is reasoned in section 3.2, the aim of the present work in the first place is to develop a methodological framework for the assessment of impacts due to oral exposure. For the tool development and case study part of the present work, consequently, a prioritisation of substances is undertaken in order to show the application of the methodological development. Chapter 3 concludes that none of the reviewed approaches fulfils the formulated requirements for impacts due to ingestion exposures towards the prioritised substances. Consequently, the needs for model development with respect to including the impacts due to oral intake of substances into the Impact Pathway Approach are identified and formulated. These will be addressed in the following methodological Chapters: on the general outline which includes the aspects of atmospheric modelling and spatial differentation of the ground into zones (Chapter 4), the environmental fate modelling of the terrestrial and aquatic environment (Chapters 5 and 6, respectively), the exposure and impact assessment (Chapter 7), and monetary valuation (Chapter 8). Note that the description especially of the environmental fate and exposure assessment parts are rather complex and are, therefore, only generally given in these Chapters. A more thorough documentation of these components is provided in Appendix A.

In Chapter 9, the developed approach for the prioritised substances will be evaluated. This will be done by means of a general discussion of the assumptions made and decisions taken, a comparison with independent data, scenario analyses, and sensitivity analyses of the key parameters.

The application of the extended Impact Pathway Approach to case studies is then presented. Principally two types of scenarios will be looked at: one dealing with marginal emission situations and the other with releases from whole economies (in Chapter 10 and 11, respectively).

The work will close with a Chapter on conclusions including perspectives (Chapter 12).

2 Assessment of human health impacts and the approach followed

Generally speaking, impacts on human health due to human activities shall be assessed and valued in the present work. Due to the spatial coverage which entails a "lack of full access ... to the phenomena of interest" (Oreskes et al., 1994, p. 644), it is necessary to perform this assessment by means of a numerical simulation model. The methodological framework to be followed consists of the *Impact Pathway Approach* which will be outlined below (section 2.2). At the onset of the present work, it focused on exposures to air pollutants via inhalation which is why the method especially needed an extension with respect to ingestion exposures via food and/or drinking water. This has brought about the necessity to introduce the media soil and water into the analysis. Furthermore, a detailed and explicit human exposure assessment needs to be set in place for the ingestion exposure route. Also for consistency reasons, the aims and requirements for the respective model development will be defined based on a general modelling review (section 2.3). The type of modelling approach to follow will then be defined. In Chapter 3, the needs for model development are formulated based on a review of existing models and according to the prioritised contaminants.

The focus is set on human health because it is known from experience that damages to human health dominate by far the external costs out of the set of receptors for which impact assessment and monetary valuation schemes are available beside global warming damages (European Commission, 1999b). It shall be noted that the evaluation of impacts on living organisms other than humans may comprise another important externality maybe even leading to a loss of species in certain settings, thereby potentially reducing biodiversity. The consideration of such impacts, however, is rather complex as one has to deal with many species showing rather different sensitivities which may even depend on the habitat in which they live. The protection of 'biodiversity' is very often formulated as a goal in the scientific as well as the political context. The definition of 'biodiversity' as an indicator, however, is rather diverse due to the fact that there are many different aspects to it (cf. Linares Llamas, 2003) all of which are quite difficult to operationalise. Examples of these aspects are diversity in genes, conservation of species where they exist or at a global level. The inclusion of impacts on other living organisms especially with respect to biodiversity is, thus, deemed a whole study area of its own which may be addressed in future investigations.

Before continuing, some definitions or considerations on some of the terms used within this study are given as follows.

2.1 Definitions and considerations of some terms

2.1.1 Nomenclature of substances of concern

In the environmental context, substances of concern are termed by notions like environmental chemical, xenobiotics, hazardous or poisonous substances, contaminants or pollutants. All of these have specific connotations. Their application shall be outlined briefly here.

Environmental chemicals, sometimes also referred to as 'man made substances' can either simply be defined as chemicals that occur in the environment (Walker et al., 2001) or as substances which enter the environment as a result of human activity and occur in concentrations or amounts that may put living organisms, in particular humans, to a risk according to Anonymous (1971) cited in Bliefert (1997) and Korte (1992). Following the second definition, environmental chemicals can furthermore be differentiated into those of natural origin and 'foreign' substances (Korte, 1992). In a strict sense, the latter are exclusively synthetic substances (Römbke and Moltmann, 1996) and are, thus, foreign to any organism, i.e., they do not play a part in their normal biochemistry. They can be termed *xenobiotics*. Environmental chemicals of natural origin may for instance be heavy metals that are enriched in the environment due to a human activity, a wide-spread example being lead in soils which has been released due to combustion of traffic fuel.

The terms *contaminant* and *pollutant* can be described separately but are often in effect synonymous. Both are used to describe chemicals that are found at levels judged to be above those that would normally be expected. Whereas the definition of 'contaminant' ends here which is simply equivalent to the second definition given for environmental chemicals above, pollution should mean contamination resulting in adverse biological effects in the environment in a scientific precise way (Chaney and Ryan, 1994; Chapman, 2001). This is, however, not an easy distinction to make. Whether or not a contaminant is a pollutant may depend on its level in the environment and the organism or system being considered

(Walker et al., 2001). Thus, one particular substance may be a contaminant relative to one species but pollutant relative to another. Even more complicated, it may be a contaminant for one individual of a population and a pollutant to a more sensitive one of the same population. Finally, the question about the existence of thresholds for an effect related to the occurrence of a contaminant is crucial. In line with the reasoning in section 7.3, in practice it is often difficult to demonstrate that harm is not being caused so that in effect pollutant and contaminant become synonymous (Walker et al., 2001). Correspondingly, the terms 'environmental chemical', 'contaminant' and 'pollutant' are used interchangeably in this work.

Some environmental chemicals are of higher concern than others. In the context of potentially toxic substances, composite terms for pollutants used in the regulatory process (e.g., of the European Union, European Commission, 2001a) are for instance: Persistent Organic Pollutants (POPs), Persistent, Bioaccumulative and Toxic (PBT) chemicals and very Persistent and very Bioaccumulative (vPvB) substances. As one can see from these notions, in any case their characteristics with respect to persistency give reason for increased attention which will have implications on the choice of contaminants on which the present study focuses (see section 3.2).

2.1.2 Nomenclature with respect to exposure

Human exposure may occur via different *routes of exposure*. The main exposure routes are inhalation of air, ingestion of food, drinking water and other matter such as soil, and dermal exposure (United States - Environmental Protection Agency, 1992, 1997c; World Health Organisation, 2000a; European Commission, 2003c). Other routes of exposure exist such as intravenous, intraperitoneal, subcutaneous and intramuscular routes (cf. United States - Environmental Protection Agency, 1994) occurring especially in the medical domain. These are, however, less important for environmental chemicals.

When assessing substances in the soil and water environment, there is no doubt that ingestion is to be included in the analysis. Inhalation may also need to be considered for instance in cases when people are exposed to substances volatilising from contaminated tap water (cf. McKone, 1993a; Finley and Paustenbach, 1994; Georgopoulos et al., 1997; Hopke et al., 2000).

Another distinction of exposures can be made according to *target populations* (e.g., workers, consumers, public, European Commission, 2003a; European Centre for Ecotoxicology and Toxicology of Chemicals, 1994). The assessment of occupational exposures as well as exposures towards consumer products is beyond the scope of the present analysis.

A third way of classifying exposures is into *direct* and *indirect*. Different definitions and distinctions are, however, made. For instance, in some regulatory risk assessment guidelines it is distinguished between direct exposures for example at the working place or through consumer products and indirect exposure via the environment, i.e., exposure via air, water, soil and food (European Centre for Ecotoxicology and Toxicology of Chemicals, 1994; European Commission, 2003a). A different distinction is made in analyses making use of environmental fate and exposure models noting that the guidelines mentioned above may involve such tools as well. In the latter context, only exposure towards exposure media that are not part of the environmental fate model is considered indirect, i.e., inhalation of air and ingestion of water are direct whereas ingestion of food is indirect (McKone, 1993a; van de Meent et al., 1996; International Council of Chemical Associations, 1998; Hertwich et al., 2000; Huijbregts et al., 2000a; Schwartz, 2000; Trapp and Schwartz, 2000). Further note that only inhalation is considered direct by United States - Environmental Protection Agency (1998) most likely because the fate analysis only covers air from which the other media's concentrations are derived.

It has been mentioned above that the assessment of exposures at the work place and due to consumer products which are classified as direct exposures among other by European Commission (2003a) is out of the scope of the present analysis. Therefore, the second approach to distinguish between direct and indirect exposure is followed. Indirect exposure, hence, means ingestion of food. As a consequence, direct exposure (of humans) principally occurs via inhalation of air, ingestion of drinking water and soil particles, and skin contact to air, water and soil.

Due to the model's spatial resolution (section 4.3), exposure is primarily assessed for diffuse inputs to the environment for example by multiple emission sources. However, one needs to be aware that exposure to contaminants in food and drinking water but also in ambient air can also originate from various other sources like

- accidental releases (Alloway and Steinnes, 1999; Buckley-Golder et al., 1999; Fiedler et al., 2000; European Commission, 2001b),
- tire-wear from vehicles (Councell et al., 2004),
- contamination of food for instance due to migration of substances from packaging into food (Harrison, 2001a; Watson, 2001), due to food processing (Büchert et al., 2001), or due to contamination of feeding stuff (Fiedler et al., 2000),
- natural background of trace elements (Kabata-Pendias and Pendias, 1992; Wedepohl, 1995; Reimann and de Caritat, 1998; Smedley and Kinniburgh, 2002),

- smoking for example in the case of cadmium (Chaney et al., 1999), nitroaromatic compounds (Purohit and Basu, 2000) and benzene (Hattemer-Frey et al., 1990),
- grilled food items (Purohit and Basu, 2000),
- tubing, especially for lead (Wilhelm and Ewers, 1999) but also other metals such as cadmium (World Health Organisation, 1992b),
- the working environment (Stern et al., 1984; Ewers and Schlipköter, 1991; Buckley-Golder et al., 1999), and
- those especially leading to indoor air contamination for example radon from soils (Davies, 1998; Hopke et al., 2000) and volatile organic compounds (VOCs) and polychlorinated biphenyls (PCBs) for instance from building materials (Brown et al., 1994; Bleeker et al., 1999).

Many of these exposures occur in a very localised area or only during short episodes. The spatial and temporal resolution of the environmental fate model brings about that such localised or temporary exposure assessments cannot be carried out. This means, for instance, that an assessment of the exposure of individuals cannot be conducted. This applies especially to those individuals with localised food supply that is produced on contaminated soils/feed (Tennant, 2001). The exposure scenario in which people eat only food that is produced in their vicinity (European Commission, 1996b) or even by themselves is also known as the *subsistence farmer* scenario (United States - Environmental Protection Agency, 1998). This approach can be extended to become a nested exposure assessment by exporting local food production surplus to regional and potentially to global levels (as done for radionuclides in European Commission, 1999a).

By *exposure pathways* the definition as given by United States - Environmental Protection Agency (1992) is adopted here which reads: "(an) exposure pathway is the course a chemical takes from its source to the person being contacted" (p. 7).

Exposure modelling is understood here as the "process of quantifying the mass flows of a chemical and calculating the resulting concentrations in the environment by means of mathematical expressions" (van de Meent et al., 1996, p. 103).

In general, exposure assessments most often build to rather large extents on results from environmental fate models. Therefore, some definitions with respect to environmental fate modelling shall be given here as well. Following the idea that a multimedia model includes the atmosphere, the aquatic ('water') and the terrestrial environment ('soil'), the term *medium* is reserved to these three 'environments' addressing them as a whole. The perception that media are distinguished according to their predominant phase is different from that of others (e.g., Cowan et al., 1995b) and at times complies with the definition of 'main compartments' (e.g., as distinguished by Trapp and Matthies (1998)). Biota could be considered as an additional medium.

Each of these media may be further distinguished into *compartments*. Compartments are boxes that are by definition homogeneous with respect to all of their properties (assumption of homogeneous mixing, Trapp and Matthies, 1998). Their properties may, therefore, serve as a basis in order to distinguish these. They are assumed to be at thermodynamic equilibrium internally. Following the Mackay level III/IV modelling approach as introduced by Mackay (1979), transfers between these compartments show resistances which are expressed as rates, i.e., following the processes' kinetics. Losses from the system such as chemical transformation or transport beyond the model's boundaries are also allowed for. The difference between level III and IV is that the one assesses steady-state situations assuming constant and continuous emissions while the other is also capable of investigating the temporal development of a substance's concentration in the distinguished compartments over time given a specified emission situation.

2.1.3 Considerations with respect to risk and impact assessment

Although also drawing to some extent on regulatory risk assessment methodologies, it shall be emphasized here that the present work aims at estimating impacts rather than risks. This statement can definitively be challenged since the impacts to be assessed are based on dose- or exposure-response functions that describe a statistical chance for an effect to occur (e.g., development of cancer or skin irritation occurrence) which is then combined with a severity measure such as Disability Adjusted Life Years to yield an impact (cf. section 7.3). Nevertheless there are differences in the approaches taken to assess either impacts or risks which shall be described in the following.

Many regulatory Risk Assessments (RAs) in the United States of America (US) and the European Union (EU, e.g., United States - Environmental Protection Agency, 1998; European Commission, 2003b) make use of so-called Risk Characterisation Ratios (RCRs). Such RCRs merely indicate whether there is concern or not by giving 'yes - no' answers. They are calculated by relating some effect measure such as the Predicted No Effect Concentration (PNEC) to a measure of exposure usually termed Predicted Environmental Concentration (PEC) yielded by an exposure model. For characterizing human exposure, no safety factors are introduced and the PNEC is divided by the PEC yielding a Margin Of Safety (MOS[1], European Commission, 2003b). This is then valued by experts in order to provide guidance whether to act from a regulatory body's point of view or during product development at company level. A fair degree of conservatism at least in the initial tiers of the assessment is introduced during the determination of the RCR components in order not to underestimate the risk (European Commission, 1996a; United States - Environmental Protection Agency, 1998; Organisation for Economic Co-operation and Development, 1999).

Olsen et al. (2001) point at the limited use of these rather qualitative RCRs in a context in which effects shall be assessed and aggregated according to their severity such as in Life Cycle Analyses (LCAs) and in externality valuation exercises. Still the authors conclude that "presently, there is no better method for a generally applicable, more quantitative risk characterisation" (ibid., p. 394). However, adopting conservative '(reasonable) worst case' assumptions reduces the validity of risk assessment approaches for LCA purposes (Olsen et al., 2001) although some authors consider the inclusion of safety factors for instance a strong point of risk assessments when compared to LCAs because they take uncertainties into account (Jørgensen and Bendoricchio, 2001).

When performing impact assessments, one needs to distinguish what impacts are tried to be estimated. Within the field of Life Cycle Impact Assessment (LCIA), for instance, it is common understanding that *potential impacts* are assessed. Unlike rather site-specific approaches such as Environmental Impact Assessments and higher tier Risk Assessments which try to estimate actual impacts, LCIAs try to characterize additional impacts by emissions taking place during the life cycle of a so-called functional unit (Guinée et al., 1996; Udo de Haes, 1996). These emissions, however, only have a potential to lead to different types of impacts which depends on several conditions (Udo de Haes, 1996). Heijungs (1995) describes it as follows: "(w)hether this potentiality becomes actuality is dependent on background concentrations and simultaneous synergistic or antagonistic concentrations, which are by their site-specific and product-unrelated character outside the scope of normal LCA, nor can they feasibly (be) included" (p. 223). This points at a shortcoming especially when evaluating toxic impacts within many present LCA methodologies that spatial and/or temporal information related to releases into the environment are lost during the data gathering step (Guinée et al., 1996; Nichols et al., 1996; Udo de Haes, 1996; Owens, 1997b; Krewitt et al., 2002) which is even stated as a limitation in the ISO norm (DIN EN ISO, 14042:2000). Furthermore, no information on other past or present emission activities or natural background concentrations (e.g., in the case of metals) is available.

While additionally assuming that there are no effect thresholds (Krewitt et al., 2002), this leads to a situation that may be perceived as if "all theoretically

---

[1] Note when evaluating pesticides according to EU legislation, the Toxicity-Exposure Ratio (TER) is defined analogously to the MOS.

possible consequences or hazards, not actual impacts or the prediction of impacts" are considered (Owens, 1997b, p. 362) extending the "worst case scenario to an impossible scenario" (ibid., p. 364).

In order to arrive at *actual impacts* of hazardous substances, it is evident that a substance must interact with an organism to exert its toxic potency leading to effects. Thus, the estimation of actual impacts necessitates information on the spatial distribution of both the change in concentration and the target organisms (Chapman, 2001; Krewitt et al., 2002) as well as their co-existence in time at the same place. One has to note that there are tendencies to make LCIAs more realistic especially in terms of the spatial distribution of releases (e.g., Potting and Hauschild, 1997; Potting et al., 1998; Nigge, 2000) partly building on the Impact Pathway Approach followed in this study (Krewitt et al., 1998, 2001; Spadaro and Rabl, 1999; cf. section 2.2).

It shall be noted that the question whether to assume threshold effect levels especially for populations will be discussed in section 7.3.

Before concluding this section, it shall, furthermore, be noted that the term 'impact' must not be understood in this document in a way to justify legal claims towards the entities responsible for the emissions investigated. To the knowledge of the author, the naming of the impact assessment step has been or was a reason why the methodology of Life Cycle Analysis has not been or was not widely used within the US.

2.2 Impact Pathway Approach

In the present work, the *Impact Pathway Approach* (IPA) is followed which has been developed within the series of ExternE Projects on 'External Costs of Energy' funded by the European Commission (1999a). It is a bottom-up approach in which the causal relationships from the release of contaminants through their interactions with the environment to a physical measure of impact (the 'impact pathway') and, where possible, a monetary valuation of the resulting welfare losses is assessed (see Fig. 2-1).

As it was the objective of the ExternE study to achieve an economic valuation of impacts, the impact assessment procedure is very much oriented to arrive at the damage level. Due to its modularity, it provides results on various intermediate levels of the environmental mechanism as well that can be used independently of any valuation methodology. According to its being a bottom-up approach, the Impact Pathway Approach strives for a high spatial resolution in order to capture the sources of the substances, i.e., human activities. Unlike regulatory risk assessments, the impacts or rather the 'risks of impacts to occur' that are assessed by the IPA are intended to be representative (so-called central or best estimate) rather than conservative or protective.

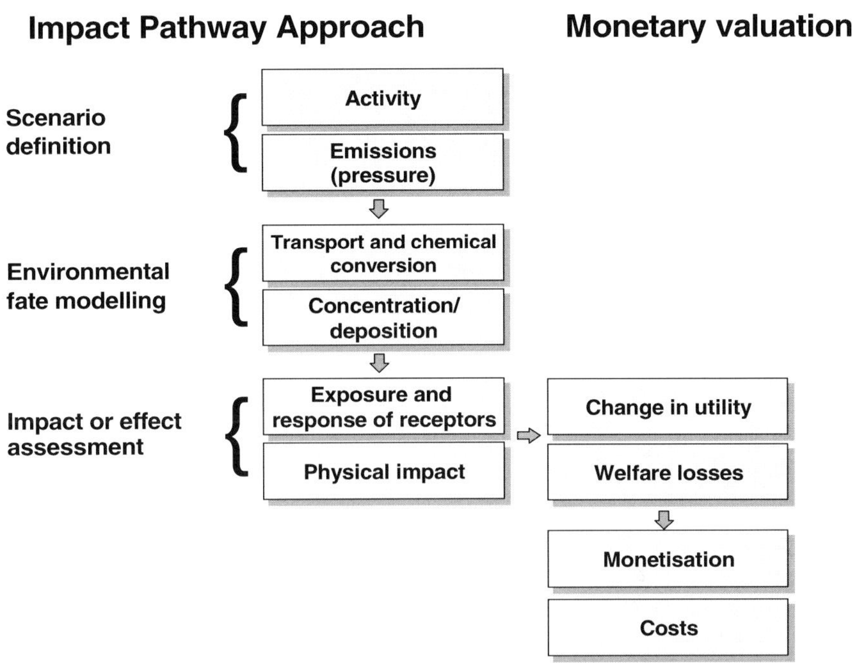

Fig. 2-1: Flowchart of the Impact Pathway Approach including monetary valuation

The Impact Pathway Approach is implemented into an integrated impact assessment and valuation tool called *EcoSense* (European Commission, 1999a). Initially, it supported the quantification of environmental impacts due to activities only at a single location such as a power plant. Further developments of the basic model led to different versions of the EcoSense model. They additionally allow the modelling of line sources and multi-sources for Europe for example from road traffic and from countries, respectively. As the emissions of the different types of sources contain different chemicals, the EcoSense transport version is capable of modelling partly different pollutants than the EcoSense single/multi source version (Table 2-1). Principally all pollutants listed in Table 2-1 (and more) can be implemented with little effort in all different EcoSense versions. Besides EcoSense Europe single/multi source versions of EcoSense have been set up for Brazil/Latin America, China/Asia, Russia and the Ukraine.

The impact assessment is performed in a spatially-resolved way. Principally one may distinguish site-generic from site-dependent and site-specific assessments (cf. Hauschild and Potting, 2003). In site-generic assessments, all sources

Table 2-1: Summary of the pollutants currently considered in different EcoSense Europe versions

Pollutants	EcoSense Europe version		
	Single source	Multi-source	Transport
SO_2	x	x	x
NO_x	x	x	x
NH_3	-	x	x
PM_{10} (primary particles)	x	x	-
Suspended particulates (particle class differentiated)	-	-	x
Non-methane volatile organic compounds (NMVOCs)	x	x	x
CO	x	-	x
As, Cd, Cr, Hg, Ni, Polycyclic Aromatic Hydrocarbons (PAHs), Pb[a], PCB[a], PCDD/F	x	-	-
Benzene, benzo(a)pyrene, 1,3-butadiene, ethene, formaldehyde	-	-	x

a.Exposure-response functions are not implemented at present.

are considered to contribute to the same generic receiving environment while a moderate to high degree of spatial differentiation in terms of emission sources and/or receiving environment is employed for site-dependent and site-generic approaches, respectively. In order to cover different substances and different scales, the EcoSense single/multi source version for Europe provides three air quality models completely integrated into the system (Table 2-2). In order to allow for this site-dependent and/or site-specific assessment, EcoSense provides a comprehensive set of relevant input data for the whole of Europe. Based on the European CORINAIR emission database, the definition of emission scenarios takes into account emission reduction measures in specific countries or more specific administrative units as well as in industry sectors.

Table 2-2: Air quality models implemented in EcoSense

Model	Application	Type	Reference
Industrial Source Complex Model (ISC)	Local transport of air pollutants from point sources (site-specific)	Gaussian plume model	Brode and Wang (1992)
ROADPOL	Local transport of air pollutants from line sources (site-specific)	Gaussian plume model	Vossiniotis et al. (1996)
Windrose Trajectory Model (WTM)	Regional (long-range) transport and chemical reaction (site-dependent)	Climatological trajectory model	Trukenmüller and Friedrich (1995) and Trukenmüller (1998) based on work done by Derwent and co-workers (Derwent and Nodop, 1986; Derwent et al., 1988)
Source Receptor Ozone Model (SROM)	Regional assessment of ozone concentrations (site-dependent)	Episodic trajectory model (country-to-grid matrices)	Simpson and Eliassen (1997), Simpson et al. (1997)

For the impact assessment and valuation step, the initial version of EcoSense already includes a large number of exposure-response functions and monetary values that were compiled and thoroughly reviewed within the ExternE projects (European Commission, 1995, 1999a).

The Impact Pathway Approach can be regarded as a particular example of Life Cycle Analysis (LCA) which is why in the following many concepts from this field of research are drawn from.

2.3 Model aim and requirements

According to Veerkamp and Wolff (1996), "(b)efore selecting a model, the fundamental problem is to define precisely the question a model is intended to answer and the level of accuracy required" (p. 94). The main aim of the present work is to extend the existing human health impact assessment and valuation approach (cf. section 2.2) to substances that reach human beings through the media soil and water. The final indicator to be estimated are the external costs

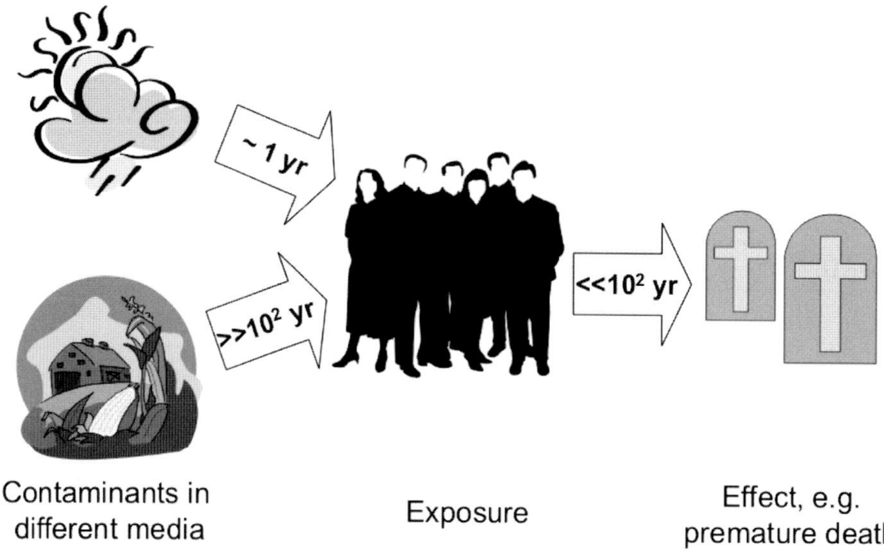

Fig. 2-2: Maximal time scales between contamination of different media leading to exposures via inhalation and/or ingestion and impacts on human health (cliparts by Corel Corporation, 1999, 2002)

related to a human activity. Due to the extending nature of the work, the methodology presented and used here needs to take into account the guiding principles and assumptions that had been followed during the series of ExternE projects for consistency reasons. According to European Commission (1999a), the guiding principles of the Impact Pathway Approach are (a) transparency, (b) consistency and (c) marginal approach.

The guiding principle of transparency is addressed by documenting precisely what was done and how in addition with an indication of the related uncertainties and methodological completeness of the assessment (cf. Chapter 9). Furthermore, the EcoSense tool has been designed to allow for any changes of the underlying data and equation formulations with respect to the impact assessment and monetisation by the (knowledgeable) user. This was achieved by the usage of a database for the storage of data as well as the equation definition (cf. section 4.4).

Consistency means that the assumptions between the different components of the Impact Pathway Approach are in line with each other. These assumptions need to apply to all of the evaluated cases (or scenarios) as well in order to allow for valid comparisons. One sub-aspect of consistency are the spatial and temporal scales that are looked at. Within the ExternE-methodology impacts are attempted to be estimated over the whole temporal and spatial scale, focusing on impacts occurring in Europe. Depending on a chemical's environmental behaviour, the lifetime between emission and exposure to a receptor may vary considerably (cf. Fig. 2-2). Whereas for example sulphur compounds in air have a residence time in the order of days (Seinfeld, 1986), persistent substances such as heavy metals may reside in soils or sediments for many years leading to rather delayed exposures to human beings (Hellweg, 2000; van den Bergh et al., 2000; Huijbregts et al., 2001). Also the time elapsed between the exposure to a pure air pollutant and an apparent corresponding impact may be in the order of decades, for instance for chronic mortality due to the exposure to fine particles (Pope et al., 1995).[2] However, the delay between emission, inhalation exposure and effect usually is at most about one generation due to the restricted residence time in air[3] of substances exerting quantifiable effects on human beings. Thus, the consideration of exposure routes due to ingestion implies the coverage of longer time horizons in order to fully assess the effects of long-lived substances. This also leads to the question how effects occurring at a very distant point in time can be valued in terms of the present value of money (cf. section 8.1 on the issue of discounting). In any case, the uncertainty about the predictability of the future is an issue that needs to be kept in mind.

Although the approach originally had been described as marginal, i.e., small additional or incremental human activities leading to emissions and, thus, effects are evaluated, also analyses of whole economies have been performed in the meantime (European Commission, 2003d).

The Impact Pathway Approach principally constitutes a methodology which can be applied to any situation/location on the globe. However, it was in the first place developed for Europe (cf. section 2.2). It is also this part of the world for which the implementation of the IPA is most advanced. Because of this and due to the fact that the present work was supported by several EC-funded projects (see Acknowledgements), the tool to be described will focus on the geographical scope of the European EcoSense versions (see Fig. B-1). This also means that the environmental fate and exposure/impact assessment to be developed needs to comply with the assumptions of the models used for the inhalation impact assessment (cf. Table 2-2). In the case of the regional air quality model

---

2 If premature death occurs in the long run (so-called chronic mortality) one may additionally distinguish between (apparent) latency times, a period with health impairments (morbidity) and years of not realized life expectancy (e.g., Years Of Life Lost, European Commission, 1999a; Hurley and Miller, 2001; cf. sections 7.3.8 and 8.2).

3 Note that the substance may be deposited to the surface and volatilise once or many times again.

WTM which is implemented in all different EcoSense versions, one main assumption in this regard is that it operates on meteorological data that are taken as representative for a one year period (section 4.1). Furthermore, the model to be developed needs to allow for a bottom-up analysis of impacts. A spatially-resolved modelling framework is adopted in order to be able to perform site-dependent impact and external costs assessments for example to identify the contribution from different countries to the overall external costs. Spatial differences were shown to be significant in terms of exposure (e.g., Krewitt et al., 2001; Nigge, 2001) although the authors focused on inhalation exposure. Hertwich et al. (1999) found that substance-specific and exposure parameters are more sensitive to the overall exposure assessment result. However, they suggested to explore the informativeness of spatially-resolved models which is also subject of the present study.

As regards the level of accuracy required, it may be obvious that the ambition of an impact assessment methodology operating at the spatial resolution and for the geographical scope outlined above cannot be as high as in a localised impact or risk assessments for instance (Hunsaker et al., 1990). Furthermore, as is discussed in Chapter 9 the assessment endpoint, i.e., the external costs defies its monitoring. Nevertheless, expectation estimates are striven for. Already the present work as such is an improvement towards more knowledge about the magnitude of the external costs occurring due to human activities as hardly any (if at all) information on the external costs for exposure routes other than inhalation had been available prior to this effort. In line with European Commission (1999a), the external costs and the exposure leading to the related impacts will be analysed at the population level, not below (e.g., individuals).

Furthermore, the model development needs to obey the mass conservation principle in order neither to miss nor to fabricate substance amounts. It has to be noted, however, that the air quality model based on which the model development will take place (cf. section 4.1) does not fully comply to this criterion.

The extension of the Impact Pathway Approach involves the four components shown in Fig. 2-1: (a) emission scenarios, (b) environmental fate modelling, (c) exposure and impact assessment, and (d) monetary valuation. The emission scenarios are subject to the cases investigated and are, thus, part of Chapters 10 and 11. Likewise, the monetary valuation will be based on the state-of-the-art suggested by latest ExternE follow-up project(s) (cf. Chapter 8). In contrast, the environmental fate analysis on the one hand and the exposure and impact assessment on the other need to be set in place. In many risk assessments, the suggested schemes and tools do not integrate these two components but follow a modular approach by first performing an analysis of the environmental fate and then assessing the exposure and potentially the impacts (cf. United States - Environmental Protection Agency, 1998, 1999b; International Atomic Energy Agency, 2001; McKone and Enoch, 2002; European Commission, 2003c). The exposure analyses, thereby, usually assess the transfers from the environmental fate media into the exposed organisms such as humans, plants and/or animals by assuming equilibrium conditions (e.g., by employing bioconcentration, bioaccumulation, or root concentration factors). Depending on whether they intend to perform a generic assessment (e.g., International Atomic Energy Agency, 2001; European Commission, 2003c) or a regionalized assessment (e.g., United States - Environmental Protection Agency, 1998, 1999b; McKone and Enoch, 2002), the exposure assessments show different degrees of complexity. This is related to the extent to which conservative assumptions are made or protective purposes are followed.

Due to the fact that the exposure assessments follow similar, equilibrium-based computational approaches, the following section 2.3.1 will focus on the different possibilities how to design an environmental fate model.

2.3.1 Modelling framework

In the following, an overview of different existing modelling approaches is given in order to elaborate which approach is most suited for the present work, concluded in section 2.3.2. The overview is structured into:

- mechanistic versus functional/box models,
- coverage, spatial scope or model extent,
- spatial aspects other than a model's spatial scope, and
- temporal aspects.

The findings influenced the compilation of Table 2-3 which tries to demonstrate in what way properties and release patterns of the substances potentially to be included in the assessment influence the model design.

The left hand side of Table 2-3 describes a chemical's characteristics and release patterns which vary to the indicated degree (e.g., a substance's persistence can vary from absolutely persistent to readily degradable). These features have an impact on the model design, as indicated on the right hand side of the Table (e.g., non-linear dose-response information for a substance brings about the need to assess the absolute concentrations and not just their increases in the environmental medium of concern).

Table 2-3: Attempt to structure the implications of different substance properties, reaction chemistry and modes-of-entry on model design

Substance characteristics and release pattern					Design of environmental fate and human exposure model			
Long range transport	not significant	vs.	significant	⇒	small scale	vs.	large scale	Spatial scope / extent
Chemical mode-of-entry	point source	vs.	multiple point sources ('diffuse emission')	⇒	small to large scale[a]	vs.	large scale	
	non-constant releases (e.g., intermittent pulses, in- or decreasing)	vs.	Continuous and constant emission	⇒	quasi dynamic[b,c]		steady-state	Temporal scope[d]
Persistence	readily degradable	vs.	persistent	⇒	quasi dynamic[e,b]	vs.	steady-state[f]	
Properties changing due to temporally varying conditions[g]	significant	vs.	not significant	⇒	('true') dynamic (if cannot be time averaged, e.g., as for rainfall in steady-state models)		steady-state appropriate, depending on application	

Table 2-3: Attempt to structure the implications of different substance properties, reaction chemistry and modes-of-entry on model design

Substance characteristics and release pattern					Design of environmental fate and human exposure model			
Sorption and reaction behaviour	approximately linear	vs.	non-linear	⇒	linear differential equations	vs.	non-linear differential equations	Formulation
				⇒	no background data needed to estimate marginal changes in concentration or exposure	vs.	background needed to estimate absolute concentrations or exposures	Background[h]
Dose-response relationship	(pseudo) linear (at least above any biological thresholds)	vs.	non-linear	⇒				
Intermedia transfer	negligible	vs.	important	⇒	single compartment[i]	vs.	several (integrated or coupled) compartments	Number of compartments
Media via which most species exposure occurs	medium of release	vs.	another medium or several media	⇒	single compartment[a]	vs.	several (integrated or coupled) compartments	
Effect of reaction products	no concern	vs.	concern	⇒	single species[j]	vs.	multi-species	Speciation or chemical forms

Table 2-3: Attempt to structure the implications of different substance properties, reaction chemistry and modes-of-entry on model design

Substance characteristics and release pattern					Design of environmental fate and human exposure model			
Effect of parent and/or of transformation substance	independent of location	vs.	dependent on location	⇒	zero dimensional	vs.	one to two dimensional	Spatial resolution[k]

a. This depends on the long range transport capabilities of the receiving medium or of the media into which intermedia transfers occur, for example.

b. 'Quasi' denotes that only the concentration of the substance varies in time (cf. Brandes et al., 1996).

c. The relationship between the steady-state solution of a linear Mackay-type multimedia model and the time-integrated exposure assessment of pulse emissions is, however, acknowledged (cf. Heijungs, 1995).

d. Suggestion: decades would be a meaningful temporal scope for today's society when computing dynamically; this could be increased significantly for sustainability considerations and when addressing intergenerational equity.

e. Dynamic approaches are suggested for substances with quick transformation and/or adsorption rates (cf. Mulkey et al., 1993; Wania and Mackay, 1999).

f. In the case of very persistent substances, it may be desirable to at least give an indication of the time horizon for the development towards the steady-state (Cowan et al., 1995a; Trapp and Matthies, 1995), for example by means of level IV calculations in the case of Mackay-type multimedia models ('response time', Mackay, 1991).

g. Like vapour pressure etc.; it shall be noted that also environmental properties or states including target organisms vary in time, potentially requiring the use of 'true' dynamic models termed 'structurally dynamic models' or 'variable parameter models' (Jørgensen and Bendoricchio, 2001, p. 315 and pp. 382ff; see main text for further explanations).

h. If (varying) background concentrations need to be taken into account due to non-linear fate mechanisms or effect measures (cf. sections 4.2.3 and 7.3, respectively), the model's scope needs to be large when not just assessing subsistence farmer exposure scenarios (cf. section 7.2) regardless of whether the substance has only localised sources and is very immobile. Depending on the variability of background concentrations and/or the characteristic travel distance of the respective substance, either a nested model set-up (like SimpleBox version 2.0, cf. Brandes et al., 1996) or a global model (e.g., GLOBOX, Wegener Sleeswijk, 2005) could be used. Furthermore, the background potentially also of reactants and competing substances needs to be included in the assessment.

i. If emission takes place into different compartments, all receiving compartments need to be considered even if no intermedia transfer occurs.

j. If reverse reaction is negligible.

k. 'Lateral spatial resolution' or 'dimensionality' according to van de Meent et al. (1996); see main text for further explanations; the nested approach followed in the SimpleBox model version 2.0 (Brandes et al., 1996) might be classified differently, as the different scales vary in their spatial resolution (note: whether a model has also vertical subdivision, e.g., layers, is not of importance here).

Mechanistic versus functional/box models

Any fate and exposure model makes the assumption of homogeneity[4] in the distinguished elementary spatial units for which balances are computed. The size of those elementary spatial units and, hence, the model formulation is what makes the difference between a mechanistic and a functional or lumped parameter model. In contrast to functional models, mechanistic models are based on rate constants and not on capacities (Hoosbeek and Bryant, 1992). Mechanistic models use ordinary (one independent variable like time) or even partial differential equations (more than one independent variable; e.g., additionally x, y and z location coordinates) and are, hence, relatively more and/ or absolutely highly data demanding. The mechanistic models which use partial differential equations would only be favoured if such a high information density on environmental state variables as well as on emissions could be provided more or less readily. This will presently at best only be the case for very localised emissions with little to no dislocation of the substances of concern (local spatial scope). However, the present work focuses on an impact assessment methodology at the European scale which is why functional models or simple mechanistic models with ordinary differential equations are to be favoured primarily due to environmental and emission data availability reasons. Examples for the latter are the multimedia models of the Mackay-type (e.g., Mackay, 1991). Despite their simplifications, functional models seem likely to be increasingly advantageous also with respect to their performance when the physical scale of the modelling exercise increases (Addiscott, 1993).

Coverage, spatial scope or model extent

Depending on a substance's mobility in and/or its diffuse release into the environment, a fate and exposure model may need to cover up to the whole world (Table 2-3). For instance, mercury has a residence time in air in the order of months to years (Lindqvist and Rodhe, 1985; United States - Environmental Protection Agency, 1997b) in which it could travel around the globe several times. Nevertheless, the appropriate spatial modelling resolution may not only be a function of fate, but also the importance of exposure levels at different locations remote to the source. Also, depending on the available information on where emissions take place which may vary from site-generic over site-dependent to site-specific, the spatial scope of the assessment needs to be adjusted (Organisation for Economic Co-operation and Development, 1999;

---

4 Be it just homogeneity in terms of degree of variability or similar stochastic behaviour.

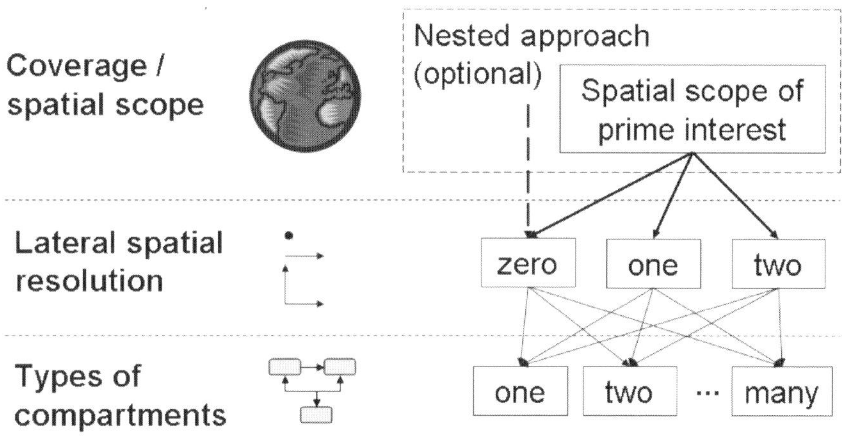

Fig. 2-3: Options for the combination of the spatial scope, lateral spatial resolution and compartmentalisation of an environmental fate (and exposure) model (clipart by Corel Corporation, 1999)

Hauschild and Potting, 2003). For instance, due to the usual lack of spatially (and temporally) resolved Life Cycle Inventory (LCI) data (e.g., Owens, 1997a), generic Life Cycle Impact Assessments should be performed at the global level. Apart from formulating a fully generic model of the whole world, there are principally two ways to take global scale distributions of chemicals into account (cf. Fig. 2-3):

- 'sub-regions interconnected by advection' (Wania, 1996): the total model's scope is divided into adjacent regions (or zones) where all regions have the same level of detail (same hierarchical level). Multimedia model examples for the global scale are the models with meridional zones described in Wania and Mackay (1995) and Scheringer et al. (2000b), and the GLOBOX model (Wegener Sleeswijk, 2005) that subdivides the whole globe by national boundaries. Many atmospheric chemistry and global oceanic models similarly exist, with various levels of complexity and demonstrated validity, and
- 'nested sub-regions' (Wania, 1996): the world is divided into areas with higher and lower levels of detail. The components with higher level of detail are contained in the ones with less details. An early example is the SimpleBox 2.0 model (Brandes et al., 1996) with a global scale represented by an arctic, a tropic and a moderate zone. There is a continental scale nested

in the latter zone, which in turn contains a regional scale. IMPACT 2002 (Pennington et al., 2005) reflects a more recent example, offering the possibility of a spatially-resolved European model nested in an a-spatial global model.

According to van de Meent et al. (1996), the nested approach could be used to combine different types of models (e.g., functional models at the larger scale with mechanistic models at the local scale). This of course depends on whether a chemical is released at only one site or diffusely at many sites and whether background concentrations need to be considered (see Table 2-3). Advantages of nesting even spatially-resolved regional models into a global model include that all the chemical releases are taken into account and that the importance of exposures outside of the modelled region can be estimated.

Both approaches apply to scales below the global scale as well. Whereas type 1 is more data demanding, the nested approach would allow to have a generic, however to some degree spatially-resolved, broad scale environmental fate and exposure model. In the context of representative impact and external cost assessments, this would bring us only a small step closer to the assessment of actual rather than potential impacts. In a comparison of regional distribution models, on the other hand, Märker et al. (2000) stress the demanding task of modelling at intermediate or regional scales. This is due to the fact that heterogeneities at intermediate scales cannot be as appropriately accounted for as at smaller scales since data is most often not available. However, the properties do not average out like at the global scale. The main question resulting from this is whether one wants to model only a portion or the full extent of the model's scope in more detail. This is again dependent on the kind of substance one wants to assess (cf. Table 2-3).

Spatial aspects other than a model's spatial scope

"Different processes and connectivities emerge as dominant as we move from the plot scale to catchment or regional scales" (Kirkby et al., 1996, p. 396) or put the other way around, as one moves from generic assessments such as status quo Life Cycle Analyses (LCAs) to local risk assessments for instance. Upscaling, and in particular downscaling, are problems that one is confronted with when developing a fate and exposure model with different spatial resolutions for a given spatial scope. From a soil science perspective, Wagenet (1998) cited in Addiscott (1998) commented that at different scales different variables are often needed to describe similar processes. Addiscott (1998) reflects further whether different models are needed, too, given the present limitations of our understanding of the processes. In line with this, van de Meent et al. (1996) recommend to use (a-spatial) multimedia box models only for screening purposes. Predictions of effects at specific times and places, on the other hand, may require the use of a more sophisticated dynamic, two or three-dimensional air, water or ground water quality model.

Some authors suggest to use (pseudo) linear formulations with parameters showing little variability when modelling at larger scales (Addiscott, 1993, 1998). Prominent examples of (pseudo) linear models in the area of environmental fate models are the multimedia box models of the Mackay-type (Mackay, 2001) that have already been used in the field of Life Cycle Impact Assessment (LCIA, e.g., Huijbregts et al., 2000b; McKone and Hertwich, 2001; Hertwich et al., 2002; Jolliet et al., 2003). As opposed to these fully integrated multimedia model mathematical solutions, it is also possible to directly link single-medium models (Margni, 2003; an example for a mechanistic very localised model: Whelan et al., 1992; Margni et al., 2004). The usage of single-medium models is also to be favoured if a pollutant does not escape from the medium into which it is exclusively released (van de Meent et al., 1996). Klepper and den Hollander (1999) come to the conclusion that the value of using single-medium models is dependent on the type of medium when dealing with chemicals that are not true multimedia substances ('multi-hop'). Whereas the applied multimedia model gives fair estimates for air and soil, a single-medium spatially-resolved model should be used to assess a substance's concentration in the water compartment in order to improve the assessment (ibid.).

In line with Hertwich et al. (2002), one of the underlying principles guiding these reflections is that the properties of the considered substances highly influence the model design related to spatial aspects in order to meaningfully assess a substance's interaction with the environment, including human beings (see Table 2-3). Here, *spatial aspects* comprise the questions about the spatial scope, the so-called *lateral spatial resolution* (or 'dimensionality' according to van de Meent et al., 1996), as well as the number of environmental compartments to be distinguished. By 'lateral spatial resolution' the different ways how to differentiate a model's geographical scope into zones is meant. Examples are many typical multimedia models without spatial differentiation into zones. A lateral spatial resolution of zero means that there is only one zone distinguished. When this resolution is unity one has to deal with a line or cascade model where one zone follows the other. Example are the GREAT-ER model (European Centre for Ecotoxicology and Toxicology of Chemicals, 1999) and the single-medium water model with sequential water stretches as applied in Trapp et al. (1994). A model with a lateral spatial resolution of two consists of zones that are added one to another to fill the entire area of a model's geographical scope by several zones. Examples are the global model with nine separate climatic zones as described by Wania and Mackay (1995), TRIM (United States - Environmental Protection Agency,

1999a), the POPCYCLING-Baltic model (Wania et al., 2000), BETR (MacLeod et al., 2001), EVn BETR (Prevedouros et al., 2004), IMPACT 2002 (Pennington et al., 2005) and GLOBOX (Wegener Sleeswijk, 2005).

One reason for conducting impact assessments in a spatially-resolved way is that the concentrations of a substance and/or the susceptibilities of target organisms can vary substantially in space. Wania (1996) differentiates between two primary causes why there is spatial variability of chemical concentrations in the environment (beside temporal variations):

- type 1 variability is due to spatial differences in source strength and the inevitable incompleteness of mixing processes; this variability is highest for immobile and reactive chemicals with localised emission patterns and
- type 2 variability is caused by the variability of the environment resulting in different intensities of various fate processes in different locations.

Apart from the release mode, hence, the main criteria for the decision whether and to what degree to model in a spatially-resolved way are a substance's dislocation behaviour and interaction with the environment.

The distinction of these two types of variability was made on the background of environmental fate modelling. For an impact assessment context, it is stressed here that type 2 should be explicitly extended to also comprise exposure, particularly in the case of humans. This variability is caused by the variability in exposure patterns resulting in different intensities of food and water supply on the one hand and population density on the other. Additionally, there might be cases where also the effect side needs to be taken into account when determining the spatial importance in a fate and exposure model. This is especially the case if sensitivities against a poisonous chemical vary substantially, for instance for different varieties of species at different locations or for the same species under different environmental conditions (e.g., temperature, salinity/hardness of waters).

The effect side also raises the question about considering transformation products of an emitted chemical. This is because the transformation product might be more toxic than the parent compound and again the organisms might show different sensitivities towards the transformation product at different locations. The issue of speciation is only taken up in Table 2-3 but will not be explicitly addressed in this work.

Temporal aspects

As regards the temporal aspects, release patterns and substance properties with respect to degradability and other environmental fate behaviour such as volatilisation may play a role in the design of an environmental fate and exposure model (cf. Table 2-3). There are principally two different temporal scopes: steady-state and dynamic.

Steady-state is the situation in which the fluxes into a spatial unit for which a mass balance is calculated equal the fluxes out of it. As a result, the inventory and, thus, the concentration in this balance unit do not change in time. It is the final situation which would occur if for example a society or a human activity proceeded to emit a substance into the environment at a given level. To assess this situation may be relevant for sustainability-related questions (e.g., European Commission, 2003d). The occurrence of a steady-state may be assumed for non-short-lived substances (Wania and Mackay, 1999) and when the assessment is applied for a short time period (Mackay, 1991). Another application is related to the assessment of pulse emissions in the context of Life Cycle Impact Assessments of hazardous substances. Heijungs (1995) has shown that the steady-state solution of a (linear) multimedia model can also help to assess the time-integrated exposure to pulse emissions under certain conditions which does not require dynamic computations. One has to note that the development towards a steady-state may take a considerable amount of time (e.g., several hundreds or even thousands of years in the case of metals, van den Bergh et al., 2000; Huijbregts et al., 2001; de Vries et al., 2004) given the potentially very long residence times of, for example, trace elements in soils (Alloway et al., 1996), also implying that initial concentrations do not play a role any more (only fluxes, not stocks are relevant). It may, therefore, be desirable to at least give an indication of the time horizon for the development to the steady-state (Cowan et al., 1995a; Trapp and Matthies, 1995) especially in the case of very persistent substances such as non-radioactive elements. This leads to the necessity for dynamic approaches. In the case of Mackay multimedia models, so-called level IV calculations constitute a means in order to provide such response times (Mackay, 1991).

Dynamic calculations should be favoured in cases in which (a) releases of substances are discontinuous or not constant (except for exposure assessments of constant pulse emissions, see above), (b) substances are dealt with whose fate is largely controlled by the transformation or sorption rates (Mulkey et al., 1993; Wania and Mackay, 1999) and/or (c) whose properties vary substantially in time (e.g., due to diurnal or seasonal temperature changes). One has to note that not only substance properties may change in time. Brandes et al. (1996) introduce the term 'quasi-dynamic' for calculations that only allow for the change of substance masses in the model while all other parameters are kept constant. If the dynamic behaviour also of environmental parameters shall be considered a 'true dynamic' model needs to be employed. Depending on the degree of variations in the considered parameters, such models may be classified as 'structurally dynamic models' or 'variable parameter models' (Jørgensen and Bendoricchio, 2001, p. 315

and pp. 382ff). Those models account for the evolutionary potential of ecosystems which is stochastic in nature. Stochastic processes not only play a role for organisms but can also be encountered in less complex model situations such as describing solute movements in soils (cf. Richter et al., 1996, pp. 6f).

Depending on the dynamics of the phenomena as such and also the spatial scale, different *temporal resolutions* need to be employed for dynamic approaches. These may range from below a day to annual time steps. When trying to cover a rather large geographical area with some degree of spatial resolution (e.g., regional), data availability is critical both in space and time. For geochemical processes, Drever (1997b) notes that "it is rarely possible to construct a meaningful catchment budget for a time-scale of less than a year" (p. 241). Water balance models operating at intermediate spatial scales usually operate at monthly to annual time scales ('seasonal scale', Blöschl, 1996) when not dealing with events such as floods. An annual temporal resolution is also used for climatological air quality models (e.g., Trukenmüller, 1998).

Depending on how detailed the impact assessment shall be conducted, also temporal aspects of the effect might need to be included. For instance, climatological models are not well suited to assess impacts on different development stages of an organism each of which might show different susceptibilities towards the chemical under study. This depends on many factors, including the release pattern of the chemical.

2.3.2 Conclusion with respect to the modelling framework

Beside the criteria mentioned in the introduction to this sub-chapter (2.3), i.e., striving for transparency, consistency and central estimates, assessing impacts at the population level, and following the mass conservation principle, several decisions with respect to the design of the environmental fate model need to be made. These concern:

- the modelling approach (e.g., capacity, mechanistic, stochastic, lumped parameter models),
- the geographical scope of the model and how this is subdivided ('spatial resolution' with respect to zones and/or land uses/compartments), and
- the temporal resolution.

A few of the various options presented in the previous sections are already decided upon. This is because the present work builds on an existing methodological framework (the Impact Pathway Approach, cf. section 2.2) with a suggested software tool (EcoSense, European Commission, 1999a). As a result, the geographical scope should be the same mostly covering Europe as presented in Fig. B-1. The Impact Pathway Approach, furthermore, constitutes a fairly detailed, site-dependent or bottom-up approach to evaluate human exposure towards contaminants. This suggests to use a rather high spatial differentiation of the geographical scope of the model, rather than employing a site-generic modelling approach. Finally, the temporal scale of the air quality model to which the soil and water model is to be connected is one year using annual average data (Trukenmüller, 1998). Another advantage of using long-term average data and annual time steps is that it facilitates the assessment of the steady-state situation. This is relevant for time-integrated exposure assessments of pulse emissions (Heijungs, 1995) and sustainability analyses of constant and continuous releases to the environment (European Commission, 2003d).

The remaining degrees of freedom are, therefore, the specific way how to spatially differentiate (which will be dealt with in sections 4.3 and 5.1) and the general modelling approach. For consistency reasons, functional models or simple mechanistic models with ordinary differential equations are to be favoured. This is primarily due to environmental and emission data availability reasons at the geographical scope at which the EcoSense model operates to which its extension shall comply. Another reason might be that these model types are increasingly advantageous for larger scale modelling (Addiscott, 1993). Examples are the multimedia models of the Mackay-type (e.g., Mackay, 1991). These have several advantages, amongst others:

- the models are "well suited for predicting average regional concentrations resulting from highly dispersed and diffused sources" (Cowan et al., 1995b, p. x); noting their use limitation to screening exposure assessments if implemented without spatial and temporal differentiation (van de Meent et al., 1996),
- the "intermediate effort and reasonable accuracy" (Tolle et al., 2001, abstract) of multimedia fate models make them well suited for Life Cycle Impact Assessments "involving comparative assertions or governmental policy decisions" (ibid.), and
- when developing the soil and water model according to this modelling approach, a potential extension towards a fully integrated multimedia model is possible in the future.

The multimedia modelling approach of the Mackay-type is, therefore, adopted here.

3 Multimedia environmental fate and/or exposure assessment of prioritised contaminants

The previous Chapter has led to the conclusion that the multimedia modelling approach of the Mackay-type is adopted (cf. Mackay, 1991). In the following, a non-exhaustive review on existing multimedia models of this kind is given in order to evaluate their applicability in the present context. These are at least used for analysing the environmental fate of substances but may comprise also exposure assessment capabilities. As was mentioned before, most of the exposure assessments rely on equilibrium distribution between environmental media and organisms (cf. introduction to section 2.3). Therefore, also some risk assessment schemes are included in the review comprising exposure assessments that follow this concept without utilizing the Mackay environmental fate approach (section 3.1.4).

Due to the fact that there are many different types of substances to which humans might be exposed via soil and water and which require different modelling approaches, a prioritisation of substances is additionally reasoned (section 3.2). Based on this selection and the findings of the model review, the model development needs are formulated (section 3.3).

Before existing modelling approaches are reviewed, it shall be noted that during the development of the present approach another multimedia model for the evaluation of external costs has been proposed (Spadaro and Rabl, 2004). This builds on the generic Uniform World Model (UWM, e.g., Rabl et al., 1998) that was extended by a multimedia exposure assessment (United States - Environmental Protection Agency, 1998). The Uniform World Model only addresses a substance's environmental fate in air which is why it is not relevant in the present context also due to its limited spatial resolution. The followed exposure assessment, in turn, is also presented in section 3.1.4.

3.1 Existing multimedia environmental fate models with or without exposure assessment

Depending on the purpose of an existing multimedia model, one may distinguish between:

- multi-zonal multimedia environmental fate models without exposure assessment,
- multi-zonal multimedia environmental fate and exposure models, and
- oligo-zonal multimedia environmental fate and exposure models.

According to the so-far open questions as regards model design (section 2.3.2), the main evaluation criteria are: geographical scope, spatial differentiation into zones and compartments, exposure assessment capabilities and applicability to the substance types of interest (cf. section 3.2). Further characteristics such as aim and application of the model as well as particularities are also contained in the Tables compiled below.

3.1.1 Multi-zonal multimedia environmental fate models without exposure assessment

There are many spatially-resolved multimedia environmental fate models differing not only with respect to their aim and applicability but also in terms of how the spatial differentiation has been realized (Wania, 1996; Wania and Mackay, 1999; Scheringer and Wania, 2003). Their spatial coverage range from water bodies (Mackay and Southwood, 1992; Wania, 1996; Mackay and Hickie, 2000) over countries (Devillers et al., 1995; Woodfine et al., 2002) to the globe (Wania and Mackay, 1993a, 1995; Scheringer et al., 2000b; Scheringer and Wania, 2003; Wania, 2003). They may comprise the full set of environmental media (i.e., soil, water and air) or just some of them (e.g., water and soil, Di Guardo et al., 1994; Barra et al., 2000). Apart from the 'water body multimedia models' (Mackay and Southwood, 1992; Wania, 1996; Mackay and Hickie, 2000), these models shall be briefly presented here.

There are principally two common criteria for the spatial differentiation of the model's geographical scope into zones. Global models usually follow the latitudes segmenting the globe into climatic bands (Wania and Mackay, 1993a, 1995; Scheringer et al., 2000b; Scheringer and Wania, 2003; Wania, 2003). These are mostly used for the evaluation of the so-called 'cold condensation' or 'global fractionation' theory of Persistent Organic Pollutants (POPs, Wania and Mackay, 1993b; Scheringer et al., 2000b; Scheringer and Wania, 2003; Table 3-1).

The other common criterion when spatially differentiating is according to watersheds (Bintein and Devillers, 1996b; Wania et al., 2000; Woodfine et al., 2001) although some of these authors also take additional criteria into account

Table 3-1: Characteristics of global multi-zonal multimedia environmental fate models without exposure assessment

Characteristics	Globo-POP	Global Multimedia Fate Model
Aim and application	estimation of environmental fate of organic chemicals on the globe that favour enrichment in arctic ecosystems	estimation of environmental fate of organic chemicals on the globe towards the poles; investigating the influence of different numbers of zones
Chemicals considered		
• chemical groups	semi-volatile, non-dissociating, Persistent Organic Pollutants (POPs)	semi-volatile to volatile, non-dissociating, persistent to moderately persistent organic chemicals
• emission to media	emissions into atmosphere, freshwater or cultivated soil	emissions into soil
Environmental fate model		
• type of model	Mackay-type fugacity model	Mackay-type model formulated as a concentration-based mass balance
• temporal scope	steady-state and dynamic (i.e., level III and IV)	steady-state and dynamic (i.e., level III and IV)
• spatial scope and differentiation	the globe is spatially differentiated into 10 latitudinal/meridional bands according to climate	variable amount of latitudinal bands covering the globe
• compartments or media considered	nine bulk compartments: four vertical layers in air, two different types of soil (cultivated and uncultivated), freshwater and freshwater sediments, and the surface ocean	three bulk compartments: soil, oceanic surface water and tropospheric air; limited number for computational efficiency reasons
Remarks on particularities	variable temperatures affecting partitioning	variable temperatures affecting partitioning; variable amount of zones
References	Wania (2003), Wania and Mackay (1995)	Scheringer et al. (2000b)

Table 3-2: Characteristics of a gridded multi-zonal multimedia environmental fate model for Europe (without exposure assessment; Prevedouros et al., 2004)

Characteristics	European gridded model
Aim and application	estimation of environmental fate of Persistent Organic Pollutants (POPs) in the European environment
Chemicals considered	
• chemical groups	Persistent Organic Pollutants (POPs)
• emission to media	at least into the atmosphere
Environmental fate model	
• type of model	Mackay-type fugacity model
• temporal scope	steady-state and dynamic (i.e., level III and IV)
• spatial scope and differentiation	Europe is spatially differentiated into 50 regions according to a 5 x 5 degree grid plus four perimetric boxes (i.e., the Atlantic, Mediterranean, Eurasian and Arctic box)
• compartments or media considered	seven bulk compartments: upper and lower atmosphere, soil, vegetation, freshwater and sediment, and coastal water
Remarks on particularities	-
References	Prevedouros et al. (2004) building on BETR North America (cf. Table 3-3)

(Table 3-3). These include climatic and ecological characteristics (Bintein and Devillers, 1996b), and biophysical geographic (temperature, precipitation, ecosystem type, soil type, land use and meteorology), social geographic (population distribution, industrial and agricultural activity) and political factors (Woodfine et al., 2001) among other, although basically only soil types seem to play a role for the delineation of the BETR North America model apart from watershed information (MacLeod et al., 2001).

Recently, a gridded multimedia Mackay model has been published (Prevedouros et al., 2004, Table 3-2). It subdivides Europe into 50 regions according to a 5 x 5 degree grid surrounded by four boxes. Water connectivities in the terrestrial environment were defined based on river discharge information.

Many of the purely environmental fate models just presented are designed to analyse the behaviour of non-ionizing, organic substances belonging to the group of Persistent Organic Pollutants (POPs). Due to their persistency, POPs may show rather long residence times in air which bring about a long-range transport potential. Therefore, several of these models at least distinguish two atmospheric layers (Wania and Mackay, 1995; MacLeod et al., 2001; Wania, 2003; Prevedouros et al., 2004).

The POPCYCLING-Baltic model (Wania et al., 2000) is special in mainly two respects. First, it shows a different spatial differentiation of the air environment from the terrestrial/marine environment. Secondly, it computes not only mass balances for the substance under investigation but also for the carrier phases air, water and particulate organic carbon in water. Furthermore, it considers sediments in the marine environment and distinguishes between coastal zones and open sea. In the case of the Baltic Sea, the term 'open sea', however, must be seen relatively.

3.1.2 Multi-zonal multimedia environmental fate and exposure models

There are only a few multi-zonal multimedia environmental fate and exposure models available at present. The main one encountered which is relevant here is IMPACT 2002 (Pennington et al., 2005; Jolliet et al., 2003). Its characteristics are presented in Table 3-4.

IMPACT 2002 comprises large parts of Europe, i.e., most of Western Europe. Similar to the POPCYCLING-Baltic model (Wania et al., 2000), it follows different delineation schemes for air and the terrestrial environment. According to a master's thesis related to the development of IMPACT 2002 (Pelichet, 2003), a segmentation of the atmosphere following irregular boundaries such as watersheds introduces errors especially when the substance to be investigated is rather short-lived in air. Therefore, a delineation of the atmosphere according to a grid is suggested which is in line with many existing air quality models for larger scales (Pekar et al., 1999; Green et al., 2000; Bey et al., 2001; Ilyin et al., 2001), global water balance models (e.g., Vörösmarty et al., 1998) and also with the European gridded model presented above (Table 3-2). While the sea environment also follows the grid delineation for air, the terrestrial environment is spatially differentiated in IMPACT 2002 according to watersheds.

Unlike the environmental fate models presented in section 3.1.1, IMPACT 2002 provides full exposure and impact assessment capabilities (Pennington et al., 2005; Jolliet et al., 2003). For human health, different exposure pathways are aggregated into the so-called Intake Fraction (Bennett et al., 2002) which assesses the portion of an emission that a population will be finally exposed to. By aggregating the exposure at the population level, a so-called 'production-

Table 3-3: Characteristics of multi-zonal multimedia environmental fate models applicable to particular regions of the world

Characteristics	CHEMFRANCE	BETR North America[a]	POPCYCLING-Baltic
Aim and application	estimation of environmental fate of organic chemicals in France	evaluating long-range transport potential of organic pollutants; formulation of continent-scale management and regulatory strategies for chemicals	non-steady state multimedia mass balance model for assessing long term fate of persistent organic pollutants (POPs) in the Baltic Sea environment
Chemicals considered			
• chemical groups	organic chemicals that may also dissociate[b]	organic pollutants	semi-volatile, non-dissociating, persistent organic chemicals (POPs)
• emission to media	emissions to air, water, soil and sediment	(not specified)	emissions to air, forest canopy[c], forest soil, agricultural soil, freshwater and coastal water
Environmental fate model			
• type of model	Mackay-type fugacity model	Mackay-type fugacity model	Mackay-type fugacity model
• temporal scope	steady-state (level III) if one region is investigated; or seasonal results for the whole modelled area (i.e., France)	steady-state and dynamic (i.e., level III and IV)	dynamic (i.e., level IV)

Table 3-3: Characteristics of multi-zonal multimedia environmental fate models applicable to particular regions of the world

Characteristics	CHEMFRANCE	BETR North America[a]	POPCYCLING-Baltic
• spatial scope and differentiation	France is differentiated into 12 regions according to hydrological (drainage basins), climatic (precipitation, temperature, wind) and ecological criteria (nature of soil and vegetation type)	the North American Continent consisting of Canada, the United States of America and Mexico is subdivided into 24 regions principally according to watersheds and soil types	the model's scope is differentiated differently for the terrestrial and sea environment (following mostly the eight aquatic sub-basins of the Baltic Sea and related drainage areas), and air (four air-sheds)
• compartments or media considered	six bulk compartments: air, fresh surface water (including fish), soil, sediment of freshwater bodies, ground water, coastal water	seven bulk compartments: two air layers, vegetation, soil, freshwater and sediment, and coastal water	ten bulk compartments: air, agricultural soil, forest soil and canopy, freshwater and sediment, coastal water and sediment, and open sea water and sediment
Remarks on particularities	dissociating organic substance can be modelled[b]	emission rates and temperatures may be allowed to vary in time	advective intercompartmental transfer fluxes of the contaminants are calculated as the product of a flux of a carrier phase (air, water and particulate organic carbon) and a contaminant concentration in that phase; mass balances calculated for carrier phase; forest canopy distinguished as a compartment; different spatial resolutions for air and the other media

Table 3-3: Characteristics of multi-zonal multimedia environmental fate models applicable to particular regions of the world

Characteristics	CHEMFRANCE	BETR North America[a]	POPCYCLING-Baltic
References	Devillers et al. (1995), Bintein and Devillers (1996b), Bintein and Devillers (1996a)	Woodfine et al. (2001), MacLeod et al. (2001)	Wania et al. (2000)

a. The latest version of ChemCAN (Woodfine et al., 2002) appears to build mostly on the BETR North America model which in turn is an expansion of an earlier version of ChemCAN (MacLeod et al., 2001, p. 2); it just has a smaller geographical scope while keeping 24 distinguished zones.

b. A pH dependency of possible ionization in fresh surface water and its sediment can be considered as was done by Bintein and Devillers (1996b).

c. The author is irritated as to how emissions directly into the leaves/needles in a forest canopy can actually be mediated/accomplished (cf. p. 44, ibid.).

Table 3-4: Characteristics of IMPACT 2002, a multi-zonal multimedia environmental fate and exposure model

Characteristics	IMPACT 2002
Aim and application	estimation of environmental fate and related effects of mostly organic chemicals in Western Europe
Chemicals considered	
• chemical groups	organic chemicals, metals
• emission to media	emissions to air, water and soil
Environmental fate model	
• type of model	Mackay-type model formulated as a mass-based mass balance
• temporal scope	steady-state and dynamic (i.e., level III and IV)
• spatial scope and differentiation	Western Europe is spatially differentiated and contained in a global box; spatial differentiation of the terrestrial environment according to drainage basins into 135 zones; air is spatially differentiated according to a 2 x 2.5 degree grid; oceanic zones follow the air grid where applicable
• compartments or media considered	seven bulk compartments: air, fresh surface water and related sediment, agricultural and natural soil, oceanic water and related sediment
Exposure model	
• target / safeguard organisms	human health, and aquatic and terrestrial ecosystems
• routes considered	inhalation and various ingestion pathways
Effect / impact model	human health: cancer and non-cancer effects considered following the Disability Adjusted Life Years (DALY) concept (Murray and Lopez, 1996a, 1996b); aquatic and terrestrial ecosystems: potentially affected fraction
Remarks on particularities	different spatial resolutions for air/sea and soil/freshwater; 'production-based' exposure assessment; different exposure pathways aggregated into the Intake Fraction (Bennett et al., 2002)
References	Jolliet et al. (2003), Pennington et al. (2005)

based' approach is realized (Pennington et al., 2005) which accounts for the division of labour and overcomes the conservative 'subsistence farmer' approach mostly followed by screening regulatory risk assessments. The effects on human health due to the estimated exposure is assessed following the Disability Adjusted Life Years (DALY) concept (Murray and Lopez, 1996a, 1996b).

Another example is the Total Risk Integrated Methodology (TRIM, United States - Environmental Protection Agency, 1999a, 1999b, 2002a, 2002b) . The TRIM design offers a rather flexible framework for the assessment of so-called hazardous and criteria air pollutants, examples for the latter are particulate matter, ozone, carbon monoxide, nitrogen oxides, sulphur dioxide and lead (United States - Environmental Protection Agency, 1999b). The flexibility is realized, for instance, by the capability of using different environmental fate models that may be based on first-order or higher order algorithms (United States - Environmental Protection Agency, 2002b). While aiming at multimedia capabilities, the modular design may even allow to use single medium models (e.g., Gaussian plume models for air, United States - Environmental Protection Agency, 1999b). It is still being developed which is why only a few of the components principally aimed at are ready for use. In the case of the fate module, only first-order models are available (United States - Environmental Protection Agency, 2002a). Also only inhalation exposures can be assessed at present. Due to its preliminary status and its principally flexible design, it is not further presented here.

The Framework for Risk Analysis in Multimedia Environmental Systems (FRAMES) is a third example of this type of models (Whelan et al., 1997). Similar to TRIM, however, it allows for the inclusion and combination of different models. Therefore, its characteristics are not well determined which is why it will not be analysed here either, noting that modularity and flexibility in terms of combinations of different models offers well-suited, task-specific assessment capabilities.

3.1.3 Oligo-zonal multimedia environmental fate and exposure models

Oligo-zonal multimedia environmental fate and exposure models shall be reviewed next. By 'oligo-zonal', it is meant that the geographical area of prime interest is not further subdivided into zones although noting that in the case of nesting different hierarchical levels may be taken into account.

All of the models presented in Table 3-5 combine at least in parts a Mackay-type multimedia model with an exposure and risk assessment (McKone, 1993a, 1993b; Brandes et al., 1996; European Commission, 1996a; Vermeire et al., 1997; Schwartz et al., 1998; Schwartz, 2000; Huijbregts, 1999, 2000; Huij-

Table 3-5: Characteristics of oligo-zonal multimedia environmental fate and exposure models

Characteristics	CalTOX	EUSES	USES-LCA	Dynabox
Aim and application	assist in health-risk assessments that address contaminated soils and the contamination of adjacent air, surface water, sediments and ground water	screening and refined quantitative risk assessment of the risks posed by new and existing chemical substances to man and the environment	performing Life Cycle Impact Assessment of toxic substances at the global scale	performing dynamic risk assessments of metals
Chemicals considered				
• chemical groups	mostly non-ionic organic chemicals, also ionic organic and inorganic chemicals such as metals	mostly non-ionic organic chemicals	mostly non-ionic organic chemicals, also ionic organic and inorganic chemicals such as metals	metals
• emission to media	originally emissions to soil ("soil-bound contaminants" McKone, 1993b, p. 8) but allowing for inputs to any of the distinguished compartments	locally: air and water; regionally and continentally: air, industrial soil, sewage treatment plant and water	emissions into air, freshwater, sea water, and agricultural and industrial soil	(not specified)

Table 3-5: Characteristics of oligo-zonal multimedia environmental fate and exposure models

Characteristics	CalTOX	EUSES	USES-LCA	Dynabox
Environmental fate model				
• type of model	Mackay-type fugacity model	local scale: different models for air, sewage treatment plant, surface water and soil; regional and continental scale: Mackay-type model formulated as a concentration-based mass balance[a]	Mackay-type model formulated as a concentration-based mass balance[a]	Mackay-type model formulated as a concentration-based mass balance[a]
• temporal scope	steady-state and dynamic (i.e., level III and IV)	regional and continental scale: steady-state (i.e., level III)	steady-state and dynamic (i.e., level III and IV)	steady-state and dynamic (i.e., level III and IV)
• spatial scope and differentiation	regional, no (lateral) differentiation	generic or standard environment (may be adapted); three nested scales, i.e., local, regional, continental, plus a personal scale (only exposure assessment)	global; two nested scales, i.e., continental and global; global scale is differentiated into three climate zones (arctic, moderate, tropic)	global; three nested scales, i.e., regional, continental and 'outside' world

Table 3-5: Characteristics of oligo-zonal multimedia environmental fate and exposure models

Characteristics	CalTOX	EUSES	USES-LCA	Dynabox
• compartments or media considered	seven bulk compartments: air, ground-surface soil, root-zone soil, vadose-zone soil, plants, surface water and sediment	local: depending on the model employed; regional and continental (six bulk compartments): air, water, sediment, and natural, agricultural and industrial soil	continental (eight bulk compartments): air, freshwater and sediment, sea water and sediment, and natural, agricultural and industrial soil; global (three bulk compartments): air, sea water, soil	regional: air, surface water, suspended matter, biota, sediment, natural soil, agricultural sand soil, agricultural peat soil, agricultural clay soil, pore water in sand soil, pore water in peat soil, pore water in clay soil, industrial soil, ground water; continental: air, surface water, suspended matter, biota, sediment, natural soil, agricultural soil, industrial soil, ground water; sea: air, sea water, suspended matter, biota, sediment; outside world: deep soil, deep sediment

Table 3-5: Characteristics of oligo-zonal multimedia environmental fate and exposure models

Characteristics	CalTOX	EUSES	USES-LCA	Dynabox
Exposure model				
• target / safe-guard organisms	human health	man: consumers, workers and man exposed through the environment; environment: sewage treatment plant populations of micro-organisms, aquatic, terrestrial and sediment ecosystems, and populations of predators	human health and environment distinguished into freshwater aquatic and sediment, sea water aquatic and sediment, and terrestrial environment	human health, and aquatic and terrestrial ecosystems
• routes considered	inhalation and various ingestion pathways (total of 23 different exposure pathways); aggregated into an average daily potential doses	man: inhalation, ingestion of food (i.e., fish, root crops, leaf crops, meat, milk) and drinking water, exposure towards consumer products and at the workplace; environment: water - fish - predators, soil - earthworm - predators	inhalation and ingestion including soil ingestion for humans; other organisms via contact with the environmental medium	(not explicitly stated)

Table 3-5: Characteristics of oligo-zonal multimedia environmental fate and exposure models

Characteristics	CalTOX	EUSES	USES-LCA	Dynabox
Effect / impact model	Human Toxicity Potentials (HTPs); based on Risk Characterisation Ratios (RCRs) relating potential dose to a measure of inherent toxicity; HTPs are the ratio of a substance's RCR and another of a reference substance; given for cancer and non-cancer effects	Risk Characterisation Ratio: man: Margin of Safety (MOS); environment: PEC/PNEC ratio	toxicity potentials based on normalized Risk Characterisation Ratios (RCRs): man: predicted daily intakes related to so-called human limit values for humans; else: PEC/PNEC ratios	Risk Characterisation Ratios (RCRs): man: predicted daily intake related to so-called Acceptable Daily Intake (ADI); else: PEC/PNEC ratios

Table 3-5: Characteristics of oligo-zonal multimedia environmental fate and exposure models

Characteristics	CalTOX	EUSES	USES-LCA	Dynabox
Remarks on particularities	vertical differentiation of the soil compartment into layers; contaminant concentrations in ground water are based on the leachate from the vadose-zone soil; uncertainty and sensitivity analysis capabilities	conservative ('reasonable worst case'), screening level; release scenarios provided; sewage treatment plant; local scale; different risk characterisation (i.e., based on acute or chronic data) depending on whether intermittent or continuous releases are considered; several features of SimpleBox 2.0 (Brandes et al., 1996) are not used in EUSES: global spatial scope by means of a moderate, an arctic and a tropic zone, variable soil depth, vegetation compartment, fish as part of suspended solids, performing a temperature correction and computing dynamically	almost closed system due to global spatial scope except for exchange with the stratosphere; worst-case estimates are replaced by realistic ones; chemical-specific penetration depths into soils; temperature dependency of hydroxyl-radical reaction rates as well as influence of pH on environmental behaviour of dissociating substances and hydrolysis rates considered	'outside' world provides only ultimate sinks; "The differentiation of agricultural soil into sand, peat and clay does not affect the overall picture. However, it introduces differences in soil concentrations of a factor up to 10." (Heijungs, 2000, p. 75)

Table 3-5: Characteristics of oligo-zonal multimedia environmental fate and exposure models

Characteristics	CalTOX	EUSES	USES-LCA	Dynabox
References	McKone (1993a), McKone (1993b), McKone and Hertwich (2001), Hertwich (1999), Hertwich et al. (2001)	Brandes et al. (1996), European Commission (1996a), Vermeire et al. (1997), Schwartz et al. (1998), Schwartz (2000)	Huijbregts (1999), Huijbregts (2000), Huijbregts et al. (2000a), Huijbregts et al. (2000b), Huijbregts et al. (2001)	Heijungs (2000)

a. The environmental fate model builds on SimpleBox (e.g., Brandes et al., 1996). The mass balance of this model is based on concentrations and not on fugacities.

bregts et al., 2000a, 2000b, 2001; Heijungs, 2000; McKone and Hertwich, 2001). Their substance coverage is mostly non-ionic organic chemicals although CalTOX (McKone, 1993b) and USES-LCA (Huijbregts et al., 2000b) also have been applied for other substances such as metals. Dynabox was explicitly developed for the application to metals (Heijungs, 2000). In order to better model dissociating substances and hydrolysis, USES-LCA introduced compartment-specific pH values (Huijbregts, 1999). Fugacity-based environmental fate model formulations are principally designed to address rather volatile substances. In order to also assess rather involatile substances, a so-called 'aquivalence approach' was developed (Mackay and Diamond, 1989) which is included in the CalTOX model. In contrast to CalTOX, the other tools show nesting of different spatial scales, thereby reaching continental (European Commission, 1996a; Heijungs, 2000) or even global coverage (Huijbregts et al., 2000b). In terms of spatial differentiation into compartments, a special feature of CalTOX is that it distinguishes three different layers in soil, a feature that was largely supported by recent findings as regards volatile organic compounds (McKone and Bennett, 2003). Dynabox, in turn, differentiates different types of agricultural soil which however "does not affect the overall picture" (Heijungs, 2000, p. 75) and also adds an outside world with a deep soil and deep sediment compartment as ultimate sinks.

CalTOX probably constitutes one of the most comprehensive models to address human exposures covering a total of 23 different exposure pathways (McKone, 1993a; McKone and Enoch, 2002). The other approaches are not as comprehensive with respect to human health noting that EUSES also assesses exposures at the work-place and via consumer products. EUSES, USES-LCA and Dynabox, however, additionally assess exposures of other safeguard objects such as terrestrial and aquatic ecosystems.

All effect assessments follow risk characterisation approaches relating an environmental medium concentration to a safe concentration such as the PEC/PNEC ratio or a dose to which an individual may be exposed to a safe dose. These are called Risk Characterisation Ratios (RCRs). In case of human health risk assessment, EUSES makes use of the Margin Of Safety (MOS, European Commission, 1996a) concept which simply relates a safe dose to the estimated exposure dose. The risk assessor might then judge whether the resulting MOS is large, i.e., protective enough or not. The Human Toxicity Potentials (HTPs) assessed by CalTOX (Hertwich, 1999; Hertwich et al., 2001; McKone and Hertwich, 2001) are based on RCRs relating a potential dose to a measure of inherent toxicity such as cancer potency and Reference Dose (RfD) or Reference Concentration (RfC) for cancer and non-cancer effects, respectively (Hertwich et al., 2001). The HTPs are yielded by dividing the RCR of a substance under study by one of a reference substance (normalization) both obtained from the same emission scenario. The toxicity potentials as used by USES-LCA are computed analogously for all safeguard objects (Huijbregts et al., 2000b). All these risk characterisations constitute threshold approaches indicating whether there is concern or not. In particular when used at screening level, EUSES is meant to be conservative (European Commission, 1996a), i.e., rather overestimating than underestimating a risk.

3.1.4 Non-Mackay-type multimedia environmental fate and exposure assessment frameworks

In this section, exposure assessment approaches and tools are presented that do not build on Mackay-type environmental fate models. Due to the usual modularity employed in the risk assessment, the exposure assessment parts can, nevertheless, be combined with the results of other types of environmental fate models. Principally, two exposure assessment tools with multimedia capabilities and applicable to trace elements (cf. section 3.2) have been encountered in the literature that have not yet been presented here: One is from the health physics (radionuclides) context suggested by the International Atomic Energy Agency (2001) and the other applies to hazardous air contaminants (United States - Environmental Protection Agency, 1998). It shall be noted that there may be other assessment frameworks and tools available not reviewed or even mentioned here.

The environmental fate models that are also provided by these assessment frameworks are detailed in Table 3-6. Most notably, the Human Health Risk Assessment Protocol (HHRAP) is intended to provide guidance for location-specific analyses of emissions to air from hazardous waste combustion facilities (United States - Environmental Protection Agency, 1998) whereas the framework suggested by the IAEA is generic concentrating on radionuclides (International Atomic Energy Agency, 2001).

Only the related exposure and risk assessment parts of these approaches shall be presented in the following. Due to the nature of the investigated substances, the simple safety assessment models for radionuclides not only include the inhalation and ingestion routes of exposure but also *external exposure* (International Atomic Energy Agency, 2001), i.e., the exposure due to staying in the vicinity of contaminated environmental media. Such induced effects due to 'remote' exposure are a particularity of radioactive substances. While both approaches cover inhalation and ingestion exposures, the degree of detail by which the HHRAP assesses ingestion is higher (United States - Environmental Protection Agency, 1998). The HHRAP takes more exposure pathways into account by distinguishing between different vegetal produces (i.e., belowground, aboveground protected and aboveground exposed produce) and including more animal produces such as poultry, eggs and pork.

Table 3-6: Characteristics of multimedia exposure approaches for trace elements/radionuclides

Characteristics	Simple safety assessment models by IAEA	Human Health Risk Assessment Protocol (HHRAP)
Aim and application	providing simple methods for calculating doses arising from radioactive discharges into the environment	providing guidance for performing risk assessments of substances being released by hazardous waste combustion units
Chemicals considered		
• chemical groups	radionuclides	hazardous organic chemicals and trace elements, so-called 'compounds of potential concern' (COPCs)
• emission to media	continuous or prolonged emissions from small scale facilities to air, water and sewage systems	emissions to air excluding accidental releases
Environmental fate model		
• type of model	first stage: 'no dilution model'; second stage: simple generic environmental models for air (Gaussian plume model), water (depending on the water body) and soil (based on atmospheric deposition and removal rates, e.g., due to decay)	different models for different media: air: Industrial Source Complex Short-Term Model (ISCST3); soil: based on atmospheric emission or deposition and removal rates, e.g., due to degradation or physical removal; water: based on atmospheric deposition, inputs from land and removal rates
• temporal scope	equilibrium conditions	equilibrium conditions

Table 3-6: Characteristics of multimedia exposure approaches for trace elements/radionuclides

Characteristics	Simple safety assessment models by IAEA	Human Health Risk Assessment Protocol (HHRAP)
• spatial scope and differentiation	generic; no differentiation	location-specific (close to a hazardous waste incinerator); no differentiation
• compartments or media considered	air, water (rivers, estuaries, coastal waters, lakes and reservoirs); soil only as part of the terrestrial food chain (derived from atmospheric deposition)	mostly air based on which other media concentrations are derived
Exposure model		
• target / safeguard organisms	human health	human health
• routes considered	inhalation (air and resuspended solids), ingestion (plants, milk, meat, fish, drinking water, and soil particles by animals and humans) and external exposure (e.g., when staying in or at radionuclides containing air, sediments etc.)	inhalation and ingestion of belowground and aboveground (protected and/or exposed) produce, beef and dairy products, pork, chicken and eggs, drinking water, and fish; note: no inhalation and drinking water exposures of farm animals considered
Effect / impact model	collective dose compared to reference level	Risk characterisation: cancer: based on slope factor and lifetime average daily dose; non-cancer: hazard quotient relating either average daily dose to the Reference Dose (RfD) or air concentration to the Reference Concentration (RfC)

Table 3-6: Characteristics of multimedia exposure approaches for trace elements/radionuclides

Characteristics	Simple safety assessment models by IAEA	Human Health Risk Assessment Protocol (HHRAP)
Remarks on particularities	conservative, screening level; assuming (quasi-) equilibrium conditions between released radionuclides and the environment	higher tier approach than screening level ("reasonable potential risk", p. 1-6), less conservative than the latter
References	International Atomic Energy Agency (2001)	United States - Environmental Protection Agency (1998)

Similar to the approaches presented in the previous section 3.1.3, both effect assessments make use of Risk Characterisation Ratios (RCRs). It is noted that the HHRAP also distinguishes between cancer and non-cancer effects similar to CalTOX (Hertwich et al., 2001). While the approach suggested by the IAEA is meant for screening level assessments (International Atomic Energy Agency, 2001) and, thus, rather overestimating than underestimating exposures and/or effects, the HHRAP is location-specific and tries to evaluate reasonable rather than theoretical worst-case maximum potential risks (United States - Environmental Protection Agency, 1998).

3.2 Selection of contaminants

Before drawing conclusions with respect to the development needs (cf. section 3.3), the scope of the substances to be covered shall be defined. It was argued in section 2.3.2 that a rather simple mathematical framework is adopted due to the spatial scale at which the model shall operate and related data availability constraints. The framework follows the multimedia type of modelling, as first suggested by Mackay (Mackay, 1979, 1991).

It is more than obvious that depending on the questions to be answered different prioritisations of substances will result. For instance, when providing decision support for the ban of substances (cf. Stockholm convention on Persistent Organic Pollutants, POPs) only substances whose production is not yet banned is of relevance. For the assessment of the welfare of societies, on the contrary, also impacts due to such banned substances need to be included in the evaluation if they still lead to impacts (European Commission, 2003d). Another example is burning wood in open fire places which may substantially contribute to a person's exposure towards particulate matter. However, this (indoor) exposure is irrelevant in terms of external cost assessments as the related costs need to be classified as internal, assuming that the person burning the wood is aware of the consequences in terms of health effects. Also the scale at which the analysis will be performed will guide the selection of sources to be considered (Reimann et al., 2000).[5]

The present work aims at elaborating and providing a methodology for the assessment of external costs due to multimedia exposures, thereby extending an existing approach for inhalation exposures (European Commission, 1999a). As a consequence, one of the main aims of the case studies to be presented in

---

5 "(O)n a regional scale mobile pollution sources such as traffic or industrial activities using large tracts of land such as agriculture and forestry may have a considerably stronger impact on environmental quality than local industrial pollution sources" (ibid., p. 168).

Chapters 10 and 11 is to demonstrate the application of the suggested approach. As there are some hundreds or even thousands of substances that may be hazardous, a limitation in the initial coverage of the model to be developed with respect to substances is necessary especially due to resource constraints.

The most important selection criterion is *relevance* for which political concern is taken as a proxy. There is public concern about long-lived substances such as heavy metals and POPs due to accumulation in the environment (e.g., Lindberg, 1989; Kabata-Pendias and Pendias, 1992; United Nations - Economic Commission for Europe, 1998; Rat von Sachverständigen für Umweltfragen, 2004) that are furthermore either poisonous or bioaccumulative or both. Such substances have influenced many legislation processes and policy initiatives for instance at the European Union level such as the Water Framework Directive (WFD, 2000/60/EC, Parliament and Council of the European Union, 2000), the preparation of the fourth Daughter Directive for the Air Quality Framework Directive (AQFD, 96/62/EC, Council of the European Union, 1996b), the Integrated Pollution Prevention and Control Directive (IPPC, 96/61/EC, Council of the European Union, 1996a), the European Environment and Health Strategy (European Commission, 2003f) and the EU Thematic Strategy on Soil (European Commission, 2003g) to name some of them. Recent evidence suggests that metal contamination via air is of high actuality in that the highest atmospheric depositions into Alpine glaciers occurred in the second half of the twentieth century since the mid seventeenth century (Barbante et al., 2004).

The project series Externalities of Energy (ExternE) has focused on external costs resulting directly or indirectly from energy conversion techniques (European Commission, 1999a). Since the present work builds on the ExternE-methodology, another selection criterion is to include only those substances in the assessment that are predominantly emitted by energy conversion techniques. A fairly recent study by the United States Environmental Protection Agency (US-EPA, French et al., 1998) quantifies the impacts of fossil fuelled power plants in the USA, thus providing valuable guidance on priorities for the analysis. The highest priority is given to mercury, followed by arsenic and by dioxins and furans. Lead, cadmium, chromium and nickel are also studied in detail but found to be less important than mercury and arsenic. In fact, US-EPA considers that lead and cadmium are not priorities. However, for lead there is a significant difference between the USA and Europe due to background exposures since in the USA leaded gasoline was phased out 10 to 20 years earlier; furthermore, even so-called unleaded gasoline contains some lead, currently about 10 % of leaded gasoline, to be reduced in future years.

3.2.1 Discussion on mercury and its compounds

The assessment of mercury is rather demanding. Mercury occurs predominantly in the gaseous phase in the atmosphere (Puxbaum, 1991) of which a lower bound share of 95 % is elemental mercury according to Fitzgerald (1994) cited in United States - Environmental Protection Agency (1997b). Due to the long residence time of elemental mercury in air (in the order of months to years, Lindqvist and Rodhe, 1985; United States - Environmental Protection Agency, 1997b), the air quality modelling should not be confined to the atmospheric boundary layer and should at least cover one hemisphere if not the globe (United States - Environmental Protection Agency, 1997b; Ryaboshapko et al., 1998) similar to many Persistent Organic Pollutants (Pekar et al., 1999). Furthermore, several species are involved. Three species may be differentiated for regional air quality purposes: elemental mercury (Hg0), divalent mercury (HgII) and particulate-bound mercury (e.g., Ryaboshapko et al., 1998 and RELMAP as described by United States - Environmental Protection Agency, 1997b). The model by EMEP additionally considers methyl mercury (MHg, Ryaboshapko et al., 1998) with a relatively short atmospheric half-life of 12 hours due to ready photochemical and chemical degradation. As methyl mercury usually only constitutes a minor fraction of the overall mercury in air, there is good reason to exclude it from air quality modelling exercises. In particular when modelling water and/or wetlands (e.g Olson and Panigrahi, 1991; United States - Environmental Protection Agency, 1997b), however, this species gains in importance and needs to be explicitly considered due to its potential toxic effects (cf. Tsiros, 2001 and model 'IEM-2M', United States - Environmental Protection Agency, 1997b). The consideration of different species and more importantly the confined spatial coverage of the existing external cost assessment tool EcoSense make the inclusion of mercury meaningless since especially the intercontinental air transport cannot be modelled appropriately. As a result, mercury is not included in the present analysis.

3.2.2 Discussion on 'dioxins'

As stated above, the US-EPA also identified dioxins as priority substances (French et al., 1998). The term 'dioxins' usually refers to a group of polychlorinated, planar aromatic compounds with similar structures, and chemical and physical properties (Anonymous, 2000). Each of these compounds is also referred to as *congener*. This group of compounds consists of 75 polychlorinated dibenzo-*p*-dioxins (PCDDs) and 135 polychlorinated dibenzofurans (PCDFs), of which 2,3,7,8-tetrachlorinated dibenzo-*p*-dioxin (TCDD) is the most toxic and most studied congener. Dioxins are lipophilic compounds that bind to sediment and organic matter in the environment and tend to be absorbed in animal and human fatty tissue. The seventeen 2,3,7,8-chlorine substituted PCDD and PCDF congeners in particular are extremely resistant towards chemical and biological degradation processes and, consequently, persist in the environment and accumulate in the food chain. There is evidence that the so-called coplanar polychlorinated biphenyl (PCB) congeners exert a similar effect on living organisms like PCDDs and PCDFs. The group of PCBs is, therefore, also counted to the 'dioxins'. It consists of 209 congeners of which 130 are likely to occur in commercial products (Anonymous, 2000) which is in contrast to the dioxins and furans which have never been produced intentionally. PCDD/Fs and PCBs belong to the group of POPs which are internationally banned according to the Stockholm convention on Persistent Organic Pollutants noting that the usage of POPs that are active ingredients of pesticides is still allowed in some countries.

As PCDD/Fs and PCBs are normally present in environmental and food samples as complex mixtures of congeners causing comparable effects, the concept of Toxic Equivalents (TEQs) has been developed. This concept uses the available toxicological and biological data to generate a series of weighting factors, called Toxic Equivalency Factors (TEFs), each of which expresses the toxicity of a 'dioxin-like' compound in terms of the equivalent amount of the most toxic dioxin congener, 2,3,7,8-TCDD (Harrison, 2001b). Multiplication of the concentration of a compound by its TEF yields a TEQ. Also the exposure-response information for ingested dioxins is given per TEQ (United States - Environmental Protection Agency, 2001) based on the World Health Organisation Toxic Equivalency Factors (WHO-TEFs, van den Berg et al., 1998) superseding a former set of so-called International Toxic Equivalency Factors (I-TEFs, North Atlantic Treaty Organization/Committee on the Challenges of Modern Society, 1988).

Apart from exposure through accidents and at the working environment, human exposure to dioxins is mostly attributable to ingestion (more than 90 %, Buckley-Golder et al., 1999; Fiedler et al., 2000; European Commission, 2001b). Hence, contaminated plants and animals that are eaten need to have become exposed prior to human exposure. Contamination of the environment with dioxins is primarily caused by the aerial transportation and deposition of emissions from various sources although dioxins with natural origin might also enter the food chain via cattle feed (Ferrario et al., 2000). In principle, plants may also accumulate pollutants via root uptake from the soil but the importance of the soil-to-plant pathway for dioxins is generally negligible (Welsch-Pausch et al., 1995; Wania and Mackay, 1999; Cousins and Mackay, 2001) and confined with respect to plant species (McLachlan, 1997).

Another possible exposure pathway may be due to sludge 'amendments' to soils. The exposure from sludge to plant into the food chain is of minor importance and depends on the level of sludge contamination, the intensity of sludge use and the agricultural practices (McLachlan et al., 1996). In Germany, sludge amendments to grassland are even prohibited (Fiedler, 2003) and food items are treated prior to consumption.

In order to allow for attributing an exposure to an emission of dioxins by a human activity (i.e., the impact pathway), in principle chemical transport models would need to be applied for each of the PCDD, PCDF and PCB congeners. Although the exposure-response information is given in an aggregated way, a differentiated modelling approach is necessary due to the fact that the congeners contributing to the toxic effects show very different dispersion behaviours in the atmosphere (Eitzer and Hites, 1989; Kaupp et al., 1994; Oh et al., 2001) with octachlorinated dibenzo-*p*-dioxin (OCDD) possibly even being built from pentachlorophenol (PCP, e.g., Baker and Hites, 2000). Additionally, it is known that vegetation considerably influences the atmospheric transport of dioxins (Bennett et al., 1998; McLachlan and Horstmann, 1998; Cousins and Mackay, 2001). Consequently, an air dispersion model considering exchange processes with vegetation is needed for the assessment of dioxins not only for inhalation but also for a considerable portion of the ingestion exposures. This is because root uptake is generally negligible (Welsch-Pausch et al., 1995; Cousins and Mackay, 2001) and the contribution of fish for instance ranges from 2 % to 63 % across the European Union depending on the consumption habits of a (sub-) population according to Anonymous (2000). Most of the fish consumed in the EU stems from sea catches (European Centre for Ecotoxicology and Toxicology of Chemicals, 1994), however, which would bring about the need to model the fate of the assessed substances also in the marine environment which is not attempted in the present study (cf. section 6.1). As a result, the necessary air quality model that includes vegetation has not been available which is why a comprehensive external cost assessment due to ingestion of dioxins remains open.

3.2.3 Trace elements and Mackay modelling

The remaining substances considered in the US-EPA report are first of all arsenic and secondly heavy metals such as cadmium and lead (French et al., 1998). Although it was concluded in that study that for example cadmium and lead are not priorities, this must be seen from a regulatory risk assessment perspective where exposure levels are compared to safe levels. While this approach is valid, for instance, when trying to protect the most exposed individual, the assessment of external costs due to effects at the population level supports the assumption that there is no safe level, i.e., that there is no effect threshold (cf. section 7.3). From an external cost point of view, hence, there is concern about each substance that has the potential to cause adverse effects.

In order to estimate external costs based on adverse effects following ingestion, corresponding dose- or exposure-response functions are required. Exposure-response information for ingestion is very scarce (cf. Searl, 2002). In order to derive slope factors from threshold information, a method has been proposed fairly recently which is adopted in this study (Crettaz, 2000; Crettaz et al., 2002; Pennington et al., 2002; cf. section 7.3.1), offering the possibility to assess not only inorganic arsenic for which exposure-response information is available only via drinking water (e.g., United States - Environmental Protection Agency, 2005) but also heavy metals such as cadmium, lead and hexavalent chromium. Note that, although arsenic as a metalloid strictly speaking does not belong to the group of heavy metals, it is common use in the scientific and the regulatory literature to consider arsenic part of the (heavy) metals (e.g., Pacyna, 1987; Berdowski et al., 1997; Buse et al., 2003; European Commission, 2003f, 2003g; Joint Research Centre of the European Commission, 2003). It may be more appropriate to call these elements *trace elements* altogether since their occurrence in the 'experienced' environment, i.e., at the earth's surface, is limited (Wedepohl, 1991, 1995).

Heavy metals including arsenic is a group that has been widely disregarded (or rather avoided) in the realm of Mackay-type multimedia modelling, one reason being that heavy metals need individual treatment (Mackay, 1991; Hertwich et al., 2000). Examples of multimedia models that were applied to heavy metals are USES-LCA (Huijbregts et al., 2000a, 2000b), the EQC (only lead, Mackay et al., 1996a) and CalTOX (e.g., Hertwich et al., 2000). As pointed out by several authors, research in multimedia modelling of metals is, however, needed (Hertwich et al., 2000; Huijbregts et al., 2001).

It is assumed here that heavy metals except for mercury do not have a significant vapour pressure so that they can be considered to be non-volatile (Lide, 2002). Due to this characteristic, multimedia models that are based on fugacity face the problem to deal with this group of substances. This is why the aquivalence approach has been introduced and employed (Mackay and Diamond, 1989; Diamond et al., 1992; Hertwich et al., 2000). However, there are other features that make heavy metals troublesome to model. First of all, they speciate which means that they exist in different chemical forms some of which may precipitate (e.g., as sulphides in sediments) and which can also be transformed back. Also, their solid-water partitioning behaviour is highly influenced by the pH, the competing ions as well as available reaction partners present in the medium considered (e.g., Anonymous, 1999b). As many of them form cations they do not only bind to the (dissociated functional groups of) organic matter for example of soils but also to clays as well as to iron and manganese oxides/hydroxides (Jenne, 1998b). The latter have the unpleasant characteristic that they are not stable when redox conditions change.

However, as typical (i.e., Mackay-type) multimedia models are evaluative or screening models, they are fairly simple in that they divide the environment into rather large homogeneous boxes whose properties are constant over time (e.g., Mackay, 1991). Temporally variable conditions are usually not accounted for although attempts to allow for stochastic processes such as intermittent rain have been undertaken (e.g., Hertwich et al., 2000; Hertwich, 2001; MacLeod et al., 2001). Different from modelling degradation products of organic compounds where usually only the concentration of the parent compound and the respective reaction half-life are needed (see Fenner et al. (2000) for a discussion and a possible way out of this situation), modelling speciation of metals including adsorption involves knowledge about the ionic strength, pH and redox conditions as well as reaction kinetics and concentrations of the potential ligands or (highly heterogeneous environmental) adsorbents which can react with the heavy metals in the different media (e.g., Hering and Morel, 1990; Morel and Hering, 1993; Tompson, 1993; Turner, 1995; Ritchie and Sposito, 1995; Zachara and Westall, 1999).

Speciation is not included in the assessment at present due to two reasons: (a) the information on the different parameters influencing speciation is not existing at the geographical scope and for the spatial resolution employed; additionally the data on the physical-chemical properties of all species will most likely not be available either (Mackay et al., 1996b) and (b) setting up a multi-regional multimedia multi-species model (cf. United States - Environmental Protection Agency, 1999b) becomes too complex in terms of computation and data storage resources. A multi-species model may be considered in the future most likely on the expense of spatial detail. However, as pH can be considered one of the single most important parameters to influence the solid-water partitioning behaviour of heavy metals (cf. Sauvé et al., 2000), its dependence on pH is implemented in WATSON, the model whose development is described in this work. USES-LCA already included different compartment pH values although only for consideration of the behaviour of dissociating organic compounds (Huijbregts et al., 2000b).

3.2.4 Selected substances

Thus, mainly three criteria suggest to focus on the non-volatile heavy metals cadmium, lead and chromium as well as arsenic in the present study:

1. mercury and POPs such as PCDD/Fs, PCBs and benzo(a)pyrene require the modelling at the hemispheric or even global level (United States - Environ-

mental Protection Agency, 1997b; Ryaboshapko et al., 1998; Pekar et al., 1999) in order to cover the full impact pathway, especially in space; this is a main requirement when following the Impact Pathway Approach (cf. introduction to section 2.3) noting that lower bound estimates might also be informative,

2. heavy metals have until now only been poorly represented in multimedia models, and
3. the limited non-threshold effect information for ingestion (cf. Crettaz, 2000; Searl, 2002) suggests to further reduce the amount of trace elements addressed.

As a result, the rest of this work will focus on these trace elements. At times, also approaches for organic compounds will be provided for comparison and possible future methodological development reasons.

3.3 Need for development

None of the models presented in section 3.1 can be used for the calculation of external costs directly. Apart from the final external cost calculation (cf. Fig. 2-1), most of the models neither have the spatial coverage and resolution required, i.e., a rather detailed representation of Europe, nor provide exposure and/or impact assessment capabilities. If they allow for the assessment of effects these are mostly relying on Risk Characterisation Ratios (RCRs) that do neither take the magnitude of the effects nor their severity into account. They basically indicate whether there is concern or not. Additionally, the tools used in regulatory risk assessments usually introduce a fair amount of conservatism which does not allow the assessment of representative estimates.

However, there is one main exception as regards environmental fate and impact assessment in Europe which has been developed only recently: IMPACT 2002 (Pennington et al., 2005; cf. section 3.1.2). Nevertheless, shortcomings with respect to the purpose of the present study are:

- it does not cover the same area as the multi-source EcoSense version for Europe (Fig. B-1). As a result, some member countries (e.g., the Baltic states, Greece, Finland) of the European Union are not included. For the purpose of the present study, another reason for covering the same area as the existing EcoSense Europe versions is to provide estimates of the external costs that are comparable particularly to those for inhalation exposures assessed by these tools,
- the spatial resolution of both the environmental fate and exposure/impact model is rather coarse allowing for little spatial differentiation below the catchment level and only providing receptor data at the country level (e.g., human population, food production),

- it was developed for Life Cycle Impact Assessment (LCIA) purposes and does not cover the monetary valuation step necessary for cost-benefit analyses, and
- heavy metals and trace elements are covered only as a first attempt. A refinement is, therefore, deemed necessary. From the development of the metal-specific Dynabox model, it may be learned that the distinction of further compartments does not seem to influence the overall risk assessment from metal exposures (Heijungs, 2000). However, differences in the predicted soil concentrations of about one order of magnitude may occur.

The description of the respective model development is provided in the following Chapters.

4 Multimedia environmental fate assessment framework: outline, atmospheric modelling and spatial differentiation

Based on the review of methods and models and the concluded needs for developments as described in the previous Chapters, the methodology that allows the assessment of exposures via soil and water which in turn lead to monetisible impacts will be described in the following. The methodology is implemented in a new module complementing the software tool EcoSense (European Commission, 1999a). This module is called 'integrated WATer and SOil environmental fate, exposure and impact assessment model of Noxious substances' (WATSON). For the easiness of referring to the new methodology, it will be referred to the implemented model name throughout this document noting that the modelling concept and its implementation into a tool are two distinct things. The way how the methodological approach taken has been implemented in order to become the WATSON tool is described in section 4.4.

The methodological approach suggested here builds on an existing air quality-related external cost assessment scheme (European Commission, 1999a). Its regional air quality model will be presented in section 4.1. WATSON is linked to this air quality model whose deposition fields serve as input to the terrestrial and aquatic environment (Fig. 4-1). Reasons under which conditions such a coupling is justified and how the coupling is performed are argued in sections 4.1.1 and 4.1.2, respectively. Based on the deposition field or on direct emission specifications to soil and/or water, the approach assesses the environmental fate in different soil and water compartments (Fig. 4-1). As was reasoned in section 2.3.2, the approach for the environmental fate model as introduced by Mackay (1979) is followed. The way how the assessment area, i.e., mostly Europe, is subdivided into zones is described in section 4.3. Their further subdivision into compartments is then subject of the subsequent Chapters. Within these, also special attention is spent on how to explicitly address metals.

In line with the suggestions given by an expert group of multimedia fate and exposure modellers (Cowan et al., 1995b), the detailed exposure assessment

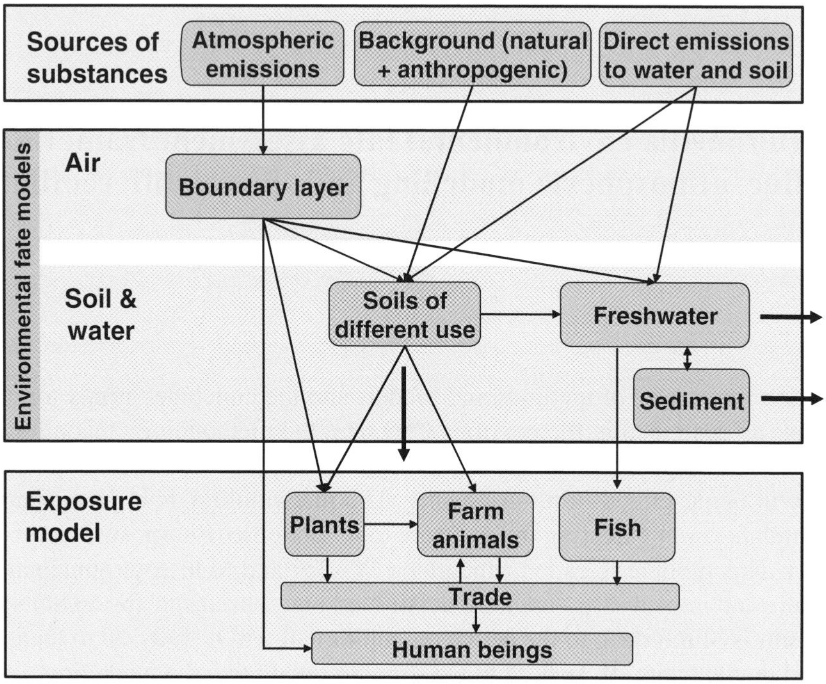

Fig. 4-1: Conceptual structure of the environmental fate and exposure assessment of the WATSON model and its linkage to the air quality model (arrows connecting boxes denote a substance's environmental pathway, arrows not connecting boxes indicate ultimate removal processes from the model's scope)

is performed separately from the environmental fate modelling although trade of food items might be considered an additional type of an environmental fate process involving rather long-range transports. The exposure together with the impact assessment are subject of Chapter 7. The approach taken for the monetisation of the effects is described in Chapter 8.

4.1 Dispersion in air and air to ground interface

In line with for example van Pul et al. (1998) and Bennett et al. (1998), atmospheric transport is modelled with the help of a Lagrangian trajectory model implemented in the EcoSense multi-source version (Windrose Trajectory Model, WTM, Trukenmüller and Friedrich, 1995). In contrast to fully integrated multimedia exposure models, the use of air dispersion models is advantageous when

Table 4-1: Treatment of different particle size classes by the Windrose Trajectory Model (WTM)

Size class [µm]	Median aero-dynamic diameter [µm]	Mass distribution scheme A [%]	scheme B [%]	Washout ratio [-]	Dry deposition velocity [m per s]
< 0.95	0.2	70	42	$5.05 \cdot 10^4$	0.00065
0.95-4	1.5	20	33	$3.78 \cdot 10^5$	0.0025
4-10	6	5	14	$3.78 \cdot 10^5$	0.0071
10-20	14	3	6	$3.78 \cdot 10^5$	0.0132
> 20	40	2	5	$3.78 \cdot 10^5$	0.067

rather complete emission information in terms of space are available (Hertwich et al., 2000). The WTM is based on work done by Derwent and co-workers (Derwent and Nodop, 1986; Derwent et al., 1988) and operates on the EMEP 50 x 50 km^2 grid (see Fig. B-1). The model is a receptor-oriented Lagrangian trajectory model employing an air parcel with a constant mixing height of 800 m moving at a representative wind speed. In contrast to forward trajectory models, the receptor-oriented backward trajectory model type is able to take reaction kinetics higher than first order into account enabling to model pollutants that are reaction products ('secondary pollutants') of reaction partners stemming from different sources (Trukenmüller, 1998). The results are obtained at each receptor point by considering the arrival of 24 trajectories weighted by the frequency of the wind in each 15° sector. The trajectory paths are assumed to be along straight lines and are started at 96 hours from the receptor end point. The meteorological data for instance for the windroses and wind speeds are annual averages which are best taken from long-term observations which makes the data representative (climatological data, Trukenmüller, 1998).

In order to allow for particulate transport which is important for rather involatile trace elements being released to air, WTM distinguishes five particle size classes (as done in van Jaarsveld, 1990) that are treated separately in terms of wet and dry deposition velocities (Table 4-1). Also, different substances follow different mass distributions. Organic substances, lead and mercury associated with particles follow scheme A whereas the other metals are assumed to follow scheme B. It needs to be noted that the suggestion with respect to the size class distributions stems from the late eighties/early nineties when most of the lead emissions in Europe occurred from the burning of leaded gasoline. Nowadays, it is, therefore, more likely that lead follows scheme B (Lee, 2003; Samara and Voutsa, 2005) which is also in line with the chemical forms mostly released from high-temperature processes (Pacyna, 1987). For arsenic and cadmium, scheme B's mass distribution is in agreement with recent findings whereas that of nickel shows a four-modal shape (European Commission, 2000b and literature cited therein).

4.1.1 Linking of an air quality model and a soil/water model

One drawback for coupling an air quality model to a multimedia (soil and water) model could be that it is not fully integrated. This means that the assumed/expected multiple intermedia exchanges of for instance the so-called multimedia organic pollutants between air on the one hand and soil and water on the other may not be allowed for. For the bulk of substances which are not true 'multi-hop pollutants' (Klepper and den Hollander, 1999), however, the intermedia exchange (or feedback) is assessed to be small (Margni, 2003; Margni et al., 2004). Heavy metals can principally re-enter the atmosphere via volatilisation and resuspension when attached to particles that were previously deposited. Apart from mercury, however, heavy metals do not have a significant vapour pressure so that volatilisation can be neglected. Suzuki et al. (2000) investigated the influence of wind erosion on the fate of rather persistent organic chemicals, i.e. PCDD/Fs, with the help of a (fully integrated) multimedia model. In a sensitivity analysis, they found that this process is negligible. It is noted that these chemicals possess remarkable vapour pressures if compared to many trace elements and especially those that are assessed in this work (cf. section 3.2.4). This could mean that the found insensitivity of dioxins to the soil wind erosion process is due to volatilisation going on to some extent. Nevertheless, this process is not considered in the methodological framework presented due to the fact that soil wind erosion mainly occurs on plain areas in arid to semi-arid climates with little to no vegetation cover (Scheffer and Schachtschabel, 1989). Within Europe, these climates can mostly be found around the Mediterranean Sea. However, the share of non-vegetated land is grossly small (cf. right of Fig. 5-2) noting that also arable land may show only a small vegetation cover under black fallow conditions or prior to total plant coverage.

Based on the findings of Margni and co-workers (Margni, 2003; Margni et al., 2004), the feedback of volatile substances can be taken into account in the present modelling framework when defining the air quality model's exchange rates with the respective ground surface for the particular 'multi-feedback' substance (see Table 4-2 for examples of feedback fractions).

Table 4-2: Feedback fractions of selected substances (Margni, 2002)

Substance	Feedback fraction [%]
Benzene to air	2
Benzene to water	1
2,3,7,8-TCDD	0.2
Benzo(a)pyrene	$9.1 \cdot 10^{-4}$ [a]

a. Value is supported by findings of Pekar et al. (1999) in that no re-emission from soil or sea water to air occurs for 11 years.

It is, therefore, concluded that the coupling of a single-medium air quality model to a water and soil multimedia type of model is a justifiable approach for assessing average environmental concentrations of non-'multi-feedback' pollutants at the regional scale.

In the next section, it is described how the linkage is performed together with the underlying assumptions.

4.1.2 Interface between air and soil/water

The results with respect to atmospheric depositions from the air quality model form the basis for the indirect input to the terrestrial and aquatic environment.[6] As the air concentrations and depositions are given on the EMEP 50 x 50 km^2 grid, this information needs to be transformed to match the regions distinguished (see Fig. 4-2 or 4-3). This is done on an area-based weighting scheme without distinguishing between different land uses. With the exception of orographic fog or cloud droplet impaction (e.g., Lovett et al., 1982), the assumption of a homogeneous deposition pattern holds for wet deposition. However, this assumption appears to underestimate or overestimate to some degree dry deposition rates at forest and non-forest sites, respectively, as expressed by filter factors which are assumed to lie in the range of 1.6 for deciduous forests to 2.1 for coniferous forests for metals (Reinds et al., 1995) especially with respect to gaseous deposition (e.g., Horstmann and McLachlan, 1998). However, it was found that forests can no longer be regarded to have a filter effect relevant to aerosols with an aerodynamic diameter of less than 5 μm (Jonas and Heinemann, 1985) with the excep-

[6] From a technical point of view, these are stored in a database as described in section 4.4.

tion of forest edges near emission sources (e.g., Hasselrot and Grennfelt, 1987) whose area share is small compared to the full forested area. Most of the metals being released in a particle-bound way fall into this particle size class (see Table 4-1). As a consequence, the values assumed by Reinds et al. (1995) are considered too large as they were also based on work done by Ivens et al. (1989) for basic cations that belong to larger particle size classes. As also the dry gaseous deposition of non-volatile substances like most trace elements can be neglected, the conversion of the deposition rates from grid cells to (undifferentiated) regions on an area-weighted basis is considered a valid approach.

4.2 General description of the soil and water environmental fate model

The fate model for the terrestrial and aquatic environment is formulated like a spatially-resolved Mackay-type multimedia model based on homogeneous compartments at equilibrium and first order kinetics for the exchange between compartments and respective loss processes. In line with Brandes et al. (1996), the mass balance is based on concentrations. In matrix notation, the respective inhomogeneous system of ordinary linear first order differential equations reads:

$$\vec{v} \cdot \frac{d\vec{c}}{dt} = A \times \vec{c} + \vec{b} \tag{4-1}$$

where

A : coefficient matrix of dimension n x n [m^3/s] (process rates are defined as described in Tables 5-5, 5-9 and 6-3 and in more detail in the sub-sections to A.3)

$\vec{b}$: perturbation vector of dimension n with exogenous inputs considering atmospheric deposition or direct emissions to the compartments [kg/s] (input rates are defined in Table 4-3 and described in more detail in the sub-sections to A.6)

$\vec{c}$: concentration vector of dimension n [kg/m^3]

t : time [s]

$\vec{v}$: volume vector of dimension n [m^3] (volumes are defined as described in more detail in the sub-sections to A.4).

In this equation, the volume vector and the coefficient matrix contain information on various process rates which depend on nature and substance-specific properties. The perturbation vector defines the emission scenario analysed. As described in section 4.4 and demonstrated in section 9.3.3, the coefficient matrix can be defined in a very flexible way which allows the inclusion or exclusion of compartments as well as of processes. Also, the spatial differentiation into zones may be varied.

This system of linear differential equations can be solved for the steady-state situation or dynamically, referred to as level III or IV, respectively (e.g., Mackay, 1979, 1991; Trapp and Matthies, 1998). 'Steady-state' means that there is no concentration change in time (any more) given a constant and continuous emission into the modelled system. Eq. (4-1) hence becomes:

$$\vec{v} \cdot \frac{d\vec{c}}{dt} = 0 = A \times \vec{c} + \vec{b} \Rightarrow \vec{c} = A^{-1} \times -\vec{b} . \qquad (4\text{-}2)$$

The steady-state solution may serve to analyse which impacts present emission levels if enduring might have on future generations in a sustainability context for instance (European Commission, 2003d) or for time-integrated exposure assessments of pulse emissions (Heijungs, 1995).

The way the dynamic solution is computed is described in section A.1.2.

4.2.1 Defining the inputs to the terrestrial and aquatic environment

In section 4.1.2, the linkage between the air quality model and the water and soil environment has been described. Beside atmospheric inputs, also direct releases to the soil and water compartments can be taken into account. The way how these inputs are modelled by the presented methodology is shown in Table 4-3 and described in more detail in sub-sections to A.6. It is distinguished into regular processes and those modifying particularly atmospheric depositions. Note that the question whether and under which conditions the removals from the atmospheric deposition might lead to erroneous negative inputs is discussed in section A.6.5 (note the negative signs for these processes in Table 4-3).

4.2.2 General remarks on processes considered in the environmental fate modelling

Processes to be considered in an environmental fate model may be distinguished into three groups:

1. removal processes,
2. transport within zones, and
3. transport between zones.

Table 4-3: Process formulations determining the (exogenous) inputs into the water and soil compartments

Name	Refer to section ... for more details	Formulation[a]	
Regular inputs			
Direct emissions into soil or water	A.6.1 (p. 421)	$S_j(s,p,i,z) = S(s,p,i,z)$	(4-3)
Wet or dry atmospheric deposition	A.6.2 (p. 421) A.6.3 (p. 422)	$S_{a\text{-}i}(z,s,p,i) = A(z)\cdot fr\_A(i,z)\cdot ATMDEP_{wet\mid dry}(s,p,z)$	(4-4)
Modifications of the regular inputs			
Wet atmospheric deposition to permeable soils considering preferential flow	A.6.4 (p. 423)	$S_{a\text{-}i}(z,s,p,i) = A(z)\cdot fr\_A(i,z)\cdot ATMDEP_{wet}(s,p,z)\cdot(1-fr\_v_{\text{pref flow/rain}}(z))$	(4-5)
Wet atmospheric deposition to the subsurface through preferential flow	A.6.4 (p. 424)	$S_{a\text{-}j}(z,s,p) = A(z)\cdot(1-fr\_A(w,z)-fr\_A(gl,z)-fr\_A(u,z))\cdot fr\_v_{\text{pref flow/rain}}(z)\cdot ATMDEP_{wet}(s,p,z)$	(4-6)

Table 4-3: Process formulations determining the (exogenous) inputs into the water and soil compartments

Name	Refer to section ... for more details	Formulation[a]
Removal from dry atmospheric deposition due to harvest of exposed above-ground produce	A.6.5 (p. 427)	$$S_{\text{a-ag}}(s,p,z,r,n,e) = -ATMDEP_{\text{dry}}(s,p,z) \cdot \frac{1-10^{-(r_{\text{plant surface loss}}(r,e)\cdot t_{\text{exposure duration}}(r,e))}}{r_{\text{plant surface loss}}(r,e)} \cdot fr\_w_{\text{intercept/deposition}}(r,e) \cdot \frac{P(r,n)}{Y\_fw(r,n,e)} \quad (4\text{-}7)$$
Removal from wet atmospheric deposition due to harvest of exposed above-ground produce	A.6.5 (p. 429)	$$S_{\text{a-ag}}(s,p,z,r,n,e) = -ATMDEP_{\text{wet}}(s,p,z) \cdot fr\_w_{\text{adhere/wet deposition}}(p,r,e) \cdot \frac{1-10^{-(r_{\text{plant surface loss}}(r,e)\cdot t_{\text{exposure duration}}(r,e))}}{r_{\text{plant surface loss}}(r,e)} \cdot fr\_w_{\text{intercept/deposition}}(r,e) \cdot \frac{P(r,n)}{Y\_fw(r,n,e)} \quad (4\text{-}8)$$

a. *A*: area of the zone [m^2]; *ATMDEP*: atmospheric deposition [$kg/m^2/s$]; *fr_A*: area fraction of a compartment within a zone [-]; *fr_v*: fraction of a process velocity [-]; *fr_w*: mass fraction of a substance [-]; *P*: annual production rate of a crop [kg FW/s]; *r*: process rate [1/s]; ρ: density [kg/m^3]; *S*: source of substances into the water and soil fate model [kg/s]; *t*: duration [s]; *Y_fw*: yield of produce [kg FW/m^2]; symbols in parentheses denote a parameter's dependency on the compartment (generic: '*i*' and specific: '*a*': air; '*ag*': arable (or agricultural) land; *gl*: glacier; *n*: (semi-) natural ecosystems; *u*: impervious surface (urban/built-up area)), exposure assessment framework ('*e*'), administrative unit ('*n*'), pollutant ('*p*'), receptor (or crop, '*r*'), emission scenario ('*s*') and/or the zone ('*z*')

There are principally two ways how substances can be removed from the mass balance: by 'degradation' and by transport beyond the model's boundaries. The latter is related to transport within or between zones.

A better notion for 'degradation' which might imply that a substance has been fully mineralised and does not pose any harm any longer could be 'chemical transformation' or 'inactivation'. In particular the latter notion might well be suited to comprise all processes that keep toxic substances from becoming effective (again). Some reflections on inactivation processes especially with respect to trace elements will be given in section 4.2.3.

In an environmental fate model consisting of water and soil compartments, transport within and between zones is mostly driven by water flows although diffusion of substances between adjacent compartments such as freshwater and sediment also occurs. The zones have been defined according to basin boundaries (cf. section 4.3). These zones are interlinked by a cascade flow from upstream areas to downstream areas making use of the Pfafstetter code (Verdin, 1997). Since each zone constitutes a separate drainage area which may principally receive water from at most two upstream zones and may deliver to one downstream zone (cf. top of Fig. 4-4), all water flows are funnelled to the outlet of the zone. It is assumed here that the outlet of a zone is the only place where exchanges between zones occur. If ground water was considered, the assumption that there is no exchange of water between ground water bodies of adjacent zones would be in line with Arnold et al. (1993) and Blöschl (1996). This means that zonal boundaries act as barriers also for subsurface flows so that exfiltration into surface freshwater bodies would only occur within one zone. The situation would of course be different if an air compartment was added in an integrated way.

Also processes that take place in terrestrial compartments do not cross zonal boundaries. For instance, processes such as erosion and overland flow only deliver to the corresponding freshwater body of the same zone. Principally these flows may also connect different terrestrial compartments of the same zone. However, information on the situation of for example arable land towards natural ecosystems gets lost according to the 'semi-distributed' approach as suggested by Becker (1995) and followed in this work (cf. section 5.1). Transport within zones, thus, primarily connects the terrestrial compartments to the aquatic environment, i.e., mostly from soils to streams and rivers but also from soils to the subsurface which may or may not be beyond the model's boundaries.

The processes will be described in the respective sections on the different compartments below. Their formulation has been guided by the SimpleBox model (Brandes et al., 1996). Before these are described some reflections on inactivation processes with respect to non-degradable substances will be given as announced above.

4.2.3 Remarks on the consideration of inactivation processes

As metals or non-radioactive elements are perfectly persistent compounds that do not degrade, their possible transformation reactions shall be looked at more closely. The following transformation reactions are principally to be considered in the terrestrial environment:

- speciation, i.e., different chemical compounds of the same element which may also be distinguished functionally (e.g. according to bioavailability) or operationally (e.g. according to separation techniques; cf. e.g. Ure and Davidson, 1995),
- inactivation due to irreversible binding (e.g., Selim and Amacher, 2001), and/or
- precipitation of insoluble minerals (e.g., Robarge, 1999).

Considering speciation is in principle possible by adding the same amount of equations per considered species in the environmental fate model as for a single species version, provided the respective information on transformation reactions are available. This may in turn lead to very large equation systems posing higher requirements on the available computer and storage resources.

Irreversible binding, however, is another issue.'Irreversible binding' means that the release of substances that are sorbed to 'geo-media' is kinetically hindered and practically impossible (Lumsdon and Evans, 1995). When discussing the fate-modelling of metals in multimedia models for use in assessments of life cycles and external costs, it should be kept in mind that the time frame may be in the order of several hundreds or even thousands of years (van den Bergh et al., 2000; Huijbregts et al., 2001) given the potentially very long residence times of these contaminants, for example, in soils (Alloway et al., 1996). Any notion about irreversible binding or precipitation becomes less important in such a very large time frame.[7] Any short term experiments that indicate that part of the substance is 'irreversibly' bound are irrelevant since on the time scales that are involved minerals can completely dissolve, be transformed etc. and all elements are in principle available. That does not mean that at any time the metals are completely available. The processes described like complexation and precipitation are at any moment in time still at work.

The suggestion is not to include the processes of 'irreversible binding' and 'insoluble' mineral formation explicitly but to use solid-water partitioning coefficients that have been measured in natural soils (not influenced by recent anthro-

---

[7] Although noting that such long time horizons potentially bring about the necessity to include geological processes.

pogenic additions of the relevant element) on the basis of total element soil concentrations (e.g., by hydrofluoric acid destruction).

There are also other reasons not to include irreversible binding into the environmental fate model even when assessing short time scales. Irreversible binding as any binding is dependent on available surfaces which is why this process is capacity-limited. The net 'irreversible' nature is due to sorption at specific sites that have a higher affinity for the respective metal (higher binding strengths). In particular these binding sites become less and less available with a higher degree of 'irreversible' binding occurring until the capacity is exhausted (Selim and Amacher, 2001). Models that are used to describe sorption processes (e.g., Langmuir and Freundlich isotherms as well as surface complexation models, Jenne, 1998a) take this binding capacity into account and are as a consequence non-linear. The degree of occupancy of the specific sorption sites is also the reason why solid-water partitioning values for some metals (like copper, cadmium and lead) are dependent on the overall metal concentration (Anonymous, 1999b; Selim and Amacher, 2001). This is also true for the dynamic equilibrium between a precipitate and the dissolved metal fraction. Introducing parameters that depend on a substance's concentration into an environmental fate model would require to formulate it with non-linearities. Thus, the approach followed in the development of the WATSON environmental fate model that is formulated as a set of ordinary first order linear differential equations would have to be abandoned. Another aspect of considering the inactivation processes explicitly is that plant uptake as used in many exposure models (e.g., United States - Environmental Protection Agency, 1998; International Atomic Energy Agency, 2001) is based on a transfer factor relating the total dry soil concentration to the plant concentration. In the analysis of the total dry soil concentrations, often strong agents like nitrohydrochloric acid ('aqua regia') or hydrofluoric acid are used which would even release at least to some degree the 'irreversibly' bound and precipitated fractions of the metals irrespective of their availability under natural conditions. Thus, there is a need to also include the inactivated metals in the bulk concentration numbers. However, if the process of inactivation of metals be it due to irreversible binding or due to precipitation was to be introduced into the steady-state environmental fate model it would need to be formulated as an overall loss from the system removing the amount of metals at the same time from the bulk soil. This, in turn, would not allow to consider this fraction in the bulk soil concentration for plant root uptake estimates. Another option would be to introduce another compartment which solely contains the highly unreactive portion of metals that is only released at an extremely low pace. This would, however, enlarge the numbers of compartments and, thus, equations to be solved. Furthermore, influences of an environmental medium's oxidative power (or redox conditions) that varies diurnally or seasonally (e.g., Bartlett, 1999; Olivie-Lauquet et al., 2001) on speciation and/or inactivation cannot be dealt with if employing a climatological model that makes use of long-term annual meteorological and hydrological information. As a result, one would have to abandon the level III (steady-state) modelling approach which would require the development of a new model in order to allow for irreversible binding and redox conditions adequately.

Irreversible binding does not only apply to metals but also to the realm of organic chemistry forming the so-called 'bound residues' (e.g., Chung and Alexander, 1998; Eschenbach et al., 1998; Karimi-Lotfabad et al., 1998). In a critical review, Luthy et al. (1997) state that the fundamental knowledge about the nature of the sequestration of hydrophobic organic chemicals by geosorbents is still lacking. In a general model, the authors distinguish between partitioning that is assumed to be linear and non-linear adsorption (see above). Sorption and desorption show reaction rates that range from minutes to even years. Although these rates are derived from macroscopic observations that lack microscopic explanations especially when considering the heterogeneous mixture of potential organic sorbents present in soils, sorption processes involving kinetic considerations are usually not included in the more advanced level III/IV multimedia models as chemical equilibria are assumed within compartments (Mackay, 1991). It might, therefore, be worth considering whether to include 'irreversible binding' of organic chemicals as a kind of degradation process rendering the respective amounts unavailable to further dispersion and potentially toxic effects. As 'degradation' is considered for organic chemicals, one may need to explore whether the formation of bound residues is already implicitly contained in the degradation indicators (e.g., half lives).

4.3 Spatial differentiation of the terrestrial and freshwater environment

The fate model for the terrestrial and aquatic environment is formulated in a spatially-resolved way. 'Spatially-resolved' means that different zones are distinguished in order to allow for a site-dependent impact assessment. The way how these zones are delimitated will be described in the following. Subsequent sections will then deal with the subdivision of the zones into compartments. It shall be noted that similar to the SoilFug model (Di Guardo et al., 1994; Barra et al., 2000), WATSON only includes terrestrial and aquatic compartments.

When dividing an area in sub-entities, one needs to select criteria how this division is performed. Different approaches and/or recommendations for spatial differentiation in multimedia modelling efforts exist (see also Wania, 1996 and a general discussion in section 2.3.1):

- Pelichet (2003) recommends to use a grid-based differentiation of the air compartment and a watershed-based differentiation for the terrestrial environment. Based on this evaluation, the earlier version of IMPACT 2002 has been modified to separate the medium air according to a 2° by 2.5° grid (cf. Pennington et al., 2005).
- GLOBOX is based on countries with only one air and water compartment which are (uni- or bidirectionally) connected to all adjacent countries irrespective of watershed borders for water flows (Wegener Sleeswijk, 2005).
- BETR (north American multi-zonal multimedia model) mostly spatially differentiates its geographical scope based on watersheds (MacLeod et al., 2001; Woodfine et al., 2001). This applies to all compartments.
- EVn BETR (European-scale multimedia model) subdivides Europe into 5° by 5° grid cells (Prevedouros et al., 2004). Connectivities for air and water exist between adjacent grid cells.
- ChemCan (Woodfine et al., 2002) divides Canada into 24 ecological regions.
- There exist other environmental fate models of different spatial resolutions (Wania and Mackay, 1995; Wania, 1996; Scheringer et al., 2000b). However, these are 'investigative' fate models that try to predict what distribution patterns different substances follow and not exposure models that are needed to arrive at impacts.
- A more general recommendation was given at the SETAC workshop on multimedia models (Cowan et al., 1995b) in that the zones investigated should cover areas with more than a few hundred square kilometres due to the assumption of uniform mixing. However, this recommendation was given for spatially unresolved models. Spatially-resolved models, in contrast, aim at distinguishing areas with different concentrations. Thus, the recommendation given is considered not applicable here.

It may be concluded that there exist several approaches for spatial differentiation in the realm of spatially-resolved multimedia modelling ranging from administrative units (i.e., nations) over regular grids to natural properties especially water divides.

Apart from air advection, water generally constitutes the main carrier for substances across the landscape. The importance of water flows further increases for substances whose environmental fate is not largely determined by the rates of transformation. In any case, lateral surface and subsurface flows need to be considered which belong to the so-called 'lateral flows domain' (Becker, 1995). Modelling of lateral flows "must principally take into account the boundaries of hydrological systems like river basins, ground water systems etc., i.e. the drainage basin water divides" (ibid., p. 138). This is in line with Hunsaker et al. (1990) who note that zones for which impacts are assessed should be functionally defined, i.e., the "boundaries should be determined by physical or biological processes that affect the impact of the hazard such as the boundaries of watersheds, airsheds, and physiographic provinces" (p. 327). This will additionally support the transferability of the approach to other regions.

Consequently, watershed or drainage basin information are used for the delimitation of the terrestrial environment. Single watersheds vary substantially in size (e.g., the Danube compared to rivers that only stretch a few kilometres inland). Treating watersheds of considerably different size in the same way, i.e., as just one zone, has bearings on the environmental fate modelling. Due to the homogeneous mixing assumption, however, an artificial effect may result which may be called the 'instant long-range mixing effect'. Consider emissions taking place near the river mouth which are instantly mixed into the entire water contained in the watershed according to the homogeneity assumption within compartments. Whereas for smaller catchments the error introduced would not be too severe, this would lead to a situation in which emissions for example occurring in the Netherlands end up in Lac de Neuchatel in Switzerland if the Rhine - as a larger river - was not further subdivided into sub-catchments. Also, when assessing rather readily degradable substances these would occur at locations where they would never arrive due to the fast chemical transformation taking place.

Consequently, there is a need for larger watersheds to be further subdivided. Beside the subdivision itself, information on how the different zones are connected to each other is needed. The subdivision adopted in WATSON follows watershed information based on the HYDRO1k Basins dataset (EROS Data Center, 1996) which provides both of these sets of information.

Connectivities are defined according to the Pfafstetter code (cf. Verdin, 1997). This code allows to identify whether and where a zone is situated within a drainage basin. According to this code, each drainage basin of larger rivers is subdivided into nine sub-basins if at least four larger tributaries can be identified. These are coded with even numbers from downstream to upstream. The drainage areas between these basins (called interbasins) assume the respective odd numbers and constitute the main stem of the subdivided river. This procedure can be repeated for each basin and interbasin if again at least four tributaries can be identified. The Pfafstetter code can also be applied starting at the continental level. For Europe, the Rhine catchment, for instance is identified at the third subdivision level by the code "914" (Fig. 4-4). A further subdivision is also possible at least at the fourth level (as indicated in Fig. 4-4) and for some (inter-) basins even below. Therefore, also the connectivities by water currents between zones are given by EROS Data Center (1996).

The zones were visually checked to Cleveland et al. (1984) and European Environment Agency Data Service (1998) and corrected where deemed necessary (cf. Table B-1).

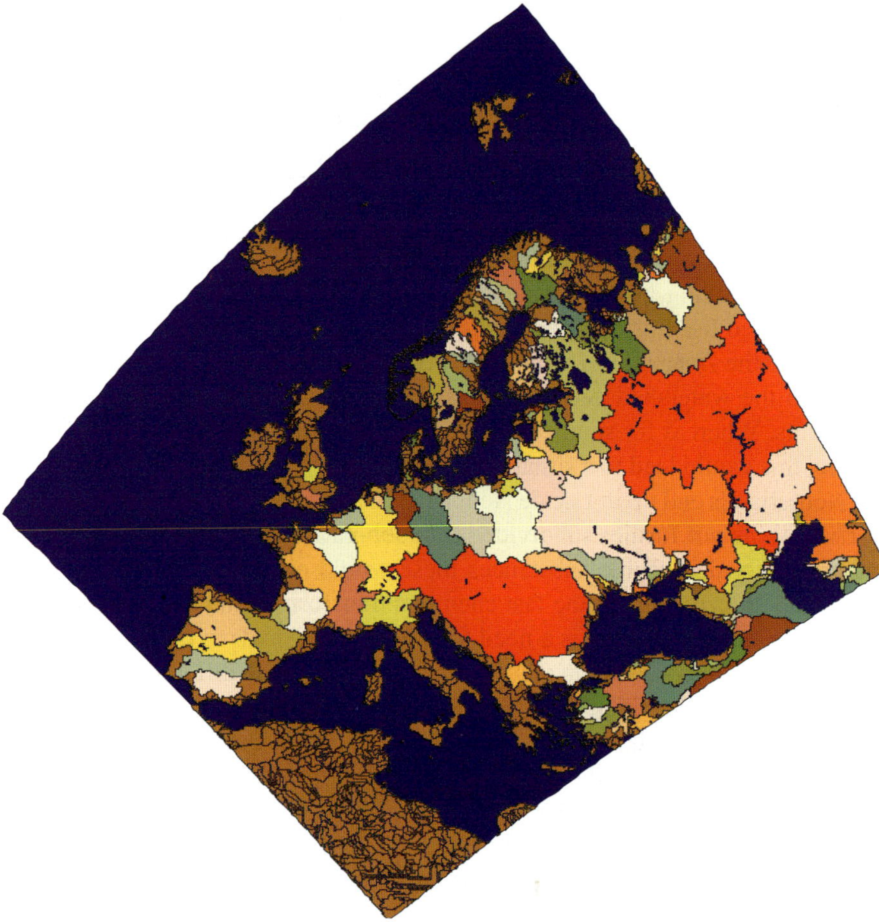

Fig. 4-2: Spatial resolution of the WATSON model based on watersheds; data taken from EROS Data Center (1996) and adjusted (see text)

A further subdivision into zones has been performed according to land cover information on freshwater bodies. In order to distinguish at least larger lakes with a potentially high water volume from rivers, lakes of an area larger than 100 km^2 were defined as described in section B.2.1. In case these are not just contained within one zone but spread over several zones, all these lake zones are allowed to also constitute separate zones.

The two presently available subdivisions of the spatial scope of the WATSON model into zones are shown in Fig. 4-2 and 4-3 (low and high resolution, respectively).

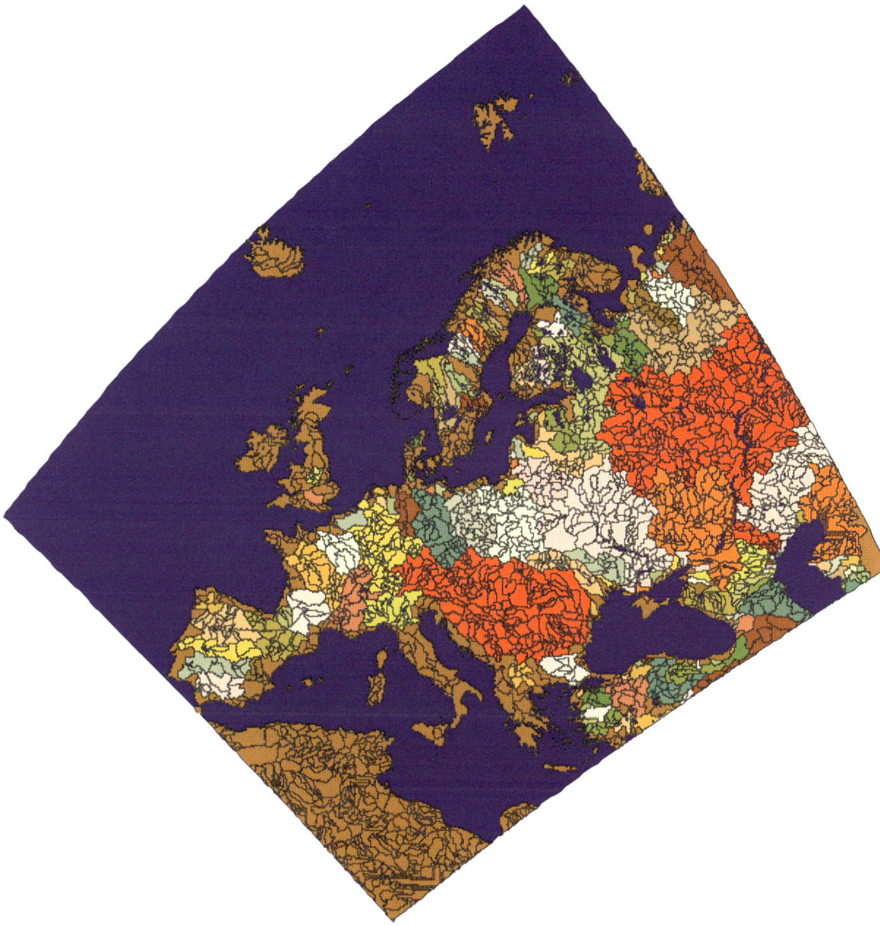

Fig. 4-3: Spatial resolution of the WATSON model based on watersheds which are further subdivided in the case of larger catchments; data taken from EROS Data Center (1996) and adjusted (see text)

4.4 Implementation

This section on the implementation of the conceptual model into a software tool shall neither serve as a manual to the usage of WATSON nor shall it provide details on the algorithms implemented. Instead, some technicalities shall be described.

In contrast to the majority of multimedia fate and exposure models which are implemented as spreadsheet models, for instance EUSES (Vermeire et al.,

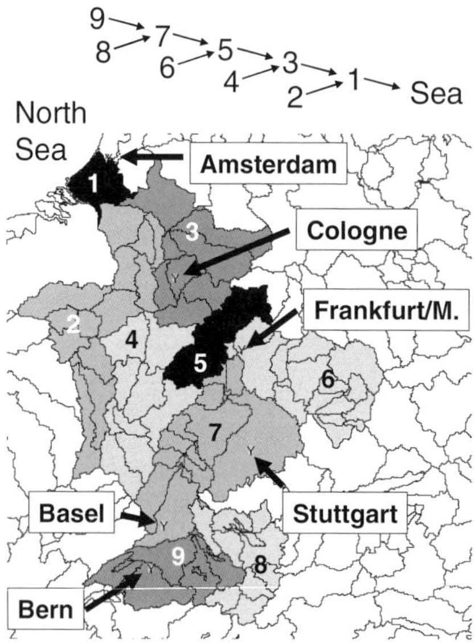

Fig. 4-4: Organisation of the Rhine catchment including the Meuse river according to the Pfafstetter code (note the Rhine catchment is identified by "914" at the continental scale, the shown digits constitute the fourth level subdivision, i.e., "914x"; the general Pfafstetter coding principle is also shown at the top)

1997), USES-LCA (Huijbregts, 1999), CalTOX (McKone, 1993b) and IMPACT 2000 (Pennington et al., 2005), the software tool developed here does not employ spreadsheets for the environmental fate and exposure assessment steps of the Impact Pathway Approach. While the existing EcoSense multi-source model is coded in C (MS Visual Studio 1.5) and the data storage is done with the help of a Paradox database, WATSON is coded in C++ (MS Visual Studio 6.0) and uses a LINUX-based Oracle database version 8.1.6i. This allows a flexible definition of process formulations and combinations as well as the use of different environmental settings (see explanation of *process sets* below). This way, data are kept separately from the simulation code (Robinson, 1999) which facilitates their changeability (Veerkamp and Wolff, 1996), however, on the expense of computation time.

Unlike many existing multimedia models, WATSON's mass balance is based on concentrations (like SimpleBox, Brandes et al., 1996) rather than on fugacities (e.g., Mackay, 1979) avoiding the aquivalence approach (Mackay and Diamond, 1989; Diamond et al., 1992). The solution of the system of linear differential equations is facilitated with the help of the NAg C library mark 6 (cf. section A.1).

Data processing of spatially distributed parameters has been done with ESRI ArcInfo version 7.1.1 and displayed with ESRI ArcView GIS version 3.1.1 employing various datasets. The datasets together with the derivation of the spatially variable parameters used in the environmental fate model are described in detail in Appendices B and C.

4.4.1 Definition of scenarios

WATSON allows the analysis of different scenarios. A *scenario* consists of the combination of several definitions:

- of emissions into different media (defined by a so-called *exogenous input type*; cf. section A.6) which may either be continuous and constant or consist of a constant pulse emission over a specified time period; WATSON allows for different allocation schemes for direct emissions to water and soil (e.g., according to population density or land uses); as with the exposure assessment, the specification especially of direct releases into water and soil follows administrative units (cf. Fig. B-4),
- of allowed environmental fate processes including the definition of the spatial differentiation in terms of compartments distinguished and degree of sub-division of the geographical scope into zones (defined by a so-called *process set*; cf. section 4.3 on spatial differentiation),
- of considered initial background concentrations, and
- of the exposure assessment to be followed (defined by a so-called *exposure frame* or expo frame).

The environmental fate matrix is, thus, defined by the process set in a very flexible way. Similar to TRIM.FaTE (United States - Environmental Protection Agency, 1999a), within WATSON the user can switch particular processes on and off rather than setting unrealistic values for example for vapour pressures of non-volatile compounds like most trace elements (as done, e.g., in Guinée et al., 1996; European Commission, 2003b). If the process set is defined in such a way that there is a compartment without any removal process the respective compartment is not further considered in the assessment.[8] The ability to change the compartmental mass balance in terms of processes combined as well as in terms of process formulations is a prerequisite in order to cover several substance classes (e.g., Trapp and Schwartz, 2000). The process set is computed and stored only once per substance and may be used by different scenarios.

---

[8] This is actually an option which can be switched on and off by the user.

Parameters, processes, process sets, receptors, exposure frames, exogenous input types and auxiliary formulae which may help to internally derive parameter values are defined based on different assumptions. These assumptions especially when they might cause conflicts are also assigned to these components so that a check can be performed as to whether a combination of these components may lead to errors (e.g., considering preferential flow in the fate (cf. section A.3.7) but not in the exogenous input part (cf. section A.6.4)).

4.4.2 Temporal modes of operation

In order to address a variety of questions, different temporal modes of operation are possible with the WATSON model:

- steady-state is a situation in which no change in concentration occurs over time. That means that all outputs of a compartment equal the inputs. This situation may, thus, be relevant for sustainability-related questions (e.g., European Commission, 2003d). Furthermore, Heijungs (1995) has shown that the steady-state situation can also be used for time-integrated exposure assessments of pulse emissions. For life cycle analysis purposes where pulse emissions are dealt with, the perception prevails that temporal discounting should not be performed that may lead to neglecting even the larger share of potential future impacts of long-lived pollutants (e.g., Udo de Haes et al., 1999), especially of metals and radionuclides. Thus, steady-state solutions are regularly computed.
- quasi-dynamic including pulse emissions: in order to evaluate the temporal development of the concentrations or the exposure of a continuous or a pulse emission, also a quasi-dynamic solution is implemented. In line with Brandes et al. (1996), the term 'quasi-dynamic' indicates that all parameters but the chemical concentrations or releases are constant over time. In principle, the user can choose the time step as (s)he likes. However, it must be kept in mind that a time step that is not given in full years is inappropriate when using this climatologically-based model.
- time to reach steady-state: Another temporal feature of WATSON is the so-called 'time to reach steady-state'. This measure indicates how far in the future the steady-state will be reached (e.g., Cowan et al., 1995a; Trapp and Matthies, 1995). Two limits can be defined by the user: the percentage of the steady-state solution and the maximum time period to be investigated. As the time to 100 % steady-state may be in the order of centuries or much longer for metals (e.g., Huijbregts et al., 2001; de Vries et al., 2004) and, thus, converges very slowly, these limits aid to run the computation more efficiently. This third mode of temporal operation comprises the two other modes. An

application of this mode of operation can be found in Bachmann et al. (2004).

For a more general discussion on steady-state and quasi-dynamic modelling as well as their computations for the mathematical approach followed, the reader is referred to sections 2.3.1 and A.1, respectively.

It shall be noted that computations with time steps that are not full years is not adequate in terms of resulting meaningful values for the eventually desired period of time (e.g., seasonal, monthly, daily variations). This is due to the use of long-term average data for the description of the environment.

5 Modelling the environmental fate in the terrestrial environment

In this Chapter, the environmental fate modelling approach for the terrestrial environment is presented. The description is generally divided into modelling of concentrations in terrestrial compartments distinguished by land uses and/or covers (such as agricultural soils; section 5.1) and modelling of contaminants in (terrestrial) plants (section 5.2).

5.1 Environmental fate modelling for different land covers

The WATSON model is primarily an exposure model with which impacts are assessed and valued. Modifying the definition given by van de Meent et al. (1996) and in line with Severinsen and Jager (1998) an exposure model is defined here more specifically as a model that describes the relationship between emissions and chemical quantities that living organisms are exposed to. Pure environmental fate models on the other hand describe the relationship between emissions and concentrations trying to quantitatively answer the question of 'how much of a substance ends up where?'. Thus, model development and set-up may require different subdivisions of the zones (cf. section 4.3) in terms of compartments distinguished and parameterisation of these compartments if one was to either develop a pure environmental fate model or an exposure model.

5.1.1 Compartments distinguished in the terrestrial environment

One may think of different criteria based on which the subdivision of the terrestrial environment can be performed. Before elaborating these criteria a short non-exhaustive overview about how the terrestrial environment is further subdivided into compartments by several existing multimedia models shall be given which builds to a large extent on the detailed description of models in section 3.1:

- a multimedia workshop organized by SETAC recommends to distinguish at least three soils of different land use/soil types (Cowan et al., 1995b). No more specific recommendations on what land uses or soil types to distinguish are made.
- EUSES and SimpleBox 2.0 distinguish between three terrestrial compartments: 'natural', 'agricultural' and 'industrial' (Brandes et al., 1996; European Commission, 1996a). Apart from their physical dimensions (i.e., mixing depths and area fractions), the only difference between these terrestrial compartments is whether they receive only inputs from air, additionally from sewage sludge or direct inputs, respectively. There is no differentiation in terms of processes taking place at varying rates (e.g., different erosion rates, infiltration capacities).
- similar to EUSES and SimpleBox 2.0, USES-LCA also distinguishes between the three terrestrial compartments stated above (Huijbregts, 1999). Furthermore, the terrestrial compartments are allowed to have different pH values in order to better account for variable solubility and, thus, the organic carbon-water partition coefficient (K_{OC}) of dissociating substances as well as hydrolysis rates in water, soil and sediments. It is stated, however, that no pH-dependency for metals is as yet considered.
- CalTOX version 4 (beta) does not (appear to) distinguish between different land uses (McKone and Enoch, 2002). However, it distinguishes between three soil layers: ground-surface soil, root-zone soil and the vadose-zone soil below the root zone. This distinction is also made by the multi-zonal multimedia model IMPACT 2002 (Pennington et al., 2005).
- similar to CalTOX, a multimedia model for the Great Lakes (CHEMGL) distinguishes between surface soil and the vadose zone, as well as ground water (Zhang et al., 2003).
- multi-zonal multimedia models usually do not distinguish between different soil compartments, for instance BETR North America (MacLeod et al., 2001; Woodfine et al., 2001), EVn BETR (Prevedouros et al., 2004), CHEMFRANCE (Devillers et al., 1995), the global model by Scheringer et al. (2000b), ChemCAN (Woodfine et al., 2002). Exceptions to this are the POPCYCLING-Baltic model (Wania et al., 2000) and Globo-POP (Wania, 2003) where the terrestrial environment is further subdivided into agricultural/cultivated and non-agricultural/non-cultivated land.
- if an urban environment is to be considered, Diamond et al. (2001) suggest to also include an organic film that coats impervious surfaces when modelling semi-volatile organic compounds. This is in line with McKone and Bennett (2003) to have a thin soil layer at the air-soil interface in order to properly consider volatilisation.

The following conclusions are drawn from this overview:

- a distinction of agricultural soils is necessary for the sake of human exposure assessment.
- soils of non-agricultural use should be included at least in order to have 100 % soil coverage.
- in principle, also natural vegetation should be included for the sake of the travelling of some (semi-) volatile substances (e.g., Bennett et al., 1998). This inclusion, however, should be realized especially in the air quality model domain (i.e., presently the WTM, cf. section 4.1) due to the exchanges taking place between air and plant material. Focusing on the media soil and water in the present work, the inclusion of plant compartments for environmental fate reasons is, therefore, left to future model developments. However, plants are also important with respect to human exposure assessment towards agricultural produce which will be dealt with in section 5.2 and Chapter 7.
- information on direct emissions to soils other than agricultural land which receive inputs for example via sewage sludge and pesticide application is rather scarce. Therefore, also the distinction of an urban/industrial soil will not be made for the sake of receiving direct inputs. Leachates from landfills are primarily considered emissions to ground water which cannot appropriately be modelled at present for even less information on ground water is available than for soils.
- the inclusion of an organic film on impervious areas (cf. Diamond et al., 2001) is considered too special for a larger scale environmental fate and exposure model.

As was discussed in section 3.2, substances to be assessed in the present work are non-radioactive, non-degradable and non-volatile trace elements. Due to these properties, the main loss mechanisms from the terrestrial environment are linked to advective transport processes by water (cf. Scudlark et al., 2005) including soil erosion. In contrast to POPs for whose environmental fate and human exposure the soil erosion process including overland flow is found to be less relevant (Fiedler et al., 2000), it is estimated that about 95 % of the heavy metals that are transported from land to the sea is particle-bound (Morgan and Stumm, 1999). Furthermore, the soil metal contents depends on the erodibility of the surface soil (Nriagu, 1978). Beside potential human exposure pathways for example via crops and animal products, thus, permeability (in line with Becker, 1995) and soil erosion which amongst others is a function of the land use or management (cf. the C-factor in the Universal Soil Loss Equation, USLE, e.g., Wischmeier and Smith (1978) and Renard et al. (1997)) will serve as the main criteria for the dif-

Table 5-1: Terrestrial compartments distinguished according to qualitative criteria; their area shares in the geographical scope of the model are also given (derived from data presented in section B.3)

Compartment	Area fraction[a] [%]	Human exposure	Permeability	Erosion potential
Arable land	29	Via crops, animals and their products	high	moderate to high
Pasture	13	Via animals and products	high	low to moderate
Semi-natural ecosystems	50	n/a	high	low to very moderate
Non-vegetated land	1.4	n/a	high	high
Impervious surfaces	1.2	n/a	n/a	n/a
Glaciers	0.9	n/a	n/a	n/a

a. The remainder of about 4 % are freshwater bodies.

ferentiation of the terrestrial environment into compartments. The resulting compartments and their qualitative features with respect to the distinction criteria are given in Table 5-1.

The real distribution of the compartments within each of the zones is not explicitly considered. Still, their distinction overcomes the critical effects of averaging their variable characteristics over large areas (similar to the 'semi-distributed' approach as suggested by Becker (1995) for large scale hydrological modelling).

As the environmental fate of hydrophobic organic pollutants is highly linked to the presence of lipophilic matter, some spatially-resolved multimedia models allow the organic carbon content to vary (e.g., Wania et al., 2000; MacLeod, 2002). For similar reasons, WATSON-Europe, furthermore, includes varying pH values for the different environmental compartments in the distinguished zones (cf. section B.5) in order to take one of the key parameters into account that influences the partitioning behaviour of trace elements and particularly of metals (Sauvé et al., 2000; Kabata-Pendias and Pendias, 2001; Sauvé 2002). The mobility of trace elements such as lead, copper and chromium in soils may also substantially depend on the presence of colloidal organic matter (e.g., Bergkvist et al., 1989). However, appreciable colloidal transport beside preferential transport in general (cf. section A.3.7) is expected only to occur under rather acidic conditions ('podzolation') for which the pH value is an indicator noting that the mobility of copper and lead may not depend so much on the pH (Bergkvist et al., 1989).

Information on land use, soil pH and organic carbon content as well as on hydrology are taken from several sources (Batjes, 1996; EROS Data Center et al., 2000; Hansen et al., 1998; New et al., 1999; European Environment Agency, 2000; Lehner and Döll, 2001; Döll et al., 2003; cf. sections B.3 and B.5).

For each of the compartments, both its dimension and the processes possibly taking place need to be defined which will be defined in the following.

5.1.2 Dimensions of the terrestrial compartments

The areas that the respective soil compartments cover are determined based on GIS datasets (cf. section B.3). Unfortunately, no such GIS dataset is available at justifiable costs for the soil depth which is especially needed for the volume calculations (cf. section A.4). Therefore, the soil depth needs to be defined in a different way.

In Table 5-2, the depth for natural soil, agricultural soil and unspecified land use is shown as assumed in some multimedia models. Note that models that purely base the soil depth on a Damkoehler number-derived effective penetration depth are not considered for the reasons given in section B.3.2.

Without considering the maximum allowable effective penetration depth of SimpleBox 2.0 (Brandes et al., 1996), the soil compartment depths range from 0.01-0.1, from 0.05-0.3 and from 0.1-0.3 m for natural, agricultural and unspecified soil, respectively.

Before deciding upon a soil depth the following arguments should be reflected:

- usually agricultural land is assumed to be ploughed. This, however, only applies to arable land. Furthermore, tillage practices show different degrees of soil reworking/disturbances. Only ploughing really homogenizes the top soil while being the most disturbing tillage practice leading to homogenized soil depth between 20 and up to 60 cm in vineyards (Schütte, 2003). Principally one can distinguish between no-inversion and inversion practices, a variant of the former being no-tillage. Thus, for no-inversion techniques principally no homogenisation takes place (as intended) and for the others the ploughing layer in central Europe is about 30 cm which is the case for instance on 60 % of the arable land in Germany (Schütte, 2003),

Table 5-2: Overview on different soil depths adopted by selected multimedia models

Soil type	Depth [m]	Reference	Remarks
Natural soil	0.01-1.0	SimpleBox 2.0 (Brandes et al., 1996)	one metre is an upper limit to the effective penetration depth
	0.05	EUSES (European Commission, 1996a)	
	0.1	POPCYCLING-Baltic model (Wania et al., 2000)	forest soil
	0.01-0.1	Wania and Mackay (1995)	soil not receiving direct input; variable values due to different zones
Agricultural soil	0.2-1.0	SimpleBox 2.0 (Brandes et al., 1996)	one metre is an upper limit to the effective penetration depth
	0.2	EUSES (European Commission, 1996a)	
	0.05-0.25	POPCYCLING-Baltic model (Wania et al., 2000)	agricultural soil; variable values due to different zones
	0.15-0.3	SoilFug (Barra et al., 2000)	values for different Uniform Geographic Units; not a fully integrated multimedia model
	0.1	Wania and Mackay (1995)	soil receiving direct input
Unspecified soils (i.e., no distinction made or no type of soil indicated)	0.15	CHEMFRANCE (Devillers et al., 1995)	
	0.1	Scheringer et al. (2000b)	
	0.2-0.3	SoilFug (Barra et al., 2000)	values for different sub-basins; not a fully integrated multimedia model

- other homogenizing processes that can in places even affect several decimetres include bioturbation (e.g., by ants, moles, earthworms, earthlings), cryoturbation (driven by the change of freezing and thawing water) and peloturbation (driven by wetting and drying of soils rich in clay, Scheffer and Schachtschabel, 1989). However, significant contributions are only expected on soils with good water, air and nutrient conditions, on soils in the tundra climate, and on soils with a high clay content and changing water contents, respectively. The available GIS datasets do not allow to distinguish these soil types appropriately. Furthermore, the delimitation of natural vs. agricultural soil does not follow any of the just stated environmental properties,
- Jury et al. (1990) have shown that volatile organic compounds that occur well below the air-soil interface would need to be buried by a soil cover several metres deep in order for some of them not to re-enter the atmosphere. This means that for the sake of reducing the potentially underestimated volatilisation of these substances a soil depth larger than 0.1 m for natural soil should be chosen,
- the organic carbon content and the pH of the soil are identified to be the two key properties which influence the mobility of organic compounds and of metals, respectively. These are considered by the environmental fate model implemented in WATSON. The best and most readily available GIS dataset on organic carbon contents and pH values of soils for the geographical scope of WATSON is provided by Batjes (1996) (see section B.5.1 on the processing of these information). Information are given for 0-30 cm and 30-100 cm. This suggests to consider a soil thickness of between 0 and 30 cm for the ease of data processing.

For WATSON, a uniform depth of 30 cm is adopted which is at the higher end of the so-far assumed soil compartment thicknesses given in Table 5-2. This is motivated by the circumstance that WATSON is an exposure model which is why deeper surface layers than the root zone are generally not of interest, apart from ground water that is not considered at present. Furthermore, the findings by Jury et al. (1990) stated above together with the data availability issue suggest to use a soil depth between 0.1 and 0.3 m. A third reason may be that except for the models by Wania and co-workers (e.g., Wania and Mackay, 1995; Wania et al., 2000), multi-zonal multimedia models usually do not allow the soil depths of different zones to vary (e.g., Devillers et al., 1995; Scheringer et al., 2000b). Note that this default depth only applies to pervious soils, i.e., arable land, pasture, semi-natural ecosystems and non-vegetated land. The compartment depths of glaciers and impervious land will be addressed below.

5.1.3 Definition of the phases of terrestrial compartments

To the knowledge of the author, there is no GIS dataset available on soil texture data from which to define the volume share of void spaces in soils. Furthermore, a water content needs to be additionally defined for example for the calculation of the equilibrium distribution coefficient (section A.2). There are two publications of a multi-zonal multimedia model where these parameters are assumed to vary (SoilFug, e.g., Barra et al., 2000 and the model described by Wania and Mackay (1995), see Table 5-3). Whereas in the model by Wania and Mackay the volume share varies between zones and land uses, the ranges of volume shares in SoilFug are 20-30 % for water and the reverse for air, always yielding 50 % void space. Similar values are used by McKone and Bennett (2003) whereas in SimpleBox 2.0 (Brandes et al., 1996) a rather sandy soil (according to void spaces) is assumed which is probably due to screening level risk assessment assumptions or might reflect the high end of properties found in Dutch soils.

Although soil texture and soil moisture will vary significantly in space and time, this is not taken into account due to lack of information. In order not to be too conservative, the volume fraction values used in SimpleBox 2.0 (Brandes et al., 1996) are not adopted. Instead, soils are assumed to have a loamy texture with 50 % void spaces. Assuming that the soils are at field capacity then means that 30 % of the volume consist of aqueous phase (water tension: pF = 2.5). One has to note, however, that for example in Spain there are areas affected by desertification for which this water content will be too high. On the other hand, wetlands are not treated as water bodies but (most likely) as natural soils having effectively no gas phase.

The volume fraction of solids in the impervious compartment is set to 1 vol.-% assuming that the surface itself does not act as an adsorbent. The glacier compartment is assumed to contain 5 vol.-% solids although no partitioning to them will take place due to the effective absence of liquid water.

Another parameter usually is held constant. This is the density of the solid phase. In multimedia models, assumed solid particle densities range from 2500 to 2600 kg/m^3 (see Table 5-3). Due to the fact that the organic carbon contents is allowed to vary within WATSON (cf. section B.5.1), the solid phase density will also vary to some extent. Since the mineral solid particles of soils usually are made up of quartz with a density of 2700 kg/m^3, a mean mineral solid density of 2650 kg/m^3 can be assumed (Scheffer and Schachtschabel, 1989) which is adopted in the present study. The organic solids are assumed to have a density of 1400 kg/m^3 (Scheffer and Schachtschabel, 1989) and consist of 50 weight-% organic carbon according to 'model' humic and fulvic acids as given by Schnitzer (1978). For impervious land uses, this value is set to 70 weight-% based on the consideration that the organic matter on roads mostly consists of soot which is richer in organic carbon (e.g., Gustafsson et al., 1997).

Table 5-3: Soil characteristics according to different multimedia models

Volume fraction			Mass fraction	ρ_{solid}	Reference	Comment
gas [-]	aqueous [-]	total void [-]	organic carbon [-]	[kg/m^3]		
0.2	0.3	0.5	0.02	2600	McKone and Bennett (2003)	
0.2-0.3	0.2-0.3	0.5	0.01-0.025	n/a	Barra et al. (2000)	coarse silty and coarse loamy soils
0.2	0.2	0.4	0.05	2500	Brandes et al. (1996)	rather sandy soils
n/a	n/a	n/a	0.03-0.05	n/a	Wania et al. (2000)	organic carbon content varies between zones
0.25-0.35	0.15-0.25	0.5	0.005 (polar)-0.02 (rest)	n/a	Wania and Mackay (1995)	natural soils; water contents: lowest in the subtropics and highest in the polar/boreal zones
0.30-0.40	0.15-0.25	0.55-0.60	0.005 (polar)-0.02 (rest)	n/a	Wania and Mackay (1995)	agricultural soils; water contents: lowest in the subtropics and highest in the polar/boreal zones; void space is highest in the tropics

5.1.4 Processes considered for the terrestrial compartments

There are different processes in the terrestrial environment implemented in existing multimedia models (Table 5-4). It is evident that the different models usually consider the same processes. The only exception is resuspension of soil particles in CalTOX (McKone, 1993b). The way the so-called process 'resuspension' is described in CalTOX it may be better termed 'wind soil erosion' due to the equilibration of particle-bound substances taking place within soils in the time between the deposition of these particles from and their resuspension into air. As a result, 'resuspension' as understood by CalTOX may have different meanings or implications (such as the substances or particles being inert) in contexts other than multimedia modelling. For the reasons why this process is not taken into account in the presented methodology refer to section 4.1.1.

Due to the effectively involatile nature of the considered trace elements, the diffusive processes will not be considered further. Furthermore, the same reasoning not to consider these processes applies as for wind soil erosion (cf. section 4.1.1). The question to what degree inactivation processes could or should be included in the environmental fate model is specifically addressed in section 4.2.3. Beside wind soil erosion, all the other advective processes as given in Table 5-4, i.e., water soil erosion, (saturated) overland flow (including interflow) and matrix leaching, are considered in the presented methodology. Their formulation is given in Table 5-5 and further discussed in separate sub-sections to A.3 also stated in the Table. Note that root uptake by plants which may constitute a further removal process from soils is part of section 5.2 and not described here.

5.1.5 Innovations as regards terrestrial compartments

There are several innovations introduced as regards the modelling of the terrestrial environment. These are

- pH-dependent partitioning,
- distinction of compartments other than natural and agricultural soils (in a spatially resolved context),
- the formulation of the soil erosion process, and
- the introduction of the preferential flow process.

These shall be presented in the following.

Table 5-4: Overview on different soil-related processes considered by selected multimedia models

Process	SimpleBox 2.0	CalTOX 3.0	POPCY-CLING-Baltic	SoilFug[a]	CHEM-FRANCE
Degradation/chemical transformation/inactivation					
overall	x	x[b]	x	x	x
Advection					
leaching/ infiltration	x	x	x[c]	(x)[d]	x
overland flow/runoff	x	x	x	x	x
erosion	x	x	x[e]	(x)[d]	x
resuspen-sion of soil particles		x			
Diffusion					
volatilisa-tion	x	x	x[f]	x	x
deposition of gases	x	x			x
Reference	Brandes et al. (1996)	McKone (1993b)[g]	Wania et al. (2000)	Di Guardo et al. (1994)	Devillers et al. (1995)

a. Mainly soil considered (no air compartment).
b. Although not treated separately, it is stated by McKone (1993b) that the overall degradation constant should reflect the rates of photolysis, hydrolysis, oxidation and reduction, and microbial transformation.
c. Together with runoff.
d. Probably together with runoff.
e. Only attached to particulate organic matter.
f. Modified two-resistance model.
g. Latest published documentation of CalTOX according to McKone (2003).

Table 5-5: Process formulations for terrestrial compartments as used in the present assessment

Name	Compartments involved[a]	Refer to section ... for more details	Formulation[b]	
Degradation	i = u, b, n, p, ag	A.3.1 (p. 395)	$k_{i,\,\mathrm{deg}}(p, i, z) = A(z) \cdot fr\_\mathrm{A}(i, z) \cdot d(i, z) \cdot \frac{\ln(2)}{t_{1/2}(p, i)}$	(5-1)
Radioactive decay	i = u, b, n, p, ag, gl	A.3.2 (p. 395)	$k_{i,\,\mathrm{decay}}(p, i, z) = A(z) \cdot fr\_\mathrm{A}(i, z) \cdot d(i, z) \cdot \frac{\ln(2)}{t_{1/2}(p, i)}$	(5-2)
Water soil erosion	i = b, n, p, ag	A.3.3 (p. 396)	$k_{i\text{-}w,\,\mathrm{erosion}}(z, i) = A(z) \cdot fr\_\mathrm{A}(i, z) \cdot v_{\mathrm{erosion}}(i)$	(5-3)
Overland flow	i = b, n, p, ag	A.3.4 (p. 398)	$k_{i\text{-}w,\,\mathrm{overland\ flow},\,pH\mid\mathrm{C_{org}}}(p, i, z) = \mathrm{A}(z) \cdot fr\_A(i, z) \cdot \frac{v_{\mathrm{runoff}}(z) \cdot fr\_\mathrm{v}_{\mathrm{quick\ flow/runoff}}(z)}{ED_{\mathrm{bulk/aqueous}\,,\,pH\mid\mathrm{C_{org}}}(p, i, z)}$	(5-4)
	u	A.3.4 (p. 398)	$k_{u-w,\,\mathrm{overland\ flow,\ pH}\mid\,\mathrm{C_{org}}}(p, u, z) = \mathrm{A}(z) \cdot fr\_A(u, z) \cdot \frac{v_{\mathrm{runoff}}(z)}{ED_{\mathrm{bulk/aqueous,\ pH}\mid\mathrm{C_{org}}}(p, u, z)}$	(5-5)
Ice melt	gl	A.3.5 (p. 400)	$k_{gl\text{-}w,\,\mathrm{ice\ melt}}(z, gl) = A(z) \cdot fr\_\mathrm{A}(gl, z) \cdot \frac{d(gl, z)}{t_{\mathrm{residence}}(gl)}$	(5-6)

Table 5-5: Process formulations for terrestrial compartments as used in the present assessment

Name	Compartments involved[a]	Refer to section ... for more details	Formulation[b]
Matrix leaching	i = b, n, p, ag	A.3.6 (p. 401)	$k_{i\text{-}gw,\ \text{leaching},\ \text{pH}\vert\text{C}_{\text{org}}}(z,i,p) = A(z)\cdot fr\_A(i,z)\cdot \frac{(1-fr\_v_{\text{quick flow/runoff}}(z))\cdot v_{\text{runoff}}(z)}{ED_{\text{bulk/aqueous},\ \text{pH}\vert\text{C}_{\text{org}}}(p,i,z)}$ (5-7)
Reduced matrix leaching due to preferential flow	i = b, n, p, ag	A.3.7 (p. 402)	$k_{i\text{-}gw,\ \text{pref flow},\ \text{pH}\vert\text{C}_{\text{org}}}(z,i,p) = -A(z)\cdot fr\_A(i,z)\cdot \frac{v_{\text{rain}}(z)\cdot fr\_v_{\text{pref flow/rain}}(z)}{ED_{\text{bulk/aqueous},\ \text{pH}\vert\text{C}_{\text{org}}}(p,i,z)}$ (5-8)
Preferential transport	i = b, n, p, ag	A.3.7 (p. 402)	$k_{i\text{-}gw,\ \text{preferential transport}}(z,i,p) = A(z)\cdot fr\_A(i,z)\cdot r_{\text{preferential transport}}(p,i)$ (5-9)

a. *ag*: arable (or agricultural) land; *b*: (bare or) non-vegetated land; *gl*: glacier; *n*: (semi-) natural ecosystems; *p*: pasture/grassland; *u*: impervious surface (urban/built-up area)

b. *A*: area of the zone [m^2]; *d*: depth of a compartment [m]; *ED*: equilibrium distribution coefficient [-]; *fr_A*: area fraction of a compartment within a zone [-]; *fr_v*: fraction of a process velocity [-]; *k*: process rate as used in the coefficient matrix [m^3/s]; *r*: process rate [1/s]; *t*: residence time or half life [s]; *v*: process velocity [m/s]; symbols in parentheses denote a parameter's dependency on the pollutant ('*p*'), the compartment (generic: '*i*' and specific: see footnote a) and/or the zone ('*z*')

pH-dependent partitioning

As discussed in section 5.1.1, WATSON takes one of the key parameters into account that influences the partitioning behaviour of the investigated trace elements. This is the pH value which is allowed to vary in space in the terrestrial environment (cf. section B.5.1 for the derivation of the respective values).

Distinction of terrestrial compartments other than natural and agricultural soils

According to the selection criteria as specified in Table 5-1, not only soils with natural vegetation and those subject to agricultural management may be distinguished as done by state-of-the-art multi-zonal multimedia models. Their influence on the exposure assessment part of the Impact Pathway Approach will be investigated in a scenario analysis in section 9.3.3.

Spatially variable water soil erosion intensities

It was also stated in section 5.1.1 that the soil erosion potential of the respective land uses are taken into account when distinguishing between compartments (cf. Table 5-1). Principally one needs to distinguish between different types of water soil erosion (e.g., sheet, rill, inter-rill, gully erosion, Shen and Julien, 1993; Morgan, 1999). However, models usually only try to estimate one to few types of erosion. For instance, the empirical Universal Soil Loss Equation (USLE, Wischmeier and Smith, 1978) or its revised version (RUSLE, Renard et al., 1997) have experienced a wide range of applications because of their simplicity (least data demanding, van der Knijff et al., 2000). They are used for on-site soil losses and have been developed for sheet and rill erosion (Wischmeier and Smith, 1978). Most erosion models are usually developed only for being applied to a certain site so that absolute values of these models at the regional scale are not reliable (van der Knijff et al., 2000). Erosion models for the regional scale itself that provide quantitative data are, however, lacking (Wickenkamp et al., 2000; Bach et al., 2001). Even simple models that only predict potential erosion rates require at least information on soil texture (Hennings, 1994), a soil property for which hardly any information is available in publicly available GIS datasets that would support regionally differentiated erosion assessments.

As indicated above, when assessing soil erosion from a soil or agricultural science perspective, usually only the loss at a given site is of interest which leads especially to a reduced soil fertility or production capacity (Morgan, 1999). As a consequence, very few of the erosion models predict how much of the soil arrives at adjacent areas or compartments. Attempts have been made to relate the results of the RUSLE to inputs into streams for example by means of the sediment delivery ratio concept (Umweltbundesamt, 1999). However, the RUSLE is still too data demanding at the regional scale and the sediment delivery ratio concept is highly questioned (Walling, 1983).

No transport of eroded soil from one terrestrial compartment to another is considered in WATSON for two reasons: (a) the compartments distinguished are assumed to be homogeneous implying that re-distribution of eroded soil within one compartment is irrelevant and (b) there is a lack of information about the situation of one compartment relative to another (cf. section 4.2.2). Rather, only the transport from the terrestrial environment into surface freshwater bodies is assessed. Zaslavsky (1979) quoted by Golubev (1982) estimated that only 10 % of the gross erosion is transported to the larger rivers, the remainder mostly being only re-distributed in the terrestrial environment (e.g., deposited on the lower parts of slopes). Walling (1983) estimates that only about 0.1 % to 38 % of the gross soil loss reach the rivers' outlets and are represented in the so-called sediment yield.

In order to allow for different erosion intensities on different soil compartments, the following approach is adopted. First, a value that is representative for European conditions is identified which corresponds to the one used by Brandes et al. (1996) and European Commission (1996a) (see section B.5.3 for the reasoning). Then, the crop management factor (C-factor) of the Universal Soil Loss Equation (USLE; Wischmeier and Smith, 1978; Renard et al., 1997) is made use of. Reported values are provided by Golubev (1982), Umweltbundesamt (1999) and Morgan (1999). The fairly simple C-factor subdivision by Golubev (1982) is followed here according to Table 5-6.

In order to maintain the overall erosion velocity as presented above, the following distribution scheme is employed:

$$
\begin{aligned}
v_{\text{erosion}} &= \sum_i v_{\text{erosion}}(i) \\
&= v_{\text{erosion}} \cdot \sum_i fr\_\text{A}_i \cdot Weight_{\text{erosion, i}} \cdot x \\
&= v_{\text{erosion}} \cdot x \cdot \sum_i fr\_\text{A}_i \cdot Weight_{\text{erosion, i}}
\end{aligned}
\tag{5-10}
$$

where

fr_A : fraction of the zonal area with water soil erosion that consists of compartment *i* [-] (defined based on Table 5-1)

v_{erosion} : overall erosion velocity [m per s]

Table 5-6: Relative erodibility of different land covers according to Golubev (1982) and their assignment to compartments as used in this study

Golubev (1982)		This study	
Land cover	C-factor range	Compartment	Relative weights
Bare tilled soil	1.0	Arable land, Non-vegetated land	1.0
Soil under crops	1.0-0.1	n/a	n/a
Soil under virgin grass	0.1-0.01	Pasture	0.05
Soil under virgin forest	0.001-0.0001	Semi-natural eco-systems	0.0005

$v_{erosion}(i)$: erosion velocity of compartment *i* [m per s]

Weight : relative erodibility weights of compartment *i* [-] (defined in Table 5-6)

x : scaling factor for water soil erosion [-].

Solving for the scaling factor, values of 3.01 and 3.10 are obtained when distinguishing four or three soil compartments with soil erosion, respectively. The compartment-specific erosion velocity is derived according to:

$$v_{erosion}(i) = v_{erosion} \cdot Weight_{erosion,\, i} \cdot x \tag{5-11}$$

yielding the values as given in Table 5-7 which depend on the number of compartments distinguished in an environmental fate assessment.

Although noting that the erosion process is selective with respect to particles of different size (e.g., Walling, 1983), it is assumed here to affect the bulk soil even including pore waters. One may argue that the process 'overland flow' is responsible for the transport of pore waters. However, overland flow is perceived here to entrain that amount of a substance contained in soils that is in equilibrium with water that flows at the surface or near the surface ('interflow') as described in section A.3.4.

It is clear that the approach selected in order to allow for spatially variable erosion intensities is not appropriate in any situation. It is considered a justified first approximation as this distinction is in line with both the considerably lower crop management factor of the Universal Soil Loss Equation (USLE) for forest and pasture soils (e.g., Golubev, 1982; Morgan, 1999; Umweltbundesamt, 1999)

Table 5-7: Compartment-specific water soil erosion weights and velocities depending on the number of soil compartments distinguished which show the related process

Compartment	Four compartments with water soil erosion are distinguished		Three compartments with water soil erosion are distinguished	
	Overall erosion weights[a]	Specific erosion velocities [m/s]	Overall erosion weights[b]	Specific erosion velocities [m/s]
Arable land	3.01	$2.86 \cdot 10^{-12}$	3.10	$2.95 \cdot 10^{-12}$
Pasture	0.15	$1.43 \cdot 10^{-13}$	0.16	$1.47 \cdot 10^{-13}$
Semi-natural ecosystems	0.0015	$1.43 \cdot 10^{-15}$	0.0016	$1.47 \cdot 10^{-15}$
Non-vegetated land	3.01	$2.86 \cdot 10^{-12}$	n/a[c]	n/a[c]

a. Relative weights as given in Table 5-6 times 3.01.
b. Relative weights as given in Table 5-6 times 3.10.
c. Not distinguished.

as well as with existing forest soil models (e.g., Reinds et al., 1995). Allowing the water soil erosion rate only to vary by compartments is, furthermore, supported by the present paucity or rather absence of regional erosion estimates for the whole of Europe or modelling capabilities even at the regional scale (Bach et al., 2001). In any case, it is novel in the realm of multimedia models in which no differentiation of the erosion rate according to zones and/or compartments has been made so far.

Consideration of preferential flow in soils

One process that is responsible for example for the transport of pesticides from soil surfaces to the subsurface and even into ground water is 'preferential flow' (Beven, 1991; Gish and Shirmohammadi, 1991) or to be more specific 'preferential transport' (Helling and Gish, 1991; Luxmoore, 1991; Stagnitti et al., 1995; Schwarz and Kaupenjohann, 2000). When preferential transport occurs, it means that the contact time between the percolating water and the soil matrix (i.e., the solid phase) is so small that no equilibrium between substances contained in the water and the surfaces of the soil particles can be achieved. Thus, the soil cannot act as a purifying filter to the extent which is expected under regular leaching processes. The preferential flow process is more the rule than the exception (Flury, 1996) and may have different causes (Wittig et al., 1985; Helling and Gish, 1991; Steenhuis and Parlange, 1991; Schwarz and Kaupenjohann, 2000) including colloidal transport (Jarvis et al., 1999; Noack et al., 2000). It even also applies to atmospheric deposition in forests (Wittig et al., 1985; Chang and Matzner, 2000). Preferential transport is potentially very important especially for the removal of non-degradable trace elements from the rooting zone. In contrast to all of the existing multimedia models known to the author, this process has not yet been included in any of these models so far.

The inclusion of preferential flow into the assessment involves the consideration of the fact that the part of the precipitation that undergoes preferential flow is not available for ordinary matrix leaching (cf. Eq. (5-8) in Table 5-5). This also implies that this portion of the wet atmospheric deposition immediately bypasses the top soil layer, reducing the input to the soil compartment (cf. Eqs. (4-5) and (4-6) in Table 4-3) which only constitutes the upper part of soils (cf. section 5.1.2). Thirdly, the preferentially flowing water also displaces parts of the soil pore water which may also contain colloids (cf. Eq. (5-9) in Table 5-5).

In order to appropriately formulate these processes, it needs to be known (a) how much of the percolating water undergoes the process of preferential flow and (b) how much of the substance contained in soils is transported to the subsurfaces.

Since preferential flow is known to also occur in arid climates with little to no runoff formation, the amount of water preferentially flowing through soils is assessed based on precipitation rather than on runoff. Preferential flow was chosen to be 1 % of the rain rate by default unless the water balance suggested to use a different value (cf. section B.5.2).

Data on the displacement of trace elements in soils due to preferential transport could not be encountered. However, it is known that the amounts of pesticides lost due to this process normally lie in the range of smaller than 0.1 % and 1 % and may reach up to 5 % under worst case conditions (Flury, 1996). When also including colloidal transport, a value for the amount to bypass the top soil layers of 0.1 %, thus, appears to be a reasonable first (conservative) estimate. In order to convert this overall mass balance into a rate, the 0.1 % are assumed to apply to an annual mass balance meaning that 0.1 % of the annual amount of substances present in the soil reaches the subsurface by preferential transport. The respective rate is, thus, 0.001 per year. One has to note, however, that this rate may be substantially higher for non-degrading substances such as trace elements. However, different volatilisation and adsorption behaviours, for instance, play a role here so that the value is adopted for the time being for any substance until more specific information becomes available.

5.1.6 Arable land compartment

Arable land is characterized by the production of crops for food or feed supply purposes, a 'normal' permeability and a substantial soil erosion potential at least due to episodic bare or dead fallow periods. At present all agricultural land that is not pasture or grassland is considered arable land (cf. section B.3 and left part of Fig. 5-1). In particular with respect to the soil erosion potential there might principally be a need to distinguish areas on which annual crops are grown from those with perennial plants (like vine, olive trees, fruit trees), respectively. This distinction is, however, not made at present.

Processes that are covered by the presented methodology and affect the arable land compartment are: degradation (section A.3.1), radioactive decay (A.3.2), water soil erosion (A.3.3), overland flow (A.3.4), matrix leaching (A.3.6), preferential transport (A.3.7) and removal by plants with subsequent harvest (A.3.8). Their formulations are also given in Table 5-5.

5.1.7 Pasture compartment

The pasture compartment is characterized by a 'normal' permeability and a reduced soil erosion potential compared to arable land and non-vegetated land due to a permanent vegetation cover. Pastures are the compartments on which grazing and free-range animals are kept. The distribution of pastures is shown to the right of Fig. 5-1.

Processes that are covered by the presented methodology and affect the pasture compartment are: degradation (section A.3.1), radioactive decay (A.3.2), water soil erosion (A.3.3), overland flow (A.3.4), matrix leaching (A.3.6) and preferential transport (A.3.7). Their formulations are also given in Table 5-5.

5.1.8 (Semi-) natural ecosystem compartment

By 'semi-natural ecosystems', any land use that is neither (heavily) influenced by human management like agricultural land (sections 5.1.6 and 5.1.7) nor is characterized analogously to one of the other terrestrial compartments, i.e., non-vegetated land (5.1.9), glaciers (5.1.11) and impervious or anthropogenically sealed soils (5.1.10). As a result, this compartment is intended to pool all those land covers that make the terrestrial area complete, i.e., adding up to 100 % (cf. to left of Fig. 5-2). One has to note that this compartment also comprises forests which are to varying degrees managed as well which is why the term 'semi' is added to the name of this compartment.

The semi-natural ecosystem compartment is characterized by a 'normal' permeability and a substantially reduced soil erosion potential compared to arable land and non-vegetated land due to a permanent vegetation cover.

Processes that are covered by the presented methodology and affect the semi-natural ecosystem compartment are: degradation (section A.3.1), radioactive decay (A.3.2), water soil erosion (A.3.3), overland flow (A.3.4), matrix leaching (A.3.6) and preferential transport (A.3.7). Their formulations are also given in Table 5-5.

5.1.9 Non-vegetated land compartment

By 'non-vegetated land', all areas are meant on which no vegetation is present and which do not classify as either built-up areas, glaciers or aquatic areas (cf. sections 5.1.10, 5.1.11 and 6.1, respectively). Examples are rocks, open-cast mining areas, dump and construction sites (cf. section B.3). The distribution of non-vegetated land is shown to the right of Fig. 5-2.

Although this compartment is rather heterogeneous in terms of the permeability of the different land uses contained (e.g., consolidated rocks vs. non-vegetated sandy areas, cf. Tables B-2 and B-3), it is assumed to show a 'normal' permeability. Due to the non-vegetated nature, the soil erosion potential is considered substantial.

Processes that are covered by the presented methodology and affect the non-vegetated land compartment are: degradation (section A.3.1), radioactive decay (A.3.2), water soil erosion (A.3.3), overland flow (A.3.4), matrix leaching (A.3.6) and preferential transport (A.3.7). Their formulations are also given in Table 5-5.

5.1.10 Impervious surface compartment

By 'impervious surfaces', only man-made areas are addressed. Notions like 'built-up areas', 'sealed soils' and 'urban areas' are used synonymously in the present study although putting emphasis on different aspects.

Impervious surfaces are assumed to be fully impermeable. As a consequence, they accelerate the transport of those substances that are deposited on these areas to streams. As the resolution of the land use geo-datasets is at least 1 km^2 (cf. section B.3), not all built-up areas or areas that are sealed are included, most notably roads. It is, thus, assumed that when adding all urban areas as given by the geo-datasets this sum constitutes a lower bound estimate of the existing impermeable areas (cf. to the left of Fig. 5-3).

It is difficult to define a volume of a compartment that does not have a depth according to the assumption of impermeability. In order to still provide a depth which is needed for volume calculations (cf. section A.4), two assumptions are made:

1. no long-term retention exists within the impervious surface compartment, and
2. no removal of substances occurs except for flushing, i.e., advection by water, and chemical transformation.

These assumptions lead to a situation where there is no sewage treatment or where it exists a pipe network that allows separate conduits to drain rain water on the one hand and domestic and/or industrial wastewater on the other. In order to allow for rapid flushing without storage longer than a year, thus, the volume is set to the annual amount of rainfall which is derived by zone as described in section B.5.2.

As a result, processes that are covered by the presented methodology and affect the impervious surface compartment are: degradation (section A.3.1), radioactive decay (A.3.2) and overland flow in its strict sense (A.3.4). Their formulations are also given in Table 5-5.

Note that no organic film compartment coating impervious surfaces as described by Diamond et al. (2001) is included at present as stated above.

5.1.11 Glacier compartment

As the presence of lakes seem to have a significant influence on the overall residence time of substances (e.g., Klepper and den Hollander, 1999) and glaciers are nothing but large frozen water bodies, these are distinguished as separate compartments noting that their overall area fraction is rather small (cf. Table 5-1 and to the right of Fig. 5-3). As the albedo, i.e., the proportion of light reflected by a surface, of glaciers is rather high and except for photodegradation chemical reactions in the terrestrial/aquatic environment are restricted to the presence of liquid water it is assumed that no degradation of organic compounds occurs. Thus, the overall residence time in glaciers is simply a function of their melting rate for any kind of (non-radioactive) substances.

The depth of glaciers is assumed to be 200 m which corresponds to mountainous glaciers in the northern hemisphere outside the polar region (Baumgartner and Liebscher, 1990, Table 9.3).

The only processes that are covered by the presented methodology and affect the glacier compartment are: radioactive decay (section A.3.2) and ice melt (A.3.5). Their formulations are also given in Table 5-5.

Note that glaciers could also be considered as part of the aquatic environment. Due to the water being mostly solid, i.e., frozen, glaciers are classified here as a terrestrial compartment.

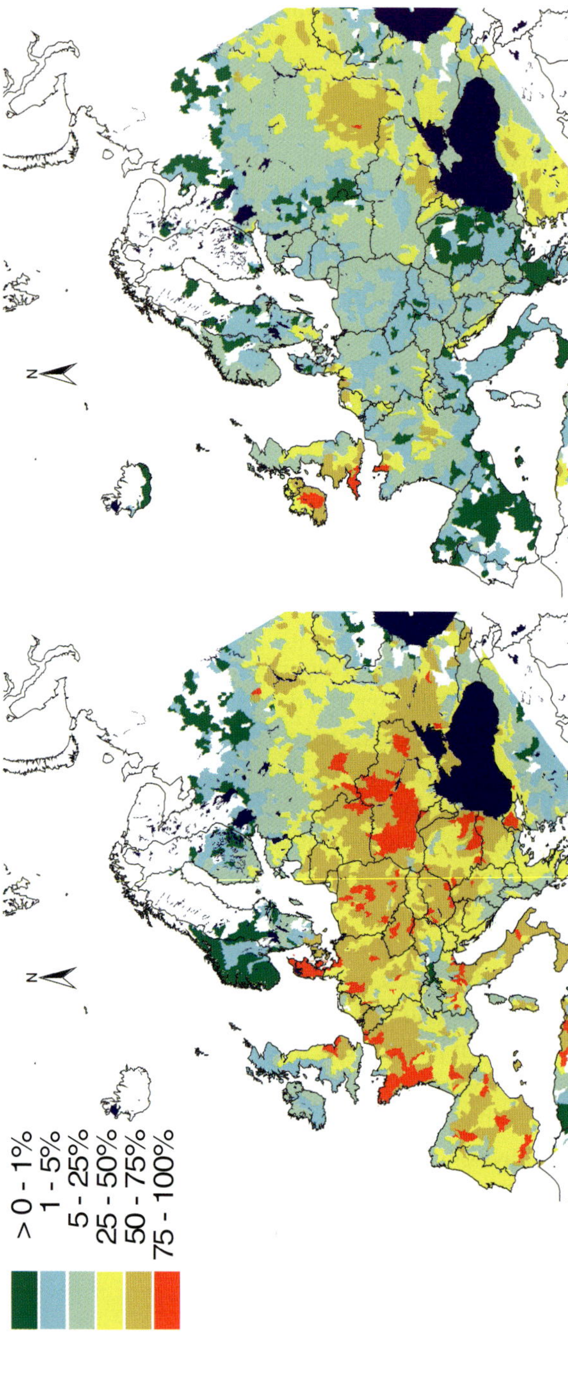

Fig. 5-1: Distribution of the predominance of arable land (left) and pastures/grasslands (right) in the different zones distinguished by WATSON

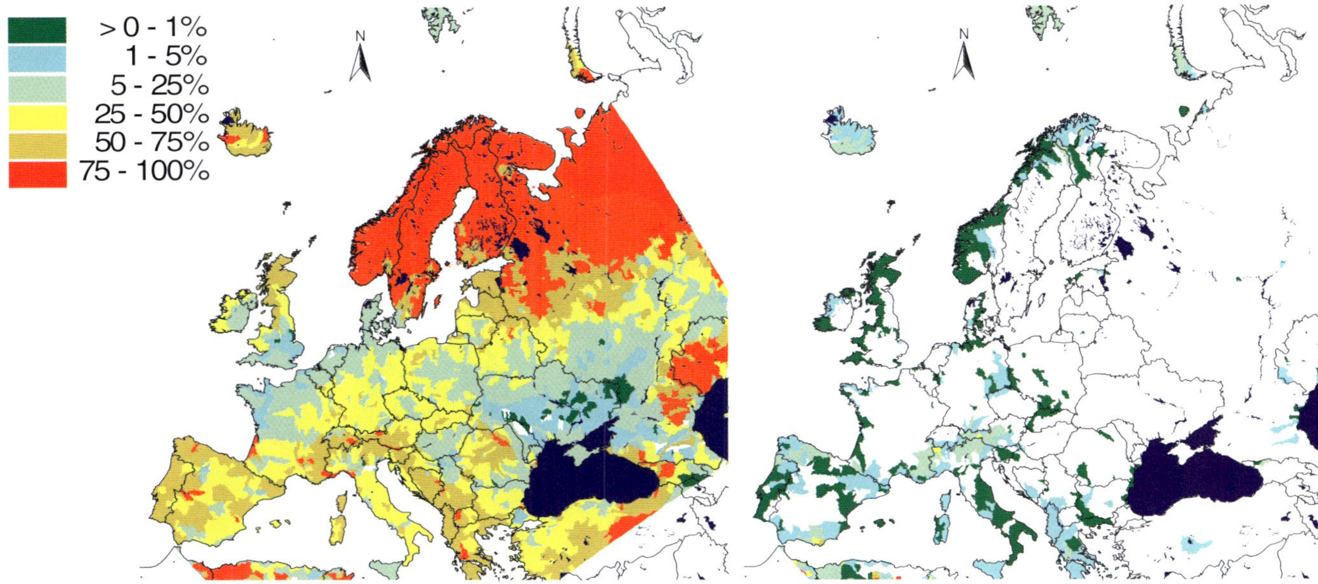

Fig. 5-2: Distribution of the predominance of (semi-) natural ecosystems (left) and non-vegetated land (right) in the different zones distinguished by WATSON

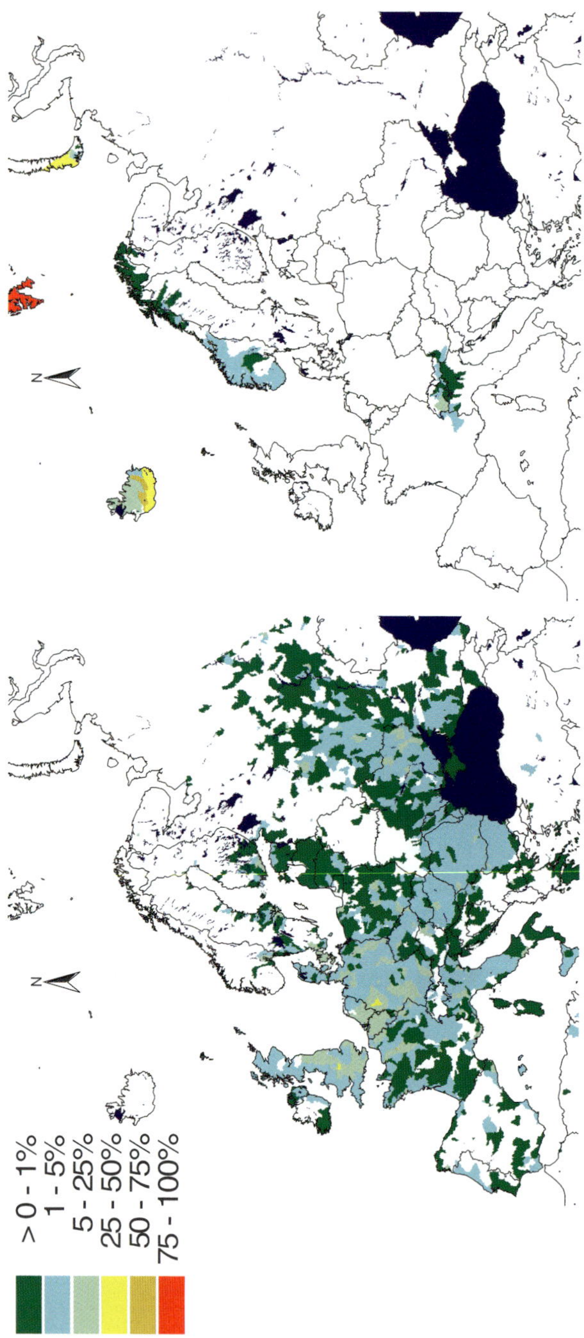

Fig. 5-3: Distribution of the predominance of impervious surfaces (left) and glaciers (right) in the different zones distinguished by WATSON

5.2 Environmental fate modelling for terrestrial plants

When assessing indirect human exposures, plants need to be considered since they form the basis of most of the food chains or webs due to their role as primary producers. How the inclusion of plants into the exposure assessment is realized, i.e., whether to include them only in the exposure part of the assessment or also in the environmental fate part or even doing without them, depends on two main factors:

1. in the case of (semi-) volatile compounds a vegetation compartment may influence the other compartments' concentrations (e.g., Severinsen and Jager, 1998) mostly sequestering these compounds (e.g., Simonich and Hites, 1994; Wagrowski and Hites, 1997) and, thus, reducing their atmospheric half-lives and consequently their characteristic travel distance (e.g., Bennett et al., 1998; McLachlan and Horstmann, 1998; Cousins and Mackay, 2001), and
2. some types of vegetation constitute food for humans or animals leading to exposure to substances entrained which for some substances dominates human exposure over inhalation (e.g., in the case of several semi-volatile organic chemicals, Bodnar et al., 2002). Apart from eastern Asian countries, aquatic plants rarely constitute a major contribution to the overall diet of the population. Therefore, only terrestrial plants will be treated in the following.

In case of 1), it is advisable to distinguish a plant compartment from soil compartment(s) if their characteristics of exchange with the air compartment are substantially different (Wania et al., 2000, as can be expressed by the filter factor, McLachlan and Horstmann, 1998). Cousins and Mackay (2001) recommend to include plant compartments into environmental fate models only when the substances are considerably taken up either via foliage or via roots. The criteria are formulated based on octanol-air and air-water partitioning coefficients. When introducing a plant compartment into an environmental fate model that is used for exposure assessments, care must be taken to make sure that this is done in a consistent way in order not to violate the mass conservation principle (cf. Hertwich et al., 2000).

When developing a concept for a plant model, the number of compartments to be considered needs to be determined. In the context of multimedia modelling frameworks, plant models of differing complexity are available. These range from single-compartment (e.g., Trapp and Matthies, 1995; McLachlan, 1996; Bennett et al., 1998; Severinsen and Jager, 1998), over two (e.g., Tolls and McLachlan, 1994), three (e.g., Paterson et al., 1994; United States - Environmental Protection Agency, 1998) to four compartment models (e.g., Trapp, 1995; United States - Environmental Protection Agency, 2002b; Charles and Jolliet,

2003). Most notably, spatially-resolved multimedia models usually only allow for one-compartment vegetation formulations (e.g., Wania et al., 2000; MacLeod et al., 2001) if at all (e.g., Scheringer and Wania, 2003). This is in line with the recommendation by Cousins and Mackay (2001) who suggest to have vegetation-soil pairs in order to allow for different vegetation types, each being represented by one aboveground compartment in addition to the soil compartment.

Reasons for distinguishing between several plant compartments either as different plant parts or as different plant species include:

- different plant parts are exposed due to different processes (especially foliar vs. root uptake, but also attachment of (particle-bound or gaseous) substances to plant aboveground surfaces),
- consumption occurs only of selected plant components (e.g., root, leafy, stem and corn produces),
- different plant parts or species are affected to different degrees by processes like harvesting, litter fall and growth, and/or
- if plants accumulate significant amounts on the expense of the amounts found/predicted in air and/or soil it is suggested to include them into multimedia models (Cousins and Mackay, 2001).

A non-exhaustive overview about existing plant models in the area of multimedia environmental fate and/or exposure modelling is given in Table 5-8. Of the models listed only two have been developed also for non-organic substances. These are United States - Environmental Protection Agency (1998) and TRIM.FaTE (United States - Environmental Protection Agency, 2002b). In the following, it will be tried to draw conclusions with respect to the different processes involved.

5.2.1 Exchange with air

Except for Reinds et al. (1995) and Trapp (2002), all models consider interactions between air and (aboveground) plants explicitly. Whereas some models assume that substances on leaves are in equilibrium with leaves (Bennett et al., 1998; Wania et al., 2000) which is debatable for some cases (e.g., due either to low cuticular permeability or to extremely low volatility and high lipophilicity of the assessed substances, Riederer, 1995) or neglect/disregard wet and/or particle-bound deposition (Paterson et al., 1994; Tolls and McLachlan, 1994; Trapp and Matthies, 1995; McLachlan, 1996; Severinsen and Jager, 1998), a few distinguish between substances in and on the leaves either as particulates (United States - Environmental Protection Agency, 2002b) or attached to the cuticle (Charles and Jolliet, 2003). United States - Environmental Protection Agency (1998) principally allows wet and dry deposition on (as well as gaseous exchange with) aboveground edible plant parts that are in immediate/intimate contact with air only (termed 'exposed produce' like leaf-vegetables, no cereals). As only the non-gaseous fraction of the chemical is allowed to undergo deposition, it can also be considered negligible for highly volatile substances. When fruits are distinguished they are not allowed to have direct exchange with air (Trapp, 1995).

The reason for excluding wet and/or particle-bound deposition onto plants by many of the models is that this process is only significant for low volatile, hydrophilic substances (Paterson et al., 1994; Trapp and Matthies, 1995). As a consequence this process cannot be neglected when having to deal with (weak) acids (many pesticides, e.g., Charles and Jolliet, 2003) and metals (e.g., Maddalena et al., 2002). Trapp and Schwartz (2000) state that it is unclear how to model particulate deposition because the chemical may remain sorbed to the particle after deposition (and washed off again), or it may migrate into the cuticle. In fact, there is some degree of contradiction whether leaf uptake is considerable for all or for some metals (Zimdahl and Koeppe, 1979; Ulrich, 1991; Weigert, 1991; Kabata-Pendias and Pendias, 1992; Greger, 1999). When not just allowing these deposits to stay on the surface but trying to define an exchange with the plant's interior, major problems in the process formulation occur (Riederer, 1995; and note in Maddalena et al., 2002). In case of TRIM.FaTE, the transfer rate needs to be provided by the user (Maddalena et al., 2002) which would require to provide hardly available values of another substance-specific parameter. Charles and Jolliet (2003) make use of an empirical relationship in order to derive a mobility rate based on a reference substance's mobility rate, a size selectivity of the cuticular membrane (which depends on the plant species) and the molar volume of the substance. They allow the exchange to occur over the full cuticle surface (expressed as the leaf area index (LAI) which is usually defined as the ratio of the area of the upper side of the leaves in a canopy projected onto a flat surface to the area of the surface under the canopy). This area appears to be too large as the deposits/residues will not cover the whole leaf surface.

It seems debatable whether to include an exchange between the deposits/residues and the leaf interior. Bromilow and Chamberlain (1995) state that uptake through the cuticle mainly concerns non-polar organic substances with a log K_{OW} in the range from 1 to 3 whereas pesticides of which many are weak acids are not taken up as readily unless applied together with surfactants. On the other hand, exposure due to particles attached to leaf surfaces may play a role for non-volatile substances. It seems clear that there is a retention mechanism for some metals by leaves (e.g., for lead by forest leaves (Zöttl, 1985; Bergkvist et al., 1989; Lindberg, 1989; Rea et al., 2001) and additionally thallium (Weigert, 1991) and vanadium (Rea et al., 2001)). This may be due to the fact that the cuticular layer functions as a weak cation exchanger (Greger, 1999) which in turn would not in-

Table 5-8: Non-exhaustive overview on existing plant models in the field of multimedia models

Model reference	Number of plant species/types and components	Processes considered
Bennett et al. (1998)	1 plant species/type, 1 aboveground component	chemical-specific vegetation/air and soil/air partitioning; kinetics of mass transfer rates among air, vegetation and soil; degradation rates in air, plant tissue and soil; litterfall (equals growth rate); explicitly neglected: harvest
Charles and Jolliet (2003)	1 plant species/type, 4 components:	
	plant surface residue	diffusive exchange between leaf and plant surface residue; degradation
	foliage	diffusive exchange with air; diffusive exchange between leaf and plant surface residue; advective transfer to stem; advective transfer from stem (unclear whether included or not); degradation
	stem	active uptake from soil based on the transpiration stream concentration factor (TSCF); advective transfer from leaf (unclear whether included or not); advective transfer to leaf; degradation
	root	active uptake from soil based on the complementary of the transpiration stream concentration factor (TSCF); diffusive uptake from soil; diffusive transfer to soil;
Critical loads of heavy metals in soils (Reinds et al., 1995)	1 plant species/type, 1 aboveground component (growing forest parts)	growth uptake from soil (i.e., net uptake considering total root uptake, litterfall and canopy interactions, i.e., foliar uptake or foliar exudation) based on transpiration stream concentration factor (TSCF)

Table 5-8: Non-exhaustive overview on existing plant models in the field of multimedia models

Model reference	Number of plant species/types and components	Processes considered
McLachlan (1996)	1 plant species/type, 1 aboveground component (forage: grass/corn)	only air-plant partitioning considered for PCDD/Fs
Paterson et al. (1994)	1 plant species/type, 3 components (root, stem, foliage)	diffusion and bulk flow of chemical between soil and root; transport within the plant in the phloem and transpiration stream between root and stem as well as between stem and foliage; exchange between foliage and air and between soil and air; metabolism and growth; no harvest considered
POPCY-CLING-Baltic (Wania et al., 2000)	2 plant species/types, 1 aboveground component: coniferous forest needles and deciduous forest leaves	foliar uptake of gaseous substances; volatilisation; foliar uptake of dry particle-bound substances and substances contained in evaporating water droplets; seasonally variable dry particle deposition; seasonally variable volume due to growth; seasonally variable litterfall; metabolism; explicitly neglected: leaching
Severinsen and Jager (1998); SimpleBox 2.0 (Brandes et al., 1996)	1 plant species/type, 1 aboveground component	diffusive exchange between air and leaves via stomata; uptake from soil based on the transpiration stream concentration factor (TSCF); stomatal uptake of fine particle-bound substances; metabolism; harvest; death; explicitly neglected: cuticle uptake, wet deposition on leaves and foliage/stem-to-root transfer
Tolls and McLachlan (1994)	1 plant species/type, 2 aboveground components (leaf-surface, leaf-interior)	only diffusive exchange between air and leaf-surface as well as between surface and interior parts of the leaves

Table 5-8: Non-exhaustive overview on existing plant models in the field of multimedia models

Model reference	Number of plant species/types and components	Processes considered
Trapp (1995)	1 plant species/type, 4 components:	
	fruit	phloem flux from stem; metabolism
	foliage	transfer from stem with transpiration stream based on stem-foliage partitioning; phloem flux to stem; diffusive exchange with air; metabolism
	stem	active uptake from soil based on the transpiration stream concentration factor (TSCF); transfer to leaves with transpiration stream based on partitioning between stem and foliage; phloem flux to fruits; phloem flux from leaves; metabolism
	root	diffusive exchange between soil and roots in water and air pores ("probably realistic only for root cortex of intact roots … upper limit for diffusive uptake into bulk root", p. 119); active uptake from soil based on the complementary of the TSCF; metabolism
Trapp (2002)	1 plant species/type; 1 belowground component (thick root)	active uptake without the help of the transpiration stream concentration factor (TSCF) or its complement; advective transfer to stem with transpiration stream; degradation; growth
Trapp and Matthies (1995)	1 plant species/type, 1 aboveground component (mainly foliage)	uptake from soil based on transpiration stream concentration factor (TSCF); gaseous deposition; volatilisation from leaves; transformation and degradation; growth; explicitly neglected: wet and particle-bound deposition

Table 5-8: Non-exhaustive overview on existing plant models in the field of multimedia models

Model reference	Number of plant species/types and components	Processes considered
TRIM.FaTE (United States - Environmental Protection Agency, 2002b)	1 plant species/type, 4 components:	
	particles on leaf	during rain: wet dry particle deposition from air; particles washed to soil; diffusive exchange between air and particles on leaf (note: not described by Maddalena et al., 2002) when no rain: dry particle deposition from air; particles re-entrained by air litter fall to soil or harvest if agricultural produce; diffusive exchange between leaf and particles on leaf; degradation
	leaf (interior)	diffusive exchange between leaf and air (note: only volatilisation but not absorption for mercury according to Maddalena et al., 2002) and between leaf and particles on leaf; litter fall to soil or harvest if agricultural produce; phloem flow to stem; xylem flow from stem; degradation
	stem	root uptake estimated by means of transpiration stream concentration factor (TSCF, in xylem) or the stem concentration factor (SCF, in bulk stem); stem to soil transfer; xylem flow to leaf; phloem flow from leaf; degradation
	root	root uptake estimated by means of root concentration factor (RCF) and a parameter describing the proportion of equilibrium value achieved; senescence (note: as mentioned in Maddalena et al., 2002); degradation

Table 5-8: Non-exhaustive overview on existing plant models in the field of multimedia models

Model reference	Number of plant species/types and components	Processes considered
United States - Environmental Protection Agency (1998)	3 plant species/types, 1 component each:	
	aboveground-exposed	direct deposition of particles; vapour transfer; root uptake based on plant-soil BCF (for organics according to Travis and Arms, 1988) for produce
	aboveground-protected	only root uptake based on plant-soil BCF (for organics according to Travis and Arms, 1988) for produce
	belowground	only root uptake based on root concentration factor (RCF; for organics according to Briggs et al., 1982), soil-water partitioning coefficient and empirical K_{ow}-dependent correction factor

fluence the environmental fate for instance of molybdenum (as molybdate), arsenic (as arsenite or asenate) and chromium (as chromium oxides). In fact, chromium does not seem to be enriched in forested ecosystems (Bergkvist et al., 1989). Unlike all other models, Severinsen and Jager (1998) allow stomatal uptake of fine particulates. However, this process does not lead to an accumulation on/in leaves that exceeds the pure deposition onto the soil and/or the leaves.

Overall, to what extent particle-bound substances will actually enter (Berrow and Burridge, 1991; Gawel et al., 2001) or just adhere to the leaves (Zimdahl and Koeppe, 1979), an issue that also depends on the metal (e.g., Bergkvist et al., 1989; Ulrich, 1991; Kabata-Pendias and Pendias, 1992; Greger, 1999; Rea et al., 2001; with contradicting evidence for lead), appears to be an unresolved question or at least one to which no generally applicable answer exists. It may, therefore, be concluded that gaseous air-leaf interactions can be neglected whereas particle deposition cannot for heavy metals that are predominantly transported in air in a particle-bound way. For gaseous mercury, the reverse conclusion applies.

The question remains to what degree the deposited metals will effectively be retained on or in the leaves[9] or even on other plant parts (e.g., the bark of trees, Schultz, 1987; Ulrich, 1991). Models apart from (measured) mass balances (e.g., Zöttl, 1985; Schultz, 1987; Lindberg, 1989; Rea et al., 2001) describing this retention are scarce. On the other hand, (heavy) metal retention by or temporary accumulation in aboveground plant parts that persist the next precipitation event may only be important if these plant parts are removed and enter the food chain as in the other case the metal amounts will be deposited to the ground due to litter fall.[10] For exposed produce, United States - Environmental Protection Agency (1998) allows for adhesion of wet deposition to the edible plant parts as well as an overall interception fraction comprising dry and wet deposition (cf. section A.6.5).

5.2.2 Exchange with soil

Principally, there are different approaches in order to model exchange processes taking place between plants and soils for organic substances and trace elements.

---

[9] According to Riederer (1995), relatively polar ($K_{ow} \leq 10$) and involatile compounds accumulate almost exclusively in the aqueous phase (95 % for log K_{aw} = -1 and 100 % for log $K_{aw} \leq -3$).

[10] One has to keep in mind, however, that in case of natural vegetation and especially with coniferous trees litter does not occur annually if one wanted to allow for dynamic calculations which preferably should be done in annual time steps due to the hydrological data available.

Organic substances

Except for the works of McLachlan and co-workers, all models addressing organic substances consider chemical exchange between soil and plant. The uptake by aboveground plant parts via xylem flow is always based on the Transpiration Stream Concentration Factor (TSCF) and the transpiration stream flux with the exception of United States - Environmental Protection Agency (1998) assuming equilibrium conditions according to Travis and Arms (1988) whereas for Bennett et al. (1998) the modelling approach is unclear. Depending on whether more than one aboveground plant compartment is distinguished, the TSCF-derived stem concentration is further transported to leaves and/or fruits by advection and/or partitioning.

The treatment of roots widely differs between the modelling approaches. While some of the models do not (explicitly) treat roots (e.g., Reinds et al., 1995; Bennett et al., 1998), the other either (a) assume the (fine) roots to be in equilibrium with soil (without distinguishing a separate root compartment: e.g., Trapp and Matthies (1995) and Severinsen and Jager (1998); considering a separate root compartment with (Maddalena et al., 2002) or without basing the transfer on the Root Concentration Factor (RCF), United States - Environmental Protection Agency, 2002b), or (b) allow for kinetic exchange between root and soil (Paterson et al., 1994) sometimes based on the 'reflection coefficient' which is the complement of the TSCF ('1-TSCF', Trapp, 1995; Charles and Jolliet, 2003). United States - Environmental Protection Agency (1998) also assumes equilibrium by using the Root Concentration Factor (RCF), however, not integrated in an environmental fate model. Although TSCF is normalized to one (e.g., Bromilow and Chamberlain, 1995), the use of the reflection coefficient appears to be debatable. When deriving a mass balance for the root this coefficient may principally result (e.g., Trapp, 1995). However, if:

$$TSCF = \frac{C_{\text{xylem}}}{C_{\text{soil solution}}} \tag{5-12}$$

then:

$$1 - TSCF = 1 - \frac{C_{\text{xylem}}}{C_{\text{soil solution}}} = \frac{C_{\text{soil solution}} - C_{\text{xylem}}}{C_{\text{soil solution}}} \tag{5-13}$$

which is postulated to equal

$$1 - TSCF \equiv \frac{C_{\text{root}}}{C_{\text{soil solution}}} \cdot \alpha = RCF \cdot \alpha \tag{5-14}$$

where

TSCF	:	Transpiration Stream Concentration Factor [-]
C	:	C_{xylem}: concentration in the xylem [kg per m^3]
	:	$C_{soil\ solution}$: concentration in soil solution [kg per m^3]
	:	C_{root}: concentration in the root [kg per m^3]
RCF	:	Root Concentration Factor relating root concentration to external solution concentration [-]
α	:	fraction of root concentration that is due to reflection of substances entrained in the (primary) transpiration stream [-].

This means that the following relationship is valid:

$$C_{\text{soil solution}} - C_{\text{xylem}} = C_{\text{root}} \cdot \alpha . \tag{5-15}$$

It is fairly dubious to assume that concentrations add up although the TSCF may be considered to 'only' constitute a dimensionless relation factor and the respective volumes involved may be similar. Anyway, it is felt here that when employing an equilibrium coefficient like the TSCF for the stem's xylem concentration one should not use this measure in order to derive the concentration in the root. Rather, one should try to aim for consistency and employ the root concentration factor (RCF) which is a result of processes at equilibrium that are both diffusive and advective in nature. Moreover, modelling exercises for organic substances have shown that the diffusive exchange with the soil dominates root uptake (Trapp, 1995). This is supported by the observation that RCFs assume values well above 1 (e.g., Bromilow and Chamberlain, 1995) rendering the fraction of the root concentration α that is due to reflection to small values. Note, that for metals as opposed to lipophilic non-dissociating organic substances, higher concentrations in roots (although not in storage organs) than in soil have also been reported (Weaver et al., 1984; Speir et al., 1992). This might also be due to the fact that cell walls of roots (and potentially other plant tissue) act as cation exchangers, a functionality that is higher in dicotyledonous (like leguminous plants, trees) than in monocotyledonous plants (like grasses including cereals, Berrow and Burridge, 1991; Greger, 1999). As is discussed below, non-essential elements might be taken up as actively as essential elements due to similar physicochemical behaviours (see below). Another detoxifying mechanism might consist of chelate-forming organic molecules (such as phytochelatins or metallothioneins) transporting metals into vacuoles[11] followed by effective sequestration (Alloway et al., 1996; Mehra and Tripathi, 2000).

All models that treat roots explicitly allow for the process of non-advective exchange with soil. Trapp (2002) has developed a model for thicker roots that assumes that only the peel is in diffusive exchange with soil with respect to organic non-dissociating substances. However, the major part of the root consists of the root core into which only uptake with the transpiration stream is allowed. The model is reported to work fairly well for substances that have a log K_{ow} of less than 2 and that neither are polar nor constitute weak acids. For lipophilic substances, the model could predict concentrations in the peel well but gave unrealistically high concentrations in the core. Comparing the work by Trapp (2002) (Eq. (5-16)) with the approach proposed by United States - Environmental Protection Agency (1998) for belowground produce (Eq. (5-17)), shows that the models are similar when equilibrium situations are assumed (i.e., neglecting the growth and metabolism factor k in Trapp, 2002):

$$
\begin{aligned}
C\_w/v_{\text{roots}} &= \frac{Q_{\text{xylem}}}{\dfrac{Q_{\text{xylem}}}{K_{\text{rw}}} + k \cdot V_{\text{roots}}} \cdot C\_w/v_{\text{soil solution}} \\
&= \frac{\dfrac{Q_{\text{xylem}}}{K_{\text{sw}}}}{\dfrac{Q_{\text{xylem}}}{K_{\text{rw}}} + k \cdot V_{\text{roots}}} \cdot C\_w/v_{\text{soil solids}} \\
&\overset{\text{equilibrium}}{\Rightarrow} \frac{K_{\text{rw}}}{K_{\text{sw}}} \cdot C\_w/v_{\text{soil solids}}
\end{aligned}
\qquad (5\text{-}16)
$$

---

[11] A vacuole is a membrane-enclosed fluid filled sac found in the cells of plants including fungi. A vacuole is often considered to be the plant equivalent of a lysosome in animal cells. From the point of view of its ability to break down large molecules under acid conditions, this is certainly the case. Furthermore, vacuoles have the facility to contribute to the rigidity of the plant; to cell elongation and to the processing and storage of waste products. Thus, it is generally assumed that vacuoles are temporary stores for reserve materials or final stores for waste products of the plant cell.

$$C\_w/w_{\text{roots}} = \frac{RCF \cdot Cor_{\text{roots}}}{K_{sw} \cdot \rho_{\text{water}}} \cdot C\_w/w_{\text{soil solids}} \tag{5-17}$$

where

C_w/x_{roots} : concentration in root on a weight by volume (x = v) or by mass (x = w) base [$kg_{substance}$ per $m^3_{produce}$] or [$kg_{substance}$ per $kg_{produce}$]

Q_{xylem} : transpiration stream flux [m^3 per day]

K_{rw} : partitioning coefficient between roots and soil water [l_{water} per $kg_{produce}$][12]

K_{sw} : partitioning coefficient between soil solid and aqueous phase [l_{water} per kg_{solid}]

k : removal rate coefficient due to growth and metabolism [day^{-1}]

V_{roots} : volume of roots [m^3]

C_w/v : concentration in soil aqueous (index 'soil solution') or solid phase (index 'soil solids') on a weight by volume base [$kg_{substance}$ per m^3_{soil}]

C_w/w : concentration in soil on a weight by weight base [$kg_{substance}$ per kg_{soil}]

RCF : Root Concentration Factor relating root concentration to external solution concentration [l_{water} per $kg_{produce}$]

ρ_{water} : density of water, i.e., 1 [kg per l]

Cor_{roots} : empirical correction factor that is 1 and 0.01 for substances with log K_{ow} less or greater than 4, respectively [-].

If RCF and K_{rw} can be considered equivalent, the main difference at steady-state is that United States - Environmental Protection Agency (1998) includes a correction factor in order to distinguish substances that are more lipophilic from those that are less, the log K_{ow} threshold being at 4. This is in line with the findings of Trapp (2002) for the dynamic case (i.e., k unequal to zero),

---

[12] Note that a check of the units for Eq. (5-16) yields some inconsistencies if K_{rw} is not unitless, i.e., the units cancel out. However, as stated in the paper by Trapp (2002), it has units l per kg (according to equation 2b in that paper).

however, at a different threshold. One may, therefore, consider to introduce a two-threshold approach where for instance at a log K_{ow} in the range of 2 to 4 a correction factor of 0.1 could be used (note that in the range between log K_{ow} from 1 or 2 to 4 the distribution behaviour of substances between aqueous phase and lipid phase of plants is in transition, cf. Figure 2 in Riederer, 1995). Another difference is that the formula by United States - Environmental Protection Agency (1998) is valid for any edible belowground plant part (including potato tubers) whereas the advective uptake process is not allowed to occur in potatoes which are considered to be part of the stem (Paterson et al., 1994; Trapp, 2002).

It appears that the kinetic approach by Trapp (2002) can reasonably well be approximated by the introduction of a correction factor to an equilibrium model as done by United States - Environmental Protection Agency (1998). If equilibration between soil solution and roots is quick (only a few hours up to 24 hours according to Bromilow and Chamberlain (1995) and Briggs et al. (1982), respectively) the assumption of equilibrium seems to be valid. Thus, there is no need to distinguish a root compartment explicitly in the case of lipophilic compounds.

Metals or trace elements

Before continuing with the consideration of how existing models treat metals, a short overview on metal uptake via roots and possible translocations within plants shall be given.

It seems that anthropogenically added metals in the environment are more readily available to plants than are those released due to weathering of rocks and/or soils (Berrow and Burridge, 1991; Alloway and Steinnes, 1999; Greger, 1999). However, factors like the metal itself (e.g., Weigert, 1991), its total amount present in soil (Berrow and Burridge, 1991; Sauerbeck and Lübben, 1991) and its speciation (Berrow and Burridge, 1991; Kabata-Pendias and Pendias, 1992; Ritchie and Sposito, 1995; Markert, 1998; Helmke, 1999) have a marked influence. Furthermore, soil conditions (like cation exchange capacity, Peterson and Alloway, 1979 and Chaney et al., 1999, and organic matter content, Berrow and Burridge, 1991), environmental factors (like temperature, Chang et al. (1987) cited in Greger (1999)), drainage status (Berrow and Burridge, 1991) or the soil reaction (pH, Bingham et al., 1986; Berrow and Burridge, 1991; Reimann and de Caritat, 1998) also have significant influences on root uptake. Their influence, however, is also intervened by the metal and plant species (e.g., Sauerbeck and Lübben, 1991), plant age and plant speciation (Zimdahl and Koeppe, 1979). Plant speciation affects root uptake to such a degree that one can even distinguish between excluders and accumulators (Greger, 1999).

This brief overview has shown that modelling root uptake may become a rather complex issue. Owing to the rather simple overall modelling approach adopted (cf. section 2.3), only more general influences of plants with respect to root uptake will, therefore, be discussed in the following.

Some macronutrients are taken up actively by plant roots (e.g., Trapp and Matthies, 1998; Strasburger, 1991). Of the metals, this applies especially to potassium and due to its association also to rubidium (Strasburger, 1991). Less specific uptake is observed for other nutrients such as some heavy metals which are needed (at least in traces) by plants for example for enzyme creation. These include iron, manganese, zinc, copper, molybdenum, cobalt and nickel (Strasburger, 1991). Cadmium shows a geochemistry that is similar to zinc although being more mobile under acid conditions and reacting more readily with sulphur (Kabata-Pendias and Pendias, 1992), as well as having a stronger affinity to manganese oxides than to iron oxides in soils (Sauerbeck and Lübben, 1991). This similar behaviour is also postulated for translocation interactions of these two heavy metals (Welch and Norvell, 1999). In general, heavy metals are mostly taken up passively by plant roots although Greger (1999) reports non-passive uptake of cadmium (e.g., by soybean, Cataldo et al., 1983, or barley, Cutler and Rains, 1974), zinc and copper (e.g., by rice, Bowen, 1987) stating at the same time that the mechanism of metal uptake is not yet known. Upon entering the root core, heavy metals may be translocated by means of the transpiration stream according to the water potential gradient and, thus, accumulate mostly in plant leaves. The degree of translocation is amongst others dependent on the heavy metal. Greger (1999) estimates that between 75 % and 90 % of the heavy metals taken up through the roots stay in root tissue (cf. Mosbaek et al., 1989). A root/shoot ratio of 100 has been found for chromium in many crops (Zayed et al., 1998).

In order to explore whether heavy metals that have been transported from roots to shoots may return to the roots, their transport in the assimilate flux (i.e., in the phloem) shall be considered next. Generally, storage organs receive substances (nutrients and xenobiotics) via the phloem flow (Sauerbeck, 1989). Cations show different mobility in the phloem. Greger (1999) considers phloem transport of heavy metals as "probably difficult" (p. 15). In fact, there is a tendency that heavy metals are more immobile than light metals and if they tend to be more mobile they are at least to some degree essential to the plant: the light metals potassium, rubidium, caesium, sodium and magnesium are relatively mobile, the essential heavy metals iron, manganese, zinc, copper, molybdenum and cobalt are moderately mobile, whereas the inhomogeneous metal group of lithium, calcium, strontium, barium, lead, polonium and silver can be considered immobile (Table 2.1.26 in Strasburger, 1991). Calcium, barium and lead (and others) are immobile in the phloem due to the formation of insoluble phosphates. Other factors may also play a role such as the relatively high pH of 8 in phloem (Bromilow and Chamberlain, 1995) and competition between cadmium and zinc (Welch and Norvell, 1999) with a usual ratio of occurrence of 1:100 (Chaney et al., 1999) which might be different in plants due to different degrees of discriminative uptake. Welch and Norvell (1999) report phloem transport of Cd but do not state to what extent this transport occurs. The immobility of some metals in the phloem leads to an accumulation in the leaves which may be responsible for the need of any perennial plant (including 'evergreens') to clear their leaves from time to time (Strasburger, 1991).

Although the picture is not absolutely clear, one may conclude that phloem flow of (cationic) heavy metals can be neglected. There are no indications made in the reviewed literature to what extent anionic heavy metal forms might be transported in the phloem. For chromium and the trace element arsenic there are some indications with respect to the behaviour of their oxo-anions in plants. For chromium, a full reduction of hexavalent chromium to less mobile trivalent chromium is postulated to occur in plant roots (Zayed et al., 1998). This reduction to the less mobile form may be responsible for the high root/shoot ratio of about 100 reported for many crop species (Zayed et al., 1998) indicating little translocation whatsoever. As arsenic behaves like phosphorus (e.g Léonhard, 1991; Efroymson et al., 1997), it is expected to be as easily translocated also in the phloem as the latter. However, as arsenic competes with phosphorus which occurs at very much higher concentrations in arable soils and as it tends to form insoluble complexes, its root uptake is highly reduced (Léonhard, 1991). This is expressed by the little soil to aboveground transfer that is reported (e.g., by Speir et al. (1992) for experiments with the wood preservative Chromated Copper Arsenate), however, contradicting results exist. Another aspect with respect to arsenic is that most of its forms present in plants are organic which are not found to be toxic to humans (Chaney and Ryan, 1994; Harrison, 2001a).

From the models presented in Table 5-8, there are only two methods that consider metal uptake. Whereas Reinds et al. (1995) only considers the root uptake process by forest canopy, United States - Environmental Protection Agency (1998) provides estimates in any edible plant part of crops assuming equilibrium between soil and the respective plant component. Due to the paucity of available models, the approach taken by United States - Environmental Protection Agency (1998) is, thus, prioritised.

5.2.3 Removal due to harvest and/or litterfall

Apart from internal plant flows, the only advective losses of plant parts are due to harvest and litterfall. Harvest leads to a net removal of substances entrained in the harvested biomass from the soil which is why it is deemed necessary to include this process in the environmental fate model also.

There are only two models of those listed in Table 5-8 that consider removal by harvest: that described by Severinsen and Jager (1998) and TRIM.FaTE (United States - Environmental Protection Agency, 2002b). A non-changing plant biomass is assumed as is done in other publications either explicitly (Reinds et al., 1995; Bennett et al., 1998; Wania et al., 2000; Charles and Jolliet, 2003) or implicitly (Maddalena et al., 2002). Therefore, the rate constant for growth equals the sum of the rate constant for harvest and the rate constant for death (Severinsen and Jager, 1998). Whereas TRIM.FaTE (United States - Environmental Protection Agency, 2002b) assumes that all of the plant biomass of agricultural produce is removed and does, hence, not contribute to the soil loading due to litterfall, Severinsen and Jager (1998) only assume a portion of the aboveground biomass to be harvested (see below).

This approach might be defendable when dealing with annual (herbal) plants. However, for perennial plants like trees which cannot be assumed to stay in the exponential growth phase (cf. Trapp and Matthies, 1995), a certain amount of the built biomass will persist into the next growing season. In order to apply a steady-state approach, both models that include forests only consider leaves (Reinds et al., 1995; Wania et al., 2000), without taking account of the annual increase in stem diameter. Also Severinsen and Jager (1998) include trees of which parts are harvested. They additionally investigate the inclusion of tree trunks but conclude that this remains an area of investigation so that tree trunks are not considered in the following due to its poorly conceived status.

In the case of the plant model by Severinsen and Jager (1998), the harvest and death rate are linked to the growth rate by means of the harvest efficiency or its complementary value, respectively. Although not explicitly explaining what this parameter describes, it is figured that it is the volume share of the aboveground plant parts that is removed from the soil within one year, the remainder undergoing litter fall. The harvest efficiency is set to 59 % for agricultural aboveground produce and 34 % for aboveground forests. To what degree nutrient and/or contaminant rich matter like leaves and bark are left in the forests upon tree cutting may need to be investigated separately.

5.2.4 Metabolism or degradation

All but a few models in Table 5-8 include explicitly the process of degradation or metabolism. The reason for leaving this process out is presumably that they are concerned with metals (Reinds et al., 1995), focus on air-leave exchange processes (Tolls and McLachlan, 1994; McLachlan, 1996), or assess equilibrium plant concentrations (United States - Environmental Protection Agency, 1998) that may implicitly take account of degradation.

Thus, degradation or metabolism is a process that needs to be considered for degradable substances. Depending on whether speciation is taken into account, chemical transformation processes may also need to be considered when modelling heavy metals.

The issue of speciation also raises the issue of bound residues when modelling organic chemicals (cf. section 4.2.3). Trapp (1995) states that "the metabolism in plants will in many cases result in bound residues" (p. 146). Bound residues are residues non-extractable (by some solvents) that are covalently bound to organic matter (either of plant tissue or soil organic matter) making them less bioavailable and/or more stable. It is beyond the scope of the present study to elaborate and suggest an approach whether and how to include these in the overall formulation of degradation and/or the following exposure/impact assessment.

5.2.5 Translocation within plants

Assuming equilibrium within plants is problematic as plants do not have blood circulation (Sharpe and Mackay, 2000). Distinguishing between different plant parts might, therefore, be desirable (Trapp, 1995; Charles and Jolliet, 2003). If one distinguishes between roots, stem and leaves there are principally two interfaces across which exchange between these components may occur: root to stem or shoot in general and redistribution in aboveground plant parts.

Exchange between root and stem/shoot

Except for Paterson et al. (1994), the models presented in Table 5-8 do not assume exchange between roots and shoots. Most of them employ the transpiration stream concentration factor (TSCF) which relates the xylem concentration in the aboveground plant parts to the soil solution concentration, thereby skipping/ jumping over/missing out the roots. One reason for disregarding the transfer from aboveground plant parts to roots is that the mass flow in the xylem is at least one order of magnitude higher than in the phloem (Trapp, 1995). Thus, a significant transport does not occur if their transport directions are opposite.

It seems debatable whether to include a transfer from roots to shoots for (heavy) metals. Greger (1999) found that during their transportation through the plant, metals get bound largely on the cell walls, which explains why most of the metal taken up is commonly found in the roots (about 90-75 %) and smaller amounts are distributed in the shoot. For further discussion on root-shoot exchange of heavy metals refer to section 5.2.2.

Exchange between aboveground plant parts

Due to the fact that there are only a few models in Table 5-8 that distinguish between stem and foliage (i.e., Paterson et al., 1994; Trapp, 1995; United States - Environmental Protection Agency, 2002b; unclear for Charles and Jolliet, 2003) and only one additionally considering fruits (Trapp, 1995), only a few descriptions are available for substance distribution in aboveground plant parts all of which, however, do not address the issue of redistribution of (heavy) metals within plants (refer to section 5.2.2 for more information about redistribution of metals). Although not explicitly distinguishing between stem and foliage but rather between protected and unprotected aboveground plant parts, the methodology by United States - Environmental Protection Agency (1998) has also been designed to include heavy metals and trace elements. It is, therefore, adopted for the assessment of these contaminants.

5.2.6 Conclusions on how to address plants in a multimedia environmental fate model and innovations

In order to conclude this sub-Chapter on modelling of terrestrial plants, first conclusions with respect to modelling of heavy metals and trace elements, i.e., the substance class prioritised in this study, will be drawn. In order to provide suggestions in terms of the assessment of 'ordinary' organic substances which may be considered in future model developments, also conclusions with respect to modelling of plants with respect to these substances are drawn.

Unlike many existing plant models (cf. Table 5-8), the harvest of agricultural produce is considered an important removal process from the environmental fate model at least for persistent substances. In section 9.3.3, it will be explored to what extent the exposure assessment in terms of the absolute exposure and its dynamics will be influenced by the inclusion of this harvest process. One has to note that if no removal by terrestrial plants was included in the environmental fate model this would mean that the total amount of a substance removed due to human food consumption is returned to the field. This could be achieved by soil amendments with sewage sludge. However, this return flow will not be complete especially because some sludges are not allowed to be spread onto the fields due to their loading with contaminants, be it the substance to be modelled or others also occurring in the sludge. Furthermore, the place where these substances return to the field will in many cases not be the same as the one where they were removed from due to the trade of food items (cf. section 7.2). This is particularly not the case if areas with an intensive agricultural production and high population density are not spatially distributed in a rather homogeneous way. This is rather often the case.

Modelling heavy metals and trace elements

In general, it appears that roots can be assumed to be in equilibrium with soil (equilibration time in the order of hours according to Briggs et al., 1982, Bromilow and Chamberlain, 1995 and Trapp, 2002). As a consequence, exchanges between shoot and root as included by Paterson et al. (1994) can be neglected. For thick roots, Trapp (2002) proposes a dynamic approach which presumably can be approximated by the inclusion of a correction factor as done by United States - Environmental Protection Agency (1998). Thus, soil and roots can be considered as one (as done, e.g., by Trapp and Matthies, 1995; Severinsen and Jager, 1998) for equilibrium is assumed to occur within compartments in level III/IV multimedia models. The only adjustment to be made is to consider harvest which is in line with Severinsen and Jager (1998) and deemed necessary to be included in the environmental fate model as it leads to a removal of substances out of the modelled system. This also applies to the aboveground plant parts that are harvested.

The treatment of aboveground plant parts is more complex. In particular the question how to treat deposits or residues on plant leaves is not yet scientifically settled although attempts have been made (e.g., United States - Environmental Protection Agency, 2002b; Charles and Jolliet, 2003). Exchange between foliage and other plant parts is basically due to phloem flow. If exchange between shoots and roots due to phloem flow can be neglected (for non-weak acid substances according to Bromilow and Chamberlain, 1995) the same may apply to foliage-stem transfers. The case seems to be different for foliage to fruit transfers mediated by phloem flow (Trapp, 1995), however, very little amounts reach the fruits.

For (heavy) metals and trace elements, there exists only one established methodology for the assessment of metals in agricultural produce in the non-exhaustive list of plant models given in Table 5-8 although attempts to model mercury have been found elsewhere as well (e.g., Maddalena et al., 2002). This was proposed by United States - Environmental Protection Agency (1998) and is recommended at least for this type of substances.

Reinds et al. (1995) provide a rather incomplete model for forests which is due to the fact that they propose a mass balance for the soil rather than for the plant biomass. Furthermore, Cousins and Mackay (2001) recommend to include plant compartments into environmental fate models only when the substances are considerably taken up either via foliage or via roots. Another criterion is to what degree a vegetation compartment influences exposure which is practically non-existing for non-agricultural vegetation. As hardly any translocation from leaves to other plant parts is assumed to occur for heavy metals (see section 5.2.2) and their distribution within plants shows considerably higher concentrations in roots (e.g., Mosbaek et al., 1989; Zayed et al., 1998; Greger, 1999) which are assumed to be in equilibrium with soil for reasons given above, it appears that there is no need to include a natural vegetation compartment into the environmental fate model for heavy metals. Accelerated atmospheric dry particle deposition due to forests ('filter factor') appears not be significant for smaller particles (< 5 μm) in which most of the metals of concern are concentrated (Jonas and Heinemann, 1985) although other authors consider the filter effect to be effective (Reinds et al., 1995; Schütze and Nagel, 1998). Thus, no attempt will be made to include natural vegetation compartments when dealing with non-volatile metals. Methyl mercury as well as elemental mercury are considered to behave like semi-volatile substances.

As a result, if plants are considered when assessing the environmental fate of trace elements this is done by means of combined uptake-removal processes without distinguishing separate compartments. Processes considered are:

- root uptake by and harvest of belowground produce,
- root uptake by and harvest of aboveground produce for non-volatile substances,
- removal from dry atmospheric deposition due to harvest of exposed aboveground produce, and
- removal from wet atmospheric deposition due to harvest of exposed aboveground produce.

Note that the former two constitute processes in the environmental fate matrix whereas the latter two influence the atmospheric deposition as an upper boundary condition. The respective formulations related to processes considered in the fate matrix are given in Table 5-9 and described in detail in section A.3.8 while the equations regarding the influence on the overall input to the water and soil environment are given in Table 4-3 (Eqs. (4-7) and (4-8)), with more details provided in section A.6.5.

Modelling non-dissociating organic substances

Based on the fact that equilibrium between soils and roots is accomplished within a few hours (Briggs et al., 1982; Bromilow and Chamberlain, 1995) and all but one of the models presented in Table 5-8 do not consider a transfer from shoots to roots, it appears that there is no need to include a separate root compartment also for organic compounds. It is, thus, proposed to follow the same approach for non-dissociating organic substances as for heavy metals and trace elements.

From what was presented in section 5.2.1, one may conclude that there is no need to distinguish a leaf surface compartment for semi-volatile organic compounds that are not applied to vegetation directly (such as pesticides). This is mainly due to the difficulties with characterizing this compartment (Riederer,

Table 5-9: Process formulations for terrestrial plants of agricultural use as used in the present assessment

Name	Refer to section ... for more details	Formulation[a]	
Root uptake by and harvest of belowground produce	A.3.8 (p. 404ff)	$k_{\text{i, uptake+harvest root crops}} = \frac{1}{fr\_V_{\text{solid phase/bulk}}(i) \cdot \rho_{\text{solid phase}}(i, z)} \cdot emp_{\text{BCF, root crops}}(p, r, e) \cdot BCF\_dw/dw_{\text{root/soil}}(p, r, e) \cdot fr\_w_{\text{solid phase/bulk}}(r, e) \cdot P(r, n)$	(5-18)
Root uptake by and harvest of aboveground produce for non-volatile sub-stances	A.3.8 (p. 404ff)	$k_{\text{i, uptake+harvest aboveground crops}} = \frac{1}{fr\_V_{\text{solid phase/bulk}}(i) \cdot \rho_{\text{solid phase}}(i, z)} \cdot BCF\_dw/dw_{\text{plant/soil}}(p, r, e) \cdot fr\_w_{\text{solid phase/bulk}}(r, e) \cdot P(r, n)$	(5-19)

a. *ATMDEP*: atmospheric deposition [kg/m^2/s]; *BCF_dw/dw*: bioconcentration factor [-]; *emp*: empirical factor [-] or [s]; *fr_V*: fraction of a volume [-]; *fr_w*: mass fraction of a substance [-]; *k*: process rate as used in the coefficient matrix [m^3/s]; *P*: annual production rate of a crop [kg FW/s]; *r*: process rate [1/s]; ρ: density [kg/m^3]; *S*: source of substances into the water and soil fate model [kg/s]; *Y_fw*: yield of produce [kg FW/m^2]; symbols in parentheses denote a parameter's dependency on the compartment ('*i*' replacing agricultural soil '*ag*' and pastures '*p*'), exposure assessment framework ('*e*'), administrative unit ('*n*'), pollutant ('*p*'), receptor (or crop, '*r*'), emission scenario ('*s*') and/or the zone ('*z*')

1995) and because wet and/or particle-bound deposition is only significant for low volatile, hydrophilic substances (Paterson et al., 1994; Trapp and Matthies, 1995). For pesticides, however, the inclusion of a 'leaf surface' compartment is only necessary if there is exchange between the surface residues on the one hand and plant interior or air on the other.

This leaves us with two compartments for most of the semi-volatile substances: the stem and the leaf compartment. There are two reasons why these may need to be distinguished:

- different parts of the plants are eaten and
- different parts of the plants exhibit different concentrations (cf. Trapp, 1995).

Although there is no 'all-in-one device suitable for every purpose'[13]-like plant meaning that usually not both the stem and the leaves of one plant are used as food, the need to distinguish between stem and leaves (as done by United States - Environmental Protection Agency, 1998) is evident and is, thus, suggested to be considered by default for all non-pesticide organic compounds.

Note that modelling degradation processes for organic substances in plants may require a re-consideration. As the equilibrium between soil and roots can be regarded as to include also degradation in the case of organic substances, it may be argued that considering an explicit degradation removal process additionally leads to double-counting of this process and should, therefore, be skipped.

---

[13] Translation for German 'Eierlegende Wollmilchsau' or literal translation 'oviparous wool-milk sow' (http://dict.leo.org/ visited as of August 2004).

6 Modelling the environmental fate in the aquatic environment

In the following, environmental fate modelling approach for the aquatic environment is described. As for the terrestrial environment, the discription is generally distinguished into modelling of concentrations in water bodies and aquatic organisms (section 6.1 and 6.2, respectively).

6.1 Environmental fate modelling of water bodies

The environmental fate assessment methodology presented covers the environmental media 'soil' and 'water'. While the terrestrial environment is subject of Chapter 5, the medium 'water' will be addressed in the following.

When talking about 'water', in principle one may distinguish it according to its:

- composition: fresh and salty water,
- phases: liquid, solid and gaseous water, and
- macroscopic occurrence, i.e., water bodies at the surface or the subsurface (e.g., groundwater).

Gaseous water or water vapour is mostly part of the atmosphere. Solid water, i.e., ice and snow, is to some extent covered by a new terrestrial compartment (cf. section 5.1.11) noting that the influence of for example sea ice cover on the global environmental fate and snow on ecotoxicology may be important for some substances (e.g., Wania, 2003; Daly and Wania, 2004). As a result, only the distinction according to its composition and its occurrence may be relevant in the following discussion. However, at present only surface freshwater bodies are included in the assessment for reasons given in Chapter 7. In particular, disregarding subsurface water, i.e., ground water, is in line with most of the multimedia models in use today.

6.1.1 Compartments distinguished

When differentiating the freshwater environment into compartments, the most common division is into the freshwater body itself and a corresponding sediment (e.g., Mackay and Diamond, 1989; 1991; Mackay and Hickie, 2000; Mackay and Southwood, 1992; Mackay et al., 1992, 1996a; McKone, 1993b; Devillers et al., 1995; Wania and Mackay, 1995; Brandes et al., 1996; Rantio and Paasivirta, 1996; Severinsen et al., 1996; Wania, 1996; Scheringer et al., 2000a; Wania et al., 2000; MacLeod et al., 2001; Prevedouros et al., 2004). For the purpose of modelling non-volatile substances directly released into surface waters, Scheringer and co-workers developed a segmented model for the river Rhine following linear algebra formulations (Beck et al., 2000; Scheringer et al., 2000a). This model distinguishes two water compartments: one containing moving waters and another representing stagnant waters just above the sediment and in shallower regions of the river. Scheringer and co-workers, however, do not state to what extent the introduction of the stagnant water compartment influences the overall results and under which conditions its distinction is recommended. Therefore, the 'ordinary' distinction into water body and bottom sediment is made. However, it shall be noted already here that a distinction of stagnant water portions from flowing waters within the overall freshwater compartment will, nevertheless, be made in this study.

When performing spatially-resolved environmental fate assessments different zones are distinguished whose freshwater and sediment compartments may be allowed to vary in terms of dimensions and properties. There are many examples of such multi-zonal models published in the context of multimedia modelling (e.g., Mackay and Southwood, 1992; Devillers et al., 1995; Wania and Mackay, 1995; Wania, 1996; Rantio and Paasivirta, 1996; Mackay and Hickie, 2000; Wania et al., 2000; Prevedouros et al., 2004). Some of these distinguish between river stretches and lakes (e.g., Mackay and Southwood, 1992; Rantio and Paasivirta, 1996) or just between different parts of lakes (e.g., Wania, 1996; Mackay and Hickie, 2000). The spatial differentiation of the presented methodology allows to distinguish larger lakes from rivers in terms of dimensions and properties as well. This is also motivated by the fact that when computing at the high resolution as shown in Fig. 4-3 about 80 % of the zones contain freshwater compartments that only consist of streams. In the following, the respective dimensions and properties of the aquatic environment are defined.

6.1.2 Dimensions of the aquatic compartments

In order to define the dimension of the freshwater and sediment compartments, one needs to know their areas covered and their average depths. The area covered

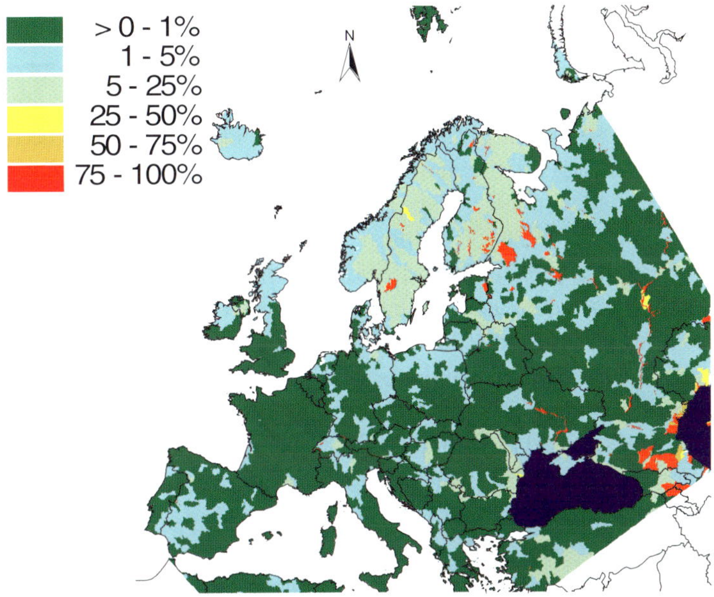

Fig. 6-1: Distribution of the predominance of freshwater bodies in the different zones distinguished by WATSON (note that the Black Sea and the Caspian Sea are presently not modelled)

by the freshwater compartment is determined by means of GIS land cover and hydrology-related datasets as presented in section B.4 and shown in Fig. 6-1. Usually, bottom sediments of freshwater bodies are perceived to have the same area as the water body as explicitly stated by Mackay et al. (1992) and Wania et al. (2000). As a result, the area fractions of freshwater bodies (cf. Fig. 6-1) also apply to their bottom sediments.

Depth of freshwater bodies

The depth of the freshwater compartment is allowed to vary (a) by following the distinction between larger lakes and other freshwater bodies and (b) according to the general observation (in humid areas) that the channel of a river will increase with increasing catchment area (Finlayson and McMahon, 1995, see also sections B.2.1 and B.4). The latter downstream-directed volume increase only applies to those rivers whose drainage basins are further subdivided into several zones, referred to as 'large rivers'.

Depth of the freshwater sediment

Most of the spatially differentiated multimedia models for which sediment depths are explicitly stated (e.g., Wania and Mackay, 1995; Wania et al., 2000) consider the depth of the active sediment layer to be invariant between zones. The depths of this layer for non-site-specific, generic or evaluative multimedia models range from 0.01 m (Mackay et al., 1992, 1996a) over 0.03 m (Mackay, 1991; Devillers et al., 1995; Brandes et al., 1996; Severinsen et al., 1996; European Commission, 2003b) to 0.05 m (Wania and Mackay, 1995; Scheringer et al., 2000a; Wania et al., 2000). It is noted that when a particular site is investigated zone-specific sediment depths may be available and, thus, used, as done in several studies (Mackay and Diamond, 1989; Mackay and Southwood, 1992; Rantio and Paasivirta, 1996; Wania, 1996; Mackay and Hickie, 2000) spanning a wider range (from 0.005 m for Lake Ontario, Mackay and Diamond, 1989, to 0.1 m for a river delta in a lake, Wania, 1996). For the purpose of the present study, a constant depth of 0.05 m is adopted for the sediment compartment.

6.1.3 Definition of the phases of aquatic compartments

Phases distinguished in freshwater bodies are usually water and abiotic suspended matter. Some environmental fate models also include fish (Mackay et al., 1992, 1996a; Mackay and Southwood, 1992; Devillers et al., 1995; Brandes et al., 1996; Severinsen et al., 1996). As noted by Mackay et al. (1992) and Brandes et al. (1996), fish usually play an insignificant role with regard to the overall fate of substances. Like suspended matter, however, these may contain appreciably high concentrations especially of less water-solvable substances. In line with many other multimedia models and chemical risk assessment frameworks (e.g., European Commission, 1996a), fish are not distinguished as phases or even as a compartment in the fate part but at least in the exposure assessment of the presented methodology. Due to the assumed equilibrium between phases within one compartment, a new process can optionally be included in the analysis which describes equilibrium partitioning of substances into freshwater fish that is caught and, thus, removed at a certain rate (cf. section 6.2). Together with other 'uptake-harvest' processes, the removal of caught freshwater fish upon exposure is part of a scenario analysis in section 9.3.3.

The composition of suspended matter as well as that of particles in the sediment varies considerably according to the information provided by several multimedia models (compiled in Table B-9 (Mackay et al., 1992, 1996a; Devillers et al., 1995; Rantio and Paasivirta, 1996) and in Table B-10 (Mackay, 1991; Mackay et al., 1992, 1996a; Devillers et al., 1995; Rantio and Paasivirta, 1996; Mackay and Hickie, 2000), respectively). Assuming that the organic carbon mass makes up 50 % of the organic matter mass (Schnitzer, 1978) with an organic matter density of 1400 kg/m^3 (Scheffer and Schachtschabel, 1989), the respective mineral matter mass fractions as well as their densities are obtained. As can be seen from both Tables, the resulting mineral matter densities tend to be lower than that of clay minerals (2200 - 2900 kg/m^3) and of quartz (2650 kg/m^3, Scheffer and Schachtschabel, 1989) ranging from 1500 to 2800 kg/m^3. While the organic carbon content of the sediment particles as given in Table B-10 spans the value range found in other publications (from 3 to 20 vol.-%, Mackay and Diamond, 1989; Mackay and Southwood, 1992; Brandes et al., 1996; Severinsen et al., 1996; Wania, 1996; Wania and Mackay, 1995), the values for the organic carbon content of suspended matter as shown in Table B-9 are located at the higher end of the range from 0.04 (Wania et al., 2000) to 0.4 in the deep water zone of a lake (Wania, 1996) or in the tropic zone (Wania and Mackay, 1995).

Like for other characteristics of the freshwater environment, a distinction of suspended solids in stream water and lakes is made. Generally, the organic matter content of suspended and deposited solids in streams is much smaller than that found in lakes. For this reason, the reported lower bound and upper bound values are used as an orientation for the characterisation of stream and lake solids, respectively (Table 6-1). The particle densities result according to the information on the respective organic carbon contents and the densities for organic and mineral matter. Two different mineral matter densities are used for the computation of suspended solid and sediment solid densities. For suspended matter, the mineral phase's density is set to that of clay minerals, i.e., 2550 kg/m^3 (Scheffer and Schachtschabel, 1989), whereas for sediment solids it is set to that of quartz, i.e., 2650 kg/m^3 (Scheffer and Schachtschabel, 1989).

Based on sediment yield data provided by Milliman and Syvitski (1992), the volume fraction of suspended solids in streams is set to $1 \cdot 10^{-3}$ vol.-% which appears to be applicable to non-Alpine mountainous, upland and lowland European rivers. As a result, the concentration of suspended matter in freshwater streams is set to 0.02469 kg/m^3. In the absence of more specific data, a value for the volume fraction of suspended matter of $1 \cdot 10^{-4}$ vol.-% is assumed for lakes which is of the same order of magnitude like the bulk of the reported values in the multimedia literature (Mackay et al., 1992, 1996a; Wania and Mackay, 1995; Rantio and Paasivirta, 1996; Mackay and Hickie, 2000).

The corresponding value for the volume fraction of solids in sediments also needs to be specified. Reported values range from 0.1 (Mackay and Hickie, 2000) to 0.4 (Mackay, 1991; Rantio and Paasivirta, 1996).[14] As the sediment compart-

Table 6-1: Characteristics of solids in the freshwater environment as used in the presented methodology

Property	Particle type	Stream	Lake
Volume fraction of ...	suspended matter	$1 \cdot 10^{-5}$ [a]	$1 \cdot 10^{-6}$ [b]
	sediment solids	0.2	0.2
Mass fraction of organic carbon in ...	suspended matter	0.02[c]	0.4[d]
	sediment solids	0.005[e]	0.3[d]
Density of solids [kg per m^3][f] of ...	suspended matter	2469	1539
	sediment solids	2627	1726

a. Selection of the value is guided by data in Milliman and Syvitski (1992).
b. Same order of magnitude like the bulk of the reported values in the multimedia literature (Mackay et al., 1992, 1996a; Wania and Mackay, 1995; Rantio and Paasivirta, 1996; Mackay and Hickie, 2000).
c. Half the value as used in Wania et al. (2000) assumed for 'pure' stream conditions.
d. In the deep water zone of a lake (Wania, 1996).
e. Although the smallest value found is 0.02 for the northern-boreal and the polar zones in Wania and Mackay (1995) an even smaller value is adopted for 'pure' stream sediments which usually have an organic matter content below 1 % (Scheffer and Schachtschabel, 1989) due to water erosion and oxic conditions.
f. Assumptions: half of the organic matter (OM) mass consists of organic carbon (Schnitzer, 1978) and taking the complement as mineral matter (MM); densities: 1400 kg_{OM}/m^3, 2550 $kg_{clay\ minerals}/m^3$ (for suspended solids) and 2650 kg_{MM}/m^3 (for sediment solids, Scheffer and Schachtschabel, 1989).

ments only comprise the active part of the overall sediments which is not as consolidated as the parts below, a value of 20 vol.-% is adopted here which corresponds to the median and the average of the volume fractions of sediments that consist of solids reported in the multimedia modelling literature.

14 Note that two values are used by Rantio and Paasivirta (1996): a value of 0.6 for sediment porosity corresponding to 40 vol.-% solids and a value of 0.05 for all segments concerning 'volume fraction of sediment solids'. It is unclear to the author how these match.

6.1.4 Processes considered for the aquatic environment

The set of processes included in the modelling exercise of multimedia models does not vary substantially between models for the aquatic environment (Table 6-2). In the presented methodology, the following processes that are not related to chemical transformation, speciation or radioactive decay are considered:

- water advection,
- sediment deposition,
- resuspension,
- sediment-water diffusive exchange, and
- sediment burial

noting that bioturbation beside resuspension may also be important for a remobilisation of heavy metals and other substances from sediments (Wania et al., 2000; Zoumis et al., 2001). Their formulation is given in Table 6-3 and further discussed in separate sub-sections to A.3 also stated in the Table. Note that degradation and radioactive decay may be defined for the aquatic environment analogously as for the terrestrial environment described in Table 5-5.

All of these processes are part of mass balances for suspended or deposited particulates or for water except for the diffusive exchange, a process which, however, may involve movement of colloidal matter as well (Mackay, 1991). The diffusive exchange between water bodies and sediments is included in the developed environmental fate model in an 'ordinary' way (cf. sections A.3.14 and A.3.15). The mass balance on water is described next while the components of the particle mass balance in the freshwater environment will be discussed in more detail in section 6.1.5.

Mass balance on water

For the mass balance on water, a harmonized set of Geographic Information System (GIS) data is used. Information on precipitation rates have been taken from New et al. (1999). Data on runoff and ground water recharge which are used to distinguish quickflow from baseflow waters have been provided by Döll et al. (2003). The quickflow waters drive the process of 'overland flow' (section A.3.4) whereas baseflow waters percolate through soil to the subsurface (section A.3.6) before exfiltrating into surface waters again. Note that except for few areas, for instance, in Spain and Africa, the general assumption of exfiltrating water flows holds.

According to the general assumptions as formulated in section 2.3, use shall be made of long-term average data. The data sources used provide average values for the period of 1961-1990 fulfilling this requirement. Due to the fact that

Table 6-2: Non-exhaustive overview about processes considered for the freshwater compartment by various multimedia models (note: chemical transformations are not listed)

Model / reference	Air-water exchange	Water advection	Sediment deposition	Resuspension	Sediment-water diffusion	Sediment burial	Bioturbation
QWASI (Mackay and Diamond, 1989)	x	x	x	x	x	x	
EQC (Mackay et al., 1996a)[a]	x	x	x	x	x	x	
POPCYCLING-Baltic (Wania et al., 2000)	x	x	x	x	x	x	x
CHEMFRANCE (Devillers et al., 1995)	x	x	x	x	x	x	
Danish model (Severinsen et al., 1996)	x	x	x	x	x		
River Rhine model (Scheringer et al., 2000a)	n/a[b]	x	x[c]	x	x[d]		
SimpleBox 2.0 (Brandes et al., 1996)	x	x	x	x	x	x	
CalTOX (McKone, 1993b)	x	x	x	x	x	x	

a. A model with at least the same water-related processes, rates and compartment properties has previously been documented in Mackay et al. (1992).
b. Not applicable for the substances investigated.
c. Only affecting suspended particulates in the stagnant water compartment.
d. There is a diffusive exchange between the moving and stagnant water compartment as well as between the stagnant water and sediment compartment.

environmental parameters are held constant during the present assessment ('quasi-dynamic' modelling), no storage change for example in soils is taken into account. The water balance is, thus, described at steady-state.

Table 6-3: Process formulations for the aquatic environment as used in the present assessment

Name	Refer to section ... for more details	Formulation[a]	
Water body and sediment compartment			
Discharge	A.3.9 (p. 409)	$k_{w,\,z1-z2,\,\text{discharge}}(z) = Q_{\text{discharge}}(z)$	(6-1)
Water circulation in large lakes	A.3.10 (p. 410)	$k_{w,\,z_{\text{down}}-z_{\text{up,i}},\,\text{lake ciculation}}(z, w) = Q_{\text{discharge}}(z_{\text{down}}, w) \cdot fr\_Q_{\text{lake circulation}}(w)$	(6-2)
Sedimentation in freshwater compartments	A.3.11 (p. 411)	$k_{w-ws,\,\text{sedimentation, pH}\lvert\text{pH inv}\rvert C_{\text{org}}}(p, w, z) = \frac{A(z) \cdot fr\_A(w, z)}{ED_{\text{bulk/aqueous, pH}\lvert\text{pH inv}\rvert C_{\text{org}}}(p, w, z)} \cdot v_{\text{sedimentation, derived}}$	(6-3)
Resuspension of bottom sediment matter	A.3.12 (p. 412)	$k_{ws\text{-w},\,\text{resuspension}}(ws, z) = A(z) \cdot fr\_A(w, z) \cdot v_{\text{resuspension, derived}}$	(6-4)
Sediment burial	A.3.13 (p. 414)	$k_{ws,\,\text{burial, pH}\lvert\text{pH}_{\text{inv}}}(p, ws, z) = \frac{\rho_{\text{solid phase}}(ws, z) \cdot Ksw(p, pH(ws, z))}{ED_{\text{bulk/aqueous, pH}\lvert\text{pH}_{\text{inv}}}(p, ws, z)} \cdot A(z) \cdot fr\_A(w, z) \cdot v_{\text{burial, derived}}$	(6-5)
Diffusion from sediment to water body	A.3.15 (p. 418)	$k_{ws-w,\,\text{diffusion, pH}\lvert\text{pH inv}\rvert C_{\text{org}}}(p, ws, z) = A(z) \cdot fr\_A(w, z) \cdot \frac{v_{\text{diffusion}}(ws)}{ED_{\text{bulk/aqueous, pH}\lvert\text{pH inv}\rvert C_{\text{org}}}(p, ws, z)}$	(6-6)

Table 6-3: Process formulations for the aquatic environment as used in the present assessment

Name	Refer to section ... for more details	Formulation[a]
Diffusion from water body to sediment	A.3.14 (p. 416)	$k_{w\text{-}ws,\ \text{diffusion, pH}\mid\text{pH}_{\text{inv}}}(p, w, z) = \frac{A(z) \cdot fr\_A(w, z)}{Ksw(p, pH(w, z)\mid pH(w))} \cdot \frac{1}{\rho_{\text{suspended matter}}(w, z)} \cdot \frac{v_{\text{diffusion}}(w)}{ED_{\text{bulk/solid, pH}\mid\text{pH}_{\text{inv}}}(p, w, z)}$ (6-7)
Freshwater fish		
Uptake by and catch of freshwater fish for non-volatile substances	A.3.8 (p. 404)	$k_{\text{w, uptake+catch fish}} = \frac{BCF\_V/fw_{\text{fish/water}}(p, r, e) \cdot P(r, n)}{Ksw \cdot ED_{\text{bulk/solid}} \cdot \rho_{\text{suspendend matter}}(w, z)}$ (6-8)

a.*A*: area of the zone [m^2]; *BCF_V/fw*: bioconcentration factor [m^3/kg]; *d*: depth of a compartment [m]; *ED*: equilibrium distribution coefficient [-]; *fr_A*: area fraction of a compartment within a zone [-]; *fr_Q*: fraction of the discharge [-]; *fr_v*: fraction of a process velocity [-]; *k*: process rate as used in the coefficient matrix [m^3/s]; *K*: solid-water partitioning coefficient [m^3/kg]; *Q*: discharge [m^3/s]; *r*: process rate [1/s]; ρ: density [kg/m^3]; *v*: process velocity [m/s] (for derived parameters: see text); symbols in parentheses denote a parameter's dependency on the exposure assessment framework ('*e*'), administrative unit ('*n*'), pollutant ('*p*'), receptor (or fish, '*r*'), compartment ('*w*' freshwater body, '*ws*': corresponding sediment) and/or the zone ('*z*')

The processing of the data related to the water balance is described in section B.5.2. The process 'discharge' or water advection is formulated based on runoff information (cf. Table 6-3 and section A.3.9).

6.1.5 Innovations as regards aquatic compartments

There are several innovations introduced as regards the modelling of the aquatic environment. These are

- the distinction of rivers from lakes in terms of the dynamics of the particles,
- the introduction of lake water circulation in those instances in which a distinction of large lakes is made; these consist of several zones that entirely consist of water.

These shall be presented in the following.

Mass balance on particulates in the freshwater environment

Mass balances focusing on suspended organic particulates are explicitly addressed for example in Mackay et al. (1992), Brandes et al. (1996) and Wania et al. (2000) to varying degrees of sophistication. For the more sophisticated mass balances, data requirements are higher and include information for instance on the primary productivity of a water body, mineralisation rates, explicit information on organic matter entering the aquatic environment from soils, or inputs from sewers. Likewise a mass balance for suspended mineral matter may be formulated. This is addressed by all consulted multimedia model descriptions according to the organic carbon mass fractions reported especially for suspended matter. When assuming that 50 weight-% of organic matter consists of organic carbon (Schnitzer, 1978), the organic carbon mass fraction of suspended matter would need to amount to 50 weight-% for the suspended particles to entirely consist of organic material. All of the reported values found in the multimedia modelling literature are below this value implying that all models consider mineral particles to be present (cf. section B.5.4). SimpleBox 2.0 even explicitly considers the overall erosion rate from soil to water although suspended matter is understood to consist of non-living organic matter only (Brandes et al., 1996). For data availability reasons, the simpler approach for suspended particulates as presented for example by Mackay et al. (1992) is followed in the present study.

The rates of the processes 'sediment deposition', 'resuspension' and 'sediment burial' of the finer particles to which most of the substances will sorb strongly depend on the flow pattern or turbulence of the water body modelled, beside particle properties and fluid density (Shen and Julien, 1993). The 'fluid' or water density is assumed to be 1000 kg/m^3 in the freshwater environment. Although noting that the properties even of the 'finer particulates' active in contaminant transport will vary considerably, no differentiation for example into mineral and organic particles and/or colloids or 'flocs' (McCutcheon et al., 1993; Nicholas and Walling, 1996; Droppo et al., 1998) will be made here in terms of process velocities. Nevertheless, the distinction into larger lakes and other freshwater bodies as well as different zones within larger catchments (sections 4.3 and 6.1.2) allows a differentiated approach towards the determination of these process rates in the spatially-resolved impact assessment methodology presented.

In line with Scheringer et al. (2000a) and Beck et al. (2000), sedimentation is only allowed to take place in stagnant waters, however, without distinguishing these as separate compartments (cf. section B.5.4). In the absence of more specific information, it is assumed that the large lakes distinguished (cf. section B.2.1) entirely consist of stagnant waters. In contrast, only 5 % of the in-stream water volumes are assumed to allow for sedimentation due to their low amount of stagnant waters. This volume fraction is substantially lower than the 25 % that have been assumed by Scheringer et al. (2000a). However, these authors have not distinguished lakes explicitly. Also, their value appears to be rather high.

Another distinction is made in that sedimentation in freshwater bodies of zones that pour directly into the sea ('river mouth') is increased due to slower flow velocities, also called aggradation zone or "area of deposition" in an idealised fluvial system (Schumm, 1977). By default, the volume share of stagnant water is set to 21 % in these zones, provided they are part of a larger drainage basin. This is guided by the idea that a smaller percentage of the deposition rate is resuspended in these areas than in other 'pure' stream zones.

The process rates relevant for the particle mass balance in surface freshwater and their relationships are given in Table 6-4 based on a literature review (cf. section B.5.4), distinguished according to pure river and pure lake situations, respectively. Large lakes are considered not to contain (significantly) flowing waters which is why the values for all of the process velocities under pure lake conditions are directly given in Table 6-4. For mixtures of stagnant and flowing conditions, the overall applicable process rates are calculated according to the Eqs. (B-17), (B-22) and (B-27) of the general form:

$$v_{\text{process, total}} = Fraction_{\text{stagnant water}} \cdot v_{\text{process, lake}} + (1 - Fraction_{\text{stagnant water}}) \cdot v_{\text{process, stream}} \qquad (6\text{-}9)$$

where

v : velocity of particles while undergoing either of the processes sedimentation, resuspension, or burial in the freshwater environment [m per s]

Fraction : volume or area fraction of stagnant waters [-].

Table 6-4: Particle mass balance for surface freshwater assumed in this study differentiated into a pure river and a pure lake situation

Characteristics	Pure river	Pure lake
Sediment deposition rate [m/s]	$0.95 \cdot 0$ [a] $+ 0.05 \cdot 3.50 \cdot 10^{-6}$ [b] $= 1.75 \cdot 10^{-7}$	$3.50 \cdot 10^{-6}$ [b]
Resuspension rate [m/s]	$0.95 \cdot 1.143 \cdot 10^{-7}$ [c] $+ 0.05 \cdot 1.156 \cdot 10^{-6}$ [d] $= 1.66 \cdot 10^{-7}$	$1.156 \cdot 10^{-6}$ [d]
Burial rate [m/s]	$0.95 \cdot -1.143 \cdot 10^{-7}$ [e] $+ 0.05 \cdot 2.35 \cdot 10^{-6}$ [f] $= 8.76 \cdot 10^{-9}$	$2.35 \cdot 10^{-6}$ [f]
Ratio resuspension / sedimentation	95.0 % [g]	33.0 %
Ratio burial / sedimentation	5.0 %	67.0 % [h]
Ratio remainder / sedimentation	0.0 % [i]	0.0 % [j]

a. As calculated for a pure in-stream sediment deposition rate by Eq. (B-20).
b. As calculated for a pure in-lake sediment deposition rate by Eq. (B-19).
c. As calculated for a pure in-stream resuspension rate by Eq. (B-26).
d. As calculated for a pure in-lake resuspension rate by Eq. (B-24).
e. As calculated for a pure in-stream burial rate by Eq. (B-31); see text for the explanation of the negative value.
f. As calculated for a pure in-lake burial rate by Eq. (B-29).
g. The highest reported value is 85 % for the shore line of a lake (Wania, 1996); due to the even higher flow rate in streams a higher value has been adopted; note that the 'effective' sedimentation is higher river mouth situations of larger rivers (Schumm, 1977) and in lakes.
h. Value selection guided by the burial at the deep water zone of a lake (Wania, 1996).
i. In case mineralization was to be considered, the value of 14 % as used in the POPCYCLING-Baltic model would be suggested to be used for organic matter in rivers (Wania et al., 2000).
j. In case mineralization was to be considered, the value of 7 % as used for the southern segment of Lac Saint Louis would be suggested to be used for organic matter in lakes (Mackay and Hickie, 2000), owing to the smaller biological activity and lower temperatures throughout the course of a year.

In section B.5.4, the mass balance for particles in the freshwater environment is discussed in more detail. In short, a value of $2.35 \cdot 10^{-6}$ metres per second for the net sedimentation (or burial) rate is identified to be appropriate for the full removal of all suspended particles from the water column of large lakes which are assumed to be 74 metres deep, disregarding the removal due to comparatively slow water advection. Following Stokes' law, this value falls in the range of velocities obtained for temperatures between 5 and 10°C for a spheric particle with a radius of 1 μm (i.e., of the clay fraction) and a density of 1539 kg/m^3 (assumed for suspended particles in lakes, cf. Table B-11). The settling velocities range from $2.21 \cdot 10^{-6}$ and $2.56 \cdot 10^{-6}$ metres per second for a temperature of 5 and 10°C and a corresponding (absolute) water viscosity of $1.518 \cdot 10^{-3}$ and $1.307 \cdot 10^{-3}$ kg/m/s (McCutcheon et al., 1993), respectively. Thus, the value appears to be reasonable.

For rivers, the same settling velocity is assumed under still-water conditions. However, it is allowed to be active only in 5 % of the water volume that are assumed to be stagnant as mentioned above. Furthermore, 95 % of the settled particles in streams are assumed to undergo resuspension so that the overall net sedimentation rate for rivers results to be $8.76 \cdot 10^{-9}$ metres per second.

Note that the value obtained for the pure in-stream sediment burial rate is negative. All of the velocities derived for streams (not only the velocity for burial, but also for sedimentation and resuspension (Eqs. (B-31), (B-20) and (B-26), respectively)) should, however, be regarded as hypothetical as these are not directly used in the process formulations (section A.3). These values are rather obtained in order to fulfil the following requirements:

- in order to provide a generally applicable computation of the overall process rates, the approach as given by Eq. (6-9) is followed which distinguishes between stagnant and non-stagnant domains within any freshwater compartment. Due to the heterogeneity of freshwater compartments ranging from pure streams over mixtures of streams and lakes to pure lakes, this methodological approach is adopted, and
- the overall in-stream net sedimentation rate, i.e., resulting sediment deposition rate minus resuspension rate as given in Table 6-4, shall amount to 5 % of the lake net sedimentation rate.

As a result, especially the negative value for the burial rate is hypothetical and is only used in order to yield a (non-negative) total process velocity. The hypothetical values for pure moving water conditions are, therefore, considered justified and scientifically defendable as long as they are consistently derived and used. As stated above, any water body is assumed to at least contain 5 vol.-% of still waters which assures that no negative end-values result.

As can be seen from Table 6-4, no mineralization is allowed to occur. In principle, one would need to distinguish between the mineral and organic phases of the respective sediment and suspended particles when taking account of mineralization. This is not done at present which is in line with Devillers et al. (1995), Severinsen et al. (1996) and Wania (1996).

Water circulation in large lakes

In contrast to the process 'discharge' which flows from an upstream zone either into a further downstream one within a catchment or into coastal waters, i.e., out of the present model's scope, there is a new process introduced into the environmental fate assessment, termed 'water circulation in large lakes' (cf. Table 6-3). This has been deemed necessary due to the distinction of larger lakes from other water bodies for reasons detailed in the following.

Some of these larger lakes are fully contained within the zones identified by the HYDRO1k basin dataset (EROS Data Center, 1996). These are only considered in terms of a larger depth. However, many of these lakes extend over different zones. Their spatial differentiation according to the HYDRO1k basin dataset resembles a rather unnatural or non-intuitive herringbone that cuts the lakes into bands (Fig. 6-2). This is due to the derivation of sub-basins according to elevation data while lakes do not show marked slopes. All of these lake portions which are connected by the downstream flow of water constitute separate zones according to the presented methodology.

If only allowing downstream-directed discharge to occur between different lake portions, there would be no water exchange between a 'downstream' and an adjacent 'upstream' lake zone due to the cascading organisation of flows between zones according to the Pfafstetter code (cf. Fig. 4-4). Therefore, water advection is allowed to also move waters 'upstream' following this code.

The process 'water circulation in large lakes' is formulated as the reverse process of discharge so that one 'downstream' zone may pour a certain amount of water into maximally two 'upstream' lake zones. The amount of water involved is set to a share of the discharge flowing out of the 'downstream' lake zone as described in section A.3.10. At the same time the same amount of water flows back in order not to violate the water mass balance. The share of discharge undergoing this process is presently set to 100 %. The influence of this process on the exposure and impact results will be analysed in a sensitivity analysis in section 9.3.3.

6.2 Environmental fate modelling for aquatic organisms

WATSON at present does not include the marine environment which is why only freshwater organisms can be considered. Similar to vegetal produce (see section 5.2), freshwater fish are neither modelled as separate compartments nor constitute phases within compartments in the environmental fate model. Rather, they may be considered by means of a combined transfer-harvest process in which freshwater fish are assumed to be in equilibrium with the freshwater compartment and removed by means of catching. Considering harvest removal of substances in a multimedia modelling context has hardly been done (cf. section 5.2.3). These

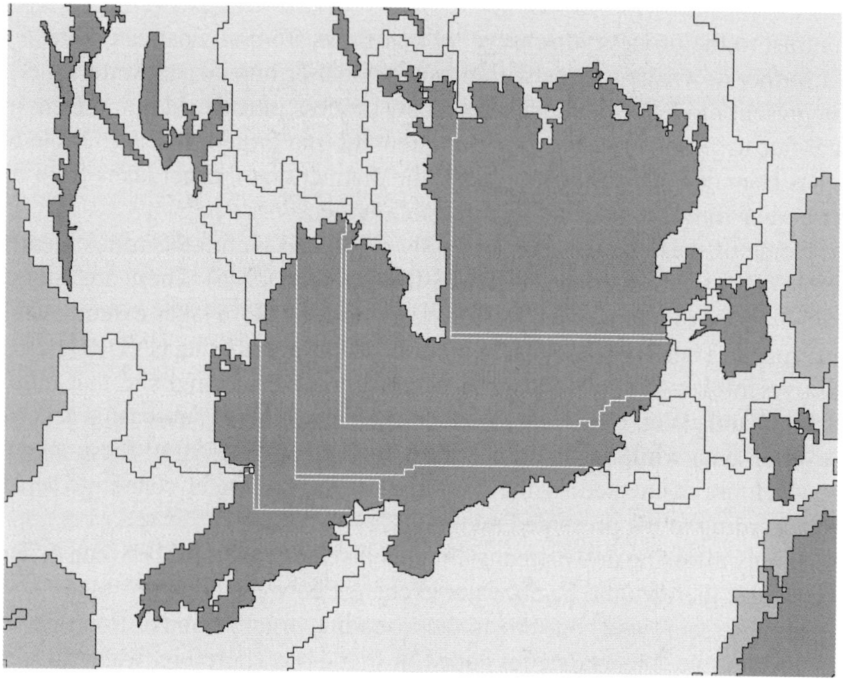

Fig. 6-2: Lake Vänern in southern Sweden as an example of a sub-division of larger lakes according to the spatial differentiation as provided by HYDRO1k basin dataset (EROS Data Center, 1996; dark grey: lakes; light grey: the Götälv catchment; water grossly flowing from north-east to south-west; lakes fully contained in one zone are also shown)

removal processes only addressed the harvest of terrestrial plants. The inclusion of a corresponding process for fish is, thus, novel in the realm of multimedia modelling. The respective equation is given in Table 6-3 (Eq. (6-8), p. 143).

In any case, human exposure towards freshwater fish consumption is part of the exposure assessment to be presented in the next Chapter (cf. section A.7.12).

7 Exposure and impact assessment

In the present work, the Impact Pathway Approach which originally focused on impacts following inhalation of toxic air pollutants by humans is extended to also cover impacts due to hazardous substances present in the media soil and water. As was argued in Chapter 2, human health impacts constitute the main component when estimating external costs. The exposure and impact assessment described in the following is, hence, exclusively addressing impacts on human beings. In contrast to the environmental fate model, the exposure as well as the impact assessment follow a spatial differentiation based on administrative units mostly according to the Nomenclature of Territorial Units for Statistics (Nomenclature des Unités Territoriales Statistiques, NUTS) used by the Statistical Office of the European Communities (EUROSTAT). Thus, the information that is available in a spatially-resolved way is attributed to the different administrative levels distinguished such as countries or municipalities (cf. section B.6).

Principally there are three main *routes of exposure*, i.e., the routes by which a chemical enters the body (United States - Environmental Protection Agency, 1992; World Health Organisation, 2000a; European Commission, 2003c):

1. inhalation: absorption through the lungs,
2. ingestion: absorption from the digestive tract, and
3. dermal absorption: penetration through the skin.

For exposure *pathways* through soil and water, the most important exposure *route* is ingestion noting that dermal exposure due to bathing and soil contact might principally also play a role (Mileson et al., 1999). In agreement with the European Union's Technical Guidance Documents (European Commission, 2003a), the dermal exposure route as well as ingestion of soil particles by humans are considered to be of importance only in the case of highly polluted soils. Only recently, however, the Directorates of Environment, Health and Research of the European Commission have jointly launched an initiative, termed 'Science, Children, Awareness, EU Legislation and Continuous Evaluation' (SCALE), in order to develop a European Environment and Health Strategy (European Commission,

2003f). As can be seen from the initiative's name, a focus is laid on children and their protection. Although mouthing behaviour is a rather normal phase of childhood development, deliberate soil ingestion also termed *pica* is considered relatively uncommon (United States - Environmental Protection Agency, 1997c). Additionally, penetration of substances through the skin is of much more concern when assessing occupational exposure (World Health Organisation, 2000a) and exposure via cosmetic products. The contribution of the dermal exposure route and soil ingestion to the overall exposure in situations of diffuse emissions is deemed negligible and, therefore, these are not further considered here.

Ingestion or the oral exposure route involves two main substrates: food and drinking water. Most (acute) heavy metal problems related to drinking water stem from the distribution system (pipes) and not from the source of the drinking water (World Health Organisation, 1992b; Becker et al., 1997; Wilhelm and Ewers, 1999; Bernigau et al., 2000). The case may be different for organic pollutants for which water treatment is not very efficient (Versteegh et al., 2001; European Commission, 2003a) and which may also lead to indoor inhalation exposure after volatilisation from tap water (e.g., McKone, 1993a; Georgopoulos et al., 1997). Nevertheless, the additional exposure due to additional human activities might still be substantial, at least in the long run. However, modelling drinking water exposure for all European residents is a task that nobody has addressed until now following a detailed site-dependent bottom-up approach that aims at giving best estimates rather than those based on conservative (reasonable) worst-case scenarios such as in European Commission (2003b) for the local scale. This is because ground water constitutes a major part of the drinking water resources (Scheidleder et al., 1999). Even at smaller scales one fails to model mass transfers in ground water aquifers due to lack of information (e.g., Eggleston and Rojstaczer, 2000). It also appears that ground water contamination due to heavy metals, for instance, is a very localised problem and is confined to areas with former or present mining activities in the case of heavy metals (Stanners and Bourdeau, 1995). Due to the lack of contamination as well as aquifer information, a modelling effort would at present result in rather unreliable concentration estimates. Thus, whereas the assessment of food ingestion is more readily feasible, the exposure via drinking water is for the moment not included in the modelling framework.

The present Chapter is divided into three parts. These describe:

1. the assessment of a substance's concentration in agricultural produce and freshwater fish,
2. the food intake, and
3. the impact assessment.

7.1 Concentration in food

In search of an existing exposure assessment scheme to be adopted for the estimation of external costs, mostly rather conservative exposure assessment frameworks have been encountered (e.g., European Commission, 2003c; International Atomic Energy Agency, 2001; cf. sections 3.1.3 and 3.1.4) which for example employ safety factors or assume protective values leading to overestimates rather than underestimates. This is desirable from a regulatory perspective. This is unacceptable, however, from a cost-benefit point of view where representative estimates are needed.

A step towards a less conservative and, thus, more representative exposure assessment is seen in the Human Health Risk Assessment Protocol (HHRAP, United States - Environmental Protection Agency, 1998). The HHRAP aims at consolidating information presented in other risk assessment guidance and methodology documents previously prepared for example by the US-EPA. Due to the fact that it constitutes a site-specific risk assessment approach, the degree of conservatism is reduced towards screening level risk assessments. Evaluating reasonable rather than theoretical worst-case maximum potential risks is recommended (United States - Environmental Protection Agency, 1998); conservative assumptions shall only be employed in order to prevent unacceptable potential damages. However, especially with respect to the exposure assessment a certain degree of conservatism is introduced: the exposure scenarios "are intended to allow standardized and reproducible evaluation of risks across most sites and land use areas, with conservatism incorporated to ensure protectiveness of potential receptors not directly evaluated, such as special sub-populations and regionally specific land uses" (p. 4-2). Thus, it is the intention of risk assessments to estimate so-called Reasonable Maximum Exposures (RME). The way how conservative elements are dealt with is described below.

United States - Environmental Protection Agency (1998) provides guidance for the assessment of ingestion exposure of

- belowground, aboveground protected and aboveground exposed produce,
- beef and dairy products, pork, chicken and eggs,
- drinking water, and
- (freshwater) fish.

Presently different types of produce (e.g., potatoes, cereals, spinach), pork, poultry, eggs, beef and dairy products, as well as freshwater fish are considered in the analysis. It has been argued above that drinking water is excluded basically due to data availability constraints. As regards fish, only freshwater fish is included albeit most of the fish eaten in Europe stems from sea catches (European Centre for Ecotoxicology and Toxicology of Chemicals, 1994). The disregard of exposure via marine fish is due to the fact that sea fish is caught at very different places which would bring about the necessity to (a) assess the environmental fate of especially long-lived chemicals at the global scale (i.e., modelling the entire oceanic system on Earth) due to marine currents and migrating animals and (b) to include rather detailed trade patterns. Disregarding sea fish consumption leads to a substantial underestimation of impacts caused by those substances whose (effective) human exposure to a rather high degree is influenced by sea fish consumption such as methyl-mercury or dioxins (e.g., French et al., 1998; Buckley-Golder et al., 1999; Anonymous, 2000). On the other hand, tentatively assuming that all fish consumed stems from freshwater bodies may overestimate the potential impacts by 1.5 orders of magnitude (Huijbregts et al., 2000b). For the presently addressed trace elements, no attempt is, therefore, made to consider exposure due to consumption of marine fish.

In contrast to the TGD (European Commission, 2003c), the assessment scheme by United States - Environmental Protection Agency (1998) includes human exposure to pork as well as poultry meat and eggs. In particular exposure to pork is relevant since this is the dominating meat type consumed in Europe (European Centre for Ecotoxicology and Toxicology of Chemicals, 1994). One has to note, however, that the availability of substance-dependent data for the transfer from feed and/or soil into pigs and poultry is rather limited.

7.1.1 Considerations with respect to animal feed and ingested soil

The proper consideration of animal feed is fairly difficult. According to United States - Environmental Protection Agency (1998), cattle are fed forage, silage and grains, swine receive silage and grains, and poultry as well as laying hens only receive grains. However, there is hardly any production data available on forage and silage whereas 'grains' that are mostly bought on the market may vary substantially with respect to its constituents. With the exception of Corn Crop Mix (CCM) that is utilized in pig keeping only in regions where corn is grown, silage and forage are only fed to cattle. It is assumed here that forage and silage are grown and utilized on or at least near the farm to such an extent as to sustain cattle keeping while pigs similar to poultry and laying hens only get fed grains.

Grains are usually administered as mixed fodder consisting for instance of cereals (e.g., wheat and barley), legumes, and oil seeds and groats (such as soy beans). Apart from forage and silage, cereals constitute the largest quantity of the animal feed. For instance, of the 67.8 million tonnes of animal feed used in 2001/2002 in Germany, there were 30 million tonnes of forage and roughage and 25 million tonnes of cereals the remainder being concentrate (Anonym, 2002). In the average mixed fodder, the share of cereals is somewhat lower (42 %) according to Deutscher Verband Tiernahrung (2003).

The most important single components in mixed fodder are wheat and soy beans (Deutscher Verband Tiernahrung, 2003). The amounts of soy beans produced in Europe compared to those imported are small (Food and Agriculture Organization of the United Nations - Statistics Division, 2003) and are, therefore, not further considered. In contrast to the oil seeds and groats, cereals for feeding purposes are exclusively grown in Europe and not imported (104 % self-supply within the EU, Anonym, 2002).[15] The average share of wheat in mixed fodder produced in Germany in 2002/2003 for instance was 19.9 % (Deutscher Verband Tiernahrung, 2003). Total grain consumption of all animals included in the assessment is scaled by this figure to yield the exposure due to uptake of wheat taken as a proxy for the grain exposure.

Accidental swallowing of soil particles by farm animals is another exposure pathway which may contribute to human exposure towards hazardous substances. This exposure pathway depends on the degree to which the animals are kept outdoors (e.g., dioxins taken up by free-foraging hens, Anonymous, 2000). In fact, the consideration of the free-range share of the total amount produced is also necessary for some of the vegetal produces such as vegetables grown in greenhouses (e.g., tomatoes).

For cattle, it is assumed that they are kept in the free-range to a very large extent such that the exposure assessment towards soil particles as suggested by United States - Environmental Protection Agency (1998) is adopted for all cattle kept in Europe, i.e., the share of beef and cow milk produced in the free-range is set to 100 %. In fact, it appears as if the soil particle intake rate is smaller for grazing milk cows than for those that are fed grass silage (Berende (1990) quoted in McLachlan (1997)). Swine and poultry, in contrast, are kept indoors to considerable amounts in Europe. This differs by region and farm animal. For instance, the share of free-range eggs in the early 2000s amounted to 6.7 % (Anonym, 2003), 20 % (Anonymous, 2004) and 25 % (Geßl, 2004) in Germany, South East United Kingdom and Austria, respectively. The amount of pigs kept outdoors in the United Kingdom is estimated to lie between 30 % for suckling pigs, 11 % for weaner pigs and 0.3 % for finishing pigs yielding a weighted average of about 10 % (Edwards, 2004).[16] This share is only 1 % in Germany (Schulz, 2004). Free-range poultry kept on organic farms in Germany which can be taken as a lower bound estimate of the overall poultry kept outdoors was 0.6 % of the total in 2000 (Anonym, 2004). This share is about 20 % in France.[17]

---

[15] Imported cereals are exclusively used for baking goods with high quality needs.

[16] The overall share of pigs kept outdoors in the UK was estimated to lie between 18 and 20 % in 1996 (Anonymous, 1996); this figure, however, most likely includes sows which constitute the largest contribution to pigs kept in the free-range (cf. the Danish situation, Temm, 2004)

The country-specific values as given above are adopted rounding the share for free-range poultry in Germany up to 1.0 % and taking 10 % for the pigs kept outdoors in the UK. For the other countries for which data are missing the default values assumed are 6.7, 1.0 and 1.0 % for free-range eggs, poultry and pigs, respectively. Although the share of free-range pigs is significant in Denmark (Geßl, 2004), the amount of fattened pigs for pork production is small while that of sows may be larger (Temm, 2004). The Danish share of free-range pigs is, therefore, also set to the default value.

7.1.2 Computation of human exposure

The concentration in food is computed according to the equations given in Table 7-2 (refer to section A.7 for more details). For the purposes of this work, the analysis is limited to the exposure pathways given there. This should not be interpreted as implying that transfers from other environmental media through alternate pathways (e.g., dermal absorption or ingestion of other food items) are unimportant. Inhalation exposure is estimated with the help of the EcoSense model (European Commission, 1999a) according to the procedure described in section A.7.2.

Generally, the values recommended by United States - Environmental Protection Agency (1998) are adopted. In case these were stated to be rather conservative, different values are assumed if provided (Table 7-1). Note that also with respect to the environmental fate assessment there are considerable deviations between the present approach and the one by the HHRAP. In particular the soil erosion and leaching to the subsurface soil layer are assumed to be zero according to the HHRAP. All these assumptions will overestimate a substance's concentration in soils. In WATSON, transport to the subsurface of soluble and (if chosen by the user) of particulate-associated substances as well as soil erosion are included for soil compartments (see sections A.3.3, A.3.7, A.3.6 and A.6.4). Due to vertical movement of substances in soils and root uptake also from the deeper parts of the soil, these soil compartments in turn are assumed to have a larger depth than one centimetre (cf. section 5.1) as assumed for untilled soil according to the HHRAP.

When determining the exposure frequency, one may need to take into account people's daily (e.g., between home and work, day care, school ...) or episodic (e.g., going on vacation, weekend trips) movement from locations with higher to lower exposure and vice versa. The difference in exposure levels in turn may depend on the emission scenario to be evaluated. Such differences will be more severe for point or (confined) line sources than for diffuse (multi-source) emissions. The differences will, furthermore, be more pronounced for inhalation

---

[17] Found at http://www.free-rangepoultry.com/ as of May 2005.

Table 7-1: Parameter values adopted in the exposure assessment deviating from those recommended by the United States - Environmental Protection Agency (1998) for ingestion

Parameter	Unit	Value		
		US-EPA		Adopted
Soil ingestion by beef cattle	[kg DW per day]	0.5	(p. 5-48)	0.3
Soil ingestion by dairy cattle	[kg DW per day]	0.4	(p. 5-52)	0.2
Exposure frequency	[days]	350	(p. 6-12)	365
Exposure duration: children	[yr]	6	(p. 6-14)	n/a
Exposure duration: adults	[yr]	30-40	(p. 6-14)	70

and ingestion of locally grown and eaten food than for consumption of traded food items. United States - Environmental Protection Agency (1998) conservatively assumes that exposed people are only two weeks absent from the geographical area for which the exposure is assessed. This is defendable since the HHRAP constitutes a risk assessment framework for point sources and two weeks is the least amount of vacation that an employee gets in the US. Unless there is a net movement of people out of the area with a higher exposure, however, setting the exposure frequency to values lower than 365 days may actually underestimate the overall exposure at the (entire) population level. Many of the pollutants investigated here may be transported over longer distances when only released high enough into the atmosphere. Thus, when evaluating inhalation and ingestion of self grown/caught food due to a single point or confined line source emitting rather close to the ground shortening the exposure frequency at the population level may be valid, especially if the source is located in an unattractive area from a tourist's and/or business traveller's point of view. However, in all other cases this does not seem to be justified.

According to United States - Environmental Protection Agency (1998), exposure duration is defined as "the length of time that a receptor is exposed via a specific exposure pathway" (p. 6-13). The recommended values are shorter than a 70-year lifetime because US Americans on average do not remain in the same area over their entire life and, thus, not (necessarily) in the vicinity of a hazardous waste combustion facility. The necessity to take an exposure duration shorter than a lifetime into account may be due to the assumption that effects show thresholds.

Table 7-2: Exposure pathway formulations for ingestion exposures as used in the exposure assessment

Name	Formulation[a]	Refer to section ... for more details
Food concentrations derived from concentrations assessed for the different compartments by the soil and water fate model		
arable land - aboveground produce	$C\_w/fw = BCF\_dw/dw_{\text{plant/soil}}(p,r,e) \cdot fr\_w_{\text{solid phase/bulk}}(r,e) \cdot C\_w/dw_{\text{ag,solid}}$	A.7.6 (p. 443)
arable land - belowground produce	$C\_w/fw = emp_{\text{BCF, root crops}}(p,r,e) \cdot BCF\_dw/dw_{\text{root/soil}}(p,r,e) \cdot fr\_w_{\text{solid phase/bulk}}(r,e) \cdot C\_w/dw_{\text{ag, solid}}$	A.7.8 (p. 444)
pasture/arable land - silage/ forage - beef/milk cattle	$C\_w/fw = \{ING_{\text{feed}}(r_{\text{animal}},e) \cdot BTF\_t/w_{\text{milk or beef/feed}}(p,r_{\text{animal}},e)\} \cdot BCF\_dw/dw_{\text{plant/soil}}(p,r_{\text{plant}},e) \cdot C\_w/dw_{\text{p\|ag,solid}}$	A.7.9 (p. 445) / A.7.10 (p. 447)
pasture/arable land - grains - beef/milk cattle	$C\_w/fw = fr\_w_{\text{wheat/total grain}}(r_{\text{animal}},e) \cdot \{ING_{\text{feed}}(r_{\text{animal}},e) \cdot BTF\_t/w_{\text{milk or beef/feed}}(p,r_{\text{animal}},e)\} \cdot BCF\_dw/dw_{\text{plant/soil}}(p,r_{\text{plant}},e) \cdot C\_w/dw_{\text{p\|ag,solid}}$	A.7.9 (p. 445) / A.7.10 (p. 447)
pasture (soil particles) - animal products	$C\_w/fw = \{BTF\_t/w_{\text{animal product/feed}}(p,r,e) \cdot ING_{\text{soil}}(r,e)\} \cdot fr\_w_{\text{free-range/total}}(r,n,e) \cdot C\_w/dw_{\text{p, solid}}$	A.7.11 (p. 447)
freshwater - fish	$C\_w/fw = BCF\_V/fw_{\text{fish/water}}(p,r,e) \cdot C\_w/v_{w\text{,aqueous}}$	A.7.12 (p. 448)

Table 7-2: Exposure pathway formulations for ingestion exposures as used in the exposure assessment

Name	Formulation[a]	Refer to section ... for more details
Food concentrations derived from exogenous inputs (i.e., atmospheric depositions)		
atmospheric deposition - aboveground exposed produce	$C\_w/fw = \frac{emp_{\text{plant surface loss}}(r,e) \cdot fr\_w_{\text{intercept/deposition}}(r,e)}{Y\_fw(r,n,e)} \cdot [ATMDEP_{\text{dry}}(s,p,z) + ATMDEP_{\text{wet}}(s,p,z) \cdot fr\_w_{\text{adhere/wet deposition}}(p,r,e)]$	A.7.4 (p. 441)

a. *ATMDEP*: atmospheric deposition [kg/m^2/s]; *BCF_V/fw*: bioconcentration factor [m^3/kg]; *BCF_dw/dw*: bioconcentration factor [-]; *BTF_t/w*: [s*capita/kg FW]; C_w/fw: estimated concentration in food [kg/kg FW]; C_w/dw: concentration in pasture soils 'p' or arable land 'ag' as predicted by the environmental fate model [kg/kg DW] (unit conversion according to the description in section A.7.1 performed); C_w/v: concentration in freshwater compartments '*w*' [kg/m^3] (unit conversion according to the description in section A.7.1 performed); *emp*: empirical factor [-] or [s]; *fr_w*: mass fraction of a substance [-]; *ING*: ingestion rate of feed taken in by an animal [kg DW/capita/s]; *Y_fw*: yield of produce [kg FW/m^2]; symbols in parentheses denote a parameter's dependency on the exposure assessment framework ('*e*'), administrative unit ('*n*'), pollutant ('*p*'), receptor (or crop, '*r*'), emission scenario ('*s*') and/or the zone ('*z*')

As a consequence, true individual exposures need to be known. However, when the effects are assumed not to show a threshold (cf. discussion in section 7.3) and the targeted quantity is the overall effect occurring at the population level, an exposure duration shorter than a lifetime is misleading provided that population mobility does not lead to a factual change in population density. The value of 70 years as used by Crettaz et al. (2002) is adopted here.

As will be presented below (section 7.2), the ingestion rates are formulated as consumption of an average individual of the population, i.e., without distinguishing between for example different age groups. Although consumption habits and amounts as well as body weight will be different between adults and children, there is no effect model available taking into account that effects occurring due to oral exposure to the substances investigated are prevalent for one population sub-group or the other (cf. section 7.3). The choice not to distinguish between different population sub-groups appears to be justified given the presently available effect information.

7.2 Trade of food, consumption and the effective Intake Fraction

In the previous section, it was explained how the food concentrations are processed. This section deals with the question: 'Who eats what and in which amounts leading to human exposure?'.

In particular unlike inhalation, the exposure via food does not exclusively lead to exposure of people living or staying in the contaminated environment. Owing to the efficient development of humankind to societies that are based on division of labour, people in the industrialised world like in Europe rely to a rather large degree, if not exclusively, on the production of the primary sector, i.e., agriculture, and to a lesser degree on homegrown products. Additionally, there is a demand to eat all different kinds of food irrespective of the season although these cannot be grown domestically in all countries throughout the year for example due to cold winters. Furthermore, some of the agricultural produces that are domestically produced have higher prices than those of food items produced abroad. All this results in a situation in which the produce is traded and transported over long distances leading to exposure of people even towards a rather localised source which live far away from the immediately affected environment.

Unless one aims at protecting the most exposed individual and especially when one tries to cover the impacts by a human activity as comprehensively as possible, such rather indirect impacts also need to be considered. In order to assess the exposure via ingestion, one, therefore, not only needs to take into account the environmental concentration of a contaminant and its transfer into plants and/or animals but also the trade of the 'carrier goods' food to the human population.

7.2.1 Consideration of trade

The approach taken in order to consider trade is in contrast to risk assessment frameworks where the conservative 'subsistence farmer exposure' scenario is often used (European Commission, 2003a). This means that food is only consumed close to where it was produced. Allowing for trade is in line with Pennington et al. (2005) who employed a 'production-based' approach where a so-called Intake Fraction (Bennett et al., 2002) assesses the portion of an emission that a population will be finally exposed to. The Intake Fraction is, thus, a good measure to base exposure-response functions on in order to get representative impact estimates (see below).

Due to the geographical scope of the approach presented, the export to regions outside of Europe as well as the import of toxic substances via food products is not addressed. Only the trade within Europe is considered. As an initial attempt, trade is assumed to lead to homogeneous food concentrations across the geographical scope of WATSON according to:

$$C\_w/fw(r, Europe, p, e)_{\text{average}} = \frac{t_{\text{year}} \cdot \sum_n C\_w/fw(r, n, p, e)_{\text{theoretical}} \cdot P(r, n)}{t_{\text{year}} \cdot \sum_n P(r, n)} \qquad (7\text{-}1)$$

where

C_w/fw : C_w/fw_{average}: average concentration of substance p in food item r in the geographical scope of the assessment ('Europe') as a result of considering production data [kg_{chemical} per kg_{food} FW]

$C\_w/fw_{\text{theoretical}}$: concentration of substance p in food item r at the administrative unit n which is theoretical as this concentration may be assessed to occur in an administrative unit in which no respective food item is produced [kg_{chemical} per kg_{food} FW] (according to Table 7-2)

P : production rate of crop r in administrative unit n [kg FW per s] (defined as described in section B.6.1)

t : time for which the production rate is given [s], i.e., corresponding to one year.

It is applied to all produce that is traded (e.g., wheat as food and/or feed, and all animal products considered; see introduction to section A.7). In future developments, a more detailed approach may be realized in which the amount that is eaten nationally is distinguished from that transported across national borders. An aggregation at least at the national level is suggested as food consumption/ supply data are only provided at this level within WATSON (see below and section B.6.2). There may be produces, however, that are not produced in one country but may as well be eaten in the respective country. This is the case for spinach for example. One cannot do without considering trade in such instances one way or the other unless one takes the risk to underestimate the overall exposure. The consideration of trade is, therefore, strongly recommended albeit its initial status of consideration at present.

7.2.2 Assessing human consumption of food

Human consumption data are given as nationally-averaged per capita values. These were taken from the FAO Food Balance Sheets ('food supply', cf. section B.6.2). Due to the fact that food supply data may overestimate the actual food consumption, a correction factor is introduced assuming that 5 % of the retailed food is not eaten for example due to loss and plate waste. No distinction between children and adults is made which seems to be appropriate as long as the effect information does not distinguish between these sub-groups of a population (cf. section 7.3).

The predicted substance concentrations in food are only valid for those food items that are produced within the geographical scope of the model. Therefore, it was checked to what degree the European food production can actually satisfy the demand of the same area. In general, the amounts produced in Europe can at least sustain consumption as regards the food groups considered in the assessment (cf. section B.6.2). Self-supply figures only consider net trade effects. Import of food (and feed) produced outside the geographical area covered by the assessment, however, leads to a 'dilution' of the predicted pollutant concentrations. This is because these imported goods are virtually unexposed due to the spatial limitation of the analysis. Nevertheless, it is assumed that people only take in food items produced within the area modelled if the self-supply at least amounts to 100 %. This is the case for all food groups analysed except spinach which shows a self-supply of only 97 %. Although the case of spinach may be regarded as insignificant, a correction factor is introduced in order for the exposure assessment to be applicable for any type of produce, regardless of the degree of self-supply. This correction factor is equal to those given in Table B-19 ('degree of self-supply') setting values larger than 100 % to unity ('value adopted').

Starting from the food concentrations as computed according to the equations given in Table 7-2, the effective personal intake rate is, thus, computed as:

$$IR\_p(r, n, p, e) = fr\_w_{\text{effective/total}}(p, r, e) \cdot ING_{\text{human supply}}(r, n) \cdot (1 - fr\_w_{\text{not consumed/food supply}}(r, e)) \cdot fr\_w_{\text{self-supply}}(r, e) \cdot C\_w/fw(r, n, p, e) \tag{7-2}$$

where

C_w/fw : concentration of substance p in food item r at the administrative unit n [$kg_{chemical}$ per kg_{food} FW] (according to Table 7-2, may consider trade of food)

fr_w : $fr\_w_{effective/total}$: mass fraction of substance p contained in food r leading to an effect [kg per kg] (defined in Table C-2)

$fr\_w_{self\text{-}supply}$: mass fraction of produce r produced in the geographical scope of the assessment [kg per kg] (defined in section B.6.2)

$fr\_w_{not\ consumed/food\ supply}$: mass fraction of (fresh) food that is produced and traded but not consumed [kg per kg] (defined in section B.6.2)

ING : ingestion of food item r by humans according to food supply information for the administrative unit n [kg FW/capita/s]

IR_p : effective personal intake rate of substance p contained in food item r by humans at the administrative unit n [kg/capita/s].

Note that the meaning of 'effective' is introduced in the following.

7.2.3 The effective Intake Fraction

As mentioned above, the overall exposure of a population is assessed by means of the population-based source-to-intake measure *Intake Fraction* (Bennett et al., 2002), sometimes also referred to as exposure efficiency (Evans et al., 2002). It is the fraction of a substance's mass released into the environment that is ultimately taken in by the human population as a result of food consumption, inhalation and dermal exposure. In case of ingestion, this implies that it aggregates the exposure towards different produces which may become contaminated due to different causes (e.g., ingestion of soil particles, forage, silage and grains by milk cattle; cf. section A.7). Each such cause-exposure chain starting at the result of the environmental fate model is termed *exposure pathway* here.

For the purpose of the present analysis, the Intake Fraction due to ingestion exposures is calculated as:

$$IF_{\text{ingestion}} = \frac{\sum_n \sum_r \sum_i IR\_p_{n,r,i} \cdot Population_n}{S} \tag{7-3}$$

where:

IF : (effective) Intake Fraction of a substance for ingestion [$kg_{\text{effective exposure}}$ per kg_{released}]

IR_p : (effective) personal Intake Rate of the respective exposure pathway i related to produce/food r at administrative unit n [kg/capita/s]; see section A.7.14 for its computation

Population : population in administrative unit n [capita]

S : source strength of a substance [kg per s].

Note that in a spatially differentiated environmental fate and exposure model the concentration as well as the source strength need to be aggregated for the geographical scope of interest. The Intake Fraction for inhalation is computed similarly (cf. section A.7.2).

The term 'ultimately' in the definition of the Intake Fraction given above implies that it is usually defined for a steady-state situation. If dynamic calculations are performed in which the mass taken in as well as the amount emitted may accumulate over time t (in full years) the mathematical definition of the Intake Fraction needs to be adapted accordingly:

$$IF_{\text{ingestion},\,t} = \frac{\sum_n \sum_r \sum_i \sum_t IR\_p_{n,r,i,t} \cdot Population_n}{\sum_t S_t}. \tag{7-4}$$

When performing the (human) impact assessment, it is of importance whether the chemical forms in the edible portions of the food items are available to humans (Markert, 1998; Welch and Norvell, 1999) and that these available forms have the potential to cause an adverse effect on a receptor. Examples are inorganic versus organic arsenic (Agency for Toxic Substances and Disease Registry, 2000b), mercury compounds (Boening, 2000) and chromium VI versus chromium III (Agency for Toxic Substances and Disease Registry, 2000a). It may even occur that the route of exposure by which most of a substance reaches a human being is not the most important one when it comes to assessing the actual impact of this substance. This could be demonstrated for marine fish and shellfish whose consumption leads to the highest exposure but not to the highest risk in the case of arsenic (Seiwert et al., 1999; Baxter and Lewis, 2002). Gebel (1999) states that arsenic taken in via ingestion of marine fish and shellfish is generally excreted indicating that this exposure pathway towards arsenic may even be irrelevant in terms of adverse effects.

The concept of the Intake Fraction is, therefore, extended here to only cover that portion of a substance to which exposure occurs which may lead to an adverse effect, termed the *effective Intake Fraction*.

In order to arrive at the effective Intake Fraction, one needs to assess the portion of the overall mass of a substance taken in that may become effective. This would at best be done by distinguishing the different chemical species in the environmental fate model. However, due to the geographical coverage and the spatial resolution aimed for (cf. section 2.3), this procedure is not feasible especially for data availability reasons. Instead, a static value is introduced in the exposure assessment. Note that the 'Personal Intake Rate' in Eq. (7-3) already is given for the effective chemical form of the substance.

According to a report issued by the British Food Standards Agency (Baxter and Lewis, 2002), inorganic arsenic usually constitutes at most 3 % of the overall occurring arsenic in the food groups investigated which is consistent with previous results on sea fish (Muñoz et al., 1999). Due to detection limit constraints, a distinction into food groups with respect to the effective fraction is deemed inappropriate. As an upper bound estimate of the potential damages caused by inorganic arsenic the fraction of 3 % is retained for all types of food products. The data situation is even worse for the other candidate for which a distinction between total and effective food contents needs to be made, chromium (Anonymous, 2002). Hexavalent chromium tends to be a strong oxidizing agent (Gauglhofer and Bianchi, 1991) which is also used in environmental chemistry in the form of potassium dichromate in order to determine the Chemical Oxygen Demand (COD) of sewage effluents (Bliefert, 1997). Because of its strongly oxidizing nature, it, thus, is readily reduced in the environment to its trivalent form with the exception of sea water (Gauglhofer and Bianchi, 1991; Agency for Toxic Substances and Disease Registry, 2000a). Furthermore, hexavalent chromium ions are assumed to be mostly reduced in human bodily fluids (Irwin et al., 1998; Anonymous, 2002) additionally decreasing the effective portion of the amount taken in. In a recent report by the Environment Agency of the United Kingdom (Anonymous, 2002), it was suggested to assume a (conservative) value of 10 % for the hexavalent state of the total chromium content in food products. This value is adopted here, again as an upper bound estimate.

Unlike the primary proposal, the (effective) Intake Fraction may also be given for sub-populations of the geographical scope of the model (like populations of different countries) and/or integrated only over a certain time period rather than over infinity. Heijungs (1995) has shown that the steady-state solution of a multimedia model can under certain conditions help to assess the time-integrated exposure to pulse emissions which does not require dynamic computations. The prerequisites are: the model must be linear, the matrix must be non-singular and the system should converge to a steady-state when integrating over infinity. Although all these prerequisites are fulfilled by the modelling approach adopted (cf. section A.1) and the processes considered, the convergence criterion is critical because the integrating time for non-degradable substances might be rather long, i.e., in the order of centuries and longer. The effective Intake Fraction of trace elements is, therefore, also computed for the dynamic case in order to get an idea of the time scales involved for the development to steady-state (see also footnote f of Table 2-3).

7.3 Impact assessment

In order to assess the impacts from exposures to substances, it is generally preferable to use dose- or exposure-response relationships in order to estimate effects that can be derived based on observations on human populations. Combining these effects with an appropriate measure of severity then yields impacts (see below). As experiments at least with human beings are not ethically defendable, the best information available is provided by epidemiological investigations. Epidemiologically derived exposure-response functions are widely used in the context of human health assessments due to inhalation for policy decision purposes (e.g., European Commission, 1999a; Friedrich and Bickel, 2001a).

In contrast to inhalation, however, the available information for exposure-response functions due to food ingestion is scarce (Searl, 2002; Agency for Toxic Substances and Disease Registry, 2003; United States - Environmental Protection Agency, 2005). Most effect information is given as thresholds like No Observed Adverse Effect Levels (NOAEL) or Lowest Observed Adverse Effect Levels (LOAEL). Such measures bring about two main problems in the context of pan-European external cost assessments:

1. during marginal external cost assessments, a threshold-based effect measure 'punishes' the human activity that emits the final amount of a substance causing the threshold to be exceeded by holding it responsible for all effects to occur. However, there were usually other human activities as well that used up the 'assimilative capacity of the environment' (Pearce and Turner, 1990) or from an exposure perspective the human population's ability to accommodate emissions, i.e., the 'erosion of the available Margin Of Exposure' (MOE, Crettaz et al., 2002). Comparative analyses are, thus, hampered.

2. in order to decide whether a threshold exceedance is likely to occur, true environmental concentrations need to be estimated. Due to limited resources and imperfect information for instance on all emissions and processes influencing the environmental fate of a substance, a modelling exercise at the regional scale needs to fail to predict true environmental concentrations if it does not succeed by accident.

It is consequently necessary to look for alternatives.

7.3.1 Approach by Crettaz and co-workers

Recently, an approach has been proposed to also convert threshold effect information into linear so-called β_{ED10} *slope factors* for cancer (Crettaz et al., 2002) and non-cancer effects (Pennington et al., 2002) based on Crettaz (2000). Drawing on the benchmark dose BMD_{10} concept (Crump, 1995) that is discussed within the US-EPA (e.g., United States - Environmental Protection Agency, 1995), the effective dose ED_{10h} is the maximum likelihood (rather than the 95 % lower confidence limit for the BMD_{10}) estimate of the dose corresponding to 10 % response of humans over background.[18] It is derived by fitting a steady model through a discrete set of measured dose-response data employing a so-called linear multistage model. The ED_{10h} is taken as the point of departure in order to extrapolate to lower doses. It is assumed that the dose-response curve is linear and crosses at the origin for substances not showing thresholds in their effects. The slope factor β_{ED10} is, thus, computed as (Crettaz et al., 2002):

---

[18] Note that Crettaz et al. (2002) use a variable with the acronym q1* when directly deriving the β_{ED10} *slope factor* from linear exposure-response information. When applying Eq. (7-12), Crettaz (2000) makes use of different kinds of linear exposure-response models, i.e., *slope factors* or *unit (lifetime) risks* in US-EPA (United States - Environmental Protection Agency, 1996b) or WHO terminology (World Health Organisation, 2000b), respectively. Both measures relate a risk or the probability of an individual to develop a disease (especially cancer) due to a lifetime exposure to a substance. The 'unit' in the WHO's name hints at the risk that a continuous exposure to one microgram per litre in water or one microgram per cubic metre in air poses. These units indicate that they need to be adjusted to match the US-EPA's slope factor (cf. Table 7-4). - The q_1* is estimated as follows: In order to fit a dose-response curve through a set of bioassay data, the US-EPA suggests the use of the linearised multistage model (LMS) which allows for non-linearities at high doses but forces a linear component at low doses. The respective linear low-dose slope is termed *slope factor* (United States - Environmental Protection Agency, 1996b) and denoted by q_1, the corresponding 95 % upper bound confidence limit by q_1*. The latter, thus, introduces an element of conservatism which the β_{ED10} *slope factor* approach intends to overcome. For more information, refer to Crettaz et al. (2002) and the literature cited therein.

$$\beta_{\mathrm{ED10}}(p) = \frac{0.1}{ED_{10\mathrm{h}}(p)} \tag{7-5}$$

where

β_{ED10} : slope factor for substance *p* based on effective dose affecting 10 % of a population over background [individual lifetime risk per mg/kg Body Weight/day]

$\mathrm{ED}_{10\mathrm{h}}$: maximum likelihood estimate of the effect dose of substance *p* inducing an added response of 10 % over background incidence for humans [mg/kg Body Weight/day]

0.1 : human response level corresponding to the dose $\mathrm{ED}_{10\mathrm{h}}$ [-].

The slope factor, thus, represents a measure for the population-averaged excess individual risk of an effect per unit daily dose for a lifetime exposure (70 years for humans). The linearisation is based on a non-threshold assumption. In contrast to non-carcinogenic effects (Pennington et al., 2002), it is generally well accepted that there is no threshold for genotoxically acting carcinogens even at the individual level (International Programme on Chemical Safety, 1999; World Health Organisation, 2000b; Tennant, 2001). On the other hand, the linearisation is considered justified irrespective of the type of effect due to the growing recognition that 'no evidence' does not necessarily mean 'no effect' and that bioassays cannot give real insights on linearity or non-linearity at low doses, which only depend on the extrapolation model adopted. While toxicologists argue that mechanistic threshold concentrations or doses may exist for human health effects for many (non-genotoxically carcinogenic) substances, usually it has not been possible to establish the existence of mechanistic thresholds in epidemiological studies (e.g., European Commission, 1999a). Populations consist of individuals that show different susceptibilities or sensitivities to develop the investigated diseases even at low ambient levels (Hurley and Miller, 2001). Additionally, it may be argued not to assume thresholds from a precautionary principle perspective which is adopted by the European Council (European Commission, 2000a). However, care must be taken not to bias the assessment through rather conservative approaches.

The ED_{10h} from which the β_{ED10} *slope factor* is derived according to Eq. (7-5) can be estimated from different threshold effect measures (Crettaz, 2000; Crettaz et al., 2002; Pennington et al., 2002). The estimation schemes employed in this study are given in Table 7-3. It must be emphasized that the derivation particularly of the LOAEL and NOAEL strongly depends on the experimental design. As a result, also the ED_{10} and, thus, the β_{ED10} are more uncertain when these are derived based on threshold effect data. It is, therefore, strongly suggested to derive the β_{ED10} from *slope factors* or *unit (lifetime) risks* in US-EPA (United States - Environmental Protection Agency, 1996b) or WHO terminology (World Health Organisation, 2000b), respectively, if sufficient data from laboratory bioassays are available. The respective equations are given in Table 7-4 which distinguishes between inhalation and ingestion exposures.

Before addressing the issue how health effects shall be quantified, a note on the consideration of mixtures in the present study shall be made. Effect assessments of mixtures still constitute a rather open field of research (e.g., Steinberg et al. 6/1995; Escher and Hermens, 2002). Therefore, the potential for more than additive or antagonistic interactions of different substances (Mücke 6/1995; Kroes, 1996) is at present not taken into account during the effect assessment of this study. As a result, the different contaminants are assumed to exert their effects in a non-interactive and additive way for example by simple similar or simple dissimilar action (Kroes, 1996).

Because 'effects' in general may lead to consequences with different severities like acute death or some short-lived skin irritation, it is necessary from a valuation perspective to distinguish between such diverse effects. In case of fatal diseases, the concept of Years of Life Lost (YOLL) is recommended in different contexts (Murray, 1994; European Commission, 1999a; Krewitt et al., 2002). The YOLL indicator measures the reduction in life expectancy resulting from an increased level of exposure to pollutants in the environment. In order to also account for effects related to morbidity, Crettaz et al. (2002) and Pennington et al. (2002) make use of the Disability Adjusted Life Years (DALY) concept (according to Murray and Lopez, 1996a, 1996b cited therein). It comprises the effects measured by the YOLL indicator and adds the measure Years of Life lived with a Disability (YLD). Although the approach has some disadvantages related to the derivation of the YLD and when applied to non-cancer effects (see below), it is deemed a step towards a more differentiated assessment of cancers for whose valuation only one generic monetary value for any type of cancer is used according to the latest ExternE methodology (European Commission, 2004).

The β_{ED10} *slope factor* is combined with the DALY concept in order to yield the *effect factor* according to the terminology of Life Cycle Impact Assessment (LCIA). As the slope factor gives the increase in risk for one 'standard' individual if he/she is continuously (i.e., daily) exposed to a given dose, one needs to divide this cumulative dose by the individual's lifetime in order to allow for analyses of an exposure situation that lasts potentially shorter than a lifetime (Hurley and Miller, 2001). This way, it is implicitly assumed that the increase in risk depends linearly on the mass of a substance taken in regardless of when and for how long the exposure takes place. In order to express the effect factor on a personal level, one needs to divide additionally by the 'standard' body weight.

Table 7-3: Estimation of ED_{10} from threshold effect measures

Threshold effect measure	Remarks	Equation[a]	
BMD_{10}	Equation 4 in Pennington et al. (2002) solved for ED_{10h}	$ED_{10h} = \frac{BMD_{10}}{0.54}$	(7-6)
BMC_{10}	Equation 4 in Pennington et al. (2002) solved for ED_{10h} and adapted to inhalation exposures	$ED_{10h} = \frac{BMD_{10}}{0.54} = \frac{INH}{BW} \cdot \frac{BMC_{10}}{0.54}$	(7-7)
LOAEL	Equation 8 in Pennington et al. (2002)	$ED_{10h} = \frac{0.3 \cdot LOAEL_{\text{animal, subchronic}}}{emp_{\text{animal} \to \text{human}} \cdot emp_{\text{subchronic} \to \text{chronic}}}$	(7-8)
NOAEL	Equation 7 in Pennington et al. (2002)	$ED_{10h} = \frac{1.6 \cdot NOAEL_{\text{animal, subchronic}}}{emp_{\text{animal} \to \text{human}} \cdot emp_{\text{subchronic} \to \text{chronic}}}$	(7-9)
TD_{50} from rats	Equation 8 in Crettaz et al. (2002) updated by Keller (2005) for application to rat bioassays	$ED_{10h} = \frac{TD_{50,\text{ rats}}}{18}$	(7-10)
TD_{50} from mice	Equation 8 in Crettaz et al. (2002) updated by Keller (2005) for application to mouse bioassays	$ED_{10h} = \frac{TD_{50,\text{ mice}}}{39}$	(7-11)

a. BMC_{10}: benchmark (air) concentration [mg/m^3]; BMD_{10}: benchmark dose [mg/kg Body Weight/day]; *BW*: body weight [kg per person], here: 70; ED_{10h}: maximum likelihood estimate of the effect dose of a substance inducing an added response of 10 % over background incidence for humans [mg/kg Body Weight/day]; *emp*: extrapolation coefficients from animal to human (if applicable: 1.6 for dogs, 6 for rats, 13 for mice, otherwise 1) and from subchronic to chronic exposures (if applicable: 3.3, otherwise 1) [-] (cf. Pennington et al. (2002)); *INH*: inhalation rate [m^3 per capita and s], here: 20 m^3 per capita and day (cf. section A.7.2); *LOAEL*: Lowest Observed Adverse Effect Level [mg/kg Body Weight/day]; *NOAEL*: No Observed Adverse Effect Level [mg/kg Body Weight/day]; TD_{50}: median Tumor Dose [mg/kg Body Weight/day]; *0.3*, *1.6*, *18*, *39*: linear regression coefficients [-]

Table 7-4: Estimation of the β_{ED10} slope factor based on linear exposure-response information (cf. footnote 18)

Route of exposure	Remarks	Equation[a]	
Ingestion, food	Equation 5 in Crettaz et al. (2002), $r^2 = 0.95$	$\beta_{ED10} = 0.5 \cdot ERF\_dose$	(7-12)
Ingestion, water	Conversion of water concentrations into dose based on average drinking rate and body weight; note that Eq. (7-15) partly reverses the conversion from *ERF_conc* into *ERF_dose*	$\beta_{ED10} = 0.5 \cdot ERF\_dose = 0.5 \cdot \frac{BW}{ING_{water}} \cdot ERF\_conc_{water}$	(7-13)
Inhalation	Conversion of air concentrations into dose based on average inhalation rate and body weight; note that Eq. (7-15) partly reverses the conversion from *ERF_conc* into *ERF_dose*	$\beta_{ED10} = 0.5 \cdot ERF\_dose = 0.5 \cdot \frac{BW}{INH} \cdot ERF\_conc_{air}$	(7-14)

a. β_{ED10}: slope factor for a substance based on effective dose affecting 10 % of a population over background [individual lifetime risk per mg/kg Body Weight/day]; *BW*: body weight [kg per person], here: 70; *ERF_conc*: linear exposure-response information for inhalation [individual lifetime risk per mg/m^3] or ingestion of water [individual lifetime risk per mg/l], usually given as *unit (lifetime) risk*; *ERF_dose*: linear exposure-response information particularly for ingestion of food [individual lifetime risk per mg/kg BW/day]; ING_{water}: drinking rate [l/day], here: 2 as for adults (United States - Environmental Protection Agency, 1997c); *INH*: inhalation rate [m^3 per capita and s], here: 20 m^3 per capita and day (cf. section A.7.2); *0.5*: linear regression coefficient [-]

Since this effect factor is usually given for the steady-state situation, the β_{ED10} slope factor needs to be adapted to allow for an exposure situation which involves an average person over his/her entire life. The effect factor is calculated as (Crettaz et al., 2002; Pennington et al., 2002):

$$EF(p) = \frac{\beta_{\mathrm{ED10}}(p)}{BW \cdot t_{\mathrm{lifetime}} \cdot 365} \cdot DALY_{\mathrm{personal}} \tag{7-15}$$

where

EF	:	effect factor of substance p [yr lost per mg intake]
β_{ED10}	:	slope factor for substance p based on effective dose affecting 10 % of a population over background [individual lifetime risk per mg/kg BW/day]
BW	:	body weight [kg per person]; here: 70
t	:	human lifetime (or 'exposure duration', cf. Table 7-1) [yr]; here: 70
365	:	conversion factor [days per yr]
DALY	:	Disability Adjusted Life Years per affected person [yr lost per incidence].

In the ExternE methodology, morbidity and mortality impacts are regularly treated separately rather than being combined in a single measure like DALYs. This is basically due to the fact that the different health states are valued differently in monetary terms. When adopting the concept of the β_{ED10} *slope factor* as a linear dose-response function and differentiating the aggregated DALY value into a mortality component (YOLL) and a morbidity component (YLD), Eq. (7-15) serves to assess human health impacts according to the following equations:

$$YOLL_{\mathrm{population}}(s,p) = S_{\mathrm{total}}(s,p) \cdot t_{\mathrm{emission\ duration}} \cdot IF(s,p) \cdot \frac{\beta_{\mathrm{ED10}}(p)}{BW \cdot t_{\mathrm{lifetime}} \cdot 365} \cdot 1000^2 \cdot YOLL_{\mathrm{personal}} \tag{7-16}$$

$$YLD_{\mathrm{population}}(s,p) = S_{\mathrm{total}}(s,p) \cdot t_{\mathrm{emission\ duration}} \cdot IF(s,p) \cdot \frac{\beta_{\mathrm{ED10}}(p)}{BW \cdot t_{\mathrm{lifetime}} \cdot 365} \cdot 1000^2 \cdot YLD_{\mathrm{personal}} \tag{7-17}$$

where

1000^2	:	conversion factor [mg per kg]
365	:	conversion factor [days per yr]
β_{ED10}	:	slope factor for substance *p* based on effective dose affecting 10 % of a population over background [individual lifetime risk of incidence per mg/kg BW/day]; defined in Tables 7-6 and 7-7
BW	:	body weight [kg per person]; here: 70
IF	:	effective Intake Fraction of substance *p* of emission scenario *s* [$kg_{effective\ exposure}$ per $kg_{released}$]; computed according to Eq. (7-3)
S	:	source strength of substance *p* for emission scenario *s* [kg per yr]
t	:	$t_{emission\ duration}$: emission duration [yr] $t_{lifetime}$: human lifetime (or 'exposure duration', cf. Table 7-1) [yr]; here: 70
YLD	:	$YLD_{population}$: overall Years of Life lived with a Disability for emission scenario *s* of substance *p* [yr lost] $YLD_{personal}$: personal Years of Life lived with a Disability due to a disease related to the slope factor β_{ED10} [yr lost per person and incidence]; defined in Tables 7-6 and 7-7
YOLL	:	$YOLL_{population}$: overall Years of Life Lost for emission scenario *s* of substance *p* [yr lost] $YOLL_{personal}$: personal Years of Life Lost due to a disease related to the slope factor β_{ED10} [yr lost per person and incidence]; defined in Tables 7-6 and 7-7.

Note that the impact per kilogram of substance released is computed by neglecting the source strength and the emission duration.

7.3.2 Dynamically computing the impact

It has been mentioned above that the Intake Fraction may not only be calculated for steady-state situations but also dynamically. When analysing an emission scenario dynamically, the amount of a substance released into the environment and also the amount taken in by the human population may vary over time. As a result,

Eqs. (7-16) and (7-17) need to be adjusted in order to allow for dynamic analyses of pulse and no-pulse emission scenarios.

The adaptation depends on the time step t_{step} chosen for the analysis and also the investigated integration time. Due to the temporal resolution especially of the employed environmental data which are given as long-term averages (section 2.3.2), only time steps may be investigated that are given in full years. Note that the time step should match the investigated substances' dynamics in terms of exposure, i.e., at least not longer than a substance's residence time in the exposure media. Further note that this may also imply that different time steps be used for ingestion and inhalation-based impact assessments. This will especially be the case for pulse emission scenarios of substances with a residence time in air of one year maximally.

Thus, when analysing the temporal development of (human) exposure towards a continuous or pulse emission of $t_{emission\ duration}$ time until the end of the investigated time horizon (n iterations times t_{step}), Eqs. (7-16) and (7-17) are reformulated according to Eqs. (7-18) and (7-19) using Eq. (7-4) in order to compute the effective Intake Fraction.

$$YOLL_{\text{population},\, i \cdot t_{\text{step}}} = \sum_{i=1}^{n} [S_{\text{total}} \cdot \min\{t_{\text{emission duration}}, i \cdot t_{\text{step}}\} \cdot (IF_{i \cdot t_{\text{step}}} - IF_{(i-1) \cdot t_{\text{step}}})] \cdot \frac{\beta_{\text{ED10}}(p)}{BW \cdot t_{\text{lifetime}} \cdot 365} \cdot 1000^2 \cdot YOLL_{\text{personal}} \tag{7-18}$$

$$YLD_{\text{population},\, i \cdot t_{\text{step}}} = \sum_{i=1}^{n} [S_{\text{total}} \cdot \min\{t_{\text{emission duration}}, i \cdot t_{\text{step}}\} \cdot (IF_{i \cdot t_{\text{step}}} - IF_{(i-1) \cdot t_{\text{step}}})] \cdot \frac{\beta_{\text{ED10}}(p)}{BW \cdot t_{\text{lifetime}} \cdot 365} \cdot 1000^2 \cdot YLD_{\text{personal}} \tag{7-19}$$

7.3.3 Distinction of severity for cancer effects

The magnitude of the personal YOLLs and YLDs depends on the severity of the disease or damage related to the slope factor. For cancers, Crettaz and co-workers (Crettaz, 2000; Crettaz et al., 2002) provide statistics on the values for the YLD and YOLL indicators per specific cancer types. The list does not contain all types of cancer which is why a $DALY_{personal}$ is also given for an average cancer case by weighting each $DALY_{personal}$ according to the prevalence of the associated cancer. The average cancer $DALY_{personal}$ is 6.7 years per person/incidence (Crettaz et al., 2002). Although the authors state that they "do not apply specific weightings to the importance of one year of life lost based on the age at which death occurs and do not discount future damages compared to the present ones" (p. 942), Keller (2005) recently found out that the personal YOLLs had in fact been provided considering these value judgements. While the personal YLDs are maintained, the personal YOLLs increase by about a factor of two towards the ones provided by Crettaz et al. (2002). The $DALY_{personal}$ value consequently increases to 12.8 years per person/incidence. When exploring the contribution of the YLD to the $DALY_{personal}$ using the data given by Keller (2005) for carcinogens, it is found that the YOLL indicator's contribution to the DALY is larger than 85 % for all types of cancer and equal or more than 95 % for more than two thirds of the cancer types. This shows that the Years of Life lived with a Disability (YLDs) are almost negligible for cancers.[19] The YOLLs and YLDs will, however, not be treated separately in the present study, i.e., the same monetary value will be used (cf. section 8.2). This is because the YLD is a measure that is supposed to be commensurate to a life year lost due to morbidity effects (Murray, 1994).

7.3.4 Distinction of severity for non-cancer effects

In order to distinguish the severity of the non-cancer effects, use will be made of a proposal by an expert panel at the International Life Science Institute (ILSI) to subdivide toxicological impacts into several subcategories (Burke et al., 1996 quoted in Owens, 2001 and Pennington et al., 2002). Three categories have been distinguished taking into account reversibility and life-shortening potentials of the respective impacts (Table 7-5). Other than for inhalation-related effects (Hofstetter, 1998; Hurley and Miller, 2001), quantitative measures such as DALYs are currently not readily available for non-cancer effects. In line with Pennington et al. (2002), the simplified classification in Table 7-5 is modified to be compatible with the DALY approach by assuming as a preliminary basis a $DALY_{personal}$ of

[19] In order to distinguish morbidity from mortality effects for unspecified, average cancers, one may choose that 97.3 % of the $DALY_{personal}$ corresponding to the median value provided by Keller (2005) are attributed to YOLLs leaving 2.7 % to YLDs, i.e., 12.5 and 0.3 years per person/incidence, respectively. The average weight for the unspecified average cancer YLD is stated to be 0.809 (Crettaz et al., 2002). This means that when assuming the generic YLD of 0.3 years per person/incidence the time duration during which the corresponding impaired health status prevails is 0.3 / 0.809 = 0.42 years. However, the value of 0.809 appears rather large when compared to the otherwise explicitly stated disability weights in Crettaz et al. (2002).

12.8 years per person/incidence for category 1. This initial value is based on the average for cancer effects (see above) given that these effects are included in this category. The ILSI panel subjectively scaled the differences between the three categories by factors of 10 (reflected in the weights in Table 7-5). Consequently, the non-cancer effects of category 2 and 3 are attributed $DALY_{personal}$ values of 1.28 and 0.128 years per person/incidence, respectively. Given the rather undefined quality of the non-cancer health endpoints, no distinction into YOLLs and YLDs is made despite the same apportionment as for the general cancer case would be straightforward.

7.3.5 β_{ED10} slope factors and physical impacts used in this study

Tables 7-6 and 7-7 summarize the slope factors either taken from Crettaz (2000) or derived according to the equations reproduced in Tables 7-3 and 7-4 for the selected trace elements as well as the $YOLL_{personal}$ and $YLD_{personal}$ values for cancer and the $DALY_{personal}$ values for non-cancer effects (Keller, 2005) employed in this study. Note that both the slope factors and the health quality measures are given per incidence.[20]

7.3.6 Value choices and DALYs

Furthermore, it needs to be noted that the DALY concept in general builds on some inherent value choices made. According to the Impact Pathway Approach, such value choices should be kept out of the determination of the physical impact to the extent possible and should instead only be applied during the valuation step. When deriving DALYs one of whose purposes it is to inform resource allocation decisions (Nord, 2002), value choices made are (Murray, 1994):

- the way how morbidity effects are converted into YOLL-equivalents,
- the assumed life expectancy which complies to the highest occurring on earth, i.e., that in Japan; the duration of time lost due to a death at each age is determined according to this life expectancy of 82.5 and 80 years for females and males, respectively,
- valuing the time lived at different ages differently according to the societal/social perception which leads to the introduction of an age-weighting function, and
- the employed discount rate of 3 %.

---

[20] Incidences should not be confounded with prevalences. These are different measures of a disease's occurrence. The *prevalence* of a condition means the number of people who currently have the condition, whereas *incidence* refers to the annual number of people who have a new case of the condition.

Table 7-5: International Life Sciences Institute classification scheme for human health impact categories (Burke et al., 1996 taken from Owens, 2001 and Pennington et al., 2002)

Criteria	Category 1 Irreversible / Life-shortening effects	Category 2 Probably irreversible / Life-shortening effects	Category 3 Reversible / Non life-shortening effects
Examples	• Cancer • Reproductive effects • Teratogenic effects (birth defects) • Acute fatal or acute severe and irreversible effects (e.g., fatal poisoning) • Mutagenicity	• Immunotoxicity • Neurotoxicity[a] • Nephrotoxicity (kidney damage) • Hepatotoxicity (liver damage) • Pulmonary toxicity (lung damage) • Cardiotoxicity (heart damage)	• Irritation (eye, skin, mucosal; that is transient) • Sensitisation (allergy) • Reversible acute organ or system effects (gastrointestinal inflammation)
Weight	1	0.1	0.01
$DALY_{personal}$	12.8	$12.8 \cdot 0.1 = 1.28$	$12.8 \cdot 0.01 = 0.128$
$YOLL_{personal}$	12.5	1.25	0.125
$YLD_{personal}$	0.3	0.03	0.003

a. Neurotoxicity may also be ranked in category 1.

First, in order to convert the time lived with a disability into years of life lost, principally different approaches can be followed (e.g., Murray, 1994, see also below). Presently, the weighting factors are yielded by employing the so-called *person trade-off* (PTO) method (Murray and Lopez, 1996a cited in Müller-Wenk and Hofstetter, 2003 and Essink-Bot, 1998). Two variants had been used in order to promote explicit deliberation within and among the subjects by framing the same question from two different viewpoints. Essink-Bot (1998) explains it in the following way: "In the first, PTO1, a respondent is asked to decide for how many N (N > 1000 persons) in health state X he would be willing to trade one year of life extension of 1000 healthy individuals for the extension of life by one year for the group in the health state X. In the second variant (PTO2), the respondent

Table 7-6: Cancer effect-related β_{ED10} slope factors and physical impacts for mortality (YOLL) and morbidity (YLD) due to inhalation and ingestion exposure of selected trace elements

Trace element	Exposure route	β_{ED10} [risk of incidence per (mg/kg BW and day)]	$YOLL_{personal}$ [years lost-equivalents per person and incidence]	$YLD_{personal}$ [a] [years lost-equivalents per person and incidence]		Remarks
Arsenic, inorganic	ingestion	0.75	6.09	$0.045 \cdot 4.2 =$	0.19	β_{ED10}: oral slope factor for skin cancer of 1.5 [risk per mg/kg-day] (United States - Environmental Protection Agency, 2005), converted according to Eq. (7-12); impact: melanoma (Keller, 2005)
	inhalation	7.5	15.95	$0.146 \cdot 1.8 =$	0.26	β_{ED10}: unit risk for lung cancer of 4.3 [risk per mg/m^3] (United States - Environmental Protection Agency, 2005), converted according to Eq. (7-14); impact: lung cancer (Keller, 2005)
Cadmium [b]	inhalation	3.2	15.95	$0.146 \cdot 1.8 =$	0.26	β_{ED10}: unit risk for lung cancer of 1.8 [risk per mg/m^3] (United States - Environmental Protection Agency, 2005), converted according to Eq. (7-14); impact: lung cancer (Keller, 2005)

Table 7-6: Cancer effect-related β_{ED10} slope factors and physical impacts for mortality (YOLL) and morbidity (YLD) due to inhalation and ingestion exposure of selected trace elements

Trace element	Exposure route	β_{ED10} [risk of incidence per (mg/kg BW and day)]	$YOLL_{personal}$ [years lost-equivalents per person and incidence]	$YLD_{personal}$[a] [years lost-equivalents per person and incidence]	Remarks
Chromium, hexavalent [b]	inhalation	21	15.95	$0.146 \cdot 1.8 = 0.26$	β_{ED10}: unit risk for lung cancer of 12 [risk per mg/m^3] (United States - Environmental Protection Agency, 2005), converted according to Eq. (7-14); impact: lung cancer (Keller, 2005)
Lead [c]	ingestion	0.039	12.5 [d]	0.3 [d]	β_{ED10}: oral median tumor dose of 46.6 [mg/kg Body Weight/day] for kidney cancer derived by administration of lead acetate to rats (Gold and Zeiger, 1997 cited in Crettaz, 2000, p. 61), converted according to Eqs. (7-5) and (7-10); impact: average cancer (Keller, 2005)

a. The YLD is yielded by multiplying a disability weight by the duration of the respective disability.
b. No cancer effect information via ingestion available.
c. No cancer effect information via inhalation available.
d. See footnote 19 for the derivation.

Table 7-7: Non-cancer effect-related β_{ED10} slope factors and aggregated physical impacts for mortality and morbidity in terms of DALYs due to inhalation and ingestion exposure of selected trace elements

Trace element	Exposure route	β_{ED10} [risk of incidence per (mg/kg BW and day)]	$DALY_{personal}$[a] [years lost-equivalents per person and incidence]		Remarks
Arsenic, inorganic	ingestion	78	$12.8 \cdot 0.1 =$	1.28	β_{ED10}: oral chronic NOAEL of 0.0008 [mg/kg BW/day] for a human population (United States - Environmental Protection Agency, 2005), converted according to Eqs. (7-9) and (7-10), extrapolation coefficients set to 1; impact: skin lesions (category 2 effect)
Cadmium	ingestion	41.5	$12.8 \cdot 0.1 =$	1.28	β_{ED10}: oral chronic BMD_{10} of 0.0013 [mg/kg BW/day] for a human population (Crump, 1998 cited in Crettaz, 2000, p. 96), converted according to Eqs. (7-5) and (7-6); impact: kidney damage (category 2 effect)
Chromium, hexavalent	ingestion	0.15	$12.8 \cdot 0.1 =$	1.28	β_{ED10}: oral chronic NOAEL of 2.5 [mg/kg Body Weight/day] derived by administration of dipotassium chromate to rats (United States - Environmental Protection Agency, 2005), converted according to Eqs. (7-9) and (7-10); impact: reduction in water consumption by rats (category 2 effect)

Table 7-7: Non-cancer effect-related β_{ED10} slope factors and aggregated physical impacts for mortality and morbidity in terms of DALYs due to inhalation and ingestion exposure of selected trace elements

Trace element	Exposure route	β_{ED10} [risk of incidence per (mg/kg BW and day)]	$DALY_{personal}$[a] [years lost-equivalents per person and incidence]	Remarks
Chromium, hexavalent (continued)	inhala-tion	39.0	$12.8 \cdot 0.01 = 0.128$	β_{ED10}: subchronic BMC_{10} of 0.016 [mg/m^3] (United States - Environmental Protection Agency, 2005), converted according to Eqs. (7-5) and (7-7) and employing a subchronic to chronic extrapolation factor of 3.3 (cf. Pennington et al., 2002); impact: enzyme (lactate dehydrogenase) affected in rats (category 3 effect)
Lead	ingestion	143	$12.8 \cdot 0.1 = 1.28$	β_{ED10}: most sensitive oral chronic LOAEL of 0.014 [mg/kg Body Weight/day] derived by administration of lead acetate to rats (Agency for Toxic Substances and Disease Registry, 1999), converted according to Eqs. (7-5) and (7-8), as United States - Environmental Protection Agency (2005) do not provide any non-cancer effect measures in spite of evidence that lead causes hypertension, the slope factor needs to be used with caution; impact: high blood pressure in rats (category 2 effect)

a. The calculations demonstrate the derivation of the final DALY value from the generic DALY value weighted by the category weight as given in Table 7-5.

is asked to estimate for how many individuals in health state X he would be prepared to surrender one year of extended life for 1000 individuals in perfect health in exchange for the complete recovery followed by one year of perfect health for the group in the given health state." (point 18). This way of determining weights does not allow for subjective valuation by (potentially) affected people like in contingent valuation studies and might, therefore, affect the stated weight. However, Hofstetter and Hammitt (2001) conclude that the difference between individual and altruistic preferences is small.

Assuming the highest life expectancy (at birth) observed on earth to be applicable to Europe's population is deemed not to introduce an unacceptable bias. Many of the countries included in the assessment can be considered as highly developed with an on average high standard of living, i.e., about or higher than 75 and 80 years for males and females, respectively (Lopez et al., 2001a; Lopez et al., 2001b). However, it is unclear how diseases or premature deaths are taken into account by the DALY concept for those people that have survived this period life expectancy at birth. The general assumption of the highest life expectancy at birth might compensate for the assumed disregard of the health effects for these age groups.

According to the age-weighting employed, the DALY concept assigns values below to life years lived before the age of 9 and after the age of 55; the ages in between receive weights larger than unity (Murray, 1994). The rationale behind this is that individuals within a society assume different roles and have changing levels of dependency with age, thus, having different social values. This, however, is in contrast to the methodological individualism which constitutes one of the bases for the theory of welfare economics (Rennings, 1994) which provides the context for the external cost assessment.

A discount rate of 3 % is selected in order to avoid "the difficulty of the time paradox and of overvaluing eradication programmes when no discount rate is used" (Murray, 1994, p. 440). By 'time paradox' it is meant in the DALY context that one would postpone investments into health projects to the future if health benefits would be discounted at a smaller rate than the monetary costs. In contrast, if it was possible to launch a project now that will eradicate a disease for good and zero-discounting was assumed one might conclude to spend a fortune to achieve this goal as this would pay-off due to efficiently avoided DALYs caused by the respective disease during the future existence of humankind. As a result, "(o)nly when costs and benefits are discounted at the same rate do we become indifferent to the time when a project is implemented" (ibid., p. 440).

It needs to be emphasized that two of these four value choices have been addressed by Crettaz and co-workers (Crettaz, 2000; Crettaz et al., 2002) and Keller (2005), namely age-weighting and discounting. These value choices are not taken into consideration in the DALYs used and published by these authors. The DALYs given in Tables 7-6 and 7-7 can, therefore, be used as traditionally done with the YOLL values within the ExternE project series when it comes to monetary valuation (cf. section 8.2).

7.3.7 Discussion on the magnitude of the assessed DALYs

For consistency and comparability reasons between the assessed trace elements, the values provided by Keller (2005) are adopted. Only one $YOLL_{personal}$ value could be found in publications of the ExternE project series. It is given for lung cancers and amounts to 16 (Table 12.8 on p. 252 in European Commission, 1999a) which compares well with the 15.95 $YOLL_{personal}$ as suggested by Keller (2005).

The disability weights given to the different years lived with a particular cancer as reproduced by Crettaz et al. (2002) appear rather small. These have been maintained by Keller (2005). At present, it is unclear whether these disability weights also take potential depressions, pain and/or suffering appropriately into account which constitute the lost utility component related to an illness (European Commission, 1999a, see section 8.2). In principle, they should do so since "scenarios to be valued were presented consistently in the form of a disease label, a brief clinical description of the disease stage, and a generic health state profile" in the case of the European Disability Weight project (Schwarzinger et al., 2003) which has been carried out similarly as in the Global Burden of Disease study. The assignment of disability weights in the Global Burden of Disease study was according to six disability classes ranging from perfect health to death. Each class represents a greater loss of welfare or increased severity than the class before (cf. Table 7-8). As regards comparability of diseases assigned to the same class, Murray (1994) states that these "may restrict different abilities or functional capacities but the impact on the individual is considered to be similar" (p. 438). This all allows the conclusion that the overall welfare of an individual that comprises physical as well as mental aspects should have been addressed by the respondents when assigning weights to different diseases. However, there are doubts on the generalisability of the disability weights computed from the person trade-off method used in the Global Burden of Disease study when compared to those according to the European Disability Weights project using a similar method (Schwarzinger et al., 2003). The results of the visual analogue and the time trade-off method which were used additionally to the person trade-off method for the derivation of disability weights employed in the latter study, furthermore, deviate rather substantially from those reproduced by Crettaz et al. (2002). For instance, the disability weight for 'Breast cancer (disease-free stage without sequelae)',

Table 7-8: Definitions of disability weighting in the Global Burden of Disease Study according to Murray (1994)

Class	Description[a]	Weight
1	Limited ability to perform at least one activity in one of the following areas: recreation, education, procreation or occupation	0.096
2	Limited ability to perform most activities in one of the following areas: recreation, education, procreation or occupation	0.220
3	Limited ability to perform in two or more of the following areas: recreation, education, procreation or occupation	0.400
4	Limited ability to perform most activities in all of the following areas: recreation, education, procreation or occupation	0.600
5	Needs assistance with instrumental activities of daily living such as meal preparation, shopping or housework	0.810
6	Needs assistance with activities of daily living such as eating, personal hygiene or toilet use	0.920

a. Limited ability has been arbitrarily defined as a 50 % or more decrease in ability.

i.e., the stage after successful treatment of breast cancer, may be as large as 0.4 (Schwarzinger et al., 2003) whereas the disability weight for breast cancer-related morbidity amounts only to 0.069 (Crettaz et al., 2002) although also comprising more severe health state stages. These disease stages are found to be most influential on the magnitude of the disability weights at least in the case of the visual analogue scale method (Essink-Bot, 1998). Thus, the disability weights as given in Tables 7-6 and 7-7 are considered to underestimate the weight of years lived with a disability to some extent. As a change of single disability weights may have an impact on the DALYs associated with an average cancer, no attempt will be made here to change the disability weights. This may need to be addressed in the future.

7.3.8 Temporal delays

There are two main time delays between the emission of a substance into the environment and its effect on human health (cf. Fig. 2-2). First, the environmental fate of the substance from the source to the medium to which a person is exposed may vary substantially depending on the medium (e.g., air vs. food) and on the persistence of the substance. This may well be in the order of millennia for persistent substances such as metals (Hellweg, 2000; van den Bergh et al., 2000; Huijbregts et al., 2001). Second, the time gap between exposure and the health effect, i.e., latency time, leads to another postponement of the effect to occur (Mücke 6/ 1995; Mersch-Sundermann, 1996; United States - Environmental Protection Agency, 1998; Hurley and Miller, 2001). In case of premature death in the long run (so-called chronic mortality), one may distinguish between a period with health impairments (morbidity, e.g., expressed in Years of Life lived with Disabilities) and years of not realized life expectancy (e.g., Years Of Life Lost, European Commission, 1999a; Hurley and Miller, 2001) in addition to these (apparent) latency times. One has to note, however, that the YLD indicator as such does not tell over which time period the health impairment occurs which may in principle be relevant when valuing the impact with a non-zero discount rate. These time spans for apparent morbidity and the respective weights are also provided in Table 7-6.

In general, there is hardly any information about time delays between exposure and impact (i.e., latency times) available with respect to the trace elements investigated (Searl, 2004). This may have an effect especially in the valuation of the impacts (discounting, cf. section 8.1 and Hammitt, 2000). When performing non-zero discounting, the distribution of when the assessed DALYs occur within a given population is rather important. By default, no (minimum) latency time is, therefore, assumed noting that delays between exposure and effect may occur due to different susceptibilities of the individuals in the population when distributing the DALYs over time (see section 8.2).

8 Valuation

The presented methodology not only tries to assess the impacts of hazardous substances on human health but also values them. The way how this valuation is performed is described in this Chapter. Principally there are different ways of valuing. In this study, valuation is performed in monetary terms in order to support cost-benefit analyses for instance. Monetised externalities are termed external costs when they are negative and external benefits when they are positive.

8.1 Temporal aspects of monetary valuation and discounting

Unless dealing with acute health effects, a delicate question arises when performing a cost-benefit analysis: how can future costs or benefits be compared with present costs or benefits? Economists usually employ discounting in order to give future benefits or costs present values. Also, the European Commission recommends the involvement of discounting "whenever positive and negative impacts can be expressed in monetary terms" (European Commission, 2002, p. 16). A generalised formula for discounting is (Pearce and Moran, 2001):

$$W_t = \frac{1}{(1+r)^{f(t)}} \qquad (8\text{-}1)$$

where

W_t : *discount factor* which is the weight to be attached to a cost or benefit in year *t*

r : *discount rate*

f(t) : function of the perception of the speed at which time *t* passes.

According to the formulation of *f*(*t*), the discount factor depends hyperbolically or exponentially on the time elapsed until an asset occurs that is to be valued. The conventional way of discounting is exponential in which case $f(t)$ is equal to the time t. The formulation of the conventional discount factor can be derived in a descriptive example considering the development of the value of one unit of a currency. For instance, 1 € next year is not worth the same as 1 € now because 1 € now can be invested at a certain interest rate $r_i > 0$ to become $1 \cdot (1+r_i)$ € next year. Consequently, 1 € next year is worth $1/(1+r_i)$ € now. Discounting, thus, is a weighting scheme to convert future costs or benefits into their present monetary values. One has to note that discounting is always conducted when valuing costs at different points in time because 'no discounting' simply means to use a discount rate of zero with a resulting discount factor of one. Thus, discounting is always performed when dealing with intertemporal matters, either explicitly or implicitly.

Discount rates exist for individuals as well as for societies. The discount rate for individuals is generally based on the Individual Time Preference (ITP) whereas for societies different approaches exist like the Social Time Preference (STP) measuring the reduction of the consumption benefit over time from a consumer perspective or the Opportunity Cost of Capital (OCC) taking the return rate of the best available alternative to an investment from a producer perspective (e.g., Rennings, 1997). Both discount rates should be identical in a perfect market. This is not the case for instance owing to the incompleteness or failures of markets and the fact that an individual experiences an increase of income due to becoming more qualified in the course of a life whereas a society does not 'grow wisdom' to the same extent.[21] Generally the social discount rate is smaller than that of an individual. However, how much smaller is it?

Another question related to this one touches upon the way of discounting in those cases where costs or benefits are to be valued that occur in the far future.

---

[21] However, also societies can principally age. The ITP and the STP principally consist of the same components (see text for the formulation of the STP). Generally it is said that the *social growth rate of real consumption per capita* is smaller than that of an individual. This is because the former results as the sum of its member's growth rates of real consumption per capita. Due to lower birth rates and a higher life expectancy, there is a shift in the age structure of the population or demographic distribution of many western industrialised countries. This will usually lead to an even lower increase in the social growth rate of real consumption per capita than presently assumed. Additionally, unless a real catastrophe of historical or even astronomical size happens, societies do not 'die' whereas individuals do. An individual's *pure time preference* is, thus, larger than that of a society due to preferring to secure benefits now rather than later. This phenomenon sometimes is also called *impatience* or *irrational behavior* or *intertemporal myopia of individuals* although personally it might be less irrational due to uncertainty about the possibility to enjoy future benefits.

There are several considerations why the valuation of deep-future costs or benefits should be valued differently from those occurring in the near future that are described in the following.

The social discount rate r_s is preferably to be based on the STP (European Commission, 1999a) which is defined as:

$$r_s \cong STP = \rho + \theta \cdot g \tag{8-2}$$

where

STP : social time preference

ρ : pure social time preference

θ : elasticity of marginal utility of consumption

g : growth rate of real consumption per capita.

The STP consists of two terms which take into account the preference for present over future consumption (pure social time preference: ρ) and the growth of the economy g, respectively. The growth of the economy is modified by θ which depends on the form of the utility function and gives the percentage fall in the *additional* utility derived from each percentage increase in consumption. A typical value would be 1 due to the fact that the utility function in many cases is assumed to be logarithmic.

With this brief introduction to the STP, the question from above shall be taken up again.

In the context of long-term impacts, Azar and Sterner (1996) conclude that there is no rationale for a constant discount factor in time. Also Weitzmann (1999) suggests different discount rates for different episodes. He explores the question "what is our best prediction of the real rate of interest into the deep future?" (p. 24). Guided by this question, Weitzmann argues that the real interest rate is based on the productivity of investment which in turn strongly depends on the technical progress. While everything in the future is uncertain, he concludes that the "most fundamental uncertainty of all concerns is the discount rate itself" (ibid., pp. 28f). He argues that it is not the discount *rate* that needs to be averaged over a period of time but the discount *factors*. This is because the effective weight to be given to future costs and benefits results from averaging the discount factors and not the discount rates (cf. illustrative example by Pearce and Moran, 2001). As regards the question which value to assume, it is obvious that costs and benefits in the far future are valued the highest when taking the lowest discount rate to be expected. Therefore, Weitzmann considers this value "the only relevant limiting scenario" since "all of the other states at that far-distant time, by comparison,

Table 8-1: Declining discount rate scheme suggested by Weitzmann (1999)

Time horizon [years]	Discount rates suggested by Weitzmann (1999)
0-25	'low-normal' real annual interest rate of around 3-4 %
25-75	within-period instantaneous interest rate of around 2 %
75-300	within-period instantaneous interest rate of around 1 %
> 300	within-period instantaneous interest rate of around 0 %

are relatively less important now" (Weitzmann, 1999, p. 29) due to the compound interest effect. The discount rate should decline depending on the period of time considered in the future due to the increasing uncertainty about the predictability of future interest rates (see Table 8-1). When assuming 3.5 % for the first 25 years, the resulting discount factors are computed according to:

$$
\begin{aligned}
W_t &= \frac{1}{(1+0.035)^t} && \text{for: } 0 < t \leq 25 \\
W_t &= \frac{1}{(1+0.035)^{25}} \cdot \frac{1}{(1+0.02)^{t-25}} && \text{for: } 25 < t \leq 75 \\
W_t &= \frac{1}{(1+0.035)^{25}} \cdot \frac{1}{(1+0.02)^{50}} \cdot \frac{1}{(1+0.01)^{t-75}} && \text{for: } 75 < t \leq 300 \\
W_t &= \frac{1}{(1+0.035)^{25}} \cdot \frac{1}{(1+0.02)^{50}} \cdot \frac{1}{(1+0.01)^{225}} \cdot 1 && \text{for: } t > 300
\end{aligned}
\tag{8-3}
$$

Such decreasing discount rates which are in line with European Commission (1999a) for long-term effects can either be formulated as a step-function (e.g., Rabl, 1996; Weitzmann, 1999) or as a hyperbolic formula (e.g., Pearce and Moran, 2001). Pearce and Moran (2001), furthermore, argue that conventional discounting is only applicable if the good to be valued is money. In agreement with Rabl (1996) and Weitzmann (1999), they recommend hyperbolic discounting for non-money goods. The use of different discounting schemes for different goods appears justified since people show different time preferences for them (Pearce and Moran, 2001). Additionally, behavioural research suggests that many people show positive discount rates, but that they attach less importance to a difference between two times the further into the future these times are moved. In line with the above mentioned discounting schemes, the individual discount rate is decreasing as a function of time (Harvey, 1994).

As just indicated, Rabl (1996) points into the same direction emphasizing that discount rates for intergenerational effects should be defined from the perspective of future generations. When conventionally relying on the STP, the pure social time preference ρ of the discount rate is treated as if it represented creation of wealth while it merely involves redistribution within the present generation (cf. Schelling, 2000). The time horizon of this redistribution is limited by the duration of market transactions, especially loans. As a result, it is suggested by Rabl to split the social time preference into two periods while disregarding the pure social time preference: 1) one for the short term in which market transactions are usually made which is about 30 years (at the most) and 2) one beyond the former time period. The suggested value for the discount rate in the short term r_{short} is equal to r_{growth}. The rate r_{growth} is derived based on long-term average Gross National Products (GNP) per capita adjusted by information on Net Economic Welfare (NEW) to account for welfare aspects not considered in the GNP. It is suggested by Rabl to assume values between 1 and 2 %. After 30 years, a range from just larger than zero to the value of r_{short} is suggested for the discount rate r_{long}. This recommendation is based on the consideration about the present value of future costs which in turn is estimated from present costs according to:

$$
\begin{aligned}
C_0(t) &= C_0(0) \cdot \frac{\exp(r_{\text{escalation}} \cdot t)}{\exp(r_{\text{discount}} \cdot t)} \\
&= C_0(0) \cdot \exp((r_{\text{escalation}} - r_{\text{discount}}) \cdot t) \\
&= C_0(0) \cdot \exp(r_{\text{effective}} \cdot t)
\end{aligned}
\tag{8-4}
$$

where

$C_0(t)$: costs occurring at time t given in present values

$C_0(0)$: present costs given in present values

t : time at which future costs occur

r : $r_{discount}$: rate at which future costs are discounted

$r_{effective}$: effective rate at which present costs are projected to present values of future costs

$r_{escalation}$: rate at which present costs are projected into the future.

The rates $r_{escalation}$ and $r_{discount}$ obtain values that are close to each other

$$r_{\text{escalation}} \approx r_{\text{growth}}$$
$$r_{\text{discount}} \approx r_{\text{growth}} \tag{8-5}$$

and, thus, $r_{effective}$ would in principle be zero. As is argued by Rabl (1996), however, $r_{effective}$ should allow for technological development and should consequently obtain positive values close but not equal to zero.

There is a problem with justifying non-zero discount rates by technical progress. This is because technical progress may affect the effects to occur either by reducing loads (e.g., new developments with respect to abatement techniques) or by providing better means to cope with adverse effects (e.g., medicine, overall better health status). So, rather than discounting the value of effects one should allow for this reduction in impacts to occur in the impact assessment itself. On the other hand, it may indeed be that future generations will have (better) means at hand to tackle problems that are caused by their ancestors. By not accounting for this potential, a misleading allocation of scarce resources may result at present. However, it is rather speculative whether they will in fact have these means available (see below).

While Rabl (1996) argues on the basis of intergenerational equity, Pearce and Moran (2001) point out that discounting is about efficiency and not about equity which should be taken into account by other measures. The question, therefore, arises how to deal with intergenerational equity with respect to intertemporal impacts on human health. Intergenerational equity from an ethical perspective should mean that any individual has equal rights irrespective of when he or she lives (see Hellweg et al. (2003) and the references quoted therein) supporting the perception that there is a "primacy of rights claims over maximizing utility" (Shrader-Frechette, 2000, p. 772). Azar and Sterner (1996) add to this by stating that the "use of a lower discount rate than that observed could be seen as a way of internalizing a market failure" which is caused by the fact that "future generations are not present in the market" (p. 177). Although introducing some elements of conservatism due to scepticism, one may agree not to overly speculate about technological progress which will definitively take place.[22] But whether this will affect the human health status of a person exposed to a substance considered in this work and by when is regarded unpredictable today and, thus, rather uncertain

[22] Even if one recognizes that, e.g., former ways of living or producing things had been better than present ones.

(termed 'factual problem' by Shrader-Frechette, 2000). As a consequence, it may be argued that the *intergenerational discount rate* be zero. On the other hand, it may be regarded as certain that any individual shows a (positive) pure time preference. It is assumed here that this pure time preference is not subject to change between generations ('proxy consent' of people living today with respect to those living in the future, cf. Shrader-Frechette, 2000). Thus, the *personal discount rate* is positive when disregarding the growth rate of real income which is uncertain due to the potentially very long time scales involved. Combining the two discount rates means that all people that are potentially affected at some time in the nearer or farther future by the release of substances today are assumed to live today, however, showing a time preference that is valid for a person's lifetime. The value of this personal discount rate remains to be defined. It will assume values presumably in the range of the ITP and STP. A value of 3 % is suggested. This approach is termed the *intergenerationally equal, positive personal discounting* scheme.

Hellweg et al. (2003) suggest the use of different discount rates for scenario analyses when dealing with long-term effects. The suggested discount rates can be attributed to different archetypes of people that vary with respect to value systems as proposed by Hofstetter (1998) based on cultural theory. While the hierarchist and the individualist would employ discount rates that are either close to zero or positive, respectively, the egalitarian would even consider to use negative discount rates. When using negative discount rates, however, a waste disposal, for instance, that leads to a slower release of toxics and that, thus, prolongs the emission process would be less favoured than uncontrolled disposal. One such example is to vitrify slags (Hellweg et al., 2003). An uncontrolled disposal can definitively not be intended and accepted by present generations, for their own sake. In line with common practice within the ExternE project series, thus, the valued results, i.e., the external costs, shall be presented for different discount rates (cf. Chapters 10 and 11). There are three sensitivity discounting schemes recommended by the ExternE project series using constant discount rates of 0 %, 1 % and 3 %, respectively (e.g., Friedrich and Bickel, 2001a). The discounting schemes by Rabl (1996) and by Weitzmann (1999) presented above show declining discount rates whose values are about in the range of these sensitivity discount rates. It is, therefore, expected for monetised long-term effects to fall in the range of the ExternE project's sensitivity results also when employing these discounting schemes as well as the *intergenerationally equal, positive personal discounting* scheme introduced above. These shall not be explored further since the external costs according to the upper boundary and lower boundary discount schemes as recommended by the ExternE project series will be given in Chapters 10 and 11.

This section shall be concluded with a note on what may be termed the *environmental protection dilemma* (Rennings, 1997) or *conservationist's dilemma*

(Norgaard and Howarth, 1991). Both high and low discount rates can lead to ecological disadvantages. Lower market discount rates usually lead to an increase in economic activity and investments which in turn will normally bring about for example additional releases of substances into the environment. Higher market discount rates, however, will lead to a lower valuation of future impacts. While the first situation is not desirable for presently living and affected humans or other organisms, the latter is not desirable from an intergenerational equity point of view.

8.2 Applied concepts for economic valuation and values used

In order to be able to value impacts due to human activities, economics provide valuation methods that can be grouped into two basic approaches: indirect or behavioural methods and direct or stated preferences methods (Haab and McConnell, 2002). With behavioural methods, individual market behaviour is observed in response to changes for instance in public goods. The preferences may be revealed by different methods such as approaches with respect to travel costs, hedonic pricing and replacement costs (Powell et al., 1997; Rennings, 1997). In the stated preferences approach, researchers directly pose contingent or hypothetical questions to respondents. The most prevalent stated preferences approach is contingent valuation. The valuation is called 'contingent' because people are asked to state their willingness to pay, contingent on a specific hypothetical scenario and description of the environmental service (Mason, 2002). Although initially being looked at as inferior to behavioural methods, contingent valuation has proved to be no less reliable than behavioural methods (Haab and McConnell, 2002).

In principle, direct and indirect methods allow for the derivation of the *willingness to pay* (WTP) for a change in the risk of death for example. A related concept is the *willingness to accept* (WTA). When dividing the WTP by the corresponding change in a mortality risk, the *value of a statistical life* (VOSL or VSL) is obtained. The VOSL has some disadvantages which is why it is recommended to convert it into the *value of a life year lost* (VLYL, European Commission, 1999a; Hunt and Markandya, 2001) that may also just be termed a *value of a life year* (VOLY). Although noting that the empirical evidence on the value of the VLYL is limited (Hunt and Markandya, 2001), it is recommended by the ExternE project series in order to account for the different ages, health states and risk contexts of the affected people (European Commission, 1999a; Hunt and Markandya, 2001). Furthermore, it shall be noted that even though the terminology of the VOSL, VLYL and VOLY seemingly point into this direction it is not a life (year) that is valued but (small) changes in risk of loosing a certain time of an average individual's life expectancy.

8.2.1 Valuation of human health-related impacts

In section 7.3, the physical impacts and their assessment have been presented. Use is made of the DALY concept (Murray and Lopez, 1996a, 1996b) that combines a morbidity component expressed in Years of Life lived with a Disability (YLDs) with a mortality component (Years of Life Lost, YOLLs). The expression of morbidity effects in terms of mortality measures is appealing from a monetary valuation point of view because it constitutes an easy way of valuing both health effects with the same measure. As discussed in section 7.3, no distinction in terms of monetary valuation will be made between the two DALY components. This is mainly due to the fact that the morbidity indicator constitutes an equivalent measure of years of life lost (e.g., Murray, 1994). Therefore, the same monetary value can be used for mortality and morbidity effects on personal health when following the DALY concept. However, external costs related to morbidity effects are considered to be composed of several aspects which do not only take personal damages into account. These are (European Commission, 1999a; Hunt and Markandya, 2001):

- the value of the time lost because of the illness (opportunity costs),
- the value of the lost utility because of the pain and suffering, and
- the costs of any expenditures (a) on averting and/or mitigating the effects of the illness and (b) due to foregone earnings or absenteeism; these expenditures are also termed *costs of illness* (COIs).

Generally, the components of the morbidity external costs other than the COI are difficult to measure which is why usually only the COI are considered (European Commission, 1999a). In the case of the YLDs, however, one could argue that the pain and suffering-related costs are included in the disability weights used, at least to some extent. Thus, these are considered to be implicitly included in the physical impact indicator. In line with common practice within the ExternE project series, the costs of illness need to be added to each of the non-fatal disease periods. In order to avoid double-counting, an extrapolation from the COI to the Willingness to Pay must not be done (e.g., for cancer-related morbidity, European Commission, 1999a) due to the consideration of the YLDs (cf. Eq. (8-6)).

Only two COI values could be found in ExternE-related project reports which are hypertension due to noise (Hunt, 2001) and cancer-related morbidity (European Commission, 1999a; Table 8-2). In the absence of more information, the COI-related external costs due to the other health effects are not included in the present assessment (cf. Table 8-6).

What needs to be defined still is the monetary value to be assigned to the DALYs associated with the physical impacts as specified in Tables 7-6 and 7-7. In the recently completed, EC-funded NewExt project (Number: ENG1-2000-

Table 8-2: Monetary values used for the valuation of the costs of illness (COI) for the endpoints considered in this study

Morbidity effect	COI [$€_{2000}$ per case]	Remarks
High blood pressure[a]	3551 [b]	analogy with noise-related hypertension; hospital and absentee costs of 1830 and 1584 $€_{1998}$/case, respectively considered (Hunt, 2001)
Skin lesions	n/a	
Kidney damage	n/a	
Reduction in water consumption[a]	n/a	
Enzyme (lactate dehydrogenase) affected[a]	n/a	
Cancer-related morbidity	320700 [c]	cancer-related costs of illness of 300000 $€_{1995}$/case without considering pain and suffering-related costs (European Commission, 1999a)

a. Evidence from laboratory tests on rats.
b. Price conversion from basis 1998 to 2000 by factor of 1.04.
c. Price conversion from basis 1995 to 2000 by factor of 1.069.

00129), a value of 50000 $€_{2000}$ per chronic YOLL has been determined by means of a contingent valuation survey carried out in France, Italy and the United Kingdom (Markandya et al., 2004). This value is assumed to contain a discount rate of 3 %. The undiscounted value for chronic mortality has been derived to be 75000 $€_{2000}$ per chronic YOLL.

8.2.2 Monetary valuation and latency

As was concluded above (cf. section 8.1), two discounting schemes will be employed using 0 and 3 %, respectively. When performing zero discounting, the monetary valuation of the physical impacts is straightforward. The just presented value of 75000 $€_{2000}$ per YOLL-equivalent will be taken. As regards the value to be used when discounting at a rate of 3 %, the main question to be answered is:

What is the average value of a life year lost in the European population due to the impacts assessed? In order to answer this question, the time structure of when the effects are expected to occur needs to be known. The approach as described by Gressmann and Bickel (1997) is followed which is similar to that by Miller (2001).

The approach compares a reference scenario in which the population develops according to the unmodified mortality probabilities with a scenario in which the survival probabilities are decreased by a certain factor for all age cohorts after an initial minimum latency time. This decreasing factor is adjusted so that the time-integrated sum of the lost life years towards the reference case equals the respective YOLLs given in Table 7-6. Only the cancer-specific YOLLs shall be investigated. This is because the non-cancer impacts are derived from those of an average cancer. Consequently, the same temporal structure of the lost life years is used. Furthermore, the approach only takes survival rates into account without considering the years lived with a disability.

The physical impacts given in Tables 7-6 and 7-7 need to be classified into acute and chronic impacts in order to appropriately apply the 3 % discounting scheme during monetary valuation. None of the impacts considered in these Tables is regarded to constitute a cause for acute mortality despite the assumption of no minimum latency (Searl, 2004). 'Minimum latency' means that no effect occurs at the population level after exposure towards hazardous substances within the specified time. However, one needs to note that the years of life lost for the diseases assessed in this study represent average values at the population level. Similar to the 'no threshold' assumption at the population level, the 'no (minimum) latency' assumption means that there are sensitive individuals that develop a disease immediately after exposure, possibly also due to previous exposure, while other individuals may be affected with a delay only. This is demonstrated in Fig. 8-1 for an integrated sum of years of life lost of 15.95 (circles) and 6.09 (triangles), respectively. If a rather young individual dies in the first year after exposure his/her life years lost show in all subsequent years until he/she would have completed his/her life expectancy. This, however, means that there are new cases of death occurring at least until the peak of each of the curves shown in Fig. 8-1, with variable durations of latency. If minimum latency for instance of 10 years is assumed to occur, the years of life lost are postponed but still quite a few individuals that die do so only with a longer duration of latency (Fig. 8-2, grey circles). If one assumed that the minimum latency time is also the maximum, i.e., the effects only occur in year 11 after the exposure, then an entirely different shape of the temporal distribution of the years of life lost would result (Fig. 8-2, white circles). This could be described as a postponed acute mortality which, however, is rather unrealistic unless the hazard to be assessed is a time bomb for instance set

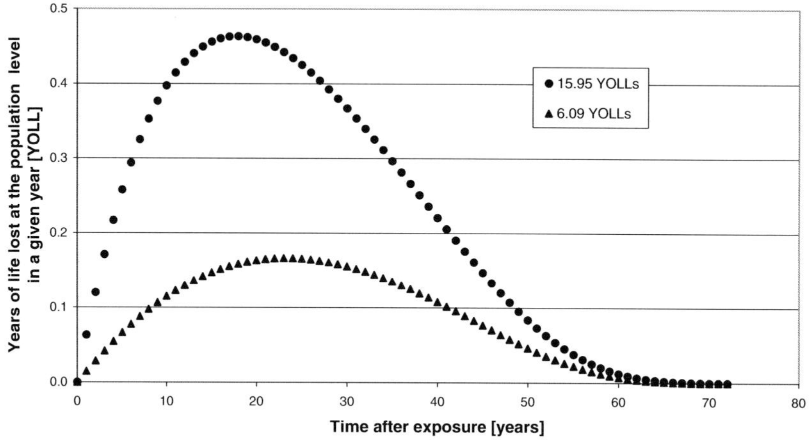

Fig. 8-1: Temporal structure of the distribution of 6.09 and 15.95 years of life lost (YOLL) due to an exposure towards a pollutant at time 0 years without a minimum latency time at the population level

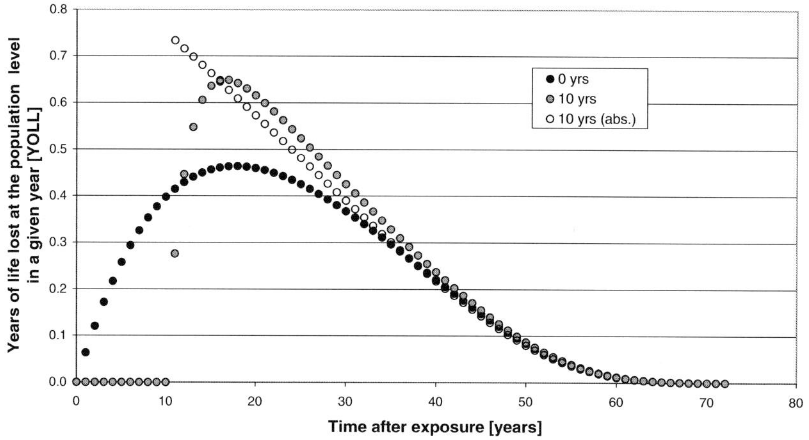

Fig. 8-2: Temporal structure of the distribution of 15.95 years of life lost (YOLL) due to an exposure towards a pollutant at time 0 years according to three different assumptions with respect to latency at the population level: no minimum latency, minimum latency of 10 years and absolute latency of 10 years (black, grey and white circles, respectively)

Table 8-3: Monetary values per YOLL when discounting at a rate of 3 % according to the approach followed in this study [$€_{2000}$ per YOLL]

Type of cancer	YOLL per incidence	Minimum latency time of ...	
		0 years	10 years
Lung	15.95	40845	37009
Skin	6.09	37788	32030
Average	12.5	39563	34627

up in year 0 and that explodes just after completion of year 10. In order to conclude this excursus on latency time, one can state that one needs to be cautious when stating that no latency time is assumed (at the population level).

To what extent does the 'no minimum latency' assumption influence the monetary value to be assigned to the DALYs when discounting at a rate of 3 %? The effect is shown in Table 8-3. Assuming a minimum latency of 10 years would lead to a reduction in the monetary value towards a situation with a minimum latency time of 0 years by between 10 and 15 % when discounting at a rate of 3 %. The values yielded without consideration of latencies suggest to use one value for all cancers investigated due to small discrepancies. The monetary value adopted in the present study for valuing DALYs when discounting at 3 % is 40000 $€_{2000}$ per DALY.

8.2.3 Impact of employing a different monetary valuation approach for morbidity effects

In section 7.3, the issue of the appropriateness of the disability weights for cancers has been identified. These disability weights are needed to aggregate the years lived with a disability (YLD) with years of life lost (YOLL) into DALYs. It shall be investigated to what extent a different approach would result in changes in the external costs quantified in Chapters 10 and 11. In the present work, the external costs related to one incidence of a disease are calculated according to:

$$\begin{aligned} Costs_{\text{external}} &= Costs(Mortality) + Costs(Morbidity) \\ &= Costs(YOLL) + Costs(YLD) + Costs(Treatment) \end{aligned} \quad (8\text{-}6)$$

Table 8-4: Implications of the pain and suffering-related monetary value for cancers according to the DALY and the ExternE approach for a discount rate of 0 %

	DALY approach				ExternE approach	
Type of cancer	Disability weight [-]	Disability duration [years with a disability per person and cancer case]	YLD per cancer case [years lost-equivalents per person and cancer case] [a]	Monetary value [$€_{2000}$ per non-fatal cancer case] [b]	Pain and suffering-related costs [$€_{2000}$ per non-fatal cancer case]	Resulting theoretical disability weights [-] [c]
Lung	0.146	1.8	0.26	19710	160350	1.19
Skin	0.045	4.2	0.19	14175	160350	0.51
Average	0.809	0.865 [d]	0.70 [d]	52500	160350	2.47

a. Note that the YLD values result when multiplying the disability duration with the disability weight.
b. Yielded by multiplying the YLDs with 75000 $€_{2000}$ per YOLL.
c. Yielded by dividing the value of 160350 $€_{2000}$ per non-fatal cancer case by the product of the disability duration and the monetary value of 75000 $€_{2000}$ per YOLL.
d. See footnote 19 for the derivation of the value.

Within this study, the YOLLs and the YLDs are aggregated into DALYs allowing the use of one monetary value for both health effects, i.e., the monetary value for mortality. According to normal practice within the ExternE project series, in contrast, only the YOLLs are valued with this monetary value while specific values for each end point are to value morbidity-related effects. At present, the value for cancer-specific morbidity effects comprises different aspects. This way of valuing morbidity aggregates treatment costs (referred to as costs of illness, COI) and the willingness to pay (WTP) to avoid pain and suffering. In order to avoid double-counting, the purely pain and suffering-related costs result as:

$$\begin{aligned} &Costs(Morbidity) = Costs(Pain + suffering) + Costs(Treatment) \\ &\Rightarrow Costs(Pain + suffering) = Costs(Morbidity) - Costs(Treatment) \end{aligned} \quad . \qquad (8\text{-}7)$$

Table 8-5: Impact of choosing the DALY or the ExternE approach with respect to valuing pain and suffering-related monetary valuation when discounting at a rate of 0 %

Type of cancer	DALY approach	ExternE approach	Ratios	
	External costs [$€_{2000}$ per case]	External costs [$€_{2000}$ per case]	$\frac{\text{ExternE}}{\text{DALY}}$	$\frac{\text{DALY}}{\text{ExternE}}$
Lung	1536660	1677300	1.09	0.92
Skin	791625	937800	1.18	0.84
Average	1280700	1415585	1.11	0.90

The presently used value for morbidity amounts to 450000 $€_{1995}$ per non-fatal cancer case (p. 257 in European Commission, 1999a). This value corresponds to 481050 € in the year 2000, the base year for valuation in the present study. The treatment costs for a non-fatal cancer case are assumed to be 320700 $€_{2000}$ (cf. Table 8-2). The difference of 160350 $€_{2000}$ per non-fatal cancer case are the purely pain and suffering-related costs according to Eq. (8-7). These shall be compared to the costs resulting from the morbidity component of the cancer-specific DALYs (Table 8-4). Only the case of discounting at a rate of 0 % is investigated as this is the upper limit scenario for the external costs to be quantified. The difference between the DALY approach and the ExternE approach in terms of valuing the pain and suffering-related effects amounts to a factor between 3 and 11. The theoretically resulting disability weights are also given in Table 8-4. Their purpose is to see which value the disability weights of the respective cancers would need to assume if one wanted to obtain the cancer-unspecific ExternE value when following the DALY approach. Except for the case of skin cancer, these would assume values larger than 1. This is not reasonable according to the underlying philosophy of the disability weights as one cannot loose more time than one possibly expects to have. If one mixed the two approaches on the expense of losing consistency particularly with the assessment of the non-cancer effects, one can see that the 'pure' DALY approach underestimates the external costs per cancer case by up to 16 % (Table 8-5). Or phrased the other way around, the external costs derived in this study might be higher by up to 18 % if one chose to use the ExternE-based valuation approach for the pain and suffering-related costs.

8.2.4 Monetary values used

In order to conclude this Chapter on monetary valuation, the monetary values as used in this study are summarized in Table 8-6. Note that the costs of illness (COI) as given in Table 8-2 are current values, i.e., intertemporally valid only when discounting at 0 %. The 3 % discounted values are derived by linear scaling with the quotient of the monetary values per YOLL of 3 % to 0 %, i.e., multiplication by 0.53. This way it is assumed that the costs of illness occurring in the future are distributed over time in the same way as the years of life lost although principally preceding these. Together with the use of one monetary value per YOLL for the 3 % discounting case (see above), this also brings about that the values for these two discounting schemes are different by a constant factor of about 2 for all human health effects considered (comparing the totals in Table 8-6).

Further note that the external costs that result from employing the *intergenerationally equal, positive personal discounting* scheme equal those according to discounting at a rate of 0 % multiplied by this factor. This is due to the fact that the value of an impact only depends on whether an incidence of a disease is assessed to occur and not on when it occurs. In contrast, when constantly discounting at a rate of 3 %, also the time lag between emission and occurrence of a disease contribute to giving a lower value to the respective impact. Thus, the intergenerationally equal, positive personal discounting scheme causes the external costs to be about half of those when 'not discounting'.

Table 8-6: Monetary values per incidence of a disease by valuation approach and discount rate as used in the present study [$€_{2000}$ per case]

Disease	0 % discounting			3 % discounting		
	WTP	COI	Total	WTP	COI	Total
Cancer						
Lung cancer	1215960	320700	1536660	648512	171040	819552
Skin cancer	470925	320700	791625	251160	171040	422200
Average cancer	960000	320700	1280700	512000	171040	683040
Non-cancer						
Skin lesions	96000	n/a	96000	51200	n/a	51200
Kidney damage	96000	n/a	96000	51200	n/a	51200
Reduction in water consumption	96000	n/a	96000	51200	n/a	51200
Enzyme affected	9600	n/a	9600	5120	n/a	5120
Hypertension	96000	3551	99551	51200	1894	53094

9 Evaluation of results

According to Beck and Chen (2000), "the public has a legitimate stake in being assured of the quality of models that are used to inform the decision-making process"[23] (p. 404). Thus, especially when developing and even more so when applying a model in a decision-support context where uncertainties are even larger than in natural sciences (e.g., Morgan and Henrion, 1990; Ragas et al., 1999), it is indispensable to give an indication of how relevant the model results are, keeping in mind that "a model is essentially a hypothesis and that no model is perfect; it would presumably cease to be a model if it were" (Addiscott, 1993, p. 17). Additionally, there is reason for evaluating model results because (United States - Environmental Protection Agency, 1997c):

- uncertain information from different sources of different quality often must be combined for the assessment;
- decisions need to be made about whether or how to expend resources to acquire additional information;
- biases may result in so-called 'best estimates' that in actuality are not very accurate; and
- important factors and potential sources of disagreement in a problem can be identified.

In the following, an overview will be given on the different concepts how to evaluate exposure and impact assessment models. Furthermore, the approach will be outlined and applied by which the reliability of the results with respect to impact assessment and their valuation at the European scale shall be assessed.

---

[23] Note that this does not just hold for computational models but of course also to any data: a "reported value whose accuracy is entirely unknown is worthless" according to Eisenhart (1968) (p. 1201) because the intended use of the value determines its accuracy. Care must, therefore, be taken when using the value in contexts other than the specified purpose.

9.1 Terminology

9.1.1 Validation, verification, evaluation ...

There are many notions around that describe the action to evaluate a mathematical model. Beside evaluation, these include verification, validation, corroboration, confirmation and quality assurance (e.g., Caswell, 1976; Oreskes et al., 1994; Addiscott et al., 1995; Rykiel (Jr.), 1996; Veerkamp and Wolff, 1996; Robinson, 1999; Beck and Chen, 2000; Schwartz, 2000). It shall not be tried here to give definitions of the different notions. The reader is asked to refer to the existing literature (e.g., Caswell, 1976; Sargent, 1984; Tsang, 1991; Oreskes et al., 1994; Rykiel (Jr.), 1996; Robinson, 1999).

There is broad consensus in the (natural) scientific and engineering literature (e.g., Oreskes et al., 1994; Addiscott et al., 1995; Rykiel (Jr.), 1996; Veerkamp and Wolff, 1996; Robinson, 1999; Beck and Chen, 2000; Schwartz, 2000) that the term *validation* should not be used in the sense that a model or theory is correct although this impression may prevail in the public (Bredehoeft and Konikow, 1993). The scientific reasoning basically builds on the work of Popper (e.g., Popper, 1968) arguing that the truth of a scientific theory cannot be justified, rather one can justify the preference for one theory or model due to its applicability being superior in a special context than that of a competitor. In contrast, a scientific theory can only be falsified or invalidated.

In this context, one needs to distinguish predictive models/theories from explanatory ones (Caswell, 1976). Whereas explanatory theories cannot be validated (but corroborated) the predictive models can with respect to their purpose (e.g., Sargent, 1984). As Caswell (1976) expresses it "the important point is that the truth or reality of the model is never at issue" (p. 319). Thus, the term 'valid' can be regarded to mean 'well founded and applicable' (Addiscott et al., 1995), 'acceptable for an intended use' (Rykiel (Jr.), 1996; see also Beck and Chen, 2000), or 'established legitimacy' (Oreskes et al., 1994) leading to 'increased' (Robinson, 1999) or 'sufficient confidence' (Sargent, 1984) for predictive models. In this case, it becomes clear that the validation of a model cannot be performed in absolute terms (Caswell, 1976; Addiscott et al., 1995; Veerkamp and Wolff, 1996): it is rather relative with respect to the test procedure and the existence of competing models both of which may be subject to change in the future. The test procedure in turn depends on the purpose of the model (see below). Following the legal and theological parlance, valid can also mean to be efficacious, i.e., producing the intended effect (Addiscott et al., 1995).

Another, more technical dimension of the evaluation of results is the quality assurance of the computer code (Tsang, 1991; Veerkamp and Wolff, 1996;

Schwartz, 2000) sometimes referred to as 'verification' (Rykiel (Jr.), 1996) by demonstrating that the modelling formalism is correct and complies to the conceptual model (Robinson, 1999).

It is stressed that the term 'validation' is used in its technical sense in this work so that confidence is gained into the applicability of the model with respect to external cost assessments.

9.1.2 Uncertainty

From an empirical science perspective, *uncertainty* may be defined as "a scientist's assessment of the probable magnitude of (an) *error*" (Henrion and Fischhoff, 1986, p. 792) which in turn is perceived as "the actual difference between a measurement and the value of the quantity it is intended to measure" which "is generally unknown at the time of measurement" (ibid.). Uncertainty may also just be defined as "essentially the absence of information, information that may or not be obtainable" (Rowe, 1994, p. 743).

It is a common perception that an error in a measurement (or an assessment) may stem from different sources or may consist of different components. In empirical science, the conventional distinction is between (according to Henrion and Fischhoff (1986) and literature cited therein):

- *random error* or *Category A uncertainty* due to uncontrolled variability among observations and which is evaluated by statistical means and
- *systematic error* or *Category B uncertainty* which is equal to the difference between the value to which the observed mean converges and the true value.

In the realm for instance of regulatory exposure assessment 'science' in which the focus is on deriving safeguard standards based on mathematical simulation models, a different distinction is widely accepted and used.[24] The United States - Environmental Protection Agency (1997c) classifies the *sources* of uncertainty into:

- uncertainty regarding parameter values (*parameter uncertainty*) which can be further subdivided into *uncertainty due to lack of knowledge* (about a value or its heterogeneity according to Finley and Paustenbach (1994) or in a statistical or scientific sense according to Bogen and Spear (1987)) and *var-*

[24] Note that there are more uncertainty classification or grouping schemes. These include the subdivision into Type A and Type B uncertainty with different meanings (according to Safety Series No. 100 of the International Atomic Energy Agency (1989) as quoted by Hoffman and Hammonds (1994)) vs. McColl et al. (2000). These will not be explained here.

iability arising from true heterogeneity across people, places or time termed inter-individual, spatial and temporal variability, respectively; whereas uncertainty may be reducible through further measurements, variability is usually not (Bogen and Spear, 1987; Burmaster and Anderson, 1994; Finley and Paustenbach, 1994),

- uncertainty regarding missing or incomplete information needed to fully define exposure and dose (*scenario uncertainty*) and
- uncertainty regarding gaps in scientific theory required to make predictions on the basis of causal inferences (*model uncertainty*).

Another aspect is not explicitly mentioned in the above list of uncertainty sources. This is the *decision-rule uncertainty*, a term proposed by Finkel (1990) which is referred to in several other publications (e.g., United States - Environmental Protection Agency, 1998; Hertwich et al., 1999, 2000; McKone and Hertwich, 2001). Hertwich et al. (2000) describe this type of uncertainty as the "uncertainty about whether the model output is a relevant representation of an issue of concern, and whether the model settings represent the conditions of concern" (p. 443). It arises "whenever there is ambiguity or controversy about how to quantify or compare social objectives" (ibid., p. 442) leading to "imprecise or inappropriate operational definitions for desired outcome criteria, value parameters, and decision variables" (McColl et al., 2000, p. 2-4) and involves value judgements or preferences. Following this description, also the *fundamental uncertainty* (Ragas et al., 1999)[25] and the uncertainty introduced by the *model context* (Rykiel (Jr.), 1996)[26] can be regarded as decision-rule uncertainty. The value judgements include the choice of the indicator, how to deal with timings of impacts (e.g., use of discounting or temporal cutoffs), formulation of an environmental fate model as an open or closed system, selection of summary statistics, choice of variables that express subjective value judgements in the form of utility functions (e.g., the monetary value attributed to loss of life), and also how (parameter) uncertainty is addressed (Hertwich et al., 2000; McColl et al., 2000). This list may be extended by the choice of whether to include certain exposure path-

[25] Fundamental uncertainty "stems from the assumptions underlying a model structure and its equations" and "was assessed tentatively on the basis of an analysis of (a multimedia fate model's) assumptions and equations and the results of a postal questionnaire among scientists and scientifically trained policy makers and representatives of interest groups" (ibid., p. 1857). Fundamental uncertainty is distinguished from what is called 'operational uncertainty' which is addressed by an output uncertainty analysis.

[26] "Context embodies all the assumptions, especially those that are unstated and relegated to the system environment of the model" (ibid., p. 242).

ways or not, a decision that may be affected by missing or incomplete information resulting in scenario uncertainty. Thus, scenario uncertainty can be regarded a sub-aspect of decision-rule uncertainty. The other uncertainty types distinguished by Finkel (1990) correspond to model and parameter uncertainty if the latter is distinguished into true uncertainty and (natural) variability. Due to the larger scope of decision-rule uncertainty as compared to scenario uncertainty, the uncertainty source classification by Finkel (1990) is adopted in this work.

Another uncertainty classification scheme has been provided by Rowe (1994) although not in terms of sources but *dimensions*. It is distinguished between

- *metrical*: uncertainty and variability in measurement,
- *structural*: uncertainty due to complexity, including models and their validation,
- *temporal*: uncertainty in future and past states,
- *translational*: uncertainty in explaining uncertain results (or communication uncertainty).

The metrical dimension of uncertainty is mostly related to both aspects of parameter uncertainty. Structural uncertainty tries to give indications about the 'usefulness of the model' and may, therefore, touch upon all different sources of uncertainty stated above. Past temporal uncertainty is exclusively related to the imperfect knowledge of past states of the 'world', i.e., true parameter uncertainty. More importantly, future temporal uncertainty refers to uncertain predictions of future states. This may result from incomplete scientific theory and/or from uncertain capabilities to predict future states due to the complexity of the world (e.g., temporal and spatial variability, vast amounts of interactions and feedback).[27] It is, thus, mostly related to model uncertainty although incomplete knowledge about all values of the most influential state variables will not be achieved either; if we tried we would take the chance to dramatically change the properties of the environmental system (cf. Tsang, 1991). Translational uncertainty occurs when (uncertain) results are communicated. It is due to the fact that the analyst or assessor as well as the decision-makers, professionals, stakeholders and the public have different levels of training and capability of understanding the results (Rowe, 1994). They also have different scientific perspectives with different terminologies. It is clear that this dimension of uncertainty cannot be analysed prior to the dissemination of results. What needs to be kept in mind, however, is that

[27] The mechanistically founded deterministic believe of Sir Isaac Newton (1642-1727) that one could predict the future if one knew all present values of the state variables has disappeared at the latest since the discovery of chaos.

the assessor has to try best to put his/her results into context and be precise about the outcome so that the audience will not be misled in perceiving the results (Chapman, 2001).

Apart from the translational uncertainty dimension, there are different relevant approaches how to evaluate the different sources of uncertainty also with respect to the different dimensions which will be presented to some extent in the following.

9.2 Approaches for the evaluation of results

Prior to conducting an evaluation of a model, there appears to exist consensus that the following topics need to be specified

- the 'purpose of the model' (Caswell, 1976; Rykiel (Jr.), 1996; Scott et al., 2000; Schwartz, 2000), 'objectives' (Robinson, 1999), or 'task specification' (Beck and Chen, 2000),
- the 'performance criteria' (Rykiel (Jr.), 1996), 'demands' (Caswell, 1976), or 'statements on undesirable outcomes' (Schwartz, 2000) for which a rigorously defined 'endpoint or target of the assessment' (Hoffman and Hammonds, 1994) is necessary and
- the 'model context' (Rykiel (Jr.), 1996), i.e., the underlying assumptions and resulting contextual 'ranges of applicability' (Tsang, 1991) or 'limitations' (Veerkamp and Wolff, 1996) of the model.

Once these topics are specified, there are different ways how to evaluate mathematical models. There exist many aspects which may be considered in the evaluation of models and their results. It might, therefore, be useful to try to group the different approaches. One way of subdividing the validation process is into the components (Rykiel (Jr.), 1996): (a) operational or whole model validation, (b) theoretical or conceptual validity, and (c) data validation of which only the operational and data components can be validated whereas theory cannot (see reasons given above). *Operational validation* (or 'black-box validation', Robinson, 1999) tries to demonstrate that the model results meet the overall performance criteria (Rykiel (Jr.), 1996) according to a model's purpose or task (Schwartz, 2000). It is most often done by comparing the model results with independent results (see section 9.2.2). *Conceptual validity* "means that the theories and assumptions underlying the conceptual model are correct, or at least justifiable, and that the model representation of the problem or system, its structure, logic, mathematical, and causal relationships, are reasonable for the model's intended use" (Rykiel (Jr.), 1996, p. 234). Conceptual validity is understood here to also include the aspect whether the conceptual model is implemented into the computational model (tool) without error. *Data validation* is understood here to indicate the quality or relevance of the data used.

One may alternatively distinguish between internal and external evaluations. *Internal* evaluations provide an assessment of the "primary, theoretical material and constituent hypotheses of which the model is composed" which is "essentially a matter of making judgements about the quality of the internal properties of the model, in particular, of whether the functions ... have been 'properly' expressed and 'realistic' values assigned to the parameters ... appearing in them" (Beck and Chen, 2000, p. 406). This description of internal evaluation complies with both concepts of *conceptual* or *theoretical validity* and *data validation* given above. *External* evaluations correspond to the definition of *operational validation* given above.

The assignment of the different approaches used for the evaluation of models and their results into the categories given above is not always straightforward (Schwartz, 2000) and presumably, therefore, not attempted by some authors (e.g., Rykiel (Jr.), 1996). Some authors give lists of possible validation or evaluation approaches (e.g., Sargent, 1984; Rykiel (Jr.), 1996) of which others even recommend to apply as many of them as possible (Tsang, 1991). This is definitely beyond the scope of the present work. In the following, some simple and/or rather common approaches will be presented and reasons given to what extent these will be employed in the present exercise.

9.2.1 Minimum requirements towards uncertainty analysis of exposure assessments according to United States - Environmental Protection Agency (1997c)

According to United States - Environmental Protection Agency (1997c), the exposure assessor should at a minimum address uncertainty qualitatively by answering questions such as (adapted from pp. 2-6f, ibid.):

- What is the basis or rationale for selecting assumptions and/or parameters, such as data, conceptual or mathematical models, exposure scenarios, scientific judgement, policies or guidance of regulatory bodies, 'what if' considerations, etc.?
- What is the range or variability of the key parameters (once identified)? How were the parameter values selected for use in the assessment? Were average, median, or upper-percentile values chosen? If other choices had been made, how would the results have differed?
- What is the assessor's confidence (including qualitative confidence aspects) in the key parameters and the overall assessment (e.g., selected exposure scenarios)? What are the quality and the extent of the data base(s) supporting the selection of the chosen values?

It is clear from the context of this guidance document, that the validation exercise stops at the exposure level and does not include the components of impact assessment and valuation. However, most of the recommendations given are applicable to the other steps of the Impact Pathway Approach as well. Whereas the first bullet point which may be referred to as decision-rule uncertainty assessment is rather qualitative, especially the second one requires the identification of key parameters first. An approach how to do this is presented in section 9.2.4 below. The third bullet point deals with confidence in the overall model which may need to be built first for example by means of other validation approaches such as comparison with reported data (section 9.2.2) or the analysis of different scenarios (section 9.2.3). Thus, in order for the presented qualitative uncertainty assessment not to become overly subjective, it is recommended here to accompany it with more quantitative assessments that are not too resource-intensive (such as probabilistic uncertainty assessments, see section 9.2.5).

9.2.2 Comparison with independent data

As stated above, operational validation tries to demonstrate that the model results meet the overall performance criteria (Rykiel (Jr.), 1996) according to a model's purpose or task (Schwartz, 2000). It is most often done by comparing the model results with independent results that are the output especially of monitoring exercises (Beck and Chen, 2000) and which can be termed *traditional validation* (Veerkamp and Wolff, 1996), but may alternatively encompass results from presumably more complex or specific models (Rykiel (Jr.), 1996). Comparing modelled data to observed ones can be referred to as *history match* (Bredehoeft and Konikow, 1993) or as part of a *historical data validation* process (Rykiel (Jr.), 1996), terms superior to just stating 'validation' as they describe more precisely what is done. It shall be noted that there is agreement that this type of validation procedure, however, is not applicable to generic or screening level exposure models for which the area of potential measurements is unspecified or the substance to be assessed is not present due to the fact that it is not yet allowed to be marketed (Veerkamp and Wolff, 1996; Schwartz, 2000).

There is a dilemma with this type of validation approach which is why "(a) neutral language is needed for the evaluation of model performance" (Oreskes et al., 1994, p. 643). If there is agreement between the simulated and the independent data in terms of the pre-defined evaluation criteria the model (result) may be judged to be 'accurate' (Caswell, 1976; Schwartz, 2000), to show 'a precise or accurate fit' (Oreskes et al., 1994), to 'increase a model's credibility' (Rykiel (Jr.), 1996), or to 'increase the confidence in a model' (Robinson, 1999). Furthermore, depending on the evaluation criteria such an accuracy may be quantitative or qualitative (Rykiel (Jr.), 1996). However, validity and accuracy are related but separate concepts (Robinson, 1999). This is because the match between model results and independent data does not prove the validity of the underlying model concept, i.e., that the model is an accurate cause-effect representation of the real system (Rykiel (Jr.), 1996). There could be other conceptual models that would produce the same output, a "situation ... referred to by scientists as nonuniqueness and by philosophers as underdetermination" (Oreskes et al., 1994, p. 642). On the other hand, if a model (result) does not compare well according to the performance criteria this does not invalidate the conceptual model (Sargent, 1984). It merely indicates that something is wrong (Oreskes et al., 1994) and be it 'just' that the data fed into the (overall) model is a worse representation of 'reality' than the underlying (conceptual) model (Rykiel (Jr.), 1996).

As a consequence, it is clear that such a comparison with independent data can increase the credibility of a model or provide evidence of a model's accuracy including the used data base.

9.2.3 Scenario analysis

With respect to model validation, scenario analyses provide point estimates while changing single components and/or assumptions in order to get an overview about the possible effect on the results albeit without indicating probabilities. Different scenarios may be analysed which differ with respect to parameter values, considered processes and their formulations, boundary conditions (e.g., open vs. closed system), emissions, or spatial and/or temporal resolution etc..[28] By means of this validation approach, also aspects of the decision-rule uncertainty can be addressed which may be supplemented by parameter sensitivity analysis (see section 9.2.4) and/or probabilistic uncertainty analysis (see section 9.2.5).

In the (regulatory) risk assessment context, some authors describe scenario analysis most useful as a screening approach (Finley and Paustenbach, 1994) especially as a *bounding estimate* or as a desirable first step prior to conducting a probabilistic uncertainty assessment (Burmaster and Anderson, 1994). The bounding estimate constitutes an upper limit of individual exposure, dose or risk and is most often used only to eliminate pathways from further consideration during screening-level assessments (United States - Environmental Protection Agency, 1992). However, care must be taken when combining parameter values selected according to worst-case assumptions. Such assessments at times substan-

---

[28] A rather advanced scenario analysis approach in terms of computational requirements according to Schwartz (2000) is the range/confidence estimate approach (Richards and Rowe, 1999).

tially overestimate the exposure even of high-end individuals (e.g., Finley and Paustenbach, 1994; Price et al., 1996; Mekel and Fehr, 2000) and, therefore, need to be classified as unrealistic. As a consequence, Schwartz (2000) calls them *cumulative worst case* scenarios. Also, the United States - Environmental Protection Agency (1992) stresses that the assessment according to the bounding estimate scenario is not apt to identify important or significant pathways since these should not be mistaken as actual exposure estimates.

Apart from the problem with respect to the cumulative worst case scenario whose risk is deemed small in this study, the discriminative power of scenario analyses is rather weak due to the fact that the results consist of point estimates without probability indications. Still, the scenario analysis provides indicative information about the importance of the varied component and/or assumption relative to the reference scenario. This is in line with United States - Environmental Protection Agency (1992) in that scenario analyses are proposed as a legitimate although more uncertain alternative to probabilistic uncertainty assessments. In this case, specific values are selected from the key parameter distributions with which scenario analyses are conducted.

9.2.4 Sensitivity analysis of parameters

The validation process of models with different spatial scale of applicability require different validation approaches (Addiscott et al., 1995; Rykiel (Jr.), 1996). This also holds for models that are very complex at least in terms of the number of variables and parameters contained (Caswell, 1976). For both categories of models, the definition of statistical criteria for evaluation purposes constitutes a problem (Caswell, 1976; Addiscott et al., 1995). For the validation of models operating at rather large scales, Addiscott et al. (1995) suggests to use approaches to test for efficacy which include sensitivity analysis although these are judged by some authors not to constitute a sufficient approach with respect to model validation (e.g., Schwartz, 2000). Additionally, sensitivity analyses most often are used to identify the most important parameters in terms of impact on the result on which to perform a probabilistic uncertainty assessment (e.g., Burmaster and Anderson, 1994; Price et al., 1996; Richards and Rowe, 1999; Schwartz, 2000). In this context, one needs to distinguish between important and sensitive parameters (Hamby, 1994). If a sensitive parameter is known precisely, it adds little to the variability of the output and, thus, its importance is restricted. Important parameters, in turn, are sensitive and rather uncertain.

According to Saltelli (2000), sensitivity analysis is “the study of how the variation in the output of a model (numerical or otherwise) can be apportioned, qualitatively or quantitatively, to different sources of variation, and of how the given model depends upon the information fed into it" (p. 3). In a more general sense, scenario analyses (see section 9.2.3) can be seen to also constitute a type of sensitivity analysis where not only the influence of variable parameters may be investigated. However, the definition of sensitivity analysis given above encompasses a variance decomposition in the results to the different influential factors ('apportioning of uncertainties') based on an uncertainty assessment for example of the Monte Carlo type (Saltelli, 2000). This is done by the class of *global sensitivity analysis* techniques (Campolongo et al., 2000b; Saltelli, 2000) which will not be considered further. The term 'sensitivity analysis' shall rather be used here in its original meaning according to Saltelli (2000) which is dealing with uncertainty in the parameters (cf. Cox and Baybutt, 1981).[29] The main purpose of sensitivity analysis in the present work is to perform a so-called *factor screening* (Campolongo et al., 2000b), i.e., the identification of 'key' (Beck and Chen, 2000), 'important' (Campolongo et al., 2000a), 'influential' (Campolongo et al., 2000b), or 'critical' (Richards and Rowe, 1999) parameters. This is done by so-called screening approaches which are computationally economical and tend to provide only qualitative sensitivity measures for instance in the form of rankings (Hamby, 1994; Campolongo et al., 2000a). Such screening approaches constitute only an early step when performing a sensitivity analysis according to its broader definition (Saltelli, 2000). Whereas scenario analyses investigate the sensitivity of factors also other than parameters (see section 9.2.3), sensitivity analysis in this context focuses on the parameter values. Their purpose is to identify the most important parameters in this work and, thus, primarily address parameter uncertainty (Hamby, 1994).

There exist a variety of screening sensitivity approaches with remarkably differing complexity (Campolongo et al., 2000a) whose appropriateness is highly model-dependent (Campolongo et al., 2000b). These can be classified as internal and as external validation tools and may allow to vary one parameter or several at a time (Schwartz, 2000). A straightforward example for those sensitivity analysis methods allowing to vary one parameter is the differential sensitivity analysis (Finley and Paustenbach, 1994; Hamby, 1994; Saltelli, 2000) which is termed 'standard one-factor-at-a-time' (OAT) or *ceteris paribus* sensitivity screening methods by Campolongo et al. (2000a). A control scenario or experiment is defined in which all parameters assume their 'nominal', 'control' or 'reference' values (Campolongo et al., 2000b; Saltelli, 2000). Then several runs are performed

---

[29] Note that the distinction into input variables and model parameters is not made here. According to Campolongo et al. (2000a) among others, "(i)nput variables are directly observable in the corresponding real system, whereas parameters are not (they may be estimated)" (p. 66).

in which only one parameter is changed at a time in a defined range. Different variations from the nominal value can be found in the literature for example 5 % (Saltelli, 2000), 10 % (Finley and Paustenbach, 1994), or 20 % (Price et al., 1996). One has to keep in mind, however, that this approach should be used only when the model to be investigated is known to be linear (Saltelli, 2000) which is the case for the linear algebra approach of the Mackay-type.

Another way of performing screening sensitivity analysis is not to just assume a fix variation employed to each parameter but to either assume probability density functions (based on parametric statistics) or ranges of variation (non-parametric statistics) for each parameter (Saltelli, 2000). In order to become even more complex, the parameter (or factor) variation can be done by random sampling or experimental design in which case not just one parameter (factor) is changed (Saltelli, 2000).

In this work, the standard OAT approach is followed whose advantage Schwartz (2000) emphasises by stating that it "always results in the same sensitivity indices, irrespective of the number of investigated variables, and is easily reproducible without further software" (p. 20). It is, therefore, selected for the identification of the most influential or key parameters which is appropriate for linear models (Campolongo et al., 2000b).

9.2.5 Probabilistic uncertainty assessment

The parameter sensitivity analysis presented in the previous section constitutes a highly useful prerequisite prior to performing a probabilistic uncertainty assessment in order to economically focus the efforts (e.g., Burmaster and Anderson, 1994; Price et al., 1996; Richards and Rowe, 1999; Schwartz, 2000). Probabilistic uncertainty assessments address the variability and uncertainty in the parameter values, preferably even separately (Burmaster and Anderson, 1994) as done for instance by Price et al. (1996) and Mekel and Fehr (2000). These are carried out by defining either ranges or probability density functions to each of the prioritised parameters (United States - Environmental Protection Agency, 1992; Saltelli, 2000). In a next step, different sets of parameter values are sampled from these ranges or distributions. Many model runs are conducted in this way in order to yield not just a range of outputs but also a probability density function of these indicating the assessed likelihood of each of the model result ranges (percentiles) to occur. There is also guidance in terms of principles of good practice available suggested in the scientific literature (Burmaster and Anderson, 1994).

Examples of such probability parameter uncertainty assessments include Monte Carlo techniques, Markov chain methods and Gibbs sampling procedures (Richards and Rowe, 1999). Of these, Monte Carlo techniques are the most commonly used methods. There are also different sampling schemes (Campolongo et al., 2000b) of which simple random or Latin hypercube sampling are generally employed in risk assessments (United States - Environmental Protection Agency, 1997d).

The main advantage of the probabilistic parameter uncertainty analysis in the context of exposure assessments is that it characterizes a range of potential risks and their likelihood of occurrence (e.g., Finley and Paustenbach, 1994). This result cannot be replaced by other techniques. Its main disadvantage is the big computational effort in terms of time and hardware (Cox and Baybutt, 1981; Burmaster and Anderson, 1994; Finley and Paustenbach, 1994; Schwartz, 2000). The assignment of an appropriate probability density function to each prioritised parameter is also a topic of its own (Finley and Paustenbach, 1994; Campolongo et al., 2000b). Cox and Baybutt (1981) term the problem of the right selection of a distribution for a parameter the 'uncertainty in the uncertainty'. However, it appears as if the selection of the distribution function as such has less an influence than for instance the choice of the allowed ranges (Finley and Paustenbach, 1994; Campolongo et al., 2000b). Another disadvantage for the present work is related to the way the model to be evaluated here is implemented (see section 4.4). There are different software products for probabilistic uncertainty assessments available for spreadsheet applications like Crystal Ball® or Risk 4.5®. However, the model developed here is not a spreadsheet model. Respective off-the-shelf probabilistic uncertainty assessment plug-ins are not available. As a consequence, a tailored probabilistic uncertainty assessment would need to be implemented which has not been possible especially due to time constraints. It is, therefore, not possible to include a probabilistic uncertainty assessment of the critical parameters in the present uncertainty analysis.

9.2.6 Expert judgement

There are several evaluation approaches which involve the judgement of (independent) experts. These include face validity, Turing test and publication of the model and its results in the open-literature or other types of peer review (Sargent, 1984; Tsang, 1991; Rykiel (Jr.), 1996; Beck and Chen, 2000). These evaluations require the availability of resources, i.e., time, on the side of the respective experts to allocate to the inspection of the model. Apart from funded model evaluation exercises and review in the open-literature this will hardly be possible to achieve so that the obvious publication in the open-literature constitutes a good alternative to allow experts to have a closer look at the model and its results.

9.3 Followed approach

A thorough in-depth evaluation of the presented external cost assessment would constitute a major task in its own right. Therefore, a more semi-quantitative approach to model evaluation is followed in the present work. The basis of the uncertainty analysis constitutes the minimum requirements articulated by United States - Environmental Protection Agency (1997c) and described in section 9.2.1. This qualitative uncertainty analysis presented in section 9.3.1 is supplemented by scenario analyses as mostly a decision-rule uncertainty assessment tool (cf. section 9.2.3) and parameter sensitivity analysis (cf. section 9.2.4). In both cases, a prioritisation of the assumptions to be varied and the parameters to be included will take place (see sections 9.3.3 and 9.3.4). In order to evaluate the model's accuracy, a comparison with reported values will be presented in section 9.3.2.

Before evaluating a model, its purpose and context needs to be defined explicitly. The purpose of the Impact Pathway Approach is to provide external cost estimates that are specific to a human activity, be it a single or a collective/societal activity. This way it supports the decision-making process with respect to conducting cost-benefit analyses of different policy options. The focus of this work is to assess the external costs resulting from human health impacts that are due to indirect exposure in order to provide decision-support at the European Union level and/or its member countries including acceding and (potential) accession countries. This implies for example that the assessment be done at the European scale. Additionally, a certain degree of spatial resolution is required in order to link the different human activities to the regionally occurring impacts. The 'context' of the model describes its applicability or limitations as a result of the underlying assumptions.

9.3.1 Qualitative uncertainty analysis according to United States - Environmental Protection Agency (1997c)

As part of the qualitative uncertainty analysis of exposure assessments, it shall be outlined to what extent the addressed assumptions or choices may influence the results of the assessment (United States - Environmental Protection Agency, 1997c).

Mathematical approach, non-linearities and equilibrium partitioning

In particular the environmental fate model is formulated as an inhomogeneous system of ordinary linear first order differential equations (cf. section 4.2) according to the Mackay-type approach (Mackay, 1979, 1991). This linear formulation has been adopted due to the ease of computation, the flexibility in terms of output, i.e., steady-state and dynamic computations which can be used for different contexts (cf. section 4.4.2 on different temporal modes of operation). This is generally oversimplifying for example environmental inhomogeneities and adsorption behaviours of trace elements (e.g., Kleeberg, 1992; Addiscott, 1993; Selim and Amacher, 2001; Smedley and Kinniburgh, 2003). However, due to the data demand of alternative modelling concepts at the scale and spatial resolution required, it is deemed a valid (at least initial) approach.

When developing a multimedia model of the Mackay-type, one has principally three options how to formulate the equations. Mackay and co-workers have based their models on fugacity (Mackay, 1979, 1991; Diamond et al., 1992; Wania and Mackay, 1995; Cousins and Mackay, 2001), whereas it is also possible to formulate them based on concentrations (Brandes et al., 1996) or mass (Pennington et al., 2005). The approaches are principally equivalent although the fugacity models have problems with substances that are rather involatile ('aquivalent' approach by Mackay and Diamond, 1989 and Diamond et al., 1992). In the end, it is a matter of preference how to formulate the mass balance.

The choice of a box model of the Mackay-type brings about the assumption of homogeneity and intra-compartmental equilibrium. While the issue of homogeneity is addressed below, it shall be noted that the assumption of equilibrium is not appropriate for substances that sorb strongly to particles and/or undergo rapid transformation (e.g., Mulkey et al., 1993). For reasons given in section 3.2.3, the assumption of equilibrium is, nevertheless, made which may lead to an overestimation or underestimation of the results, depending on the effective mobility of the substance (cf. United States - Environmental Protection Agency, 1996a), its characteristics in terms of most important exposure pathways, and the time horizon analysed or the discount rate chosen.

Worst case vs. representative estimates

It has been the intention within this study to avoid the use of conservative or worst-case data and assumptions. The problem to arrive at a so-called "cumulative worst case" (Schwartz, 2000, p. 21) where the combination of several worst-case parameter values turns the assessment overly conservative (cf. Price et al., 1996) is, therefore, expected to be highly reduced. As it has been made use of expectation values (e.g., averages) the assessment is rather believed to result in reasonable or representative estimates. However, the present methodology partly draws on approaches whose objective it is to provide assistance in the regulatory safeguard standard setting process which are targeted for example at the Maximally Exposed Individual (MEI) or the Reasonable Maximal Exposure (RME, Finley and Paustenbach, 1994; Richards and Rowe, 1999; Schwartz, 2000). This is especially the case for the exposure assessment for which it has been tried to modify worst-case assumptions to meet the purpose of this work (cf. section 7.1). However, there is still a chance that at times the mean exposure is significantly higher than the point estimate based on mean parameter values (McKone and Ryan, 1989; Hertwich et al., 2000). Due to this circumstance, even the present assessment may result in overestimated exposures, impacts and external costs.

Consideration of background and speciation

At present, no background concentration of the trace elements analysed is taken into account. As long as the model is linear and no comparison with scientific or regulatory standards is to be made, there is no need for the inclusion of any background concentration information. This is because the background cancels down when performing scenario comparisons (e.g., with and without a given emission). Furthermore, it is the anthropogenically added fraction that is more (bio-) available than the naturally occurring amounts (Berrow and Burridge, 1991; Alloway and Steinnes, 1999; Greger, 1999). Not considering releases from the natural background of heavy metals is additionally supported by de Vries et al. (2004) who argue that "weathering causes only a minor flux of metals, while uncertainties of such calculations are very high" (p. 10).

Note that when keeping the assumption of linearity but still trying to consider the natural background it does not suffice to introduce it as an initial condition for steady-state analyses. This is because it is only the fluxes that matter in this situation. Rather one would have to define a new process which may be termed 'weathering' which releases the natural background into the active pool to be modelled. This is, however, a rather slow process (Colman, 1981; Drever and Clow, 1995; Greger, 1999). One could, therefore, also consider to add a new compartment into which trace elements might be transferred by 'irreversible binding' and released (again) due to weathering. For the modelling of weathering, the reader is referred to the literature (e.g., Hoosbeek and Bryant, 1992; Drever and Clow, 1995; Drever, 1997a; Lasaga, 1995; White and Brantley, 1995; Trudgill, 2000).

It is not only that the background of the same contaminant is not taken into account but also the presence of other pollutants is not considered ('mixtures'). In particular the important effect of competing ions for adsorption sites and ligands in the environment (Bolt and van Riemsdijk, 1987; Hering and Morel, 1990; Schmitt and Sticher, 1991; Borkovec et al., 1998; Jenne, 1998a; Anonymous, 1999b; Vulava et al., 2000; Aboul-Kassim and Simoneit, 2001b; Sauvé 2002) as well as for example in human bodies (Choudhury et al., 2000) is not taken into account except for protons in the different environmental media (pH-dependent partitioning). This may lead to an overestimation of the adsorption of the modelled metals (which may be regarded as non-conservative, United States - Environmental Protection Agency, 1996a) and, thus, to longer residence times. This might have a pronounced effect on the assessment of external costs especially when employing non-zero discounting schemes. The competition for ligands, in turn, might result in a higher portion of the metal that is present as a free ion which is usually more bioavailable and can, thus, act in a more toxic way than complexes with ligands other than water molecules (McBride, 1994; Wolt, 1994; Ritchie and Sposito, 1995; Schnoor, 1996). The distinction between different complexes would involve the modelling of different species which is at present not implemented in the software tool WATSON.

When talking about different ligands the issue of speciation needs to be addressed as well. As stated in section 4.2.3, speciation is not taken into account, but phase partitioning according to the linear K_d value concept (Anonymous, 1999a; Aboul-Kassim and Simoneit, 2001b). Depending on how the employed bioconcentration factors are determined, the disregard of speciation may lead to overestimations of the food concentrations since differing susceptibilities of different substance species towards transfer into living tissues are not taken into account (Berrow and Burridge, 1991; Kabata-Pendias and Pendias, 1992; Ritchie and Sposito, 1995; Markert, 1998; Helmke, 1999). The uncertainty introduced of course also depends on the substance to be assessed. For instance, it was shown that cadmium in freshwater mostly occurs as the free metal ion (Vuceta and Morgan, 1978). This, however, strongly depends on the availability of dissolved organic compounds (e.g., fulvic acids) which is also relevant for soils (Bergkvist et al., 1989; Stoeppler, 1992; Otto et al., 2001).

Furthermore, the disregard of mixtures may lead to an underestimation or overestimation of effects if two or more substances interact in a more than additive (or synergistic) or antagonistic way, respectively (Mücke 6/1995; Kroes, 1996). Thus, the different contaminants are assumed to exert their effects in a non-interactive way for example by simple similar or simple dissimilar action (Kroes, 1996). Effect assessments of mixtures still constitutes a rather open field of research (e.g., Steinberg et al. 6/1995; Escher and Hermens, 2002) which is also why current approaches to assessing the toxic effects of mixtures still treat effects as essentially being additive (Choudhury et al., 2000) in the absence of clear evidence of antagonistic effects.

Spatial differentiation into zones and compartments

Externalities are a concept within welfare economics which is mostly of interest to policy makers. For substances that undergo long-range transport by advection in air or water, externalities may not only occur in the vicinity of the source but also in rather distant places where substances arrive at (European Commission, 1999a; Barbante et al., 2001; Friedrich and Bickel, 2001a; Scheringer and Wania, 2003; Wania, 2003). These substances may, thus, undergo transboundary transport which is why such externalities are mostly of interest to national authorities and/or governments in charge of international affairs. As a result, the assessment of externalities of such substances requires the operation at rather large scales. Furthermore, they should be rather spatially-resolved in order to allow for the discrimination of effects to occur at different administrative units. This means, for instance, that releases of rather involatile substances into a freshwater body should not lead to in-stream concentrations upstream of the release site (e.g., emissions into the Dutch part of the Rhine show up in Swiss Alpine lakes within the catchment when only discriminating according to watersheds, cf. Fig. 4-2). Therefore, a rather high degree of spatial differentiation should not only be assured during the impact assessment but also during the environmental fate assessment. The influence of choosing different spatial resolutions when delimiting according to watersheds will be explored by a scenario analysis in section 9.3.3.

The geographical scope is mostly confined to Europe (cf. Fig. 4-3). The present modelling framework is set up as a system with open boundaries. Exports of substances occur via air and water flows or sediment burial. However, there is no import included since neither intercontinental water and air advection nor (re-)imports of substances (e.g., contained in food) from outside Europe are considered. Thus, substances with the potential to undergo for instance intercontinental transport via air, ocean currents or migrating species cannot properly be addressed leading to an underestimation of effects due to the open system boundaries. Such intercontinental transport is even observed for particle-bound trace elements (Church et al., 1990).

The geographical scope of WATSON has been spatially differentiated into zones according to watersheds (cf. section 4.3). Other delineation criteria exist including a regular grid (e.g., Prevedouros et al., 2004) and combinations of watersheds with other criteria (e.g., Devillers et al., 1995; MacLeod et al., 2001). The influence of the selection of one such delineation scheme on model results is not known.

WATSON allows the distinction of several compartments (sections 5.1 and 6.1). These are assumed to be internally homogeneous and to have temporally constant properties except for the substance amounts contained. The influence of the choice of which compartments to consider is evaluated by means of a scenario analysis below.

As described in section B.4.3, the water volume of a zone consists of streams and lakes fully contained in that zone. If both streams and lakes are present, this means that virtually all water entering the zone is assumed to flow through the lake(s) with longer residence times as well although only parts may actually pass through the lake (e.g., small lake to the East of lake Vänern within the Götälv catchment, Fig. 6-2). This may lead to higher concentrations in the freshwater body of this zone while reducing the input to downstream freshwater bodies. The net effect on human exposure and finally impact depends on the distribution of the freshwater fish production intensities and is, thus, not unambiguous.

Although the presented methodology is site-dependent, some non-substance-dependent properties especially influencing a substance's environmental fate and exposure are treated as if they do not vary in space. Such property values will not be representative for all locations to which they are applied. For instance, the depths of the sediment, glacier and soil compartments are invariant between zones. This may underestimate for example the root uptake by those crops whose roots reach further into the ground than the assumed soil depth, provided the substances reach this depth to considerable amounts. This may not so much affect lead, for instance, as it appears to be concentrated in the top most centimetres (Nriagu, 1978; Rickard and Nriagu, 1978) although contradicting evidence exists (Martínez García et al., 1999). The constant water volume content is deemed not to affect the results as long as the homogeneity assumption for within soils and the linear relationship between the pore water concentration and the plant concentration according to the bioconcentration factor (BCF) are maintained. However, the constant volume fraction of solids in soils has some implications when allowing the organic carbon content to vary. This will lead to varying densities of the overall solid phase in soils (cf. Eq. (B-10)). The way the equilibrium distribution coefficient is defined (cf. section A.2) this means that the smaller the solid phase density the less of the substance is associated with the solid phase. However, it is the organic matter phase which is highly relevant not only for hydrophobic substances but also for many trace elements in terms of the solid-water partitioning (Nriagu, 1978; McCutcheon et al., 1993; Aboul-Kassim and Simoneit, 2001a). A lower solid phase density will lead to a smaller fraction adsorbed and, thus, to an increased mobility and bioavailability of the respective substance in those areas where high organic carbon contents exist. As a result, the retention of the substance in the respective soil compartments is reduced which may potentially mean an earlier exposure when compared to those soil compartment with lower organic carbon contents. For the uncertainties associated with the exposure-related parameters refer to United States - Environmental Protection Agency (1998).

There are parts of the environment which are not included entirely, i.e., they are not part of or constitute own compartments. First, the marine environment is not included which brings about that exposure is underestimated due to lack of inclusion of sea fish and shellfish consumption. The same applies to exposures via drinking water which to rather large degrees originates from ground water bodies. A more detailed discussion why the marine environment and ground water, and the related exposure pathways have been excluded from the assessment is given in section 7.3. Furthermore, the inhalation exposure of farm animals is not considered. This is believed not to cause a substantial underestimation of the exposure results which is in line with Ewers and Wilhelm (1995) and Wilhelm and Ewers (1999) for cadmium and lead, respectively.

Implications of the coupling of an air quality model to a water-soil environmental fate model

The coupling of an air quality model to an environmental fate model comprising the media soil and water limits the amount of substances that can possibly be assessed (cf. section 4.1.1). If substances are rather volatile an assessment is to be favoured in which either all media are fully integrated into one model or in which several subsequent iterative computations of both models are performed. This also holds if wind soil erosion (e.g., Nriagu, 1989; Alloway and Steinnes, 1999) leads to a substantial redistribution of substances which is at present not taken into account.

The use of air dispersion models has advantages over multimedia models of the Mackay-type if spatially differentiated emission information is available (Hertwich et al., 2000). Whether this advantage will lead to a higher or a lower estimate of the external costs largely depends on the distribution of both the substance sources and the population density.

Selection of processes and their formulation

It is not the intention here to review all processes, their formulation and the specific data used. The reasoning for the selection of the respective environmental and substance data is provided in Appendices B and C while the formulation of the processes is described in Appendix A following the mathematical approach as specified in section 2.3.2. Some of the process-related uncertainties will be addressed semi-quantitatively by means of scenario analyses and sensitivity analyses of supposedly important parameters in sections 9.3.3 and 9.3.4, respectively. Some related aspects not taken up again later will, nevertheless, be addressed in the following.

All environmental processes are kept constant in time mostly according to long-term average conditions. As a result, variability within one year and between years are not taken into account, such as changes in redox potentials, acidification, discharge, rain rates and distributions thereof, and temperature. Computations with time steps that are not full years are, therefore, not adequate in terms of resulting meaningful values for the respective period of time (e.g., seasonal, monthly, daily variations). Furthermore, predictions into the future are hampered due to the fact that "natural systems are dynamic and may change in unanticipated ways" (Oreskes et al., 1994, p. 643). Additionally, active management of the environment is not considered either. This may apply to changes in land uses, management of rivers in terms of dams as well as sedimentation and erosion control, and irrigation.

According to the *concept of geomorphic thresholds*, processes such as erosion, sediment and dissolved substance transport in rivers are not associated with average conditions but with single events (Schumm, 1977; Neal et al., 1997). These may occur even just once in a hundred or more years and may, therefore, not be contained even in long-term average data that are based on observations of a few decades time (see sections 2.3 and B.5.2). These processes will lead to a redistribution of substances from soils to surface waters and partly also to soils on floodplains.

The process of wind soil erosion is not included in the assessment for reasons given in section 4.1.1. Depending on for instance the climatic conditions, the common agricultural practice and the most relevant food item in terms of human exposure, this process may lead to higher or lower concentrations in the environmental compartments most important for human exposure. As a result, the exposure may be overestimated or underestimated due to the disregard of this process especially according to a spatially-resolved assessment that takes spatial variability for example in terms of areas potentially prone to this process and distribution of food production into account.

As stated above, irrigation is not considered. This may not be too significant in the large basins of central Europe but, for instance, in Spain (Döll et al., 2003). Similar to flooding, irrigation may influence the concentration of substances (a) in freshwater bodies due to transfer of these onto land and due to reduced water volumes and (b) in soils which receive the irrigation water.

Depending on the most important exposure pathway of the substance to be assessed, thus, the disregard of event-based (extreme) situations and the management of the environment by humans may lead to an overestimation or underestimation of the exposure.

In the case of intermittent rain, Hertwich et al. (2000) conclude that rain is important in multimedia models due to substantially prolonging the residence time in air for chemicals with a low Henry's Law constant as well as for non-volatile metals, residing only in the particle phase. When analysing the potential dose, however, the only remarkably affected chemicals were those for which most exposure occurs through inhalation (Hertwich et al., 2000). This shows that first the selection of the evaluated endpoint (here: residence time vs. potential or time-integrated dose) is relevant when assessing the importance of an assumption. Secondly, the assumption of steady rainfall in the air quality model WTM is likely not to affect the overall exposure estimate in the present assessment substantially.

The approach to model rivers differently from lakes is considered an improvement towards screening risk assessments in which water bodies are usually modelled to entirely behave like lakes, i.e., showing long residence times of water and, hence, substances (cf. section 6.1.5). This will on the one hand accelerate inputs into lakes but on the other hand also accelerate transport beyond the model's boundary downstream from lakes, i.e., into the sea. Assuming that not only the sediment particles are resuspended but also the substances present in the pore water, furthermore, increases the backflow to the water column. Although the modifications do not result in a reduced overall exposure towards freshwater fish when compared to the approach taken by screening risk assessments (cf. section 9.3.3), the way the particle dynamics in freshwater bodies is modelled as introduced here is deemed more appropriate.

As stated in section B.5.2, evaporation and consumptive water abstraction from larger water bodies are not considered due to data processing problems. This results in an overestimation of runoff and discharge. Due to the higher flushing rates, lower concentrations are estimated for some freshwater bodies which will also lower the concentration in fish following equilibrium partitioning according to bioconcentration factors.

Exposure assessment

The exposure assessment is incomplete in terms of the exposure pathways considered. Generally direct exposures in the sense of the definition used by European Centre for Ecotoxicology and Toxicology of Chemicals (1994) and European Commission (2003a) are not taken into account, i.e., exposures for example at the working place or through consumer products. This includes contamination of food and drinking water due to packaging and food preparation.

Beside exposure to drinking water and sea food, especially unintentional soil ingestion by humans is not included in the assessment which may have a substantial impact on the overall exposure situation towards rather persistent substances that are directly released into soils (Huijbregts, 1999; Huijbregts et al., 2000b). This will underestimate the overall exposure. Furthermore, food preparation such as milling, washing, peeling and cooking especially of vegetables may reduce more or less appreciably the concentrations of some substances (World Health Organisation, 1992b; Harrison, 2001a) which has not been taken into account.

The issue of worst-case assumptions has been addressed above and will not be repeated here. The application of the exposure part of a risk assessment framework developed in the US to European conditions is considered defendable. Potentially hidden obstacles may exist, for instance, with regard to different susceptibilities of the cultivated plants and/or kept farm animals in terms of uptake of substances. Also the selection of the exposure assessment scheme followed will influence the results. This will be analysed by means of a scenario analysis (cf. Table 9-4).

Receptor information is distributed according to different schemes if the data are provided at an administrative level that does not correspond to the lowest distinguished level (cf. section B.6). This means that, for instance, German annual production data on freshwater fish are distributed to the municipal level according to the freshwater volume present in the different municipalities. Depending on the resulting distribution of the food production and the assessed emissions, and the exposure pathway contributing most to the overall exposure, this may lead to an overestimation or underestimation of the exposure.

Sticking to the freshwater fish example, the freshwater volume may, furthermore, not be a good indicator for the distribution of the places where freshwater fish are kept and/or caught. It has been necessary for this particular example to additionally assume that freshwater fish are kept in water whose composition is equal to that of the freshwater bodies estimated by the fate model. This disregards the circumstance that people are not just angling in natural waters but that there is also aquaculture going on in separate lakes and/or ponds. Due to the presumably smaller water volume with potentially less inputs than into naturally occurring lake-stream networks, however, this may lead to both overestimations or underestimations of the exposure towards diffuse emissions. In the case of direct releases into freshwater bodies, the exposure assessed according to the presented approach will most likely be overestimated.

Trade is presently considered in a rather simple way. Whereas for the environmental fate assessment the system boundaries are open, these are assumed to be closed for the exposure assessment. This will overestimate the exposure within Europe that is attributable to European human activities due to export of contaminated food and import of mostly uncontaminated food, at least with respect to substances from European sources.[30] Additionally, it is obvious from trade statistics (Food and Agriculture Organization of the United Nations - Statistics Division, 2002a) that the net trade of certain food products is different between countries. This may lead to higher exposures even at the society level if the food items produced in the respective country show a higher load with respect to certain substances while at the same being exported to a lesser extent.

[30] Note that some degree of re-import may occur.

The exposure assessment allows to distinguish between different produce in terms of species. However, there are different susceptibilities not only in terms of species but also for instance in terms of different varieties of the same species and different climatic conditions (e.g., in the case of cadmium, Ursínyová and Hladíová, 2000a) beside other influences. This may over- or underestimate the presently undifferentiated exposure.

As with the environmental properties, the production, consumption and human population data are assumed to be constant with time. Whether this assumption leads to an overestimation or underestimation cannot be clearly stated. The development of the population, for instance, is uncertain. There appears to be a large probability about humankind to exist in the future (Daly and Cobb (1989) quoted in Hellweg et al. (2003)). However, the size of the population living for example in Europe is not known.

No distinction is made with respect to different population sub-groups in terms of exposure such as adults vs. children or smokers vs. non-smokers. The choice not to distinguish between different population sub-groups appears to be justified given the presently available effect information and the circumstance that a very localised exposure assessment such as towards indoor air is not intended by the developed methodology.

It shall, furthermore, be noted that the exposure via ingestion is generally more uncertain than that via inhalation in multi-pathway exposure assessments (e.g., MacLeod et al., 2004).

Impact assessment

As noted by Finley and Paustenbach (1994), the total variability in the exposure variables may be much less than the total variability in the toxicity values emphasizing the importance of reliable impact assessment approaches. Also Rabl and Spadaro (1999) and Droste-Franke et al. (2003) find that effect-related uncertainties are largest.

There is little epidemiological dose- or exposure-response information available for toxic effects following indirect exposures (cf. review by Searl, 2002). As a consequence, the use of the approach as suggested by Crettaz and coworkers (Crettaz, 2000; Crettaz et al., 2002; Pennington et al., 2002; section 7.3.1) is the only approach that is known to the author. Crettaz (2000) discusses the uncertainty sources related to the β_{ED10} slope factor approach which shall not be repeated here. Sources of uncertainty that are addressed include animal to human extrapolation in terms of effects, exposure and/or kinetics, high to low dose extrapolation (without assuming thresholds), subchronic to lifetime exposure extrapolation, inter-individual variability and data quality including experimental design (e.g., number of animals studied). In case that the true dose-response curve has a sigmoidal shape, the linear extrapolation towards lower doses will overestimate the effects (World Health Organisation, 2000b).

There is no scientific basis for assuming a threshold or no-effect level for chemical carcinogens (World Health Organisation, 2000b). This is because most agents that cause cancer also cause irreversible damage to deoxyribonucleic acid (DNA). The linear extrapolation approach can basically be justified in light of the similarities between carcinogenesis and mutagenesis as processes that both have DNA as target molecules with strong evidence for linear dose–response relationships for mutagenesis (World Health Organisation, 2000b). Furthermore, the susceptibility towards effects due to exposure to substances varies between individuals (inter-individual variability) which supports the assumption of having a non-threshold effect situation at the population level (cf. section 7.3).

The situation is different for non-carcinogens for which there exists an unresolved debate on the existence of or ability to measure thresholds and on the extrapolation of the dose-effect curve towards low doses (e.g., Krewitt et al., 2002). Therefore, external cost results due to carcinogenic effects will be stated separately from non-carcinogenic effects. Generally, if the non-threshold assumption was not tenable effects that are assessed at exposure levels below the respective threshold value would lead to an overestimation of the external costs.

The assumptions related to the human health impact indicator DALY are discussed in section 7.3. The use of the highest life expectancy at birth observed on earth is considered not to introduce an unacceptable bias when applied to the European population. The discussion on the disability weights in section 7.3.7 concludes that the disability weights for cancers as given by Crettaz et al. (2002) are considered to underestimate the years lived with a disability to some extent. In fact, the variation in the disability weight may span a few orders of magnitude depending on the method employed to determine them and the people that are involved (Schwarzinger et al., 2003). As also noted by Crettaz (2000), the uncertainties associated with the DALYp approach for non-carcinogenic effects is, furthermore, higher than for carcinogenic effects due to the subjective classification of the effects into default effect categories.

Valuation

During the valuation step different value choices are expected to be made. As noted in section 8.1, discounting is always performed when one has to deal with intertemporal effects that may or may not be valued in monetary terms. Different discounting schemes may have a profound effect on the present valuation of future impacts (Weitzmann, 1999) which may even outweigh all other influencing factors (Hellweg et al., 2003). Also the way how the Monetary value of a life year lost (VLYL) is determined may not allow for its applicability to any person living in the scope of the assessment, opening room to both ends of the scale.

As it is tried to communicate the external costs as explicitly and transparently as possible and due to the provision of sensitivity results of different discount rates, it is believed that the present study gives a good idea of the range of possible outcomes.

The potential effect of considering latency times and using a different approach to value pain and suffering-related external costs has already been discussed in section 8.2.

Miscellaneous assumptions and choices

In the following, some miscellaneous assumptions and choices shall be evaluated affecting the outcome of the assessment:

- at present the air quality model WTM provides the upper boundary condition with respect to indirect inputs into the aquatic and terrestrial environment following emissions to air (cf. section 4.1). Those portions of a substance that remain in air are not considered in the further analysis especially when assessing pulse emissions. This leads to an underestimation of impacts and, thus, external costs. The same applies to those substance amounts that are transported beyond the system boundary of the air quality model.
- information on emissions that directly enter the media soil and/or water is rather scarce and is, therefore, not considered at present. As stated in section 4.4.1, WATSON offers the possibility to distribute aggregated emission information if available. Distribution schemes according to population densities or land uses will only approximately match the true distribution of sources. Depending on the distribution of the food production and the relevant exposure pathways, this may lead to higher or lower exposure estimates.
- potentially occurring effects on organisms do not show a feedback on the environmental fate of the substance causing this effect. For instance, if concentrations became elevated enough for substantial amounts of a forest to die or causing a shift from macrophytes to phytoplankton in rivers the changes in the dynamics of these ecosystems would not appropriately be taken into account.
- due to the spatial resolution of both the air quality model used and WATSON, localised contaminations such as along roads and on floodplains cannot be assessed appropriately (cf. sections 2.1.2 and 2.3). Due to the homogeneity assumption for compartments, elevated concentrations will be diluted unless the compartment area matches the area affected by the elevated

concentrations. Diluted concentrations mean a smaller uptake into the food chain and, hence, a smaller exposure.

9.3.2 Comparison with independent data

When defining the performance criterion for the compliance of the model results with independent data, one needs to define at what stage a model whose purpose is to assess external costs from indirect exposures shall be compared to independent data. The end point of the assessment are the external costs. However, the external costs due to health impacts of a particular substance are not measured themselves; neither are the substance-induced health impacts. If they were the modelling exercise in this work would be obsolete apart from the linkage between human activity and exposure. What remains for the comparison are the exposure levels of the different routes of exposure and the concentrations in the environmental media air, soil and water further up the assessment. Thus, only intermediate results can be compared to observed values in order to operationally validate the model (Rykiel (Jr.), 1996). Such partial analysis of an overall model is also advocated by Caswell (1976).

The model to be analysed here operates at the European scale in a spatially explicit way. The spatial coverage of monitoring activities, however, is usually confined to smaller geographical scopes with an appropriate sampling density. Additionally, the investigated substances are rather persistent and have been released into the environment due to human activities for centuries (e.g., Ryaboshapko et al., 1998; Brännvall et al., 1999), however, with incomplete records. As a consequence, even if the distinction of the metals occurring in the different media into a portion of natural origin and another that was introduced by human activities is made (as tried, e.g., by the FORum of European Geological Surveys (FOREGS) project to be finalized in 2005), the match between model results and observed data will merely be indicative unless some effort is spent to set up a historical emission scenario including for example localised mining activities and past and/or present agricultural practices (e.g., arsenic-containing pesticides, Gebel, 1999, or cadmium in phosphate fertilizers, Ewers and Wilhelm, 1995). This is a task of its own and will not be tried here. Any mismatch between observed values and estimated ones, therefore, does not mean that the model itself is unreliable or inapplicable to the actual context ('operational vs. data validity' as differentiated by Rykiel (Jr.) (1996) or 'check on output space or model as a whole vs. parameter space or parts of the model' as distinguished by Beck and Chen (2000)).

As a result, only the environmental media and food concentrations as estimated by the model can be compared to independent data. When looking for observed environmental media concentrations covering large parts of Europe, it is found that the most comprehensive dataset for trace elements is available for the HELCOM area, i.e., the countries and/or river catchments adjacent to the Baltic Sea (Reimann et al., 2003). Furthermore, there is ongoing effort to extend the Convention on Long-Range Transboundary Air Pollution (CLRTAP) under the umbrella of the United Nations Economic Commission for Europe (UN/ECE) from NO_x and SO_2 emissions to also cover POPs and heavy metals (Reinds et al., 1995; de Vries and Bakker, 1998; de Vries et al., 1998a, 1998b; de Vries, 1999; United Nations - Economic Commission for Europe, 1998; Schütze, 1999; Hettelingh et al., 2002). In this frame the International Cooperative Programme on Effects of Air Pollution on Natural Vegetation and Crops (ICP Vegetation) has issued moss monitoring results (Buse et al., 2003) which may serve to perform a pattern match between the atmospheric deposition fields as calculated by the air quality model WTM and the measured moss concentrations of the respective heavy metals and trace elements.

For food concentrations, there exist some information at the national level (Stoeppler, 1991, 1992; Ewers and Wilhelm, 1995; Wilhelm and Ewers, 1999; Ursínyová and Hladíová, 2000a, 2000b; Harrison, 2001a) and generically (Gebel, 1999; Hertl and Merk, 1999). These will be presented after the comparison of the moss survey results with the atmospheric deposition as assessed by the air quality model employed in this study.

Evaluation of atmospheric deposition fields

In order to evaluate the input data on which the WATSON model operates, the deposition fields as calculated by the air quality model WTM ('Windrose Trajectory Model') would best be compared to monitoring data. However, the data availability with respect to trace element concentrations and depositions is rather poor (cf. Droste-Franke et al., 2003). Recently a monitoring study has been published employing mosses as time-integrating collectors (Buse et al., 2003). The technique of moss analysis provides a surrogate measure of the spatial patterns of heavy metal deposition from the atmosphere to terrestrial systems. A shortcoming, however, is that moss monitoring results do not allow quantitative comparisons with real atmospheric depositions (Schmid-Grob et al., 1993) which is to a very large extent due to the non-standardisible collector 'moss'. Therefore, only a pattern match will be performed.

In the study, only naturally occurring mosses were sampled that were at most three years old and growing at least 300 metres from main roads and populated areas (Buse et al., 2003). Several countries were participating. Thus, the moss survey provides the most comprehensive dataset presently available in order to evaluate atmospheric depositions of trace elements to the terrestrial environment in Europe.

The sampling period in the moss survey was 2000/2001 (Buse et al., 2003). Therefore, the 1998 emission scenario as described and used by Droste-Franke et al. (2003) was used to conduct a pattern match between the moss monitoring results and the total atmospheric deposition fields based on the EMEP 50 x 50 km grid. Due to the uncertain nature of the emission extrapolations from 1990 to 1998 for lead, only arsenic, cadmium and chromium will be compared. Note that the units of the two datasets do not match: WTM results are given in micrograms per square metre and year whereas the moss concentrations are given in microgram per gram. Due to the fact that the integration time of the mosses for the collection of the respective samples is variable and may be as long as three years, no unit conversion is tried here.

The WTM results appear to predict elevated depositions of arsenic in the United Kingdom, Belgium and the so-called 'second black triangle of Europe' on the Czech Republic/Slovakian/Polish border in accordance with the moss survey (top of Fig. 9-1). The higher depositions in the 'black triangle' on the German/Czech Republic/Polish border may be due to a former hot spot of lignite power plants in a lignite mine area in the Czech Republic according to Buse et al. (2003) which is assumed to have been active in 1990, the year based on which the 1998 emission scenario was extrapolated (Droste-Franke et al., 2003). Buse et al. (2003) report that the main sources of heavy metals to the atmosphere in Italy are located in the north which conforms with the hot spot predicted by the WTM. However, this hot spot does not clearly show in the moss monitoring. According to the latter, the biggest hot spot occurs in the southern Romanian and Bulgarian area which only shows rudimentarily in the WTM results.

The atmospheric depositions for cadmium as predicted by the WTM comply with the moss monitoring results to a rather large degree with respect to the hot spots (bottom of Fig. 9-1): Depositions are highest in the so-called 'second black triangle of Europe', east of the Picardie area (northern France), in northern Italy and in southern Romania. The elevated moss concentrations in Portugal and in Bulgaria were partly due to forest fires and geochemical anomalies, respectively (Buse et al., 2003).

Both data sources show matching elevated depositions of chromium in the area of Belgium (metal production) and around Marseille (refineries and metallurgical industry, Fig. 9-2). As with arsenic, there is a hot spot of chromium predicted by the WTM in northern Italy which is to some extent reflected in the moss concentrations. Discrepancies between the two datasets occurring in Galicia (north-western Spain) and Bulgaria can be explained by elevated soil content and serpentine bedrock/old mines, respectively (Buse et al., 2003). The WTM results especially do not capture the area of elevated moss concentrations in Romania.

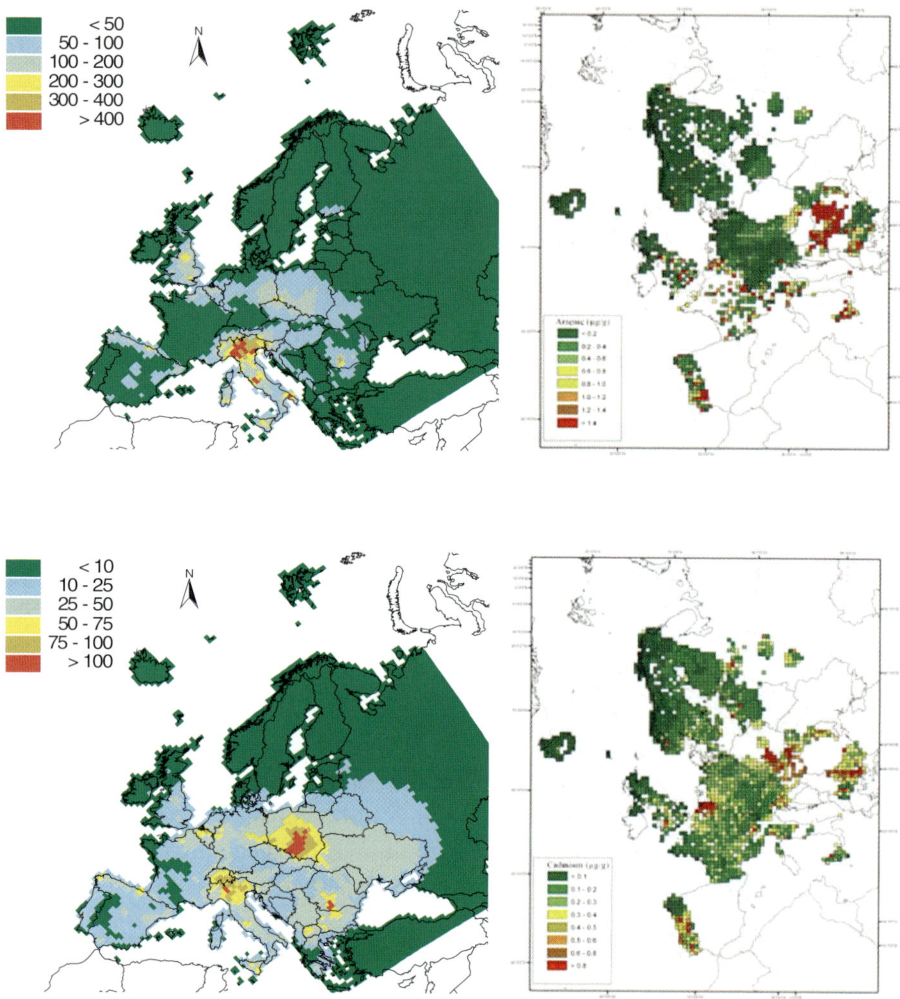

Fig. 9-1: Comparison of atmospheric depositions in micrograms per square metre and year based on air quality modelling by the Windrose Trajectory Model for emissions in year 1998 (left) and moss concentrations in micrograms per gram for the years 2000/2001 (right, taken from Buse et al. (2003) and including data for Iceland, with permission) for arsenic (top) and cadmium (bottom)

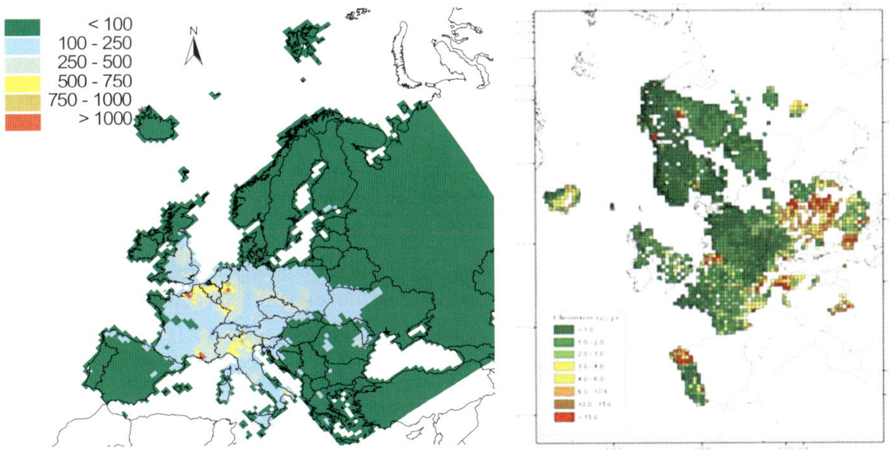

Fig. 9-2: Comparison of atmospheric depositions in micrograms per square metre and year based on air quality modelling by the Windrose Trajectory Model for emissions in year 1998 (left) and moss concentrations in micrograms per gram for the years 2000/2001 (right, taken from Buse et al. (2003) and including data for Iceland, with permission) for chromium

The comparison with the moss monitoring data reveals that the best match occurs for cadmium which is in line with a previous finding for air concentrations of these trace elements (Droste-Franke et al., 2003). This data validation exercise shows that a comparison of the environmental and food concentration data predicted by the WATSON model is only tentatively possible due to the rather poor input data in terms of atmospheric depositions. Whether this data quality issue is due to the emission data and/or the air quality model will not be further explored here.

Comparison with media and food concentration data

The concentrations in the different environmental media including food that are assessed by the presented methodology only take into account that fraction of the trace elements that was released into the environment by the human activities considered in the emission scenarios. Thus, neither the spatially variable natural background levels nor the historic anthropogenic releases and the resulting anthropogenic concentration levels can be considered. Due to lack of data, furthermore, no direct releases into the media soil and water could be included in the emission scenarios. In the absence of spatially-resolved monitoring data, merely a screening comparison of the respective media or food concentrations shall be carried out. These are compared to the concentrations assessed by the pan-European emission scenario for the year 1990 after a continuous release of 100 years (cf. section 11.2). Due to lack of a comprehensive time series on emission data, this scenario is perceived as a proxy for historic emissions since the industrial revolution. In the following, the trace elements shall be compared one by one.

The monitoring data found in the literature are given in Tables C-9, C-10, C-11 and C-12 in Appendix C for arsenic, cadmium, chromium and lead, respectively. These data serve the basis for the indication of ranges and median values to which the predicted concentrations are compared in the following Figures (Fig. 9-3 through 9-6). The predicted concentration values of soils and sediments are converted from kilogram per cubic metre bulk compartment to milligram per kilogram solid phase using spatially resolved solid phase densities and the default volume fractions of the bulk compartments that are solid phase (cf. section 5.1.3). If the lower boundary concentrations of the monitoring data are stated to be below the detection limit, half of the given detection limit is assumed as the observed concentration. In such cases, also the detection limit itself is shown in Fig. 9-3 through 9-6 (denoted as bars). Note that only values of uncontaminated samples are taken into account to the extent that these could be distinguished from contaminated ones. Further note that an attempt is made to consider the natural background. For this, the average concentrations in the upper continental crust are used as provided by Wedepohl (1995), also reproduced in Tables C-9 through C-12. These values are added to the predicted soil and sediment concentrations for the so-called '+ background' cases. In order to also assess the consequently higher concentrations in foodstuff, scaling factors are derived by relating the minimum, median and maximum values predicted in agricultural soils when considering background to those without taking background into account, respectively. These factors are then applied to the minimum, median and maximum values of all land-based produce, respectively, except for spinach. This way, it is assumed that the most contaminated foodstuff is related to the most contaminated agricultural soils and vice versa.

Without considering background, all environmental media concentrations tend to be at the lower end of or below than the (detectable) monitored concentrations (top of Fig. 9-3 through 9-6). For sediments, the discrepancy always amounts to at least two orders of magnitude. When adding the average natural background to these rather low predicted concentrations, it is not surprising that the resulting soil and sediment concentrations fall into the range of concentrations monitored for uncontaminated soils and sediments.

As regards the assessment of food concentrations, a similar picture is observed in that the predicted concentrations tend to be below those monitored without considering the natural average background in soils (bottom of Fig. 9-3 through 9-6). The difference is, however, less pronounced so that, for instance, the median spinach concentrations of lead and chromium are about the same as the expectation values of the used monitoring data. Note that there are no spinach-specific monitoring data available for lead and chromium so that the comparison can only be conducted with 'generic' vegetable monitoring data (cf. Tables C-11 and C-12). Further note that it does not become clear whether the chromium levels in several food groups including vegetables as reported by Hertl and Merk (1999) have been measured in samples of contaminated or pristine origin (cf. Table C-11). This could mean that uncontaminated samples may have smaller concentrations so that the predicted chromium concentrations also of other food groups may be in the same range as the measured concentrations.

When scaling the concentrations of those food items that are exclusively exposed via soil in order to consider the natural average background (see above), the predicted food concentrations are still lower than or compare well with those observed. The only food concentrations that are predicted to be higher than the expectation range of those measured are chromium in cereals and potatoes (cf. bottom of Fig. 9-5). The difference with respect to the median values amount to a factor of 16 and 25, respectively. In general, however, this comparison is flawed particularly by the circumstance that bioconcentration factors are used for the reactive or available portion of the trace elements in soils ("applied" contaminant, cf. United States - Environmental Protection Agency (1998) pp. A-3-18 ff.) to which by far not all of the natural background can be accounted (cf. Berrow and Burridge, 1991; Alloway and Steinnes, 1999; Greger, 1999). The '+ background' estimates, therefore, should have preferably been assessed based on the bioavailable amounts stemming from the natural background. This, however, brings about the necessity to consider the process of weathering whose modelling introduces rather large uncertainties (de Vries et al., 2004) which is why it is not done in the present study. Consequently, the comparison of the monitored levels with the predicted concentrations considering the average natural background is hampered and shall only serve illustrative purposes. Note that fish and spinach are not included in this background consideration exercise due to data availability constraints or the additional contamination pathway via air which does not allow simple scaling, respectively.

When analysing the contribution of different exposure pathways to the contamination of different food groups and in particular cattle products, it is interesting to note that soil ingestion by cattle may be rather dominant. The contribution by this exposure pathway may hold a share of at least 34 % up to 80 % of the chro-

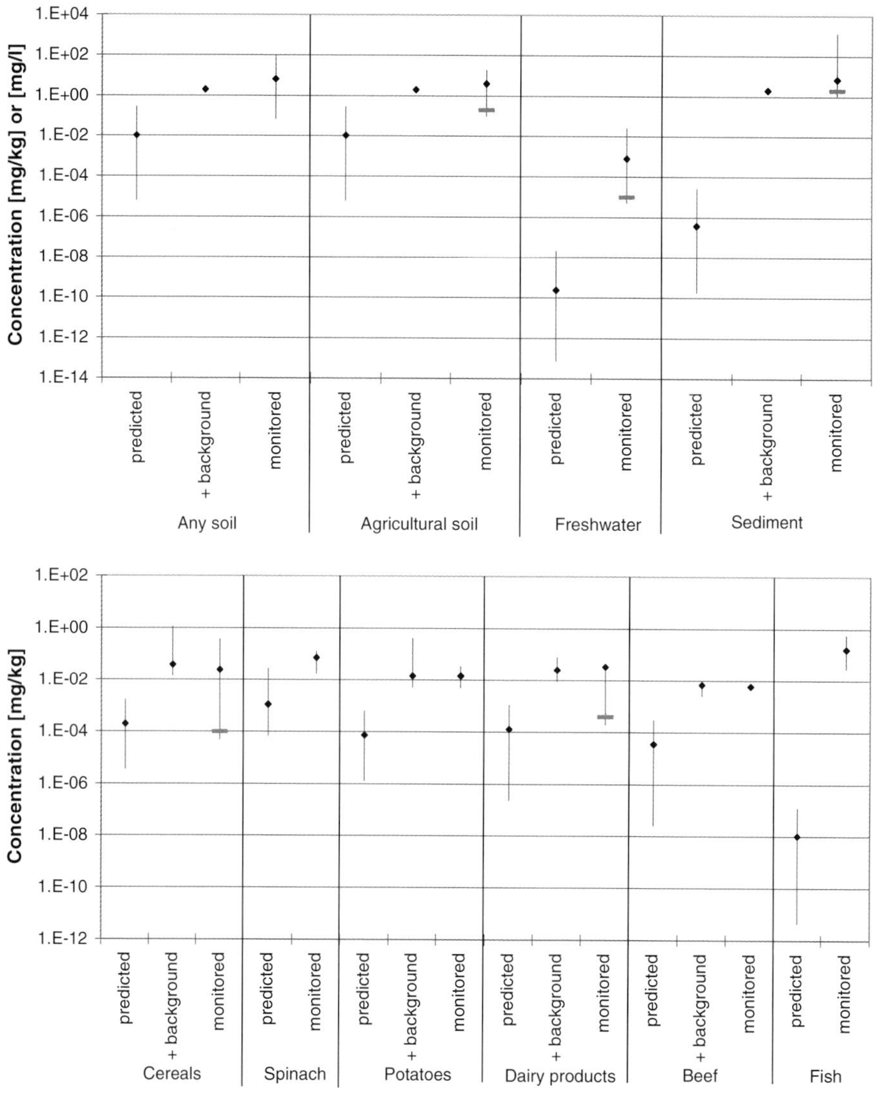

Fig. 9-3: Comparison of arsenic minimum, median and maximum concentrations as predicted by the environmental fate and exposure sub-models with reported concentrations in environmental media (top) and foodstuff (bottom, cf. Table C-9); model estimates based on the 'food removal' scenario described in Table 9-1 resulting from a 100 year continuous release according to the pan-European emission scenario for 1990 (cf. sections 11.1 and 11.2; different units; note the logarithmic scale, horizontal bars indicate reported detection limits)

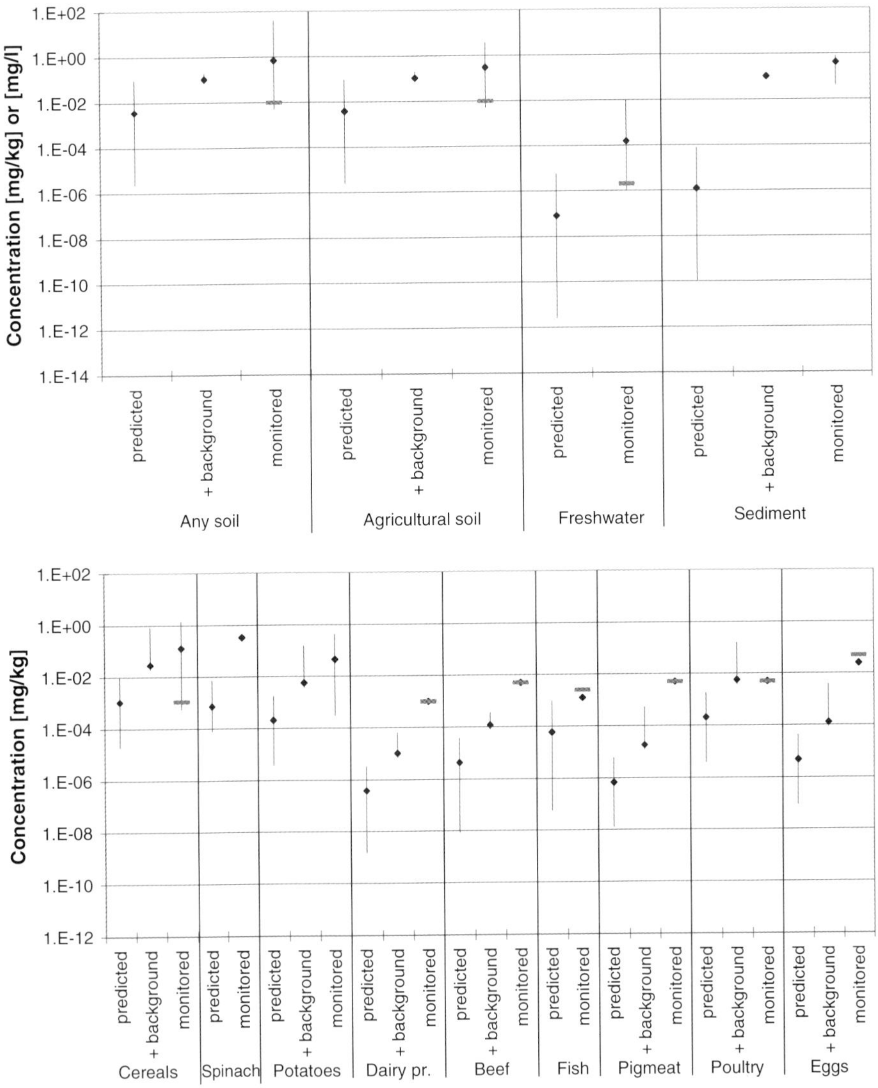

Fig. 9-4: Comparison of cadmium minimum, median and maximum concentrations as predicted by the environmental fate and exposure models with reported concentrations in environmental media (top) and foodstuff (bottom, cf. Table C-10); model estimates based on the 'food removal' scenario described in Table 9-1 resulting from a 100 year continuous release according to the pan-European emission scenario for 1990 (cf. sections 11.1 and 11.2; different units; note the logarithmic scale, horizontal bars indicate reported detection limits)

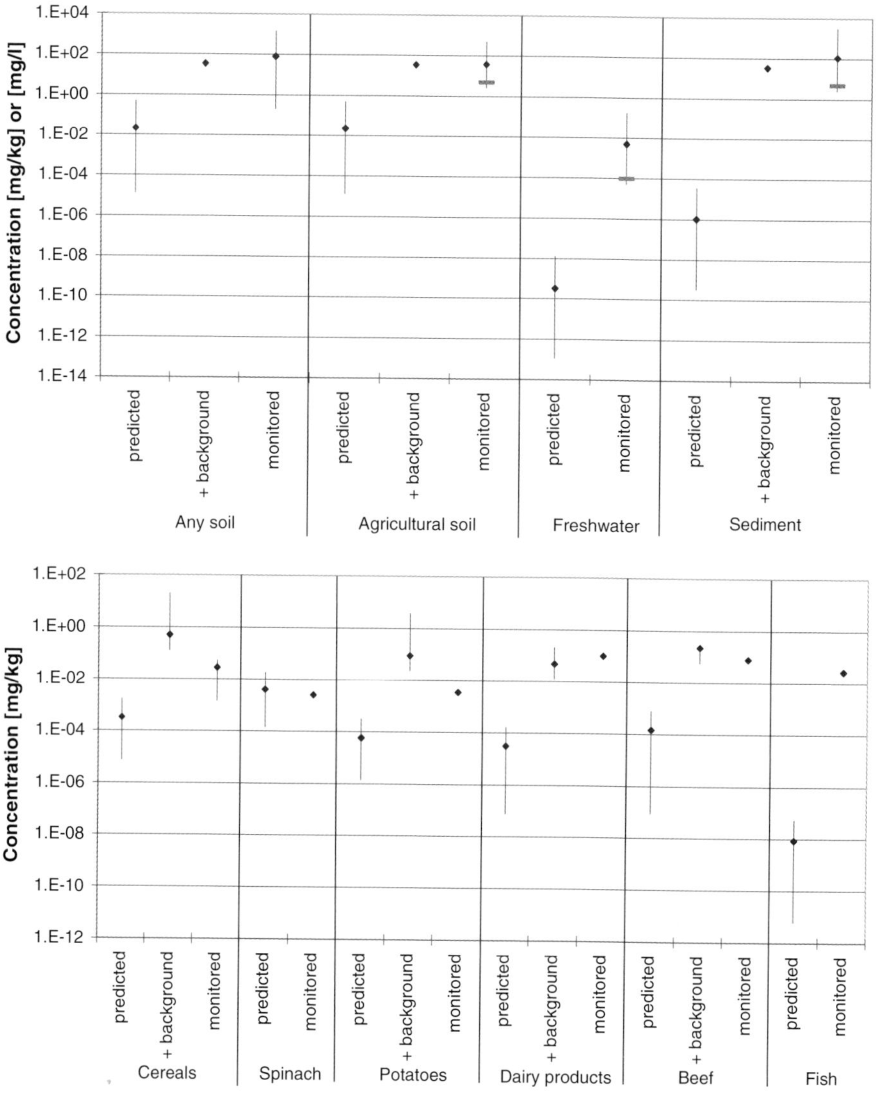

Fig. 9-5: Comparison of chromium minimum, median and maximum concentrations as predicted by the environmental fate and exposure models with reported concentrations in environmental media (top) and foodstuff (bottom, cf. Table C-11); model estimates based on the 'food removal' scenario described in Table 9-1 resulting from a 100 year continuous release according to the pan-European emission scenario for 1990 (cf. sections 11.1 and 11.2; different units; note the logarithmic scale, horizontal bars indicate reported detection limits)

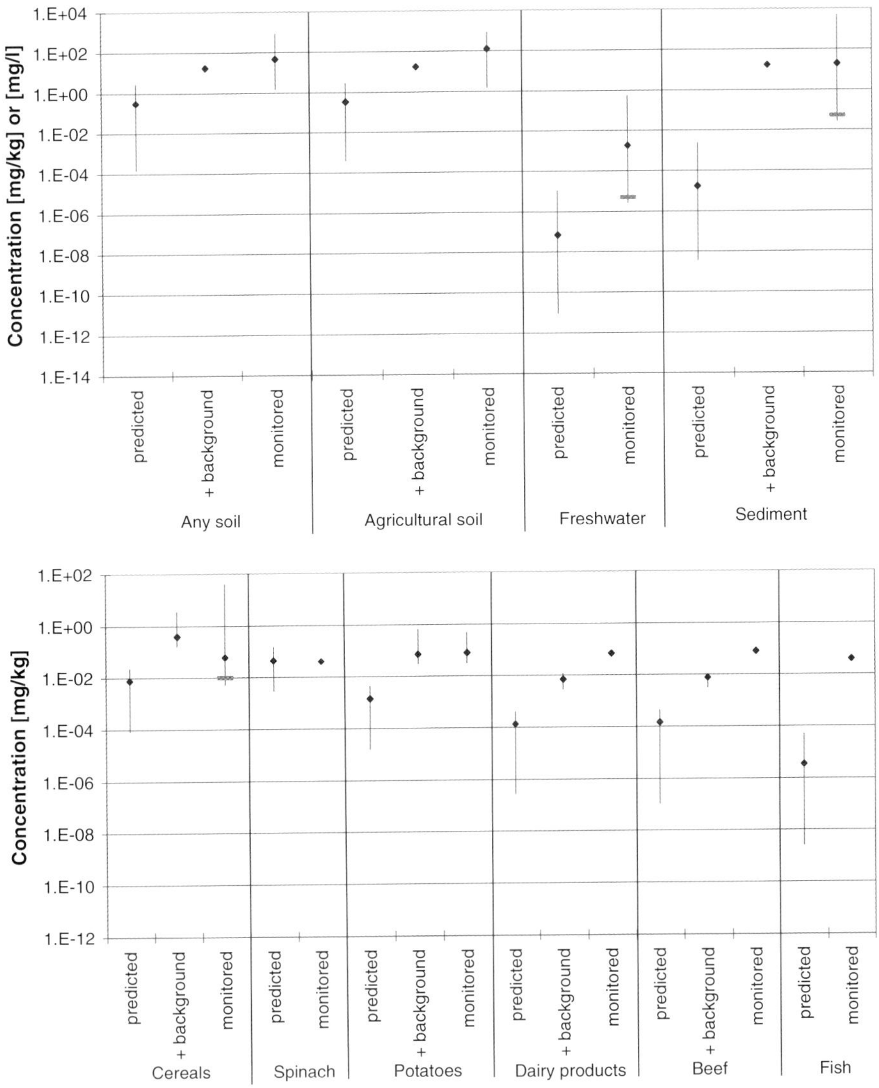

Fig. 9-6: Comparison of lead minimum, median and maximum concentrations as predicted by the environmental fate and exposure models with reported concentrations in environmental media (top) and foodstuff (bottom, cf. Table C-12); model estimates based on the 'food removal' scenario described in Table 9-1 resulting from a 100 year continuous release according to the pan-European emission scenario for 1990 (cf. sections 11.1 and 11.2; different units; note the logarithmic scale, horizontal bars indicate reported detection limits; predicted beef concentrations are compared to a measured value for pork)

mium exposure through cattle-based products, i.e., milk and beef. These shares are typically about 25 % and 50 % for arsenic exposures due to dairy products and beef, respectively. This hints at the importance of including the exposure pathway of soil ingestion by farm animals beside regular feed intake in the assessment as suggested by United States - Environmental Protection Agency (1998). It also emphasizes the need to improve the knowledge on the share of farm animals kept outdoors especially if pigs and poultry were to be included in the assessment of chromium (and arsenic). Such information is not officially available so that the assessor needs to mostly rely on expert judgement (cf. section 7.1.1).

Generally, the concentrations assessed to occur in the freshwater environment, i.e., the water bodies, sediments and fish, are well below the expectation values, regularly by at least two orders of magnitude. The processes ruling the concentrations in freshwater bodies will be subject of a discussion in section 9.3.3. It will be concluded that the processes involved in the particle dynamics in freshwater bodies need further improvement beyond the development done in this work. One may argue that no input from the subsurface by means of ground water discharge is taken into account which may lead to an underestimation of the concentrations in the freshwater environment. However, this flow entrains mostly if not exclusively heavy metals of natural origin at present (e.g., Umweltbundesamt, 2000) unless one has to deal with rather localised contaminations such as mine tailings. Consequently, the disregard of this process is not considered to be the main reason for the assessed concentrations to be that low. With respect to the concentrations in the sediments, one has to note, furthermore, that only the active sediment layer is taken into account in the present assessment (cf. section 6.1.2). This may additionally lead to lower assessed concentrations as compared to measured ones.

It can be concluded from this comparison with reported concentrations that the results of the present assessment are usually within or below the ranges of expected values. However, generally a comparison with spatially-resolved monitored concentrations would be desirable. This also applies to the natural background tentatively considered in the above evaluation.

9.3.3 Scenario analysis

Scenario analysis is considered here to constitute a model evaluation method in order to address decision-rule uncertainties. This means that assumptions are varied rather than parameter values ('non-parameter-related sensitivity analysis'). The latter will be addressed by the screening parameter sensitivity analysis presented in section 9.3.4. The focus of the scenario analysis will be on those model components that are novel. An overview on the different scenarios related to the environmental fate modelling is given in Table 9-1. Note that the sensitivity analysis of the monetary valuation is part of the regular external cost assessment in Chapters 10 and 11. The end point to be investigated is the Intake Fraction and the different contributions to it (e.g., fish, cereals, potatoes, meat, milk). Additionally the influence of the employed exposure assessment on the selected food concentrations shall be evaluated. The scenario analysis focuses on the pan-European emission scenario of cadmium for the year 1990 which is described in more detail in section 11.1. The reason for selecting cadmium is basically that all exposure pathways can be investigated including those related to farm animals other than cattle. This is due to data availability reasons (cf. section C.2).

Although scenario analyses or screening sensitivity analyses primarily provide rather qualitative rankings with respect to a factor's influence (Hamby, 1994; Campolongo et al., 2000a), a varied component is considered influential here if the analysed end-point in a case scenario deviates from the corresponding reference scenario by more than 50 %.

The scenarios given in Table 9-1 shall first be described qualitatively before presenting the results in a joint analysis.

Spatial resolution

While keeping the principal criterion for spatial differentiation, i.e., according to watersheds, the number of zones will be varied (cf. Fig. 4-2 vs. 4-3). In the 'low resolution' scenario, all river basins are treated as a whole irrespective of their size. This means for instance that no tributaries are distinguished in the Danube and the Rhine catchments. In contrast, river basins are further subdivided if respective information has been available for the 'simple high resolution' scenario (and all other scenarios given in Table 9-1). The types of processes and compartments distinguished is equal for both scenarios.

Distinction of further compartments

Another aspect to spatial differentiation apart from spatial resolution into zones is the number of compartments generically distinguished in each of the zones. Principally the number of compartments should be kept as small as possible (Trapp and Matthies, 1998). It shall, therefore, be analysed to what extent the selection of the compartments to be distinguished during the assessment influences the results.

Compared to existing multi-zonal multimedia models which usually only distinguish agricultural from natural soils in the terrestrial environment (Wania et al., 2000; Wania, 2003) if at all (Devillers et al., 1995; Scheringer et al., 2000b; MacLeod et al., 2001; Woodfine et al., 2001, 2002), the database of the

Table 9-1: Scenarios evaluated with respect to the spatial resolution, the compartments distinguished and adapted processes

Scenario	Zones		Compartments distinguished			Process modifications[a]					
	low spatial resolution	high spatial resolution	four[b]	five[c]	eight[d]	lake circulation	different particle dynamics in rivers and lakes	different soil erosion rates	ice melt, overland flow on impervious soils	preferential flow[e]	food removal[f]
Low resolution	X		X								
Simple high resolution		X	X								
Lake circulation		X	X			X					
Rivers from lakes distinguished		X	X			X	X				
Eight compartments		X			X	X	X	X	X		
Five compartments		X		X		X	X	X			
Preferential flow		X		X		X	X	X		X	
Food removal		X		X		X	X	X			X

a. For processes that are included by default refer to main text.
b. Freshwater, sediment, agricultural soil and other land uses.
c. As with the four compartment setting but distinguishing arable land from pastures.
d. As with the five compartment setting but further distinguishing (semi-) natural ecosystems, non-vegetated soils/rocks, impervious land and glaciers.
e. Related processes as described in sections A.3.7 and A.6.4.
f. Related processes as described in section A.3.8.

WATSON tool contains information on land uses such as glaciers/permanent snow, urban or impervious areas, non-vegetated land and pastures as distinguished from arable land. The scenario 'eight compartments' makes use of all of the terrestrial compartment information available (cf. section 5.1). This shall be compared to the 'rivers from lakes distinguished' scenario (see below). Similar to the 'high resolution' scenario, the area shares of the compartments glaciers/permanent snow, impervious soils or sealed areas, and non-vegetated land are added to the semi-natural ecosystem compartment while assuming the properties of the latter for the 'rivers from lakes distinguished' scenario. The same applies to pastures which are merged with the arable land compartment. The processes considered by both scenarios are basically the same. However, impervious soils and glaciers need special processes due to their properties so that neither matrix leaching nor soil erosion occurs with both compartments. Instead, all runoff water is assumed to undergo overland flow in the case of impervious soils (cf. sections A.3.4 and A.3.6) whereas glaciers only show the process 'ice melt' (section A.3.5). Additionally, soil erosion rates are a function of the compartment in the scenario 'eight compartments' leading to varying velocities of this process on different compartments which are affected by this process (cf. section B.5.3). The comparison of the 'eight compartment' scenario to the 'rivers from lakes distinguished' scenario will primarily elucidate the influence of different erosion rates on the overall exposure results.

In order to find out to what extent the distinction of pastures from arable land explains the changes caused by the introduction of all of the compartments according to the 'eight compartment' scenario, another scenario is investigated. While aggregating all other terrestrial compartments into the semi-natural ecosystem compartment (as in the scenario above), arable land and pastures will be treated separately in the 'five compartments' scenario rather than being aggregated into a generic agricultural soil compartment whose properties correspond to those of the arable land compartment.

Inclusion of processes

WATSON offers the opportunity to switch processes on and off (see section 4.4) rather than assigning unrealistic values to parameters (e.g., Guinée et al., 1996; European Commission, 2003b). Many processes considered in the environmental fate module of the WATSON model are common to multimedia models. By default, the following processes are included: soil erosion without distinguishing between compartments, discharge, matrix leaching, overland flow, sedimentation, resuspension and sediment burial without distinguishing between streams and lakes, diffusive exchange between freshwater and sediment.[31] In some scenarios, these may be replaced by newly developed processes (see above and below). However, some processes have been introduced that could not be found in other models. This may be due to the fact that the degree of spatial differentiation followed is rather different from other spatially-resolved or a-spatial multimedia models. For instance, glaciers and, thus, ice melt or the distinction of large lakes, i.e., freshwater bodies that show also 'upstream' flow as part of the lake circulation process have not yet been included elsewhere. The distinction of glaciers only makes sense if also ice melt is considered. Thus, the evaluation of this process will not take place here but is part of the 'eight compartment' scenario described above.

At least three more processes are novel in this context. The first one is circulation in large lakes which has been deemed necessary to be included due to the separation of large lakes into zones (cf. Fig. 6-2 in section 6.1.5). The results of this scenario will be compared to the 'simple high resolution' scenario. Also the influence of the preferential flow process will be investigated by a scenario having the same name. This process describes a non-equilibrium flow (Schwarz and Kaupenjohann, 2000) leading to an accelerated transfer of the substances contained in wet deposition and/or dissolved or suspended in colloidal form in the soil pore water (Jarvis et al., 1999; Noack et al., 2000) to below the surface soil (cf. section A.3.7). The third newly introduced process is a combination of plant exposure via root uptake or atmospheric deposition and plant removal due to harvest (cf. sections A.3.8 and A.6.5). An analogous removal process is also formulated for (freshwater) fish. The 'preferential flow' and the 'food removal' scenarios are compared to the 'five compartments' scenario.

Formulation of processes

Apart from the evaluation of processes by means of their inclusion or exclusion, one can also vary their formulations. The freshwater compartments in multimedia models are usually treated as if they behaved like lakes (e.g., Brandes et al., 1996). This may be justified since the freshwater volume contained in lakes is more than 40 times larger than that of freshwater streams at the global scale (Korzun et al., 1974 cited in Baumgartner and Liebscher, 1990). Considering the difference in dynamics between lakes and streams, it is also obvious that lakes will rather substantially prolong the residence time of substances contained in them. Assuming, however, that all freshwater bodies behave like lakes is rather conservative in a spatially-resolved multimedia model since the removal by freshwater flow is

---

[31] Note that partitioning is dependent on zonally-variable pH in the respective compartments except for freshwater and sediment

highly underestimated in areas where hardly any still waters exist. Under still water conditions the processes of sedimentation and resuspension will be slower or faster than under flowing water conditions, respectively. The degree of conservatism introduced will be investigated by comparing the scenario 'rivers from lakes distinguished' towards the 'lake circulation' scenario described above. The sedimentation rate in any freshwater body used in the 'low resolution', 'simple high resolution' and 'lake circulation' scenarios is set to pure lake conditions as described in Table 6-4 according to the alternative process formulations as stated in sections A.3.11, A.3.12 and A.3.13.

Results of the scenario analysis

The aggregated results of the scenario analysis for the emission situation in Europe in 1990 are shown in Fig. 9-7 in terms of the time-integrated (effective) Intake Fraction of cadmium for the ingestion exposures considered. Overall, one can note that the differences between the scenarios are rather small and mostly lie within a factor of two when comparing the aggregated Intake Fractions due to ingestion for the respective time horizons (see discussion on the special case of the 'preferential flow' scenario below). Also when looking at the contributions of the different food items to the overall result, the differences are rather small (Tables 9-2 and 9-3). The Intake Fraction of ingestion is dominated by the uptake of cereals. Generally, the cereal-related exposure amounts to about 81 % of the Intake Fraction due to ingestion assessed to occur for a given time horizon in the case of cadmium. For this heavy metal, also exposure through potatoes in general is substantial, i.e., about 18 % of the Intake Fraction due to ingestion. It shall be noted that also spinach, dairy products and beef are especially important for arsenic and chromium (see Chapters 10 and 11). The contribution of freshwater fish is generally insubstantial when compared to the other food items. Exposure via aboveground exposed produce becomes more relevant for cadmium when including the combined atmospheric deposition and harvest removal process especially in the short term when analysing pulse emissions (see value for spinach for scenario 'food removal' in Table 9-3). This has implications especially on the valuation results when dealing with shorter integration times and also when performing non-zero discounting.

All investigated scenarios show similar dynamics (bottom of Fig. 9-7). However marked differences exist between the scenario with and those without the process of preferential flow. The 'preferential flow' scenario leads to ingestion exposures that are about half of the those for the other scenarios at steady-state. The inclusion of this process can, therefore, be considered influential. In all cases, the development over time sets on with a steep change in the Intake Frac-

Table 9-2: Contribution of the different food items to the Intake Fraction (last row) of cadmium for time-integrated ingestion exposures according to the sensitivity scenarios (pan-European emissions to air in 1990)

Contribution to Intake Fraction	Low resolution	Simple high resolution	Lake circulation	Rivers from lakes distinguished	Eight compart-ments	Five compart-ments	Preferential flow	Food removal
Cereals	80.6%	81.5%	81.5%	81.5%	81.5%	81.5%	81.2%	81.5%
Potatoes	18.8%	18.0%	18.0%	18.0%	17.9%	17.9%	18.2%	17.9%
Spinach	0.087%	0.080%	0.080%	0.080%	0.081%	0.081%	0.099%	0.14%
Dairy products	0.038%	0.036%	0.036%	0.036%	0.039%	0.039%	0.038%	0.039%
Beef	0.030%	0.029%	0.029%	0.029%	0.031%	0.031%	0.031%	0.032%
Fish	0.0017%	0.00065%	0.00065%	0.0056%	0.0058%	0.0055%	0.0083%	0.0056%
Pork, poultry, eggs	0.38%	0.39%	0.39%	0.39%	0.40%	0.40%	0.40%	0.40%
Intake Fraction [$kg_{ingested}$ / $kg_{released}$]	$1.04 \cdot 10^{-3}$	$1.26 \cdot 10^{-3}$	$1.26 \cdot 10^{-3}$	$1.26 \cdot 10^{-3}$	$1.27 \cdot 10^{-3}$	$1.26 \cdot 10^{-3}$	$5.57 \cdot 10^{-4}$	$1.24 \cdot 10^{-3}$

Table 9-3: Contribution of the different food items to the Intake Fraction (last row) of cadmium for ingestion exposures after 25 years according to the sensitivity scenarios (pan-European emissions to air in 1990, only taking place in the first year)

Contribution to Intake Fraction	Low resolution	Simple high resolution	Lake circulation	Rivers from lakes distinguished	Eight compart-ments	Five compart-ments	Preferential flow	Food removal
Cereals	81.7%	81.5%	81.5%	81.5%	81.5%	81.5%	81.5%	80.9%
Potatoes	17.7%	17.9%	17.9%	17.9%	17.8%	17.8%	17.8%	17.7%
Spinach	0.12%	0.12%	0.12%	0.12%	0.12%	0.12%	0.12%	0.95%
Dairy products	0.044%	0.042%	0.042%	0.042%	0.042%	0.042%	0.042%	0.041%
Beef	0.036%	0.036%	0.036%	0.036%	0.035%	0.035%	0.035%	0.035%
Fish	0.0031%	0.0017%	0.0017%	0.012%	0.014%	0.012%	0.012%	0.011%
Pork, poultry, eggs	0.41%	0.41%	0.41%	0.41%	0.40%	0.40%	0.40%	0.40%
Intake Fraction [$kg_{ingested}$ / $kg_{released}$]	$8.80 \cdot 10^{-5}$	$8.97 \cdot 10^{-5}$	$8.97 \cdot 10^{-5}$	$8.98 \cdot 10^{-5}$	$9.02 \cdot 10^{-5}$	$9.02 \cdot 10^{-5}$	$8.98 \cdot 10^{-5}$	$9.09 \cdot 10^{-5}$

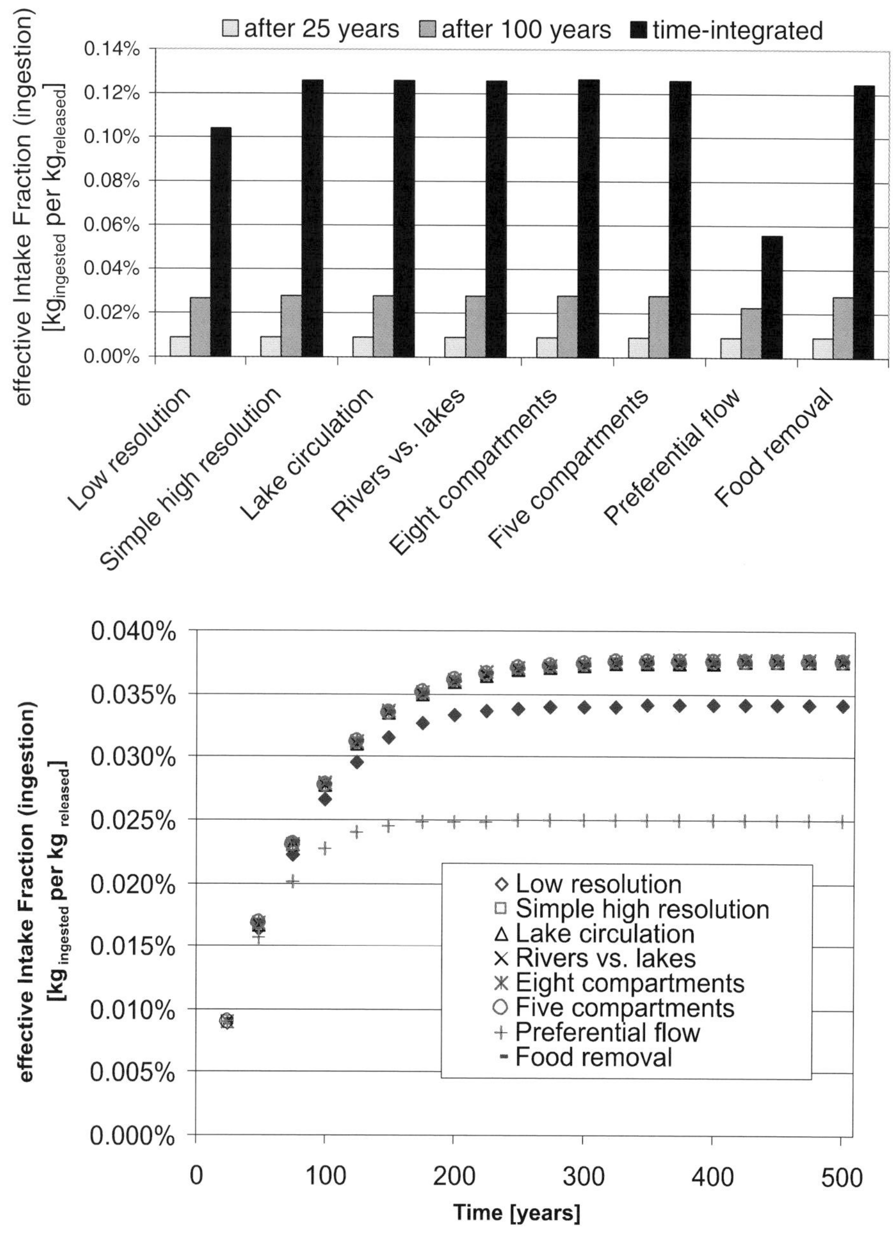

Fig. 9-7: Effective Intake Fraction for cadmium due to the ingestion of food according to the sensitivity scenarios after 25 years, 100 years and at steady state (top) and the development within the first 500 years after the pulse emission (bottom); pan-European emissions to air in 1990

tion followed by a slow approximation towards the aggregated result at steady-state. The duration of the initial fast Intake Fraction accumulation lasts about 100 and 120 years with and without the process of preferential flow, respectively. The 'preferential flow' scenario will, thus, lead to smaller exposures and damages not only in the long-run but also in the short term. The impact of preferential flow on the results will be borne in mind when concluding the case study results (section 12.3.2).

Despite similar dynamics and the small difference in terms of the overall Intake Fraction due to ingestion, there are slight variations between the scenarios not considering preferential flow. The 'low resolution' scenario leads to a smaller overall Intake Fraction for cadmium than the other non-preferential flow scenarios. This is due to lower assessed exposures via many food groups in absolute terms (multiplying the overall Intake Fractions with the corresponding food group shares in Tables 9-2 and 9-3). Most notably, freshwater fish exposures are higher by a factor of about two than in the 'simple high resolution' and 'lake circulation' scenarios which will be discussed below. When comparing the environmental concentrations of cadmium of the exposure-related media agricultural soil and freshwater of the 'low resolution' scenario with those of the 'simple high resolution' scenario, for instance, different extensions of elevated concentrations combined with different peak concentrations become obvious at steady-state (Fig. 9-8 and 9-9). The differences become more apparent when relating the corresponding media concentrations to one another. The factors thus derived are given in Fig. 9-10 for freshwater and agricultural soil to the left and to the right, respectively. The category with factors between 0.98 and 1.02, i.e., practically no change, mostly contains those areas for which no information on subdivisions below the drainage basin level are provided. These are predominantly located along the sea coasts. The areas with lower factors show smaller concentrations for the 'low resolution' scenario.

The difference in terms of exposure is the result of the interplay of the distribution of elevated depositions (Fig. 9-12), the spatial distribution of the food production (cf. Table B-16) and its allocation to agricultural soils (added area shares of arable land and pastures in this case, left and right Fig. 5-1, respectively) or freshwater bodies amongst others. The elevated cadmium concentrations assessed to occur especially in central Poland for the 'simple high resolution' scenario are averaged over the entire catchments of the Odra and Wisla rivers in the 'low resolution' case. The aggregation of catchments, thus, allows higher depositions to occur over less intensively cultivated parts of the country. Similar situations result for the catchments of the Po and Rhine river. Another factor adds to the setting of the Dniepr and Don river in the eastern Ukraine and adjacent Russian areas. The effect of lower runoff on parts of the catchments (cf. Fig. B-3)

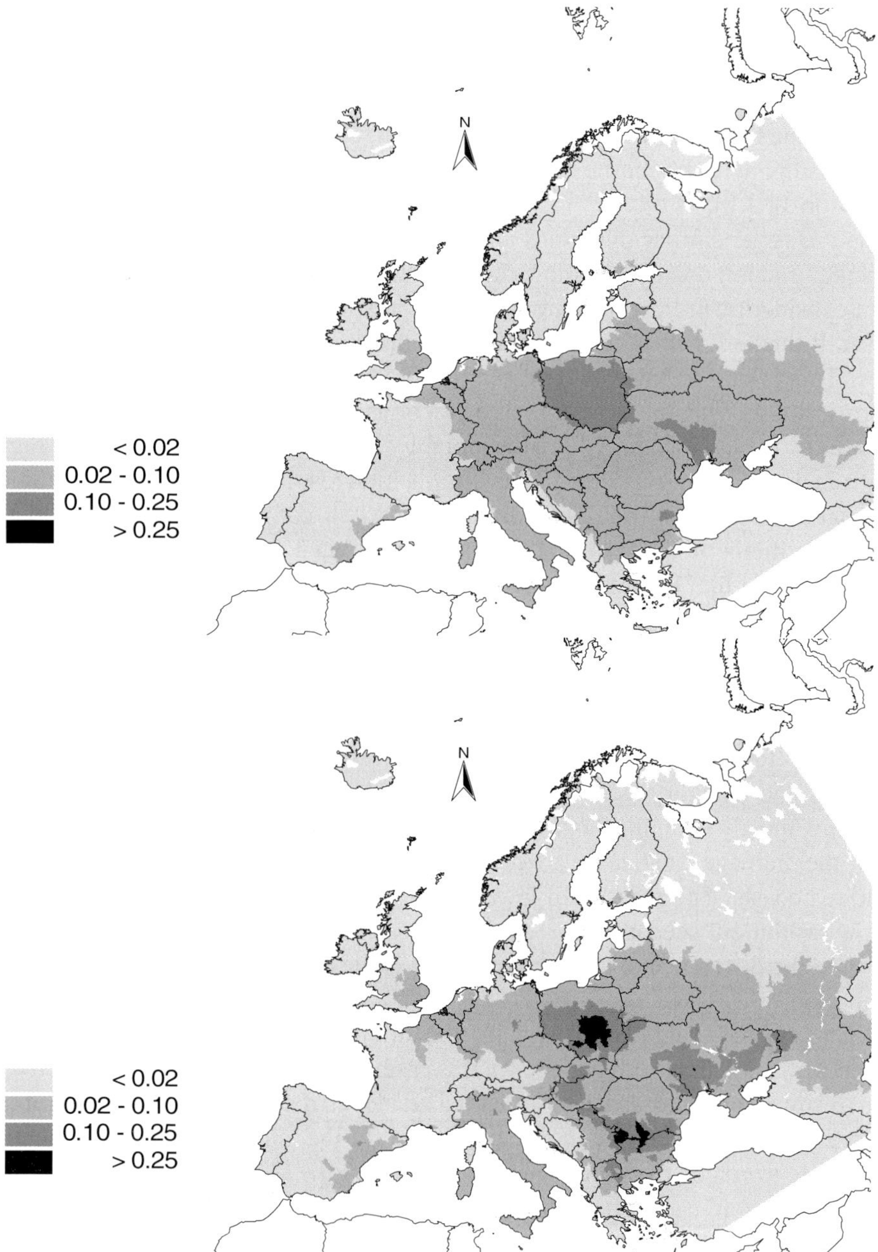

Fig. 9-8: Concentration distribution of cadmium in agricultural soil at steady-state due to 1990 pan-European emissions to air according to the 'low resolution' (top) and 'simple high resolution' (bottom) scenarios [mg/kg]

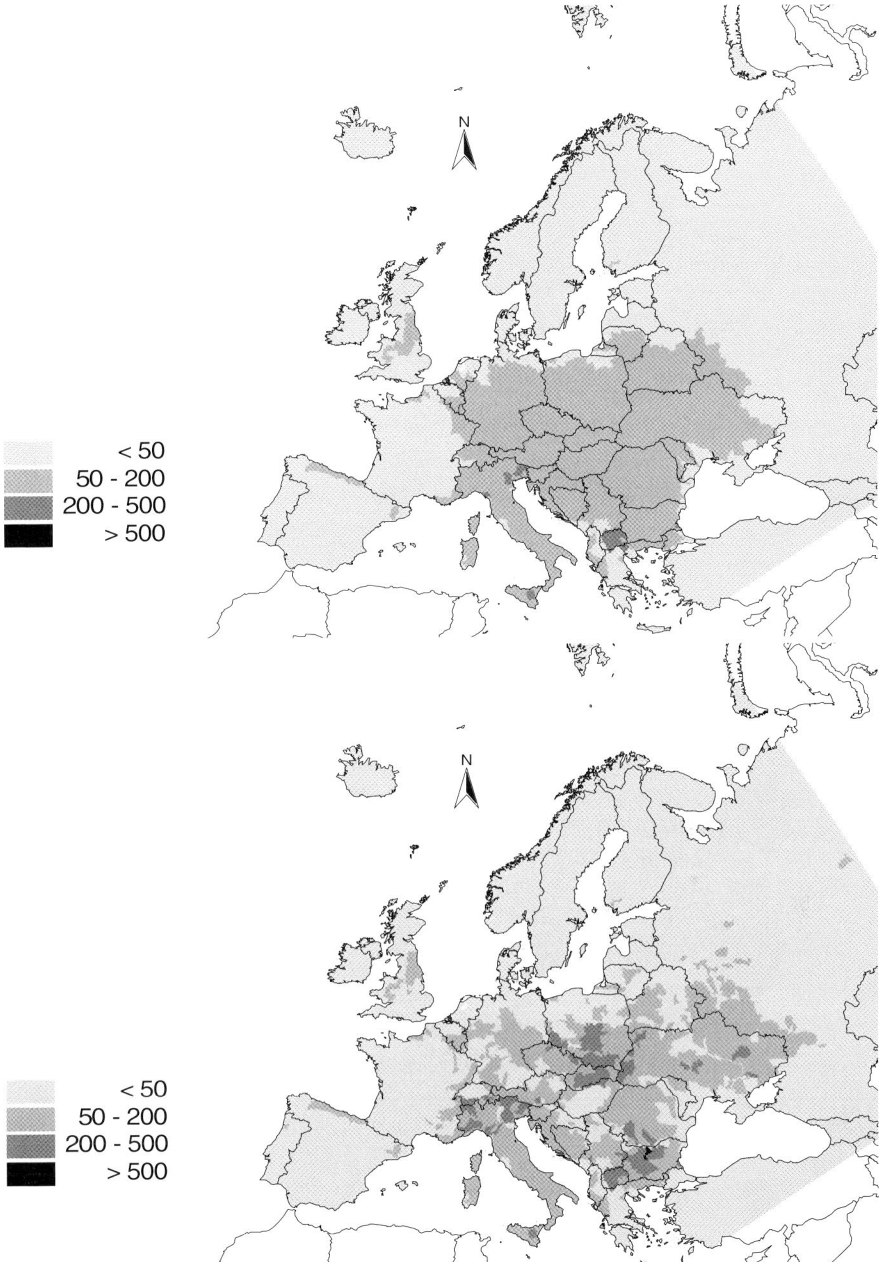

Fig. 9-9: Concentration distribution of cadmium in freshwater at steady-state due to 1990 pan-European emissions to air according to the 'low resolution' (top) and 'simple high resolution' (bottom) scenarios [mg/l]

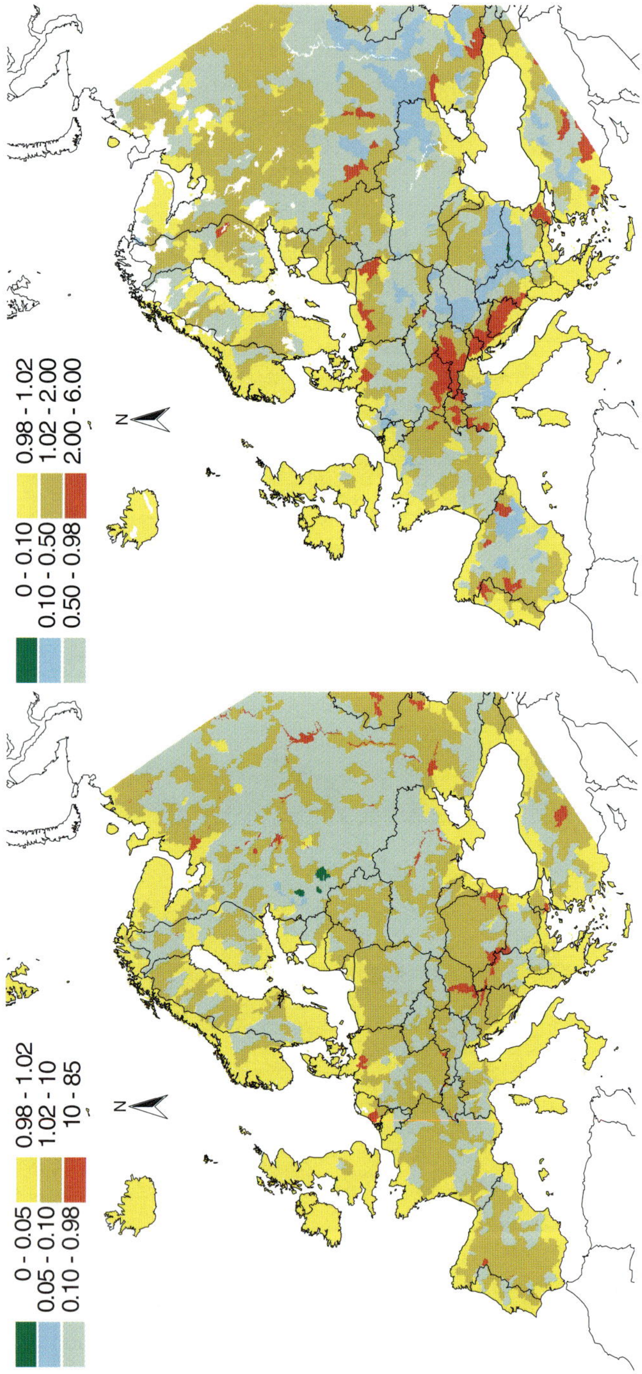

Fig. 9-10: Factors obtained by relating the concentrations of cadmium according to the 'low resolution' scenario to those assessed by the 'simple high resolution' scenario at steady-state in the freshwater (left) and agricultural soil compartments (right) [-] (pan-European emissions to air in 1990)

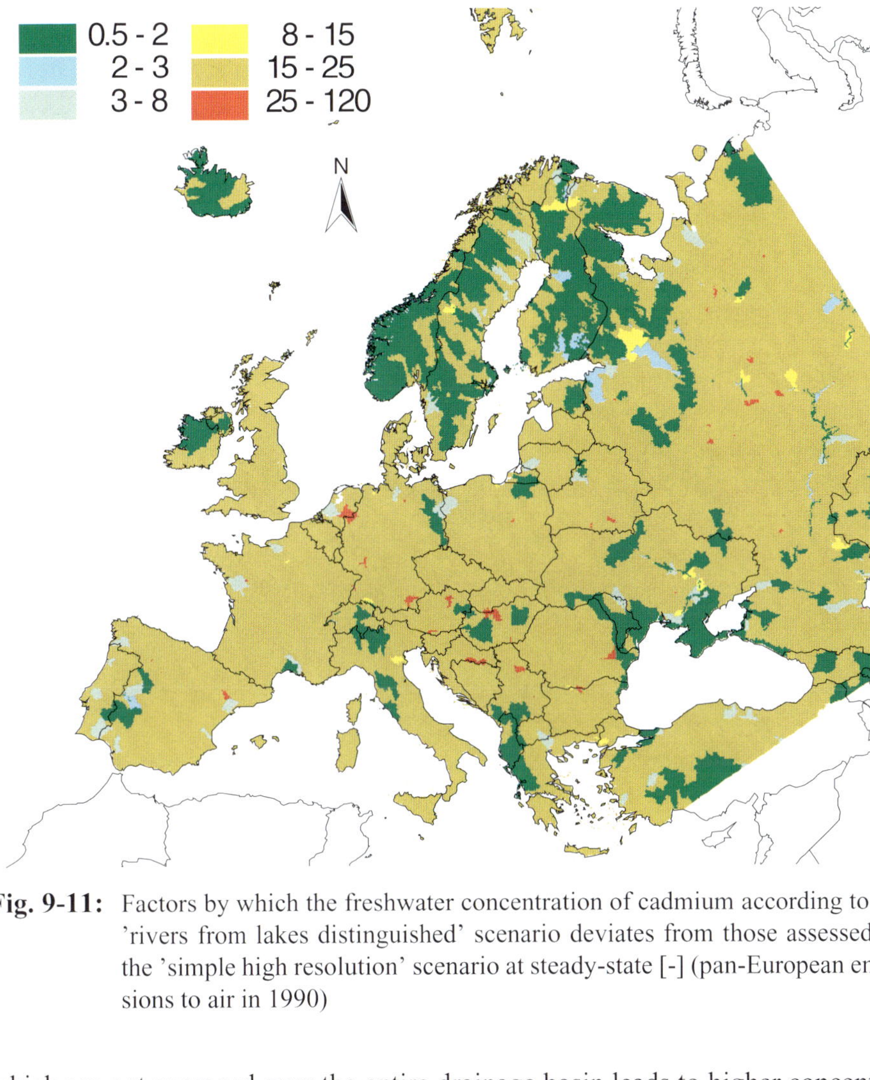

Fig. 9-11: Factors by which the freshwater concentration of cadmium according to the 'rivers from lakes distinguished' scenario deviates from those assessed by the 'simple high resolution' scenario at steady-state [-] (pan-European emissions to air in 1990)

which are not averaged over the entire drainage basin leads to higher concentrations in the 'simple high resolution' scenario in those areas with a high density of agricultural soil which is accompanied with a high production of cereals and to some degree potatoes.

There is a decrease in the contribution of freshwater fish exposure by about a factor of two when changing the environmental fate model from the low to the high spatial resolution setting. This decrease is attributable to higher concentrations predicted in many of the lakes in the 'low resolution' scenario (manifest in

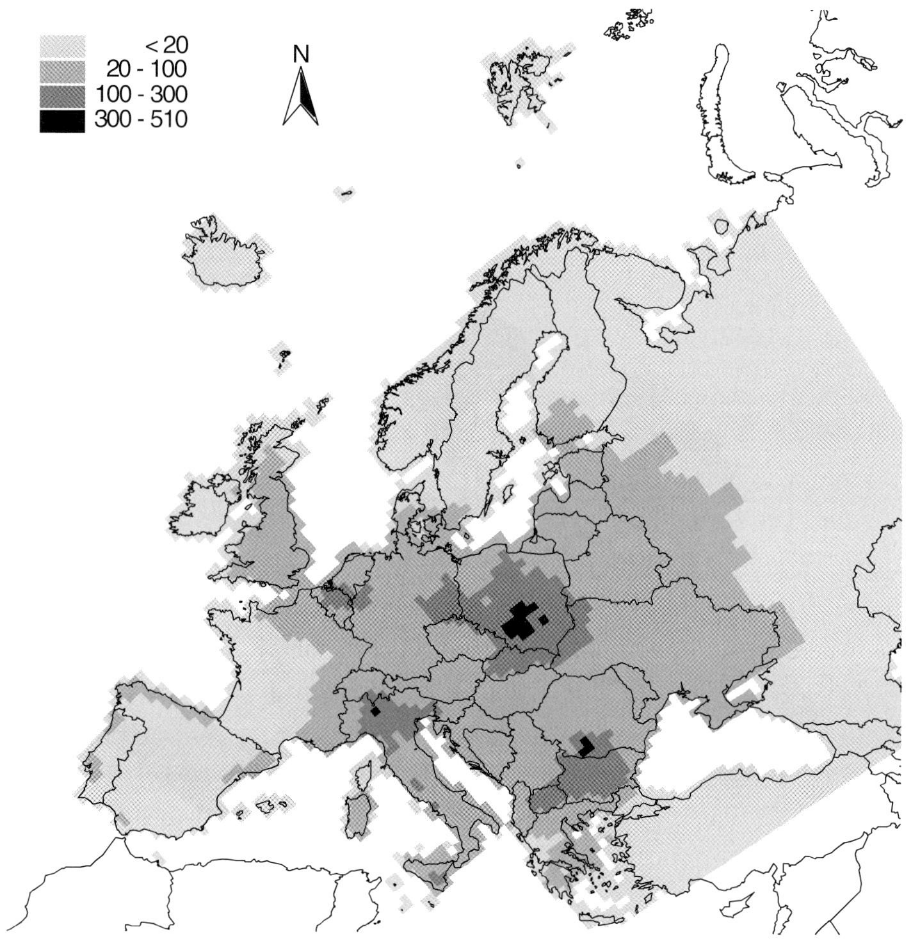

Fig. 9-12: Atmospheric deposition of cadmium according to the pan-European emission scenario for 1990 [$\mu g/m^2/yr$]

the higher exposure) that are due to the circumstance that depositions occurring in one part of the catchment are homogeneously distributed across the drainage basin. For instance, the distribution of the atmospheric deposition (Fig. 9-12) shows that especially the western parts of the Volga and Don rivers receive higher inputs than the rest. However, these depositions also reach to larger freshwater bodies in parts of the catchments that under (physically correct) downstream flow conditions are not affected by these inputs. This applies to the Rybinsk reservoir of the Volga river and the Proletarskoye reservoir of the Don river as well as for other parts of the geographical area covered such as the Rhine river and the Tagus river. In the case of the 'low resolution' scenario, however, these water bodies also receive higher inputs. As described in section B.6.1, the national fish production figures (cf. Table B-16) are distributed according to a distribution scheme that takes water volumes into account. Due to the fact that lakes hold most of the freshwater among the surface freshwater bodies, it is not surprising that higher concentrations in lakes also lead to higher fish exposures. As a result, the deviations in terms of concentrations and exposure in the short term are mostly due to the upstream transport of inputs to catchments caused by the homogeneous mixing within compartments of large sized zones.

The 'lake circulation' scenario does not lead to notable changes towards the 'simple high resolution' scenario indicating that the inclusion of circulation in large lakes is rather irrelevant for larger scale emission scenarios without direct releases into water.

The distinction of rivers from lakes in terms of the processes related to particle transport leads to smaller exposures through freshwater fish in the long run by about one order of magnitude ('rivers from lakes distinguished' vs. 'lake circulation' or 'simple high resolution' scenarios in Table 9-2). Fig. 9-11 shows the influence of the inclusion of this process on the freshwater concentrations of cadmium at steady-state. The colours dark green, light green and brown indicate areas where the deviation amounts to about a factor of two, five and twenty, respectively. While a factor of two is considered tolerable, the other two factors are due to the volume shares of stagnant waters assumed to occur under pure river conditions and in zones of large rivers that pour into the sea with 5 and 21 vol.-% of stagnant waters, respectively (cf. section 6.1.4). Surprisingly, the sedimentation process rather than the discharge seems to dominate the dynamics of freshwater streams with respect to even rather soluble trace elements such as cadmium as compared to lead, chromium and arsenic (cf. Table C-1). Otherwise the reduction in the sedimentation rate particularly in rivers would not have had such a pronounced effect on the concentrations assessed to such a large extent. Thus, a formulation of this process which is even more adequate to running waters than the attempt undertaken here appears necessary. Nevertheless, the process formulation as suggested and used in this study leads to higher contributions of the freshwater fish consumption to the overall ingestion-related Intake Fraction by at least about a factor of seven for the emission scenario analysed.

When comparing the 'rivers from lakes distinguished' to the 'eight compartments' scenario, again a revaluation of some of the less contributing food items takes place. The contribution of those food items related to pasture-based food chains (especially meat and dairy products) increase by about 10 % in the long-run when distinguishing more compartments. This can be attributed to the reduced water soil erosion rate on pastures assumed to prevail (cf. introduction to section 5.1) which leads to a slower removal out of this compartment and, thus, a slower decline in concentration. The increase in exposure via fish occurring in the short term is especially explicable by the fast transport from sealed surfaces to the freshwater environment. This is supported by the lower fish exposure of the 'five compartments' scenario when compared to that with eight compartments. This is the only notable difference when distinguishing impervious land, glaciers and non-vegetated land from natural soils for the emission scenario analysed. Owing to the observation that exposure through dairy products and beef is considerable for the trace elements arsenic and chromium (cf. Fig. 11-6), the distinction between pastures and arable land is made in the following.

When comparing the 'five compartments' scenario to the 'food removal' scenario the main difference lies in the contribution of the aboveground exposed produce, i.e., spinach, to the overall ingestion-related Intake Fraction in the short run. The inclusion of food removal can be considered influential in the case of spinach which increases by more than 50 % in the short term. Due to the fact that harvest is modelled as an ultimate removal process from the environment, the time-integrated ingestion-related Intake Fraction even slightly decreases by about 1 %.

Having analysed cadmium in more detail, the question arises to what extent the exposure towards the other three trace elements is affected by the variation of the respective components. As particularly arsenic and chromium are less mobile than cadmium, it is expected that the consideration of processes involving the particle-bound fraction of the trace elements in soils will have a more pronounced on the overall exposure and the most contributing food items. This will most notably be the case for the distinction of different erosion rates on different land uses and the preferential flow process. Allowing lower erosion rates to occur on pastures than on arable land will increase the contribution of cattle produce to the aggregated effective Intake Fraction for arsenic and chromium. The steady removal by means of preferential flow will lead to a more substantial reduction of the effective Intake Fraction for arsenic and chromium than for cadmium, given the long time scales involved when integrating the exposure over time (e.g., Fig. 11-5). For lead, the difference to the scenario analysis results presented for cadmium are not expected to be remarkable.

Variable results due to the employed exposure assessment scheme

Another question is related to the influence of the employed exposure assessment scheme. Two exposure assessment schemes especially with respect to heavy metals/trace elements have been encountered: one by the International Atomic Ener-

Table 9-4: Maximum concentrations in agricultural produce at steady-state for air emissions in 1990 according to the exposure assessments as given by International Atomic Energy Agency (2001) and United States - Environmental Protection Agency (1998) for Europe

Food concentration [mg/kg FW]	IAEA	US-EPA
Cadmium		
cereals	0.19	0.03
beef	0.025	0.0002
Lead		
cereals	1.30	0.65
milk	0.11	0.04
beef	0.20	0.04

gy Agency (2001) and another by the United States - Environmental Protection Agency (1998). These vary in terms of process formulation (cf. section A.7), parameter values and exposure pathways considered. Additionally, the IAEA exposure assessment framework is meant to be used at a screening level whereas the US-EPA's is more advanced/detailed, i.e., less conservative (cf. Chapter 7).

An analysis of these two exposure assessment schemes has been undertaken taking into account the food items cereals, beef and dairy products for cadmium and lead (Table 9-4). As this has been done early in the course of the development of the present methodology some components of the assessment could not be taken into account. The following parameter must, therefore, be regarded to be set to unity: $fr\_w_{effective/total}$, $fr\_w_{not\ consumed/food\ supply}$ and $fr\_w_{self\text{-}supply}$. For their meaning, refer to section A.7.

It can be seen that the IAEA exposure assessment overestimates the exposure to the respective food items by about an order of magnitude as compared to the one by the US-EPA. This is, in fact, not surprising due to its intended use for screening purposes. From this rough comparison, it appears justified to follow the exposure assessment as suggested by the United States - Environmental Protection Agency (1998) unless more realistic exposure assessments become available.

9.3.4 Sensitivity analysis of the parameters

As stated above, the sensitivity analysis of the parameters to be presented in the following constitutes a screening parameter sensitivity analysis. This is used in order to identify the most important parameters in the sense of Hamby (1994).

It remains to be defined when a parameter is judged to be important. This can be done in different ways. When constantly increasing one parameter after another by 20 %, Price et al. (1996) defined a change in the result of 1 % as an indication that a parameter "significantly contributed to the uncertainty and variation of the dose rate estimates" (p. 265). The relationship between model output and parameter variation is adopted as the evaluation criterion according to:

$$\text{abs}\left(\frac{\dfrac{(IF_{\text{sens}} - IF_{\text{ref}})}{IF_{\text{ref}}}}{\dfrac{(x_{\text{sens}} - x_{\text{ref}})}{x_{\text{ref}}}}\right) \geq \frac{0.01}{0.2} = 0.05 \qquad (9\text{-}1)$$

where

IF : Intake Fraction due to ingestion of single food items and/or the aggregated ingestion exposures according to the reference sensitivity case ('ref') or a parameter variation case ('sens') [kg_{ingested} per kg_{released}]

x : parameter value as used in the reference sensitivity case ('ref') or during a parameter variation case ('sens') [variable units].

There are many parameters included in the assessment whose comprehensive evaluation is beyond the scope of the present study. A prioritisation of the parameters for which a sensitivity analysis shall be carried out is, therefore, performed according to findings in the literature.

Generally, substance-specific properties appear to be most relevant (Blanchard and Lerch, 2000; Huijbregts et al., 2000a) especially when releases into air are investigated (Hertwich et al., 1999). These may be related to the environmental fate, exposure, or effect/impact assessment. For degrading substances, the persistence in the release compartment appears to be most important (Hertwich et al., 1999; Huijbregts et al., 2000a). However, chemical transformation is not considered at present for the trace elements investigated. The solid-water partitioning coefficient (K_d) is, thus, deemed to be the most important parameter with regard to the environmental fate of non-volatile substances (Blanchard and Lerch, 2000; Huijbregts et al., 2000a).

Table 9-5: Assigned pH values in the 'compartmental pH variation' sensitivity case

Compartment in this study	pH	Compartment according to Huijbregts (1999)
Freshwater	7	Continental freshwater bodies
Sediment	7	Continental freshwater sediments
Glaciers[a]	7	Continental freshwater bodies (analogy assumption)
Impervious areas[a]	6	Continental industrial soils
Non-vegetated land[a]	6	Continental natural soil
(Semi-) natural ecosystems	6	Continental natural soil
Arable land	7	Continental agricultural soil
Pastures/grassland	7	Continental agricultural soil

a.Compartment not analysed when only distinguishing five compartments.

The influence of the solid-water partitioning coefficient on the overall results shall be analysed in two ways: first, by varying the parameter values themselves and secondly, by varying the pH values of the compartments upon which the solid-water partitioning coefficient is allowed to depend. In the proposed external cost assessment framework, several parameters vary in space (cf. Appendix B) to which the pH of the different compartments belongs. It is a key variable influencing the partitioning of non-volatile trace elements (Wolt, 1994; United States - Environmental Protection Agency, 1998; Anonymous, 1999b) and their mobility in watersheds (e.g., Scudlark et al., 2005). Although the substance-specific partitioning coefficient may also vary by orders of magnitude for a certain pH range (e.g., Anonymous, 1999b) which will be investigated by the first sensitivity analysis related to the K_d value, the influence of assuming variable pH values especially for soils will be analysed. In most scenarios, the pH value of the compartments are allowed to vary by zone[32] and compartments whereas it only varies by compartments for the sensitivity case 'compartmental pH variation' mostly according to the values specified in Huijbregts (1999) that are given in Table 9-5. However, the latter sensitivity case merely serves illustrative purposes since no change in the parameter values can be computed according to the denominator on the left hand side of Eq. (9-1). Thus, this sensitivity case will be analysed in the same way as the sensitivity scenarios of section 9.3.3.

[32]Except for freshwater bodies and corresponding sediments.

Exposure-related parameters are especially influential for releases into water and for the indirect exposure routes according to Hertwich et al. (1999). According to the emission scenarios analysed in Chapters 10 and 11, considerable contributions to the time-integrated exposure stem from cereals, potatoes, dairy products and beef for the contaminants investigated. Therefore, the sensitivity of the results towards the respective bioconcentration factors and biotransfer factors shall be analysed.

Depending on the particular situation, the uncertainty related to effect information may dominate the overall uncertainties (Finley and Paustenbach, 1994; Rabl and Spadaro, 1999; Huijbregts et al., 2000a; Droste-Franke et al., 2003). The impact assessment of both ingestion and inhalation exposures is performed in a site-generic way, i.e., using the same dose-response relationships and severity measures throughout the model's geographical scope and for all individuals exposed. Its influence is qualitatively discussed in section 9.3.1 above and will be taken into account during the presentation of the case study results (Chapters 10 and 11) and the conclusions drawn.

The scenario analysis presented above (section 9.3.3) has shown that some variations in the formulation of the environmental fate model changes the relative importance of the food items contributing to the overall exposure. In particular the influence of the water soil erosion process shall be analysed which constitutes one criterion according to which the terrestrial compartments have been distinguished from each other (cf. section 5.1).

The sensitivity analysis of the parameters focuses on the pan-European emission scenario of chromium for the year 1990 which is described in more detail in section 11.1. The reason for selecting chromium is that different food items substantially contribute to its overall exposure. Furthermore, it shows the most pronounced variability in terms of its solid-water partitioning coefficient in the pH range prevailing at least in agricultural soils (i.e., a pH between 5 and 7, Scheffer and Schachtschabel, 1989) among the trace elements analysed (Table C-1).

Results of the sensitivity analysis of the parameters

The sensitivity analysis of the parameters is performed based on the environmental settings of the 'food removal' scenario (see section 9.3.3) which will be used for the assessment of external costs in Chapters 10 and 11. The development of the effective Intake Fraction for ingestion over time is displayed in Fig. 9-13 for all sensitivity cases analysed. The differences appear to occur only in the intermediate to long run except for the 'BCF above -90%' scenario due to the reduced contamination of cereals (cf. Table 9-6) dominating in the short run (cf. Fig. 9-14).

The assessed values of the ingestion-related effective Intake Fractions after 25 years and time-integrated are given by food item in Table 9-6. In order to identify significant changes, the numbers resulting according to the term in brackets of Eq. (9-1) are presented in Table 9-7. Note that exposure through pork, poultry and eggs cannot be assessed for chromium due to data availability constraints (cf. Table C-5).

The indicator values for the aggregated effective Intake Fractions for ingestion ('sum' in Table 9-7) show that all parameters significantly influence the exposure situation of the human population at least in the long run. It needs to be noted, however, that if the K_d value of chromium is increased by one order of magnitude this significance does not show in the aggregated effective Intake Fraction for ingestion but only in that for cattle exposure and fish (parameter sensitivity 'Kd +900%'). This can be attributed to the very high K_d values of chromium at higher pH values (cf. Table C-1). In contrast, the lower K_d values will only prevail in non-agricultural areas due to the minimal pH values allowed to occur owing to management practices in pasture soils which is 5.5 whereas for arable land it is 6.0 (cf. section B.5.1). It appears as if the behaviour of chromium is only highly affected in those compartments that have pH values about or below 6. This is the pH range where the most substantial changes in the pH-dependent partitioning behaviour of chromium occurs. At or below a pH value of 6, a higher share of chromium is, therefore, present in the soil pore water. In this dissolved state, chromium may increasingly undergo the processes of matrix leaching and/or overland flow leading to a quicker decline of its concentration in soils with lower pH values and, thus, to a lower exposure through food produced on these soils. As a result, also the exposure via fish increases. When decreasing the K_d values of chromium by one order of magnitude, in turn, the effect becomes significant at the aggregated exposure level. This also indicates that it does not seem to make a remarkable difference whether a substance's K_d value is in the order of 10^3 or 10^4 m^3 per kg.

In the short term, i.e., after 25 years, only the variation in terms of the bioconcentration factors of aboveground ('BCF above -90%') and belowground produce ('BCF below -90%'), and the biotransfer factor for milk cattle ('BTF dairy -90%') leads to significant changes in the aggregated effective Intake Fraction for ingestion. This is due to the marginal contribution of beef to the overall ingestion exposure in the short term (top vs. bottom of Fig. 9-14). The overall higher contribution of cattle produce in the long term is attributable to the reduced water soil erosion rate on pastures compared to arable land (cf. Table 5-7) leading to a slower removal of the trace elements out of this compartment and, thus, to a higher exposure of terrestrial food items in the long run. In general, the influence of parameters mostly or exclusively involved in the environmental fate assessment,

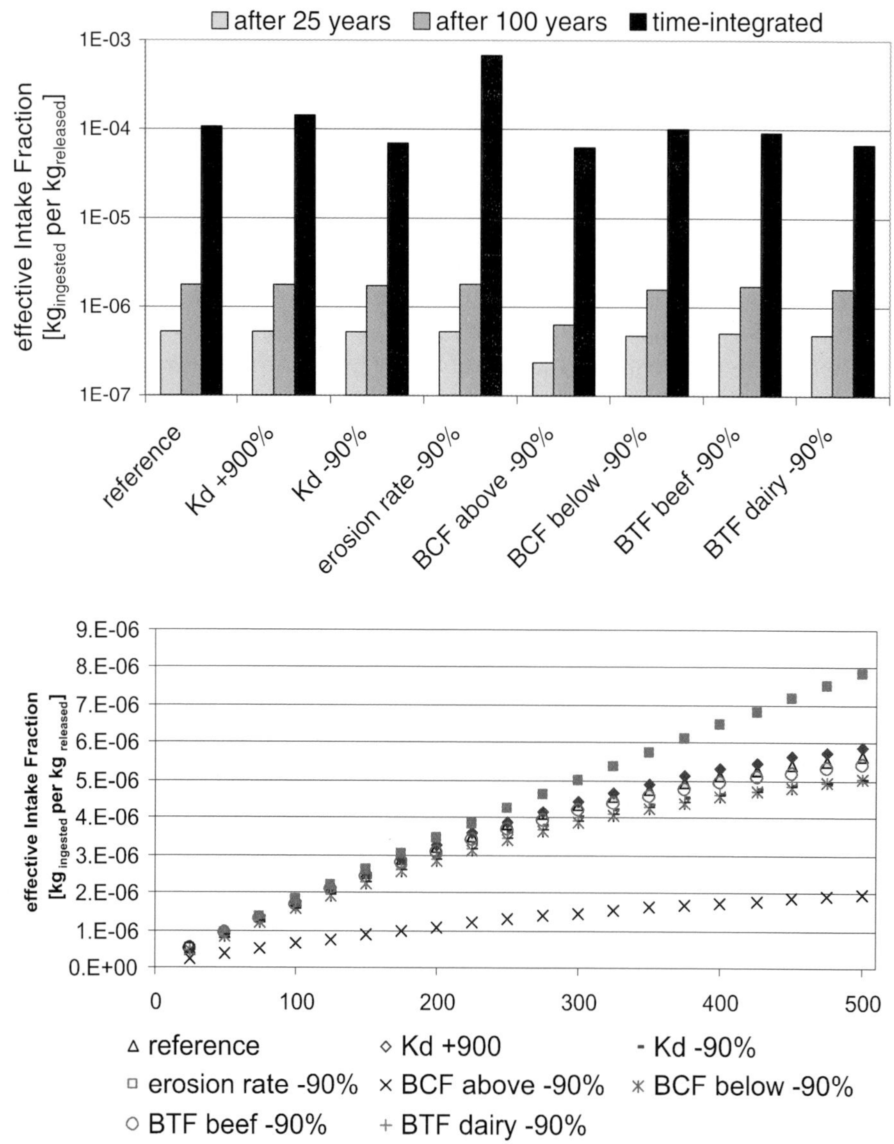

Fig. 9-13: Effective Intake Fraction for chromium due to ingestion of food according to the sensitivity analysis after 25 years, 100 years and at steady state (top) and the development within the first 500 years after the pulse emission (bottom); pan-European emissions to air in 1990

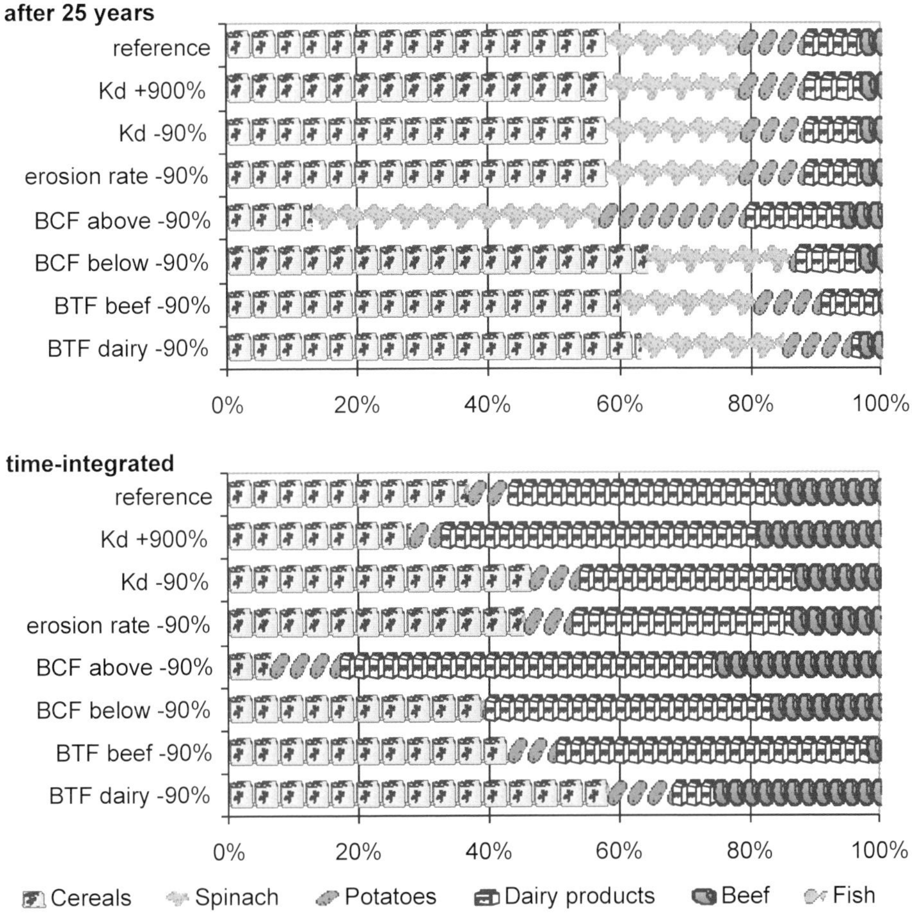

Fig. 9-14: Relative contribution of the different food items to the effective Intake Fraction (ingestion) of chromium after 25 years (top) and time-integrated (bottom) for a one year pulse emission according to the pan-European emission scenario to air in 1990 (cliparts by Corel Corporation, 2002)

i.e., the solid-water partitioning coefficient K_d and the soil erosion rate, only occurs to be significant in the long run. This indicates that the dynamics of chromium in the environment are rather slow. Thus, only the parameters involved in the exposure assessment of those food items remarkably contributing in the short term (cf. reference case in Fig. 9-14) show significant changes in the aggregated effective Intake Fraction for ingestion when integrating over shorter time horizons.

Table 9-6: Components of the effective Intake Fraction for chromium due to the ingestion of different food items according to the considered sensitivity cases after 25 years and time-integrated for the pan-European emission scenario to air in 1990 (emissions only take place in the first year) [$kg_{ingested}$ / $kg_{released}$]

Sensitivity scenario	Cereals	Spinach	Potatoes	Dairy products	Beef	Fish	Sum
after 25 years							
reference	$3.04 \cdot 10^{-7}$	$1.05 \cdot 10^{-7}$	$5.29 \cdot 10^{-8}$	$4.52 \cdot 10^{-8}$	$1.63 \cdot 10^{-8}$	$1.33 \cdot 10^{-14}$	$5.24 \cdot 10^{-7}$
Kd +900%	$3.04 \cdot 10^{-7}$	$1.05 \cdot 10^{-7}$	$5.29 \cdot 10^{-8}$	$4.52 \cdot 10^{-8}$	$1.63 \cdot 10^{-8}$	$9.54 \cdot 10^{-16}$	$5.24 \cdot 10^{-7}$
Kd -90%	$3.04 \cdot 10^{-7}$	$1.05 \cdot 10^{-7}$	$5.29 \cdot 10^{-8}$	$4.46 \cdot 10^{-8}$	$1.60 \cdot 10^{-8}$	$4.82 \cdot 10^{-13}$	$5.23 \cdot 10^{-7}$
erosion rate -90%	$3.04 \cdot 10^{-7}$	$1.05 \cdot 10^{-7}$	$5.29 \cdot 10^{-8}$	$4.52 \cdot 10^{-8}$	$1.63 \cdot 10^{-8}$	$5.10 \cdot 10^{-15}$	$5.24 \cdot 10^{-7}$
BCF above -90%	$3.04 \cdot 10^{-8}$	$1.05 \cdot 10^{-7}$	$5.29 \cdot 10^{-8}$	$3.52 \cdot 10^{-8}$	$1.46 \cdot 10^{-8}$	$1.33 \cdot 10^{-14}$	$2.38 \cdot 10^{-7}$
BCF below -90%	$3.04 \cdot 10^{-7}$	$1.05 \cdot 10^{-7}$	$5.29 \cdot 10^{-8}$	$4.52 \cdot 10^{-8}$	$1.63 \cdot 10^{-8}$	$1.33 \cdot 10^{-14}$	$4.77 \cdot 10^{-7}$
BTF beef -90%	$3.04 \cdot 10^{-7}$	$1.05 \cdot 10^{-7}$	$5.29 \cdot 10^{-8}$	$4.52 \cdot 10^{-8}$	$1.63 \cdot 10^{-9}$	$1.33 \cdot 10^{-14}$	$5.10 \cdot 10^{-7}$
BTF dairy -90%	$3.04 \cdot 10^{-7}$	$1.05 \cdot 10^{-7}$	$5.29 \cdot 10^{-8}$	$4.52 \cdot 10^{-9}$	$1.63 \cdot 10^{-8}$	$1.33 \cdot 10^{-14}$	$4.84 \cdot 10^{-7}$

Table 9-6: Components of the effective Intake Fraction for chromium due to the ingestion of different food items according to the considered sensitivity cases after 25 years and time-integrated for the pan-European emission scenario to air in 1990 (emissions only take place in the first year) [$kg_{ingested} / kg_{released}$]

Sensitivity scenario	Cereals	Spinach	Potatoes	Dairy products	Beef	Fish	Sum
time-integrated							
reference	$3.88 \cdot 10^{-5}$	$1.48 \cdot 10^{-7}$	$6.71 \cdot 10^{-6}$	$4.35 \cdot 10^{-5}$	$1.71 \cdot 10^{-5}$	$1.70 \cdot 10^{-12}$	$1.06 \cdot 10^{-4}$
Kd +900%	$3.98 \cdot 10^{-5}$	$1.49 \cdot 10^{-7}$	$6.92 \cdot 10^{-6}$	$6.97 \cdot 10^{-5}$	$2.69 \cdot 10^{-5}$	$1.80 \cdot 10^{-13}$	$1.44 \cdot 10^{-4}$
Kd -90%	$3.19 \cdot 10^{-5}$	$1.36 \cdot 10^{-7}$	$5.33 \cdot 10^{-6}$	$2.28 \cdot 10^{-5}$	$9.12 \cdot 10^{-6}$	$1.47 \cdot 10^{-11}$	$6.93 \cdot 10^{-5}$
erosion rate -90%	$3.05 \cdot 10^{-4}$	$4.07 \cdot 10^{-7}$	$5.11 \cdot 10^{-5}$	$2.28 \cdot 10^{-4}$	$9.12 \cdot 10^{-5}$	$1.44 \cdot 10^{-12}$	$6.75 \cdot 10^{-4}$
BCF above -90%	$3.90 \cdot 10^{-6}$	$1.09 \cdot 10^{-7}$	$6.74 \cdot 10^{-6}$	$3.58 \cdot 10^{-5}$	$1.57 \cdot 10^{-5}$	$1.71 \cdot 10^{-12}$	$6.22 \cdot 10^{-5}$
BCF below -90%	$3.88 \cdot 10^{-5}$	$1.48 \cdot 10^{-7}$	$6.72 \cdot 10^{-7}$	$4.35 \cdot 10^{-5}$	$1.71 \cdot 10^{-5}$	$1.70 \cdot 10^{-12}$	$1.00 \cdot 10^{-4}$
BTF beef -90%	$3.88 \cdot 10^{-5}$	$1.48 \cdot 10^{-7}$	$6.71 \cdot 10^{-6}$	$4.35 \cdot 10^{-5}$	$1.71 \cdot 10^{-6}$	$1.70 \cdot 10^{-12}$	$9.08 \cdot 10^{-5}$
BTF dairy -90%	$3.88 \cdot 10^{-5}$	$1.48 \cdot 10^{-7}$	$6.71 \cdot 10^{-6}$	$4.35 \cdot 10^{-6}$	$1.71 \cdot 10^{-5}$	$1.70 \cdot 10^{-12}$	$6.70 \cdot 10^{-5}$

Table 9-7: Values of the parameter sensitivity evaluation measure (term in brackets of Eq. (9-1)) for pan-European emissions of chromium to air in 1990 for time horizons of 25 years and time-integrated (emissions only take place in the first year)

Sensitivity scenario relative to reference	Parameter variation	Cereals [%]	Spinach [%]	Potatoes [%]	Dairy products [%]	Beef [%]	Fish [%]	Sum [%]
after 25 years								
Kd +900%	9	0	0	0	0.003	0	-10.3	0
Kd -90%	-0.9	0.005	0	0.005	1.58	1.8	-3917	0.20
erosion rate -90%	-0.9	-0.014	0	-0.014	-0.001	-0.001	68.5	-0.010
BCF above -90%	-0.9	100	0.32	0	24.6	11.04	0	60.6
BCF below -90%	-0.9	0	0	100	0	0	0	10.1
BTF beef -90%	-0.9	0	0	0	0	100	0	3.10
BTF dairy -90%	-0.9	0	0	0	100	0	0	8.62

Table 9-7: Values of the parameter sensitivity evaluation measure (term in brackets of Eq. (9-1)) for pan-European emissions of chromium to air in 1990 for time horizons of 25 years and time-integrated (emissions only take place in the first year)

Sensitivity scenario relative to reference	Parameter variation	Cereals [%]	Spinach [%]	Potatoes [%]	Dairy products [%]	Beef [%]	Fish [%]	Sum [%]
time-integrated								
Kd +900%	9	0.30	0.14	0.34	6.70	6.43	-9.94	3.91
Kd -90%	-0.9	19.7	8.4	22.8	52.8	51.7	-849	38.57
erosion rate -90%	-0.9	-762	-196	-734	-471	-483	17.5	-595
BCF above -90%	-0.9	99.9	28.7	-0.48	19.6	8.96	-0.36	46.0
BCF below -90%	-0.9	-0.06	-0.023	100	-0.001	0	-0.04	6.30
BTF beef -90%	-0.9	0	0	0	0	100	0	16.07
BTF dairy -90%	-0.9	0	0	0	100	0	0	41.0

The number of food items on which the varied parameters may have a significant influence varies from one to all. Due to the fact that the biotransfer factors (BTFs) are not involved in the environmental fate assessment, their variation only influences the exposure towards dairy products and beef. Given that the BTFs are included in all related exposure pathway computations in a linear way (cf. sections A.7.9, A.7.10 and A.7.11), their variation translates one to one into the exposure assessment of the respective food item (100 % in Table 9-7).

A similar finding is observed for the bioconcentration factor of belowground produce where merely the exposure towards the analysed crop is significantly influenced (i.e., potatoes). Due to the inclusion of the harvest removal process in the environmental fate model according to the 'food removal' environmental setting, however, the chromium concentrations are increased in those arable land compartments with joint cultivation of aboveground and belowground produce. The reduced uptake by potatoes in the 'BCF below -90%' sensitivity case leads to a higher exposure through aboveground produce at least in the long run (bottom of Fig. 9-14).

The variation of the bioconcentration factor of aboveground produce, in turn, significantly influences the human exposure towards several food items. Cereals as well as spinach classify as aboveground produce. Furthermore, farm animals are fed cereals to differing degrees. According to the 'BCF above -90%' sensitivity case, thus, the contribution not only of cereals and spinach but also of dairy products and beef to the human ingestion exposure is significantly influenced when varying the bioconcentration factor of aboveground produce. While cereals are regarded as being protected towards atmospheric depositions, spinach leaves are exposed. The contribution of spinach to the effective Intake Fraction is not significantly affected in the short term when reducing the BCF of aboveground crops due to the inclusion of the exposure pathway directly via the atmosphere. This stresses the importance of the atmospheric exposure of leafy vegetables which also shows in Fig. 9-14 and in the case studies presented in Chapters 10 and 11.

The 'Kd -90%' and the 'erosion rate -90%' sensitivity cases affect all food items significantly in the long run. Only the freshwater fish Intake Fraction after 25 years already indicates substantial changes in the short term for these two sensitivity cases. However, freshwater fish exposure is insubstantial (cf. Fig. 9-14). The decreased water soil erosion rate leads to smaller transfers of pollutants from the terrestrial compartments that show water soil erosion to the freshwater environment (section A.3.3), thereby increasing the concentrations in the arable land and pasture compartments and decreasing those in the freshwater bodies. This is reflected in the signs of the sensitivity evaluation measure in Table 9-7. This finding supports the need to appropriately represent the water soil erosion process for non-degrading and non-volatile substances, at least for long term assessments. This has already been postulated in the present work with respect to the spatial differentiation in terms of compartments (see section 5.1). The exposure through freshwater fish is also inversely correlated to the decrease in the K_d values. This result is due to two effects. First, the share of dissolved chromium in the freshwater environment is increased which leads to higher fish exposure. Second, also the total amount of chromium present in the freshwater environment is larger which can be attributed to a higher influx from the terrestrial compartments via the process of overland flow (section A.3.4) which depends on the amount of chromium present in the soil solution. The shift in the equilibrium distribution coefficient relating the aqueous phase concentration to the bulk concentration due to the change in the K_d value also translates into the process of matrix leaching. This again leads to a faster reduction of the chromium concentration in permeable soils (section A.3.6) and, thus, to a lower exposure through terrestrial plants and farm animals.

The influence of different assumptions with respect to the pH values of terrestrial compartments on the partitioning behaviour of chromium has also been investigated (Table 9-8). The effect of letting the K_d value depend on either a zonally variable pH value or just on a compartmentally variable pH value mostly shows in the long run for this metal. Two aspects can be noted. First, the aggregated effective Intake Fraction for ingestion exposures increases by 84 % when comparing the 'compartmental pH variation' to the 'zonal pH variation' scenario. This change fulfils the evaluation criterion with respect to the scenario analysis performed above where the variation in one component is classified influential if it leads to a change by more than 50 % with respect to a reference scenario (cf. section 9.3.3). Second, the contribution of different food items to the aggregated effective Intake Fraction for ingestion also changes remarkably in the long run. While there are higher exposures through all food items at least by a few percent, the exposures through dairy products and beef increase by more than a factor of two when integrating over time for the 'compartmental pH variation' scenario. These additional exposures appear to occur only in the long run as the effective Intake Fraction due to ingestion are practically equal for both sensitivity cases analysed after 25 and 100 years. The increases in the absolute value of this exposure measure are only 0.004 % and 0.4 %, respectively. The remarkable increase in the exposures through pasture-related food items can again be explained by the minimal pH values occurring in this compartment when allowing the pH to zonally vary. The invariant pH values representing neutral conditions (cf. Table 9-5) lead to a slower decline of the chromium concentrations in pasture soils and, thus, to a higher overall exposure through dairy products and cattle (see also the discussion above).

Table 9-8: Contribution of the different food items to the Intake Fraction (last row) of chromium for ingestion exposures after 25 years and time-integrated according to the sensitivity cases with respect to pH variability (pan-European emissions to air in 1990, only taking place in the first year)

Contribution to Intake Fraction for ingestion	After 25 years		Time-integrated	
	Zonal pH variation[a]	Compartmental pH variation	Zonal pH variation[a]	Compartmental pH variation
Cereals	58.1%	58.1%	36.5%	20.5%
Potatoes	10.1%	10.1%	6.3%	3.6%
Spinach	20.1%	20.1%	0.14%	0.077%
Dairy products	8.6%	8.6%	41.0%	55.2%
Beef	3.1%	3.1%	16.1%	20.7%
Fish	$2.5 \cdot 10^{-8}$	$1.8 \cdot 10^{-8}$	$1.6 \cdot 10^{-8}$	$9.3 \cdot 10^{-9}$
Intake Fraction [$kg_{ingested}$ per $kg_{released}$]	$5.24 \cdot 10^{-7}$	$5.24 \cdot 10^{-7}$	$1.06 \cdot 10^{-4}$	$1.95 \cdot 10^{-4}$

a.Previously termed 'reference' sensitivity case.

Above, significant sensitivities of different parameters have been identified. However, if the sensitive parameters are known rather precisely these parameters' sensitivities are not considered important (Hamby, 1994) which shall be discussed next.

In section B.5.3, it is discussed that the water soil erosion rate is a function of several site-specific parameters such as rainfall erosivity and crop management amongst others. The absolute value of the water soil erosion rate 'naturally' varies by two orders of magnitude across Europe (Milliman and Meade, 1983; Walling and Webb, 1983) when taking the sediment yield as an approximate indicator to the net erosion process which is in line with Morgan (1999). When operating at the regional scale and employing long-term average values, the water soil erosion rate may, therefore, be known rather precisely. However, it merely depends on compartments according to the methodological approach proposed here. Thus, the erosion rate contributes rather substantially to the overall uncertainty of the assessment. Whether the impacts according to the scenarios analysed in

Chapters 10 and 11 are overestimated or underestimated depends on the interplay of the spatial variability of several parameters such as atmospheric deposition, food production and erosion-prone areas and needs further investigations.

The concept of the solid-water partitioning coefficient K_d relies on a linearisation of the sorption behaviour of a chemical compound (Anonymous, 1999a; Aboul-Kassim and Simoneit, 2001b). The partitioning of a substance may, however, be influenced by several conditions of the environmental system for which a substance's behaviour shall be assessed. Influential factors may be the binding capacity of the solid phase, the total concentration of the substance present in the system, the pH, the organic carbon content especially in colloidal form and potential reaction partners amongst others. Although the present assessment allows to consider a pH-dependency of the partitioning of substances, the K_d value of a substance and a given pH range may still vary by one order of magnitude or more (Anonymous, 1999b). The introduction of pH-dependency could be demonstrated to decrease the sensitivity of the K_d value in the case of chromium at least when increasing its values. However, the consideration of further dependencies appears to be necessary to more reliably assess the considered substances. As a result, the K_d needs to be classified as contributing substantially to the overall uncertainty.

The transfer of substances into plants and/or animals according to a linear relationship between soil or feed concentrations on the one hand and living tissue concentrations on the other is deemed to be especially uncertain (e.g., by Vermeire et al., 1997). The reasons for this are similar to those related to the K_d concept in that the linearisation does not take into account all relevant aspects on which the BCFs and BTFs may depend such as plant or animal species variety, diet, solid and/or climatic conditions, age of the plant or animal (e.g., McLachlan, 1994). Due to the strong dependency of the exposure results on these parameters even already in the short term, they also contribute to the uncertainty of the estimated exposure.

Having analysed chromium in more detail, the question arises to what extent the exposure towards the other three trace elements is affected by the variation of the respective parameters. The solid-water partitioning coefficient of chromium in the neutral to alkaline range is the highest among the trace elements investigated (cf. Table C-1). According to the reasoning given above, it is evident that not only a decrease but also an increase of the respective K_d values will have a pronounced effect on the results for arsenic, cadmium and lead. The behaviour of chromium upon variation of its solid-water partitioning coefficients additionally suggests that the time-integrated Intake Fraction of the more mobile trace elements cadmium and lead will not only be lower but will also approach its final value quicker when decreasing the K_d values due to accelerated removal of these metals from the arable land compartment through which most of the human exposure occurs (cf. Fig. 10-3, 10-4 and 11-6). A pronounced effect will also be observed for all of the other substance-dependent parameters, provided these are related to food items through which a considerable amount of the exposure occurs. For instance, the exposure through animal products is rather small for cadmium and lead according to the case studies investigated (cf. Fig. 10-3, 10-4 and 11-6). Consequently, the variation of the biotransfer factors are expected to exert a less pronounced effect on the aggregated ingestion exposure estimates for these two heavy metals. The impact of the water soil erosion rate on the environmental fate at least of cadmium and lead is expected to be less significant, owing to their higher mobility reflected in their smaller K_d values. The higher mobility of these two metals also shows in the percentage of the ingestion-related effective Intake Fraction estimated for the case studies to occur after 10 and 100 years. These are at least a factor of four higher for cadmium and lead than for chromium and arsenic (cf. sections 10.3 and 11.4).

9.4 Concluding remarks on the evaluation of results

Overall, there exist many uncertainties associated with the presented exposure assessment methodology as presented in section 9.3. The uncertainties related to the impact assessment tend to be even larger (Finley and Paustenbach, 1994) especially due to the unavailability of reliable epidemiological dose-response functions. The appropriate evaluation of large scale multimedia exposure and impact assessment models is generally hindered due to the process of policy decision-making related to their application (Ragas et al., 1999), lack of data (Hunsaker et al., 1990) and/or adequate evaluation criteria (Rykiel (Jr.), 1996) at the respective scale.

Data quality is one of the major limiting factors in model development and model quality assurance (e.g., Addiscott et al., 1995; Beck and Chen, 2000). Regarding particularly the spatially distributed parameters, the selection of appropriate values could not always be guided by data quality but was rather constraint by data availability. Therefore, the influence of choosing other datasets e.g. for the hydrological cycle could not be evaluated.

Other uncertainty analyses have shown that especially emission information is crucial for site-dependent assessments of environmental media concentrations (Price et al., 1996; United States - Environmental Protection Agency, 1998; Vink and Peters, 2003). The comparison of the atmospheric deposition data with moss monitoring data points into the same direction but may also partly be due to the employed air quality model. It is, furthermore, supported by an EU position paper (European Commission, 2000b) emphasizing that one of the presently best available pan-European emission estimates for 1990 (Berdowski et al., 1997) in parts considerably overestimates emissions.

Trapp and Matthies (1998) have formulated as one goal in the modelling of compartment systems to keep the number of compartments as low as possible. It has been shown in the conducted scenario analysis that the distinction of pastures from arable land leads to an increase of exposure due to pasture-based food chains such as dairy products and beef. Depending on the emission scenario and the substance investigated, this may be important. Also the distinction of rivers from lakes especially with respect to the particle mass balance has a pronounced effect on the freshwater fish exposure estimates. In contrast to the differentiation of the agricultural soils into arable land and pastures, the distinction of flowing from stagnant water bodies in the way it is performed here, however, does not increase the number of compartments but merely changes compartmental characteristics. The most significant increase in compartments is related to the spatial differentiation of the model's geographical scope into zones. It appears as if the lower spatial resolution does not change the overall exposure estimates substantially for the pan-European emission to air scenario analysed. However, analyses of more localised emission sources including direct discharges into water may reveal more pronounced differences as discussed above.

The scenario analysis performed addressing different environmental settings in terms of spatial differentiation, process formulations and process inclusions supports the findings by Hertwich et al. (2000) in that the variation in the spatial resolution and/or spatial differentiation does not affect the overall exposure results of large scale contamination scenarios to a substantial degree, for instance by more than a factor of two. However, these may cause a shift in the relative importance of the different food items contributing to the overall human exposure.

The sensitivity analysis of the parameters has identified the water soil erosion rate as one non-substance-specific parameter that is significantly influential on the exposure results at least of rather immobile substances such as chromium, beside substance-specific parameters such as the solid-water partitioning coefficient, bioconcentration factors and biotransfer factors. Having used the water soil erosion as one key criterion for the distinction of compartments in an exposure assessment of rather persistent and non-volatile substances is, therefore, supported.

Regardless of the magnitude of the uncertainties, the present work as such is an improvement towards more knowledge about the magnitude of the external costs occurring due to human activities. Before this contribution hardly any (if at all) information on the external costs for exposure routes other than inhalation had been available. Therefore, the uncertainty is considered acceptable given the model's purpose (Eisenhart, 1968; Scott et al., 2000). Furthermore, the approach is adequate in that the model design has been orientated at the 'availability of parameter values' and the 'acceptability of the goals with the budget' (Draper and

Smith, 1966 cited in Caswell, 1976). Given that "the modeller and the users may have different thresholds for confidence" (Robinson, 1999, p. 68), it has been tried to document the methodological approach as explicit as possible taking account of the suggestion "that the manner in which a study is performed is more important in forming a user's quality perception than the quality (or validity) of the model and its results" (ibid., p. 68). This is in line with one of the good-practice principles to show all formula used in the model (Burmaster and Anderson, 1994; Veerkamp and Wolff, 1996) which is done in Chapters 4, 5, 6 and 7, and Appendix A of the present work.

10 Case studies on emissions from single facilities

In the following, the Impact Pathway Approach which is extended by ingestion exposures according to the methodology developed in this work shall be applied to case studies. Two different kinds of case studies will be performed. The first kind addresses the derivation of marginal external costs due to the operation of single power plants (this Chapter). The other assesses the overall quantifiable external costs due to pan-European emissions into air for the situation in 1990 which will be presented in a separate Chapter (11).

10.1 Definition of marginal emission-related case studies

The marginal emission-related case studies investigate the influence of the location of point sources on the marginal external costs due to the exposure towards the trace elements under study. The resulting, quantifiable marginal external costs will be put into perspective by comparing them to those caused by the emission of the classical air pollutants such as SO_2, NO_x, NH_3, NMVOC and primary particles previously reported.

In order to define the scope of the respective case studies, one needs to specify (European Commission, 1999a):

- the technology to be assessed,
- the location of emissions (e.g., at the power plant, supporting activities), and
- the fuel (type, source and composition).

According to the context in which this study is conducted, the techniques of prime interest are related to energy conversion (European Commission, 1999a). Generally, the combustion of hard coals and lignite leads to the highest emissions of heavy metals when compared to oil and natural gas used in the energy sector (Joint Research Centre of the European Commission, 2003). While most trace elements are emitted at amounts several orders of magnitude higher for coal than for the other fossil fuels, the combustion of heavy fuel oil may lead to

Table 10-1: Characteristics of the investigated power plants

Characteristic	Belgium	France	Germany	UK
Location	Genk-Langerlo	Cordemais, near Nantes	Lauffen	West Burton
Latitude [°]	50.97	47.18	49.08	53.38
Longitude [°]	5.50	-1.48	9.18	-1.50
Stack height [m]	140	220	240	230
Net efficiency [%]	37	38	43	38
Electricity generation [GWh_{el}/yr]	1472	2100	3900	11700

releases of nickel and vanadium in larger quantities. However, these elements are not subject of the analysis due to data availability constraints primarily related to the impact assessment (cf. section 7.3).

Consequently, the technology to be assessed are coal-fired power plants. The investigated trace elements are mostly released into air in association with particles (Joint Research Centre of the European Commission, 2003). The amounts emitted depend to a large extent on the flue gas treatment in use and the coals employed (e.g., Rentz and Martel, 1998; Joint Research Centre of the European Commission, 2003). For instance, the reduction rates from flue gas of high performance electrostatic (dust) precipitators and fabric filters lie above 99.9 %. Principally one can distinguish between three groups of trace elements in terms of their mass balance during combustion and flue gas cleaning (Joint Research Centre of the European Commission, 2003). Chromium belongs to one of these groups whose elements leave the stack to 0.1 %. Arsenic, cadmium and lead being part of another group are lost to air with the cleaned flue gas to 0.07 %. These values will be used to determine the amounts of trace elements emitted by power plants equipped with Best Available Techniques (BAT). Further information needed in order to determine the total emissions of trace elements into air during a one year period are the total annual electricity sent-out and the efficiency of the power plant the concentrations of the trace elements in the coals burnt and their lower heating value.

Four sites have been selected for the investigation that are taken from the recently completed EC-funded NewExt project (Number: ENG1-2000-00129). All facilities are coal-fired power plants. The locations and some characteristics of the power plants are given in Table 10-1.,According to the stack heights, only

Table 10-2: Ranges of trace element concentrations in coals of different origin as quoted in Joint Research Centre of the European Commission (2003) [mg/kg]

Trace element	Minimum value	Maximum value
Arsenic	1.4	18.5
Cadmium	0.06	0.73
Chromium	7.4	40
Lead	4.8	32

Table 10-3: Theoretical emission ranges of the investigated trace elements for the respective facilities [t/yr]

Plant	Estimate	Arsenic	Cadmium	Chromium	Lead
Belgium	minimum	$4.13 \cdot 10^{-4}$	$1.77 \cdot 10^{-5}$	$3.12 \cdot 10^{-3}$	$1.42 \cdot 10^{-3}$
	maximum	$6.87 \cdot 10^{-3}$	$2.71 \cdot 10^{-4}$	$2.12 \cdot 10^{-2}$	$1.19 \cdot 10^{-2}$
France	minimum	$5.73 \cdot 10^{-4}$	$2.46 \cdot 10^{-5}$	$4.33 \cdot 10^{-3}$	$1.97 \cdot 10^{-3}$
	maximum	$9.54 \cdot 10^{-3}$	$3.77 \cdot 10^{-4}$	$2.95 \cdot 10^{-2}$	$1.65 \cdot 10^{-2}$
Germany	minimum	$9.41 \cdot 10^{-4}$	$4.03 \cdot 10^{-5}$	$7.11 \cdot 10^{-3}$	$3.23 \cdot 10^{-3}$
	maximum	$1.57 \cdot 10^{-2}$	$6.18 \cdot 10^{-4}$	$4.84 \cdot 10^{-2}$	$2.71 \cdot 10^{-2}$
UK	minimum	$3.19 \cdot 10^{-3}$	$1.37 \cdot 10^{-4}$	$2.41 \cdot 10^{-2}$	$1.10 \cdot 10^{-2}$
	maximum	$5.32 \cdot 10^{-2}$	$2.10 \cdot 10^{-3}$	$1.64 \cdot 10^{-1}$	$9.20 \cdot 10^{-2}$

so-called 'high' emissions, i.e., those above 100 metres have been considered. No plant-specific information on the coals burnt are available which is why default values will be used. Table 10-2 gives the ranges of trace element concentrations in coal stemming from different mines of the world. The lower heating values of hard coals are assumed to range from 27 to 34 MJ per kilogram (Beitz and Küttner, 1995).

The upper and lower bound in terms of trace element emissions are given in Table 10-3 for the respective power plants. The minimum and maximum values are obtained by combining the upper bound lower heating value with the trace element contents of the less contaminated coals and vice versa.

Table 10-4: Effective Intake Fractions due to inhalation of selected trace elements for a one year pulse emission into air at different sites [$kg_{inhaled}$ per $kg_{released}$]

Trace element	Belgium	France	Germany	UK
Arsenic	$8.7 \cdot 10^{-6}$	$4.8 \cdot 10^{-6}$	$7.2 \cdot 10^{-6}$	$4.6 \cdot 10^{-6}$
Cadmium	$8.7 \cdot 10^{-6}$	$4.8 \cdot 10^{-6}$	$7.2 \cdot 10^{-6}$	$4.6 \cdot 10^{-6}$
Chromium	$8.7 \cdot 10^{-7}$	$4.8 \cdot 10^{-7}$	$7.2 \cdot 10^{-7}$	$4.6 \cdot 10^{-7}$
Lead	$8.7 \cdot 10^{-6}$	$4.8 \cdot 10^{-6}$	$7.2 \cdot 10^{-6}$	$4.6 \cdot 10^{-6}$

Default emission scenarios have been run with the help of the EcoSense model for all facilities by assuming that 1000 kilogram of a trace element are emitted during a one year period. The effective Intake Fractions for inhalation and ingestion exposures are derived separately based on these pulse emission scenarios. The properties of the investigated contaminants are given in Appendix C.

10.2 Impacts due to inhalation exposure

The impact assessment due to inhalation is based on the respective (effective) Intake Fraction. Its contribution to the quantifiable overall Intake Fraction ceases after one year for substances that are short-lived in air under pulse emission conditions of the same duration. The respective values due to inhalation exposures are given in Table 10-4. It can be noted that all elements emitted at one site show the same environmental dispersion. This is due to the way the trace elements are assumed to be distributed on the different particle size classes in air (Table 4-1 and Lee, 2003). Note that lead stemming from an emission source other than traffic also follows the same particle size distribution scheme in air like the other trace elements in this case. The difference by one order of magnitude between the values for arsenic, cadmium and lead on the one hand and for chromium on the other is due to the assumption that 10 % of the chromium amounts emitted are in the hexavalent state (cf. Table C-2). The Intake Fractions for the power plant in Belgium are the highest indicating that more people are affected. This is due to the prevailing westerly winds which lead to a higher exposure of the Ruhr catchment in Germany, an area with a high population density (agglomeration). A higher population density of the area affected also applies to the German emission scenario, however, to a lesser extent.

The Disability Adjusted Life Years (DALYs) due to cancer and non-cancer effects related to the release of one kilogram of the respective trace element are

Table 10-5: Disability Adjusted Life Years (DALYs) per kilogram of selected trace elements released due to cancer and non-cancer effects upon inhalation exposure caused by a one year pulse emission from selected power plant sites [years lost-equivalents per $kg_{released}$]

Trace element	Type of effect	Belgium	France	Germany	UK
Arsenic	cancer	$5.95 \cdot 10^{-4}$	$3.26 \cdot 10^{-4}$	$4.94 \cdot 10^{-4}$	$3.15 \cdot 10^{-4}$
	non-cancer	n/a	n/a	n/a	n/a
Cadmium	cancer	$2.49 \cdot 10^{-4}$	$1.37 \cdot 10^{-4}$	$2.07 \cdot 10^{-4}$	$1.32 \cdot 10^{-4}$
	non-cancer	n/a	n/a	n/a	n/a
Chromium	cancer	$1.66 \cdot 10^{-4}$	$9.11 \cdot 10^{-5}$	$1.38 \cdot 10^{-4}$	$8.79 \cdot 10^{-5}$
	non-cancer	$2.43 \cdot 10^{-6}$	$1.33 \cdot 10^{-6}$	$2.02 \cdot 10^{-6}$	$1.29 \cdot 10^{-6}$
Lead	cancer	n/a	n/a	n/a	n/a
	non-cancer	n/a	n/a	n/a	n/a

given in Table 10-5. No non-cancer effect information for inhalation exposures is available for arsenic, cadmium and lead (cf. section 7.3). The same applies to cancer effects due to inhalation of lead which means that no inhalation-related effects for lead can be assessed at present. The cancer-related DALYs per kilogram released are about in the same order of magnitude for all trace elements, owing to comparable slope factors and associated DALYs. The steeper slope factor for cancer due to inhalation of chromium is counterbalanced by the lower amount of hexavalent chromium assumed to be present in air. The non-cancer effect caused by inhalation of hexavalent chromium is classified as a category 3 effect with little years lost-equivalents associated (cf. Table 7-7) leading to a reduced contribution to the overall impact. As discussed in section 9.3.1, the assumption of a linear exposure-response function without thresholds is still a matter for debate with respect to non-cancer effects at least at the individual level. However, the non-cancer associated DALYs caused by chromium are smaller by about two orders of magnitude than those due to cancer. Also the contribution of the non-cancer effects to the overall damage costs caused by inhalation exposures are negligible (see Table 10-6).

Valuing the substance-specific inhalation-caused impacts leads to damage factors in external costs per kilogram of pollutant emitted (Table 10-6). The monetary values used are given in section 8.2.4. The external costs yielded are smaller by up to a factor of about seven when compared to those provided by European

Commission (2004). The discrepancy can be attributed to the different concentration-response model, to the different monetary values chosen and partly the different air quality models used. The effect information employed differs by a factor of two corresponding to the modification of the 95th upper limit estimate to become a maximum likelihood slope factor according to Eq. (7-14). The monetary valuation of cancer cases at a discount rate of 3 % is also different by a factor of two, using $2 \cdot 10^6$ €$_{2000}$ per generic cancer case (European Commission, 2004) and 819552 €$_{2000}$ per lung cancer case in this study (cf. Table 8-6), respectively. This means that the contribution of the trace elements investigated to the overall external damage costs due to the operation of power plants is even less substantial than according to European Commission (2004).

The damage factors for classical air pollutants such as NO_x, SO_2 and primary particles may range from 3 to 27 €$_{2000}$ per kilogram emitted (discounted at 3 %, European Commission, 2004). These values are about in the same order of magnitude as those estimated here, noting that the classical air pollutants are emitted in much larger quantities.

Ranges of annual external costs due to the operation of the four facilities investigated are obtained by scaling the damage factors (Table 10-6) with the theoretical minimum and maximum annual emission values (Table 10-3). The resulting figures in Euro per year are given in Tables 10-7 and 10-8 for a discount rate of 0 and 3 %, respectively. The external costs indicate that the use of different coals with variable degrees of contamination and (lower) heating values may have a pronounced effect of more than one order of magnitude on the external costs assessed to occur. However, usually the characteristics of the coals employed at a given plant can be known exactly so that this source of variability of the results can substantially be reduced. It shows, furthermore, that the plant with the largest electricity generation is situated in the UK leading to the highest external costs due to a one-year operation. This reflects the highest annual emissions (cf. Table 10-3) despite its smallest damage factors among the facilities analysed (cf. Table 10-6). The ranking of the other facilities is Germany, Belgium and France in descending order.

The external costs per kilowatt hour of electricity generated are also given in Tables 10-7 and 10-8. The external costs of the classical air pollutants per kilowatt hour are in the €-cent range according to European Commission (2004) whereas those computed for the trace elements in total are about five orders of magnitude smaller which is due to them being emitted to a lesser extent.

Table 10-6: Damage factors due to inhalation for a one year pulse emission from different sites discounted at a rate of 0 and 3 % [$€_{2000}$ per $kg_{released}$]

Trace element[a]	Type of effect	Type of monetary value	Belgium		France		Germany		UK	
			0 %	3 %	0 %	3 %	0 %	3 %	0 %	3 %
Arsenic[b]	cancer	WTP	44.6	23.8	24.5	13.1	37.1	19.8	23.6	12.6
		COI	11.8	6.3	6.5	3.4	9.8	5.2	6.2	3.3
Cadmium[b]	cancer	WTP	18.7	10.0	10.2	5.5	15.5	8.3	9.9	5.3
		COI	4.9	2.6	2.7	1.4	4.1	2.2	2.6	1.4
Chromium	cancer	WTP	12.4	6.6	6.8	3.6	10.3	5.5	6.6	3.5
		COI	3.3	1.8	1.8	0.96	2.7	1.5	1.7	0.93
	non-cancer	WTP	0.182	0.097	0.100	0.053	0.152	0.081	0.097	0.052
		COI	n/a	n/a	n/a	n/a	n/a	n/a	n/a	n/a

a.No effect information available for lead.
b.No non-cancer effect information available.

Table 10-7: Ranges of quantifiable external costs discounted at 0 % due to inhalation of selected trace elements and in total caused by a one year pulse emission from different sites (variable units, base year 2000)

Trace element[a]	Type of effect	Type of monetary value	Belgium		France		Germany		UK	
			[€/yr]	[10^{-9} €/kWh$_{el}$]	[€/yr]	[10^{-9} €/kWh$_{el}$]	[€/yr]	[10^{-9} €/kWh$_{el}$]	[€/yr]	[10^{-9} €/kWh$_{el}$]
Arsenic[b]	cancer	WTP	18-306	13-208	14-234	6.7-111	35-581	8.9-149	75-1256	6.4-107
		COI	4.9-81	3.3-55	3.7-62	1.8-29	9.2-153	2.4-39	20-331	1.7-28
Cadmium[b]	cancer	WTP	0.33-5.1	0.22-3.4	0.25-3.9	0.12-1.8	0.63-10	0.16-2.5	1.4-21	0.12-1.8
		COI	0.087-1.3	0.059-0.91	0.066-1.0	0.032-0.48	0.17-2.5	0.042-0.65	0.36-5.5	0.031-0.47
Chromium	cancer	WTP	39-264	26-179	30-201	14-96	74-501	19-128	159-1082	14-93
		COI	10-70	7.0-47	7.8-53	3.7-25	19-132	5.0-34	42-285	3.6-24
	non-cancer	WTP	0.57-3.9	0.39-2.6	0.43-3.0	0.21-1.4	1.1-7.3	0.28-1.9	2.3-16	0.20-1.4
		COI	n/a	n/a	n/a	n/a	n/a	n/a	n/a	n/a
Sum			*73-731*	*50-497*	*56-558*	*27-265*	*139-1390*	*36-355*	*300-3000*	*26-256*

a.No effect information available for lead.
b.No non-cancer effect information available.

Table 10-8: Ranges of quantifiable external costs discounted at 3 % due to inhalation of selected trace elements and in total caused by a one year pulse emission from different sites (variable units, base year 2000)

Trace element[a]	Type of effect	Type of monetary value	Belgium [€/yr]	Belgium [10^{-9} €/kWh$_{el}$]	France [€/yr]	France [10^{-9} €/kWh$_{el}$]	Germany [€/yr]	Germany [10^{-9} €/kWh$_{el}$]	UK [€/yr]	UK [10^{-9} €/kWh$_{el}$]
Arsenic[b]	cancer	WTP	9.8-163	6.7-110	7.5-125	3.6-59	19-310	4.8-79	40-670	3.4-57
		COI	2.6-43	1.8-29	2.0-33	0.94-16	4.9-82	1.3-21	11-177	0.91-15
Cadmium[b]	cancer	WTP	0.18-2.7	0.12-1.8	0.13-2.1	0.064-0.98	0.33-5.1	0.086-1.3	0.7-11	0.062-0.95
		COI	0.046-0.7	0.032-0.48	0.035-0.54	0.017-0.26	0.088-1.3	0.023-0.35	0.19-2.9	0.016-0.25
Chromium	cancer	WTP	21-141	14-96	16-107	7.5-51	39-267	10-68	85-577	7.2-49
		COI	5.5-37	3.7-25	4.2-28	2.0-13	10-70	2.7-18	22-152	1.9-13
	non-cancer	WTP	0.30-2.1	0.21-1.4	0.23-1.6	0.11-0.75	0.57-3.9	0.15-1.0	1.2-8.5	0.11-0.72
		COI	n/a	n/a	n/a	n/a	n/a	n/a	n/a	n/a
Sum			*39-390*	*27-265*	*30-297*	*14-142*	*74-739*	*19-190*	*160-1600*	*14-137*

a.No effect information available for lead.
b.No non-cancer effect information available.

10.3 Impacts due to ingestion exposure

The assessment of the ingestion-related human exposures is performed based on the environmental settings of the 'food removal' scenario (see section 9.3.3). The four trace elements analysed show marked differences in terms of both the absolute value of the effective Intake Fraction due to ingestion exposures and the temporal development of this measure (Fig. 10-1 and Fig. 10-2, note the logarithmic scale). The amount of cadmium taken in is highest for releases from all sites reaching 0.25 % of the overall amount released in the Belgian case. Arsenic and chromium show effective Intake Fractions due to ingestion of about one order of magnitude less than cadmium in the long run. The effective Intake Fraction due to ingestion of lead is about one third of that for cadmium. According to the present assessment, there will be a relatively and absolutely higher exposure of cadmium and lead within the next 100 years upon release of the trace elements. This means that 23.2-25.6 %, 9.6-10.6 %, 1.4-2.1 % and 1.0-1.3 % of the time-integrated effective Intake Fraction due to ingestion will have been reached within this period of time for cadmium, lead, chromium and arsenic, respectively. These figures are substantially smaller for the first 10 year period (4.3-5.0 %, 1.4-2.1 %, 0.2-0.5 % and 0.12-0.14 %, respectively). The contribution of the inhalation-related Intake Fraction is insignificant in the long run (when performing non-zero discounting, Fig. 10-1 and Fig. 10-2). This also holds for the short and intermediate term, except for arsenic. This indicates that the exposure through the media soil and water are most significant at least in the intermediate to long term.

The differences between the sites in terms of the absolute time-integrated Intake Fractions due to ingestion are within a factor of 1.3 for chromium to 2.6 for arsenic, with Belgian emissions leading to the highest specific ingestion exposures investigated and those from the UK site to the lowest. This ranking is equal to that of the inhalation Intake Fractions. Also the variation between sites is similar to the inhalation Intake Fractions despite the homogenizing effect of food concentrations due to trade. This homogenizing effect of trade has especially been postulated by Spadaro and Rabl (2004) which is demonstrated not to be the case to the extent expected by these authors. It is reflected in all subsequently derived measures such as damage costs per contaminant emitted (see below). Moreover, the dynamics for the different trace elements vary for the different sites. For instance, the development of the ingestion exposure with respect to cadmium is quickest in the UK (25.6 % of the time-integrated situation reached after 100 years) that of chromium is about the slowest at the same site (1.5 %).

Not only the total amounts taken in vary considerably in time and space but also the most contributing food items (Fig. 10-3 and Fig. 10-4). This variation may even lead to entirely different patterns in terms of the dominating food items at different integration times. For instance, the long-term exposure towards arsenic is dominated by dairy products (more than 74 %) while in the short term the composition of the ingestion exposure is more balanced. Also, the exposure through aboveground exposed produce such as spinach contributes more substantially in the near future alongside with the occurring emissions while in the long run its contribution to the effective Intake Fraction may be insubstantial (top vs. bottom for a given site in Fig. 10-3 and Fig. 10-4). The contribution of aboveground exposed produce through interception of atmospheric deposition, thus, appears to be similar to inhalation-related exposures in terms of their intertemporal significance for human exposure towards pulse emissions.

The ingestion of cadmium and lead primarily occurs contained in cereals (more than 77 % in the long run) while dairy products are also important for chromium and even more so for arsenic. Beef only constitutes a significant share of chromium's Intake Fraction in the long run according to this assessment (Fig. 10-3 and Fig. 10-4). Freshwater fish and other animal products such as pork, poultry and eggs contribute less than one percent of the Intake Fraction due to ingestion, partly owing to non-available substance-specific transfer data (Table C-5). Depending on the place of emission, the shares of the different food items contributing to the aggregated ingestion exposure also vary. For instance, cereals are more important for emissions taking place in France and in the UK while the exposure through potatoes grows in importance for emissions occurring in Belgium and Germany. This is mainly explainable by differences in the intensity of the cultivation of these two staple food products in different countries (cf. Table B-16). Differences between aboveground protected and belowground produce in terms of the bioconcentration factors are insubstantial except for arsenic (cf. Table C-4).

In the long run, the impacts due to ingestion in terms of DALYs per emitted amount of trace element tend to be larger than those due to inhalation for a one year pulse emission except for chromium (Table 10-9 vs. Table 10-5). These impacts are assessed by employing the approach described in section 7.3.1 which is based on the Intake Fractions presented above. Generally, non-cancer effects dominate the DALYs assessed via ingestion exposures (Table 10-9). Only non-cancer effect information is available for cadmium and chromium through this exposure route according to Crettaz (2000). While the DALYs due to non-cancer effects are about one order of magnitude larger than due to cancer for arsenic, this discrepancy amounts to more than two orders of magnitude for lead (refer to section 9.3.1 with respect to a discussion on the uncertainty of the effect assessment for both effect types).

Valuing the impacts assessed to occur via ingestion yields the damage factors expressed in external costs per kilogram of pollutant emitted (Table 10-10 through to Table 10-13). These are given for two different discount rates. The highest specific damage costs are estimated for emissions stemming from the Bel-

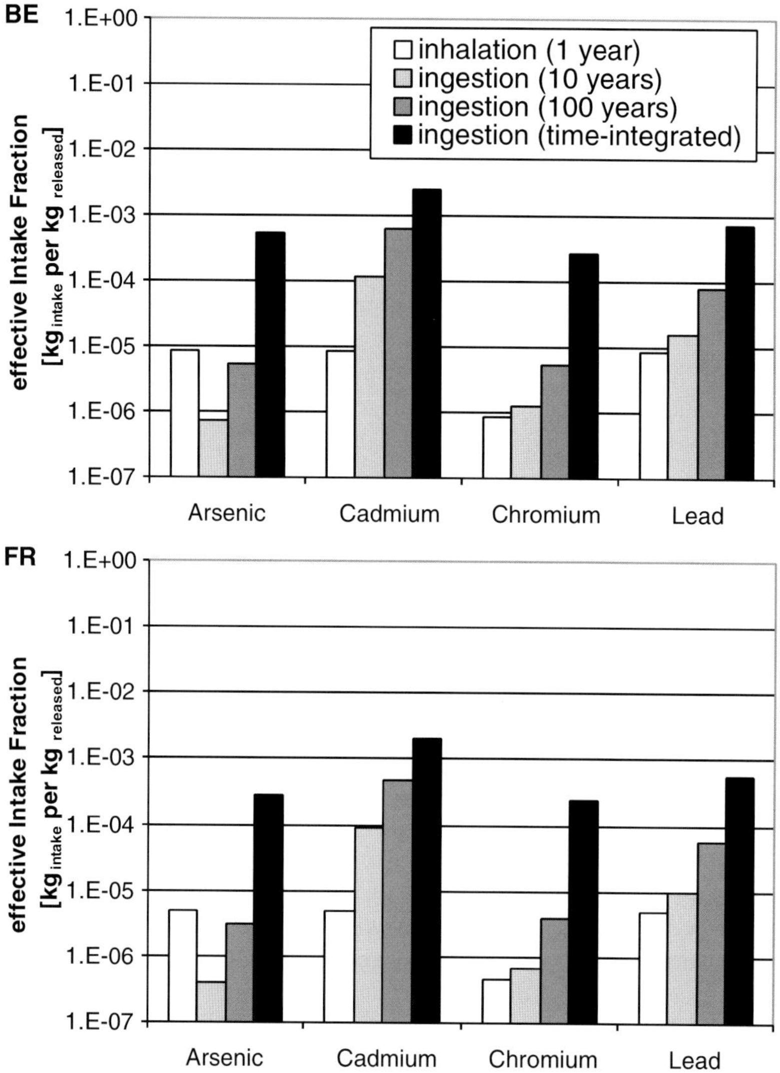

Fig. 10-1: Effective Intake Fraction of selected trace elements via inhalation after one year and via ingestion of food after 10 and 100 years, and time-integrated for a one year pulse emission from the Belgian ('BE', top) and French site ('FR', bottom); note the logarithmic scale [kg_{intake} per $kg_{released}$]

gian power plant followed by the facilities in Germany, France and the UK in descending order. In all cases, the highest damage factors are estimated to be caused by non-cancer effects due to cadmium and lead ingestion ranging from 3488 to

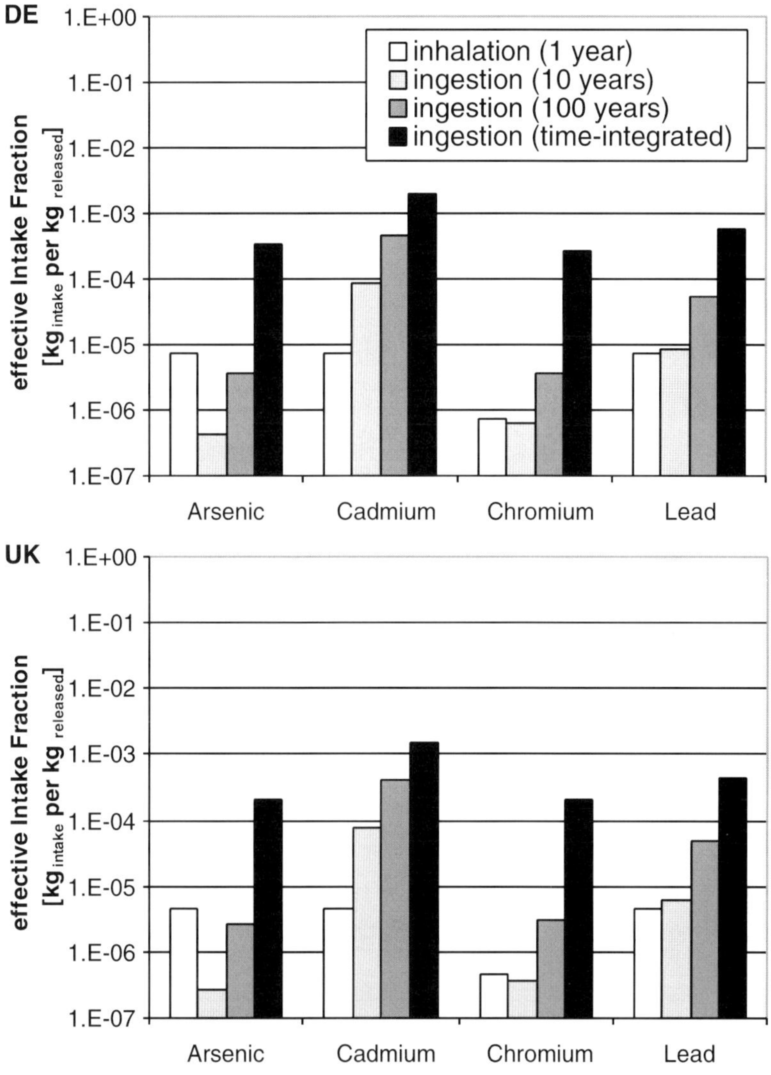

Fig. 10-2: Effective Intake Fraction of selected trace elements via inhalation after one year and via ingestion of food after 10 and 100 years, and time-integrated for a one year pulse emission from the German ('DE', top) and UK site ('UK', bottom); note the logarithmic scale [kg_{intake} per $kg_{released}$]

5642 $€_{2000}$ per kilogram of cadmium released and from 3500 to 5658 $€_{2000}$ per kilogram of lead released, respectively, when discounting at a rate of 0 %. The corresponding costs for arsenic amount to some ten percent of those for lead or

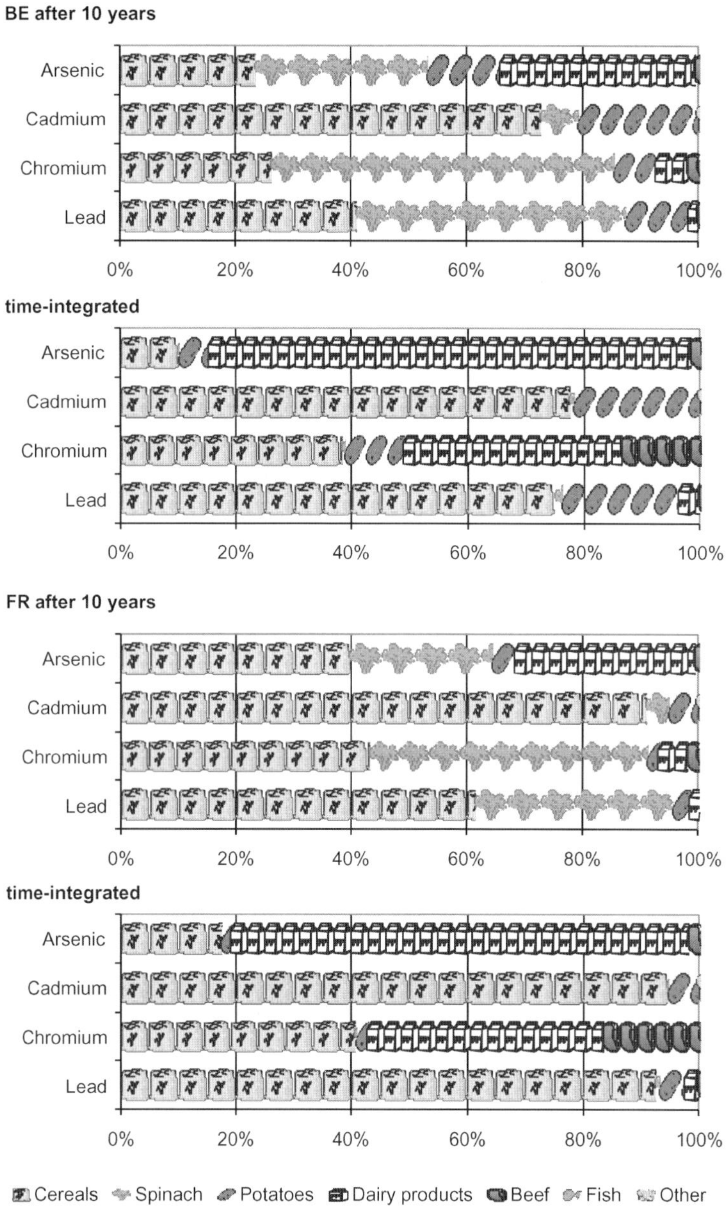

Fig. 10-3: Relative contribution of the different food items to the effective Intake Fraction (ingestion) of selected trace elements after 10 years and time-integrated for a one year pulse emission from the Belgian ('BE', top) and French site ('FR', bottom, cliparts by Corel Corporation, 2002)

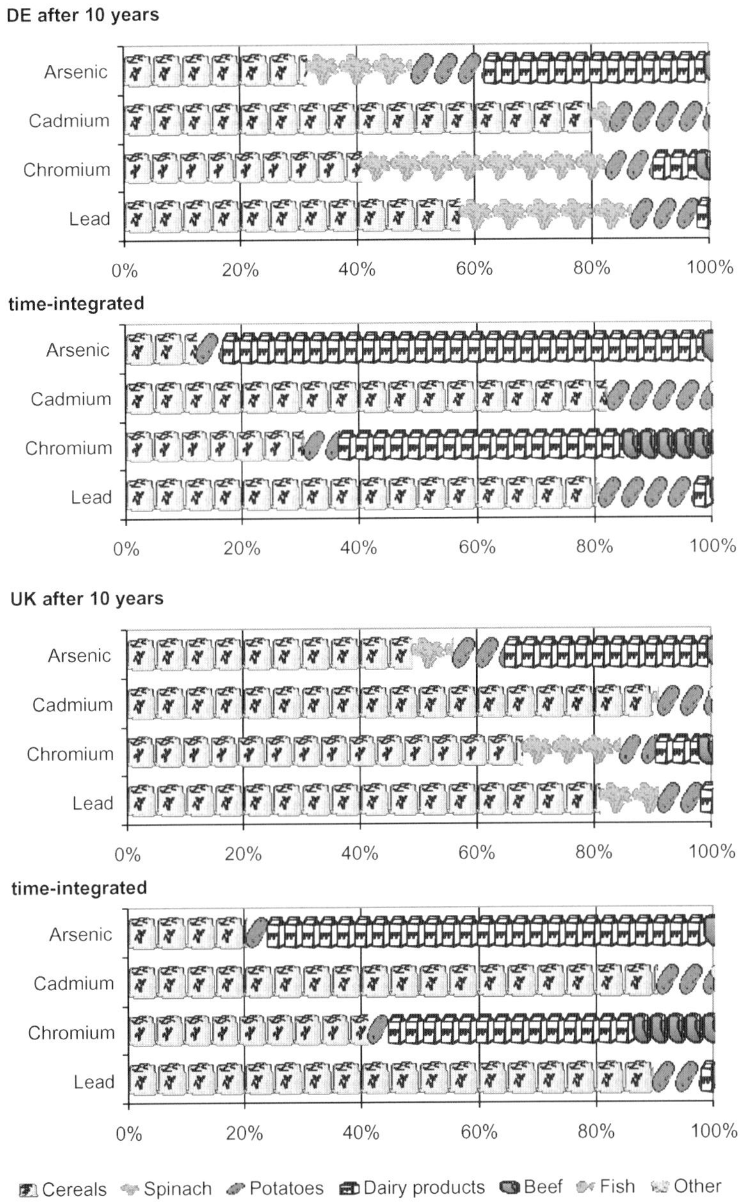

Fig. 10-4: Relative contribution of the different food items to the effective Intake Fraction (ingestion) of selected trace elements after 10 years and time-integrated for a one year pulse emission from the German ('DE', top) and the UK site ('UK', bottom, cliparts by Corel Corporation, 2002)

Table 10-9: Time-integrated Disability Adjusted Life Years (DALYs) per kilogram of trace element released due to cancer and non-cancer effects upon ingestion exposure caused by a one year pulse emission from single sites [years lost-equivalents per $kg_{released}$]

Trace element	Type of effect	Belgium	France	Germany	UK
Arsenic	Cancer	$1.39 \cdot 10^{-3}$	$7.41 \cdot 10^{-4}$	$9.12 \cdot 10^{-4}$	$5.36 \cdot 10^{-4}$
	Non-cancer	$2.94 \cdot 10^{-2}$	$1.57 \cdot 10^{-2}$	$1.94 \cdot 10^{-2}$	$1.14 \cdot 10^{-2}$
Cadmium	Cancer	n/a	n/a	n/a	n/a
	Non-cancer	$7.52 \cdot 10^{-2}$	$5.98 \cdot 10^{-2}$	$6.02 \cdot 10^{-2}$	$4.65 \cdot 10^{-2}$
Chromium	Cancer	n/a	n/a	n/a	n/a
	Non-cancer	$2.89 \cdot 10^{-5}$	$2.53 \cdot 10^{-5}$	$2.90 \cdot 10^{-5}$	$2.23 \cdot 10^{-5}$
Lead	Cancer	$2.04 \cdot 10^{-4}$	$1.58 \cdot 10^{-4}$	$1.59 \cdot 10^{-4}$	$1.26 \cdot 10^{-4}$
	Non-cancer	$7.54 \cdot 10^{-2}$	$5.85 \cdot 10^{-2}$	$5.86 \cdot 10^{-2}$	$4.67 \cdot 10^{-2}$

cadmium at the respective site. The analogous relation for chromium is below the per mill range.

There is only one ingestion-related damage factor available in the literature for the trace elements analysed (European Commission, 2004). It is given for arsenic and amounts to a value of 33.6 $€_{2000}$ per kilogram of arsenic emitted by taking only cancer effects into account and discounting at a rate of 3 %. This value is larger by two orders of magnitude and more when only comparing it to the cancer effect-related damage costs of arsenic in the present assessment. It needs to be noted that (a) no distinction is made in European Commission (2004) with respect to the toxicity of different arsenic species via ingestion exposures (only 3 % of the contents in food is assumed to be in the toxic inorganic form here, cf. Table C-2), (b) the monetary value assigned to cancers caused by ingestion of (inorganic) arsenic is different in the two studies ($2 \cdot 10^6$ $€_{2000}$ per generic cancer case according to European Commission (2004) and 422200 $€_{2000}$ per skin cancer case in this study, cf. Table 8-6, discounting at 3 %), and (c) the slope factor for ingestion exposures related to undifferentiated arsenic species is larger in European Commission (2004) by a factor of two according to Eq. (7-13). All of these issues, thus, lead to lower external costs by a factor of about 0.003 only due to the assessment and valuation of cancers per kilogram of arsenic released when following the methodology proposed in the present study. This is, however, modified by the use

Table 10-10: Damage factors due to ingestion for a one year pulse emission according to emissions from the Belgian power plant [$€_{2000}$ per $kg_{released}$]

Trace element	Type of effect	Type of monetary value	Discount rate 0 %	3 %
Arsenic	cancer	WTP	104	0.19
		COI[a]	71	0.13
	non-cancer	WTP	2207	4.1
		COI	n/a	n/a
Cadmium[b]	non-cancer	WTP	5642	337
		COI	n/a	n/a
Chromium[b]	non-cancer	WTP	2.2	0.0095
		COI	n/a	n/a
Lead	cancer	WTP	15	0.34
		COI[a]	5.1	0.12
	non-cancer	WTP	5658	128
		COI[c]	209	4.7

a.COI for average cancer.
b.Cancer effect information not available.
c.COI for hypertension.

of an environmental fate and exposure assessment model that differs from the Uniform World Model employed in European Commission (2004) leading to less pronounced discrepancies between the two approaches than the factor of 0.003. Additionally, also non-cancer effects can be valued according to the approach taken here. The consideration of these effects substantially increases the damage costs due to the ingestion of inorganic arsenic. This is also the case for lead. No impact assessment would have been possible for cadmium and chromium via ingestion exposures towards these heavy metals without non-cancer effects according to the approach followed. The significance of the non-cancer impacts stems from the steeper slope factors despite the smaller severity in terms of DALYs per person (Table 7-7) as compared to the cancer impacts (Table 7-6).

Table 10-11: Damage factors due to ingestion for a one year pulse emission according to emissions from the French power plant [$€_{2000}$ per $kg_{released}$]

Trace element	Type of effect	Type of monetary value	Discount rate 0 %	Discount rate 3 %
Arsenic	cancer	WTP	56	0.11
		COI[a]	38	0.075
	non-cancer	WTP	1180	2.3
		COI	n/a	n/a
Cadmium[b]	non-cancer	WTP	4483	255
		COI	n/a	n/a
Chromium[b]	non-cancer	WTP	1.9	0.0061
		COI	n/a	n/a
Lead	cancer	WTP	11.9	0.24
		COI[a]	4.0	0.080
	non-cancer	WTP	4388	89
		COI[c]	162	3.3

a.COI for average cancer.
b.Cancer effect information not available.
c.COI for hypertension.

The damage factors are significantly smaller when non-zero discounting is performed, owing to the long-lived nature of these pollutants (cf. Hellweg, 2000; van den Bergh et al., 2000; Huijbregts et al., 2001; de Vries et al., 2004). Depending on the dynamics of the respective pollutant (cf. Fig. 10-1 and Fig. 10-2), the effect is more (e.g., arsenic) or less (e.g., cadmium) pronounced.

Multiplying the damage factors due to ingestion exposures with the theoretical annual emission ranges given in Table 10-3 yields the annual external costs in Euro per year via this exposure route (Tables 10-14 through 10-17). The ranking of the facilities according to the resulting values for a one year pulse emission is the same as for inhalation: UK, Germany, Belgium and France in descending

Table 10-12: Damage factors due to ingestion for a one year pulse emission according to emissions from the German power plant [$€_{2000}$ per $kg_{released}$]

Trace element	Type of effect	Type of monetary value	Discount rate 0 %	3 %
Arsenic	cancer	WTP	68	0.13
		COI[a]	47	0.086
	non-cancer	WTP	1452	2.7
		COI	n/a	n/a
Cadmium[b]	non-cancer	WTP	4516	250
		COI	n/a	n/a
Chromium[b]	non-cancer	WTP	2.2	0.0059
		COI	n/a	n/a
Lead	cancer	WTP	12	0.23
		COI[a]	4.0	0.077
	non-cancer	WTP	4397	85
		COI[c]	163	3.1

a. COI for average cancer.
b. Cancer effect information not available.
c. COI for hypertension.

order. Generally, one can note that the quantified external costs due to lead by far exceed those caused by the other trace elements. A more thorough discussion on the absolute values will be done for the pan-European emission scenario which is to be presented in Chapter 11.

The external costs are also provided related to a kilowatt hour of electricity produced in Tables 10-14 through 10-17 by dividing those per year by the annual electricity sent-out as given in Table 10-1. When comparing these costs to those for the classical air pollutants as given in European Commission (2004), the conclusion is the same as for inhalation in that the external costs of the classical air pollutants exceed those of the trace elements investigated here by at least four orders of magnitude when equally discounting at 3 %.

Table 10-13: Damage factors due to ingestion for a one year pulse emission according to emissions from the power plant in the UK [$€_{2000}$ per $kg_{released}$]

Trace element	Type of effect	Type of monetary value	Discount rate	
			0 %	3 %
Arsenic	cancer	WTP	40	0.090
		COI[a]	27	0.061
	non-cancer	WTP	854	1.9
		COI	n/a	n/a
Cadmium[b]	non-cancer	WTP	3488	222
		COI	n/a	n/a
Chromium[b]	non-cancer	WTP	1.7	0.013
		COI	n/a	n/a
Lead	cancer	WTP	9.5	0.19
		COI[a]	3.2	0.065
	non-cancer	WTP	3500	71
		COI[c]	129	2.6

a.COI for average cancer.
b.Cancer effect information not available.
c.COI for hypertension.

Some general concluding remarks on the estimated DALYs and external costs for both case studies will be given in sections 12.3.2 and 12.4.

Table 10-14: Ranges of quantifiable external costs due to ingestion caused by a one year pulse emission of selected trace elements and in total according to theoretical minimum and maximum emission values from the Belgian power plant (variable units)

Trace element	Type of effect	Type of value	Discount rate 0 % [$€_{2000}$/yr]	0 % [10^{-9} $€_{2000}$/ kWh_{el}]	3 % [$€_{2000}$/yr]	3 % [10^{-9} $€_{2000}$/ kWh_{el}]
Arsenic	cancer	WTP	43-714	29-485	0.080-1.3	0.054-0.90
		COI[a]	29-486	20-330	0.054-0.91	0.037-0.62
	non-cancer	WTP	911-15160	619-10299	1.7-28	1.2-19
		COI	n/a	n/a	n/a	n/a
Cadmium[b]	non-cancer	WTP	100-1529	1582-26328	6.0-91	95-1574
		COI	n/a	n/a	n/a	n/a
Chromium[b]	non-cancer	WTP	6.8-46	0.61-10	0.029-0.20	0.0027-0.044
		COI	n/a	n/a	n/a	n/a
Lead	cancer	WTP	22-182	4.3-71	0.49-4.1	0.097-1.6
		COI[a]	7-61	1.4-24	0.16-1.4	0.032-0.54
	non-cancer	WTP	8008-67224	1587-26402	181-1515	36-595
		COI[c]	296-2486	59-976	6.7-56	1.3-22
Sum			*9420-87900*	*3902-64926*	*196-1700*	*133-2214*

a. COI for average cancer.
b. Cancer effect information not available.
c. COI for hypertension.

Table 10-15: Ranges of quantifiable external costs due to ingestion caused by a one year pulse emission of selected trace elements and in total according to theoretical minimum and maximum emission values from the French power plant (variable units)

Trace element	Type of effect	Type of value	Discount rate 0 % [$€_{2000}$/yr]	0 % [10^{-9} $€_{2000}$/kWh$_{el}$]	3 % [$€_{2000}$/yr]	3 % [10^{-9} $€_{2000}$/kWh$_{el}$]
Arsenic	cancer	WTP	32-530	15-252	0.063-1.0	0.030-0.50
		COI[a]	22-361	10-172	0.043-0.71	0.020-0.34
	non-cancer	WTP	677-11258	322-5361	1.3-22	0.64-11
		COI	n/a	n/a	n/a	n/a
Cadmium[b]	non-cancer	WTP	110-1688	1224-20368	6.3-96	70-1160
		COI	n/a	n/a	n/a	n/a
Chromium[b]	non-cancer	WTP	8.2-56	0.52-8.6	0.026-0.18	0.0017-0.028
		COI	n/a	n/a	n/a	n/a
Lead	cancer	WTP	23-196	3.2-54	0.47-4.0	0.065-1.1
		COI[a]	8.0-65	1.1-18	0.16-1.3	0.022-0.36
	non-cancer	WTP	8628-72432	1198-19940	174-1464	24-403
		COI[c]	319-2679	44-737	6.4-54	0.90-15
Sum			*9827-89266*	*2819-46912*	*189-1643*	*96-1591*

a. COI for average cancer.
b. Cancer effect information not available.
c. COI for hypertension.

Table 10-16: Ranges of quantifiable external costs due to ingestion caused by a one year pulse emission of selected trace elements and in total according to theoretical minimum and maximum emission values from the German power plant (variable units)

Trace element	Type of effect	Type of value	Discount rate 0 % [$€_{2000}$/yr]	0 % [10^{-9} $€_{2000}$/kWh$_{el}$]	3 % [$€_{2000}$/yr]	3 % [10^{-9} $€_{2000}$/kWh$_{el}$]
Arsenic	cancer	WTP	64-1071	17-275	0.12-2.0	0.030-0.51
		COI[a]	44-729	11-187	0.081-1.3	0.021-0.34
	non-cancer	WTP	1367-22741	350-5831	2.5-42	0.65-11
		COI	n/a	n/a	n/a	n/a
Cadmium[b]	non-cancer	WTP	182-2791	1090-18133	10-154	60-1003
		COI	n/a	n/a	n/a	n/a
Chromium[b]	non-cancer	WTP	15-105	0.52-8.7	0.042-0.28	0.0014-0.024
		COI	n/a	n/a	n/a	n/a
Lead	cancer	WTP	38-322	2.9-48	0.74-6.2	0.055-0.92
		COI[a]	13-108	0.96-16	0.25-2.1	0.018-0.31
	non-cancer	WTP	14189-119117	1061-17658	274-2299	20-341
		COI[c]	525-4406	39-653	10-85	0.76-13
Sum			*16437-151389*	*2573-42809*	*298-2592*	*82-1369*

a. COI for average cancer.
b. Cancer effect information not available.
c. COI for hypertension.

Table 10-17: Quantifiable external costs due to ingestion caused by a one year pulse emission of selected trace elements and in total according to theoretical minimum and maximum emission values from the power plant in the UK (variable units)

Trace element	Type of effect	Type of value	Discount rate 0 % [$€_{2000}$/yr]	0 % [10^{-9} $€_{2000}$/ kWh_{el}]	3 % [$€_{2000}$/yr]	3 % [10^{-9} $€_{2000}$/ kWh_{el}]
Arsenic	cancer	WTP	129-2138	11-183	0.29-4.8	0.025-0.41
		COI[a]	88-1456	7.5-124	0.20-3.3	0.017-0.28
	non-cancer	WTP	2729-45407	233-3881	6.1-102	0.52-8.7
		COI	n/a	n/a	n/a	n/a
Cadmium[b]	non-cancer	WTP	478-7317	952-15849	30-466	61-1009
		COI	n/a	n/a	n/a	n/a
Chromium[b]	non-cancer	WTP	40-275	0.46-7.6	0.32-2.2	0.0036-0.060
		COI	n/a	n/a	n/a	n/a
Lead	cancer	WTP	104-870	2.6-43	2.1-18	0.053-0.88
		COI[a]	35-291	0.86-14	0.71-5.9	0.018-0.29
	non-cancer	WTP	38340-321866	956-15904	782-6568	20-325
		COI[c]	1418-11904	35-588	29-243	0.72-12
Sum			*43359-391525*	*2199-36594*	*851-7413*	*81-1356*

a.COI for average cancer.
b.Cancer effect information not available.
c.COI for hypertension.

11 Whole economy case study

In the previous Chapter, emissions from single facilities have been investigated. The second case study considers pan-European emissions into air for the situation in the year 1990. Beside the derivation of damage factors, this scenario investigates the overall external costs resulting from activities of whole societies or economies which will be described in the following.

11.1 Pan-European emission scenario for 1990

In order to be able to follow the Impact Pathway Approach for a whole economy, information on all releases of the contaminants to be assessed into the environment is needed. However, information on emissions that directly enter the media soil and/or water is rather scarce. A European-wide inventory of direct emissions to water and soil is planned by the European Union but is unfortunately not yet available. In the case of Germany, for instance, there are data available on releases of some heavy metals but only aggregated at the catchment scale (Umweltbundesamt, 2000). Therefore, only emissions into air will be analysed in the following.

The air emission scenario is defined as described in Droste-Franke et al. (2003). The air emission inventory provided by the German Federal Environment Agency and TNO for Europe (Berdowski et al., 1997) constitutes the base information. Where possible, these emissions are updated by using more actual data from EMEP (United Nations - Economic Commission for Europe and Co-operative programme for monitoring and evaluation of long range transmission of air pollutants in Europe, 2002). The data are spatially distributed using the scenario on air pollution emissions for 1990 by assuming that within each main source sector the emissions of the selected trace elements have the same distribution as particle emissions. The totals of the emission values used in the analysis thus obtained are given in Table 11-8.

As for the single facility scenarios, pulse emissions of a one year duration are analysed. The effective Intake Fractions for inhalation and ingestion exposures are derived separately in sections 11.3 and 11.4, respectively. The properties of the investigated contaminants are given in Appendix C. But before that, the development of the concentrations over the course of time under continuous emissions shall be demonstrated.

11.2 Tentative historic emission scenario and contamination increase in time

Records on historic emissions that have led to the present contamination of environmental media and food items are non-existing to the extent necessary for an appropriate assessment of anthropogenic emissions for instance since the industrial revolution. Recent findings indicate that emissions having occurred in the second half of the twentieth century have been the highest in the period of the modern times (Barbante et al., 2004). According to the concentrations in the investigated ice cores, the emissions of cadmium and chromium for the 1990ies even belong to the highest among the entire time period covered (ibid.). Arsenic and lead were not included in the analysis. An upper bound emission scenario shall be investigated assuming that releases took place for a one hundred year period at the level of the pan-European emission scenario for 1990 described above (section 11.1). This scenario serves two purposes. First, it may give an idea of the present contamination level of environmental media that can be attributed to trace element releases from larger facilities which occurred since the advent of industrialisation. The resulting concentrations in the environmental media and food items have been compared to reported values in section 9.3.2. Second, it shall provide insight into the dynamics related to trace element releases into the environment. This shall be done in the following for selected trace elements and compartments and/or zones. For information reasons, also the potential concentrations after 1000 years and at steady-state will be given. As for the case studies, the environmental setting is according to the 'food removal' scenario (see section 9.3.3), however, not investigating pulse-emissions but continuous releases as stated above.

The development towards the steady-state situation is fastest for cadmium and slowest for arsenic of the investigated trace elements (cf. sections 10.3 and 11.4) which is why these two elements will be analysed here. From Fig. 11-1 and 11-2, it can be seen that the concentrations of cadmium and arsenic in the arable land compartment approach slowly towards the steady-state. While the situation after a 1000 year release of cadmium already fairly well approximates the situation at steady-state, the degree of contamination by arsenic changes substantially between these two points in time. These differences can be attributed to the distinct behaviour of cadmium and arsenic in terms of their mobility in the environment, manifested in their solid-water partitioning coefficients (cf. Table C-1).

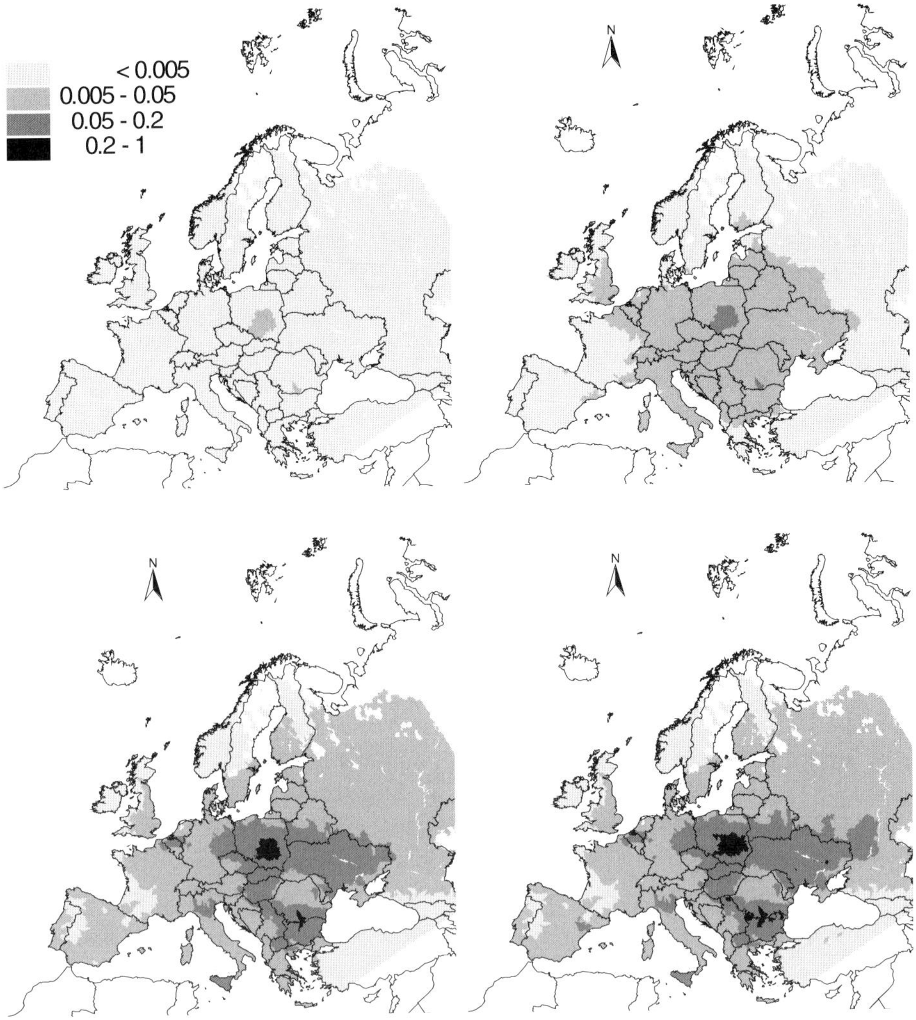

Fig. 11-1: Cadmium concentrations in arable land after 10 years (top left), 100 years (top right), 1000 years (bottom left) and at steady-state (bottom right) according to the pan-European emission scenario for 1990 (continuous releases) [mg/kg]

In order to demonstrate that the development towards the steady-state is rather different between the environmental compartments, the concentrations of arsenic in freshwater bodies are also given at different points in time (Fig. 11-3). It may be surprising to see that not only the concentrations in the arable land compartment rather slowly approach towards the steady-state situation but also those

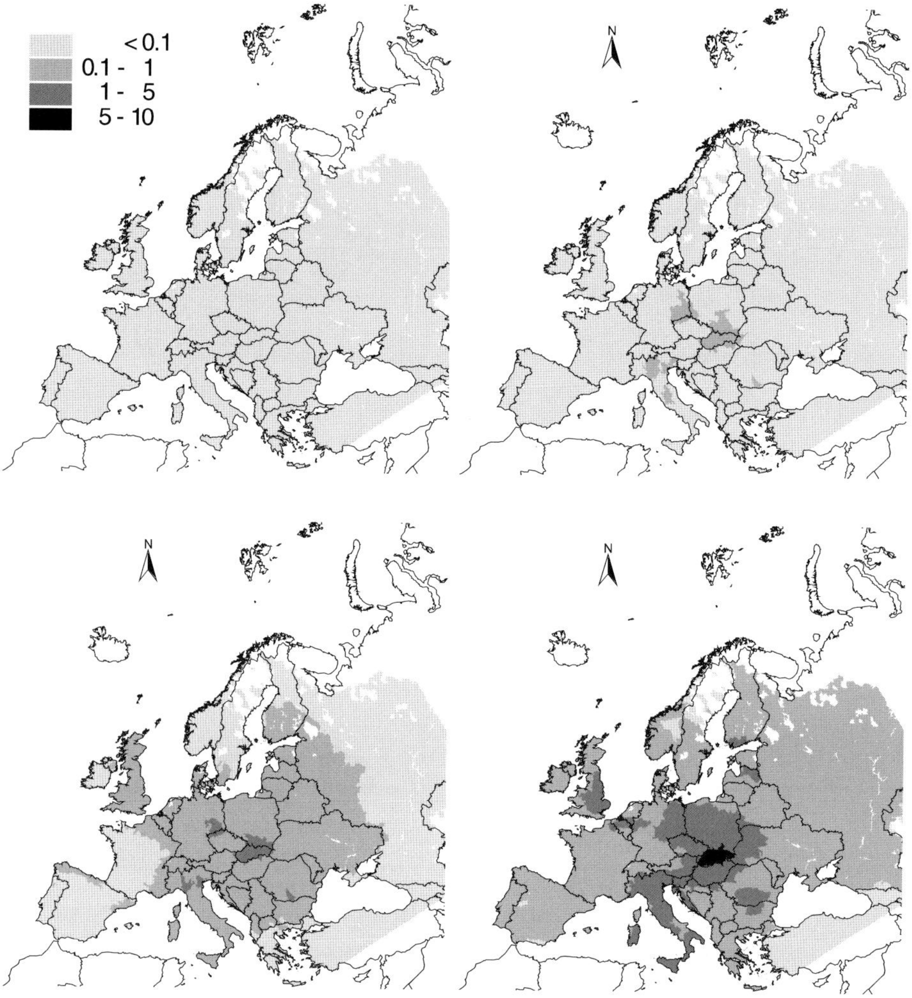

Fig. 11-2: Arsenic concentrations in arable land after 10 years (top left), 100 years (top right), 1000 years (bottom left) and at steady-state (bottom right) according to the pan-European emission scenario for 1990 (continuous releases) [mg/kg]

in freshwater bodies. In fact, substances in freshwater bodies usually have shorter residence times than in soils. However, these may only reach a steady-state once all the other compartments that deliver to the freshwater bodies are in this state. This is visualized for the temporal development of arsenic concentrations in one

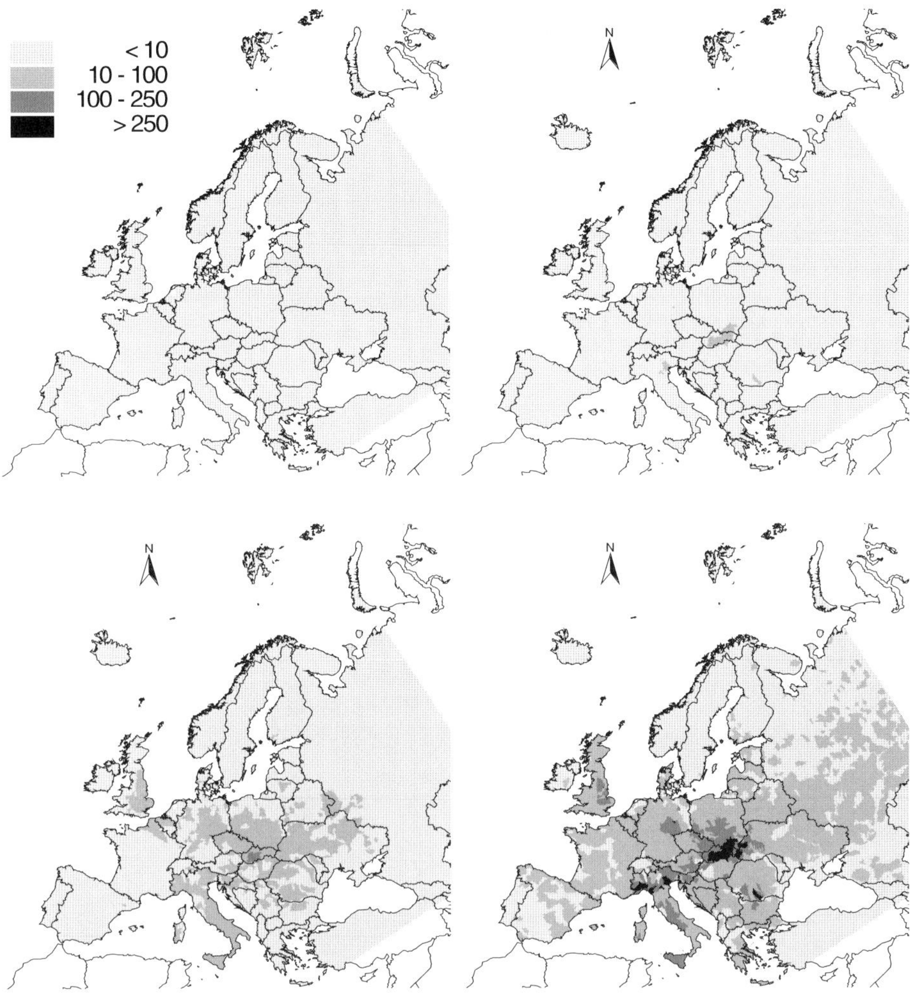

Fig. 11-3: Arsenic concentrations in freshwater bodies after 10 years (top left), 100 years (top right), 1000 years (bottom left) and at steady-state (bottom right) according to the pan-European emission scenario for 1990 (continuous releases) [pg/l]

zone. The zone selected is the Hron River, a tributary to the Danube located in the centre of the Slovakian Republic, for which the highest arsenic concentrations in both the arable land and freshwater compartment are assessed (cf. Fig. 11-2 and 11-3, respectively). The temporal development of the arsenic concentrations is

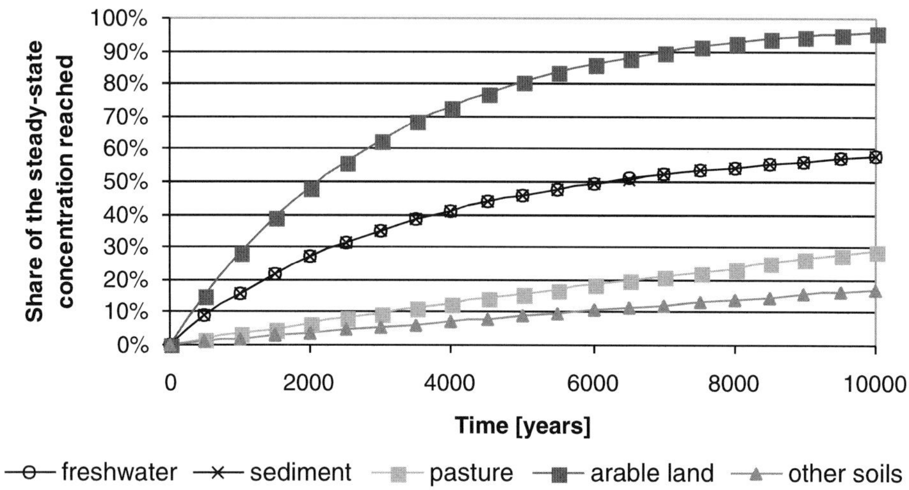

Fig. 11-4: Development of arsenic concentrations towards the steady-state in the Hron River catchment in central Slovakia according to the pan-European emission scenario for 1990 (continuous releases); the values are given relative to the steady-state situation (cf. Table 11-1) [-]

Table 11-1: Arsenic concentrations at steady-state in the Hron River catchment in central Slovakia according to the pan-European emission scenario for 1990 (continuous releases)

Compartment	Unit	Concentration
Freshwater	[ng/l]	0.72
Sediment	[µg/kg]	0.89
(Semi-) natural ecosystems ('other soils')	[mg/kg]	146
Pasture	[mg/kg]	80
Arable land	[mg/kg]	8.2

given in relation to the corresponding concentrations at steady-state in Fig. 11-4. This is because the concentrations at steady-state span orders of magnitude in this situation according to the analysed scenario (Table 11-1).

Table 11-2: Effective Intake Fractions [$kg_{inhaled}$ per $kg_{released}$] and resulting cancer and non-cancer associated Disability Adjusted Life Years (DALYs) per kilogram of a trace element released [years lost-equivalents per $kg_{released}$] due to inhalation caused by a one year pulse emission into air according to the pan-European emission scenario for 1990

Trace element	Effective Intake Fraction [$kg_{inhaled}$ per $kg_{released}$]	DALYs [years lost-equivalents per $kg_{released}$]	
		cancer	non-cancer
Arsenic	$3.2 \cdot 10^{-6}$	$2.20 \cdot 10^{-4}$	n/a
Cadmium	$1.5 \cdot 10^{-5}$	$4.41 \cdot 10^{-4}$	n/a
Chromium	$7.2 \cdot 10^{-8}$	$1.37 \cdot 10^{-5}$	$2.00 \cdot 10^{-7}$
Lead	$4.4 \cdot 10^{-6}$	n/a	n/a

Again the different dynamics between the different compartments become obvious. In the terrestrial environment, the arable land compartment is the quickest in approaching towards the steady-state. This is due to a higher outflow by means of the water soil erosion process out of this compartment followed by pastures and other land uses. In general, less than 5 % of the steady-state concentrations are reached within the first 100 years of continuous releases. While this is still the case for pastures and semi-natural ecosystems after 1000 years of continuous emissions, the share of the steady-state concentrations may amount to 16 % in the freshwater environment and up to 28 % for arable soils. After 2000 years, none of the compartments will have exceeded concentration levels that are half of those at steady-state.

Fig. 11-4 may help to explain why the influence of non-zero discounting on the case study results especially of arsenic is rather substantial (cf. sections 10.3 and 11.4) although different types of emission scenarios are investigated (continuous releases vs. pulse emission). While the arsenic concentrations in pasture soils develop rather slowly towards the steady-state situation, pasture-based food items, i.e., especially beef and dairy products, dominate the ingestion exposure towards arsenic in the long run (cf. Fig. 10-3, 10-4 and 11-6). Exactly these exposures are not taken into consideration when performing non-zero discounting owing to quasi-zero discount factors applicable to damages occurring in the intermediate to long term.

Table 11-3: Damage factors due to inhalation for a one year pulse emission according to the pan-European emission scenario for 1990 [$€_{2000}$ per $kg_{released}$]

Trace element[a]	Type of effect	Type of monetary value	Discount rate	
			0 %	3 %
Arsenic[b]	cancer	WTP	16.5	8.78
		COI	4.34	2.32
Cadmium[b]	cancer	WTP	33.1	17.6
		COI	8.72	4.65
Chromium	cancer	WTP	1.02	0.546
		COI	0.27	0.144
	non-cancer	WTP	0.015	0.00801
		COI	n/a	n/a

a.No effect information available for lead.
b.No non-cancer effect information available.

As a result, the analysis of the contamination development emphasizes the long time scales potentially involved when releasing persistent substances such as trace elements.

11.3 Impacts due to inhalation exposure

The impact assessment due to inhalation is based on the corresponding (effective) Intake Fractions. The values are given in Table 11-2. The values for arsenic and lead are in the same range as for the single facilities investigated in the previous section (Table 10-4). The reason why the Intake Fraction for cadmium and chromium tend to be larger or smaller, respectively, than for the single facility emission scenarios is seen in the distribution of hot-spot concentrations entirely over land or to some degree over the sea. According to Figure 9.2 as given in Droste-Franke et al. (2003), areas with the highest cadmium concentrations in air are located in central eastern Europe, west of the Black Sea, and along the Po river. Figure 9.3 (ibid.) shows that the highest air concentrations of chromium are on the French coast around Marseilles so that much of the chromium present in air is deposited into the Mediterranean Sea without leading to human inhalation expo-

Table 11-4: Quantifiable external costs due to inhalation of selected trace elements and in total caused by a one year pulse emission according to the pan-European emission scenario for 1990 [10^6 €$_{2000}$/yr]

Trace element[a]	Type of effect	Type of monetary value	Discount rate	
			0 %	3 %
Arsenic[b]	cancer	WTP	19.5	10.4
		COI	5.14	2.74
Cadmium[b]	cancer	WTP	16.8	8.95
		COI	4.43	2.36
Chromium	cancer	WTP	2.29	1.22
		COI	0.605	0.322
	non-cancer	WTP	0.034	0.018
		COI	n/a	n/a
Sum			*48.8*	*26.0*

a. No effect information available for lead.
b. No non-cancer effect information available.

sures. This explains the lower (effective) Intake Fraction for chromium inhalation exposures according to the pan-European emission scenario. This effect may actually be counterbalanced by tourists temporarily staying in this area especially in summer. However, migration of people is not taken into account which would also lead to some absenteeism among the local population. The difference between the pan-European scenario and those for the single facilities presented in section 10.1 carries on through the steps from exposure to impact and to valued damages in the following.

The effective Intake Fraction due to inhalation translates into DALYs (Table 11-2) according to the respective cancer and non-cancer slope factors. Missing effect information is indicated as not available ('n/a'; for further discussion refer to section 10.2). Based on the DALYs per emitted kilogram of the respective trace element, the external costs are derived next.

The external costs per kilogram emitted and those for the overall pan-European emission situation are given in Tables 11-3 and 11-4, respectively. As for the single facilities (cf. section 10.2), the damage factors estimated here are about in the same order of magnitude as those for the classical air pollutants, noting that the classical air pollutants are emitted in much larger quantities. There is, however, a change in the ranking of the trace elements in terms of leading to the highest quantifiable specific external costs via inhalation (cf. Table 10-6 and 11-3).

The total quantifiable external costs due to inhalation of the classical air pollutants released according to a pan-European emission scenario amount to about $210 \cdot 10^9$ €$_{2000}$ in EU15 when discounted at 3 % (Droste-Franke and Friedrich, 2003). One has to note that the assessment performed by Droste-Franke and Friedrich (2003) has experienced an update in terms of both the dose-response functions and the monetary valuation (European Commission, 2004). This update leads to even higher estimates by about 10 %. Comparing the resulting $230 \cdot 10^9$ €$_{2000}$ to the high-end total quantifiable external costs due to the inhalation of arsenic and cadmium which are in the order of 10^7 €$_{2000}$ shows that the inhalation-induced human health damages due to the release of the investigated trace elements contribute only marginally.

11.4 Impacts due to ingestion exposure

The assessment of the ingestion-related human exposures is performed based on the environmental settings of the 'food removal' scenario (see section 9.3.3). As for the single facilities, the four trace elements analysed show marked differences in terms of both the absolute value of the effective Intake Fraction due to ingestion exposures and the temporal development of this measure (Fig. 11-5, note the logarithmic scale). The amount of cadmium taken in is highest reaching 0.12 % of the overall amount released. Arsenic, chromium and lead show effective Intake Fractions due to ingestion of about one order of magnitude less than cadmium in the long run. According to the present assessment, there will be a relatively and absolutely higher exposure of cadmium and lead within the next 100 years upon release of the trace elements. This means that 17.7 %, 8.2 %, 1.6 % and 1.0 % of the time-integrated effective Intake Fraction due to ingestion will have been obtained within this period of time for cadmium, lead, chromium and arsenic, respectively. These figures are much smaller for the first 10 year period (2.9 %, 1.3 %, 0.25 % and 0.12 %, respectively). The contribution of the inhalation-related Intake Fraction is insignificant in the long run (Fig. 11-5). This also holds for the short term except for arsenic and lead, indicating once more that the exposure through the media soil and water are most significant at least in the intermediate to long term.

As could already be demonstrated for the single facilities, not only the total amounts taken in vary considerably in time but also the most contributing food items (top vs. bottom of Fig. 11-6). Again note the different contributions of cattle

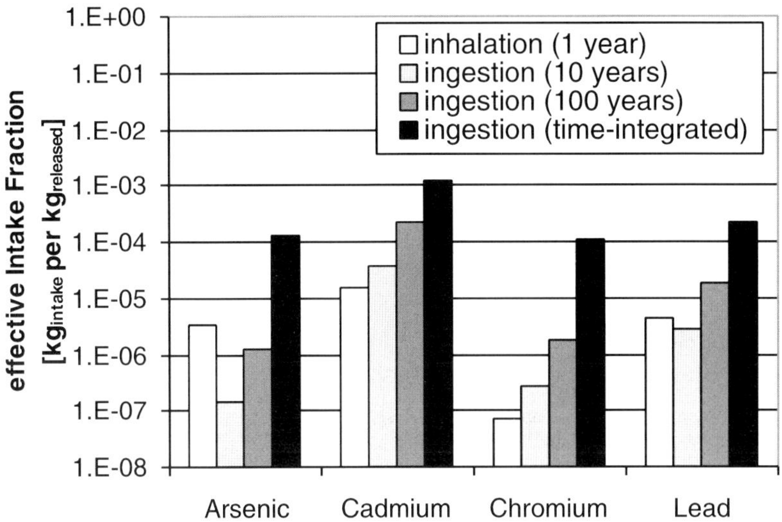

Fig. 11-5: Effective Intake Fraction of selected trace elements via inhalation after one year and via ingestion of food after 10 and 100 years, and time-integrated for a one year pulse emission according to the pan-European emission scenario in 1990 (note the logarithmic scale) [kg_{intake} per $kg_{released}$]

products and spinach for the situations after 10 years and when integrating exposure over infinite time. The human exposure towards cadmium and lead primarily occurs primarily through cereals and to some extent through potatoes while dairy products are also important for chromium and even more so for arsenic parallelling the picture for the single facilities. Beef only constitutes a remarkable share of chromium's Intake Fraction in the long run (Fig. 11-6) while freshwater fish and other animal products such as pork, poultry and eggs contribute insubstantially.

Generally, non-cancer effects dominate the DALYs assessed due to ingestion (Table 11-5) which is also due to lack of cancer effect information (cf. section 7.3). While the DALYs due to non-cancer effects are more than one order of magnitude larger than due to cancer for arsenic, this discrepancy amounts to about three orders of magnitude for lead. Exposure towards lead and cadmium leads to the highest human health impacts amounting to about 22 and 37 year lost-equivalents per tonne emitted, respectively.

Valuing the impacts assessed to occur via ingestion yields the damage factors (Table 11-6). These vary considerably according to the different discount rates employed due to the slow dynamics and long persistency of the substances investigated. The damage factors are at the lower end of those for the single facil-

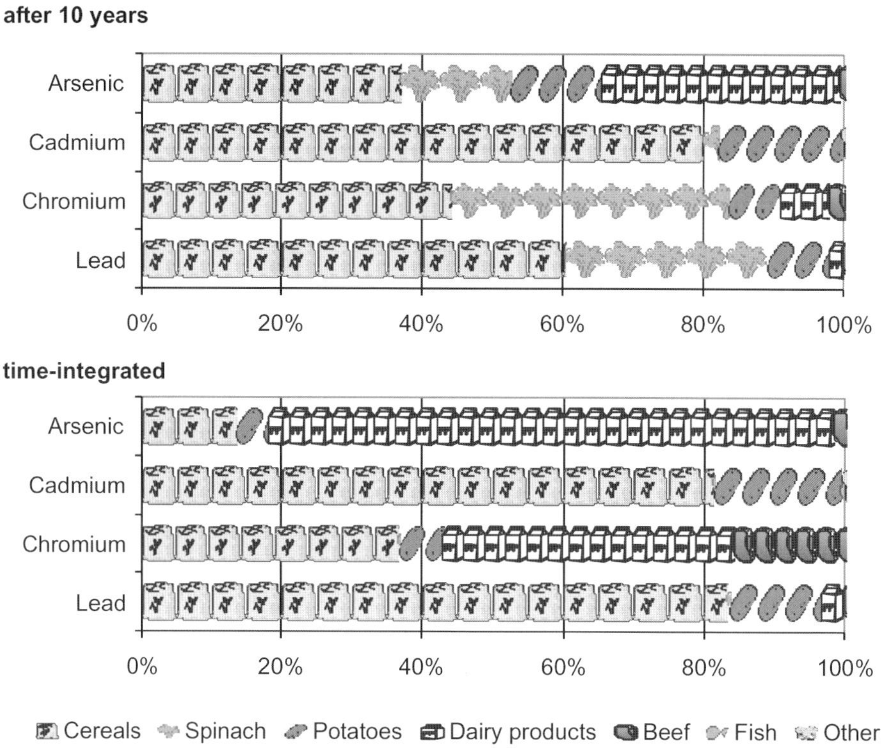

Fig. 11-6: Relative contribution of the different food items to the effective Intake Fraction (ingestion) of selected trace elements after 10 years (top) and time-integrated (bottom) for a one year pulse emission according to the pan-European emission scenario to air in 1990 (cliparts by Corel Corporation, 2002)

Table 11-5: Time-integrated Disability Adjusted Life Years (DALYs) per kilogram of trace element released due to cancer and non-cancer effects upon ingestion exposure caused by a one year pulse emission according to the pan-European emission scenario for 1990 [years lost-equivalents per $kg_{released}$]

Trace element	Cancer effect	Non-cancer effect
Arsenic	$3.35 \cdot 10^{-4}$	$7.11 \cdot 10^{-3}$
Cadmium	n/a	$3.71 \cdot 10^{-2}$
Chromium	n/a	$1.14 \cdot 10^{-5}$
Lead	$6.06 \cdot 10^{-5}$	$2.24 \cdot 10^{-2}$

ities, i.e., equal or below those for the power plant in the UK (cf. Table 10-13). This is also reflected in the estimated DALY values (Table 10-9 vs. Table 11-5). This can partly be explained by depositions taking place into the sea to a large extent (especially for chromium). The impact pathway cannot be followed through the marine environment at present as discussed in section 7.1. Additionally, the smaller impact of the pan-European emission scenario may be explained by the 'mismatch' of elevated atmospheric depositions and highly productive agricultural areas. In line with the findings by MacLeod et al. (2004), this has been identified to be one reason why, for instance, exposure through potatoes are more substantial for the emission sites in Germany and in Belgium as compared to those in the UK and France (cf. section 10.3).

The damage factors are significantly smaller when non-zero discounting is performed, owing to the long-lived nature of these pollutants (cf. Hellweg, 2000; van den Bergh et al., 2000; Huijbregts et al., 2001; de Vries et al., 2004). Depending on the dynamics of the respective pollutant (cf. Fig. 11-5), the effect is more (e.g., arsenic) or less (e.g., cadmium) pronounced. Related to the issue of discounting, it is interesting to see that its impact is variable for the investigated scenarios. For instance, when computing the ratio between the 3 % discounted and 0 % discounted damage factors for cadmium of the facility in the UK and the pan-European scenario, these ratios amount to 6.4 % and 4.0 %, respectively. This difference hints at different temporal distributions of impacts attributable to variable properties of the receiving environments leading to different dynamics for the metal to reach the human population from different release sites. This stresses once more that it does not mean that the site of release is almost irrelevant as argued by Spadaro and Rabl (2004) despite trade may lead to homogeneous levels in the food items under consideration.

A comparison of the damage factors to the one for arsenic found in the literature has been performed in a previous section (10.3) and shall thus not be repeated here.

The quantifiable external costs through ingestion exposures due to the emissions of the considered trace elements to air in 1990 range from about two million to some ten billion Euros when discounting at a rate of 0 % (Table 11-7). The highest values are obtained for lead caused by hypertension followed by those for cadmium due to kidney damage which are about a factor of 40 smaller. The damages due to arsenic and chromium contribute about a factor of two and about three orders of magnitude less than those for cadmium, respectively. When comparing the total quantifiable external costs due to ingestion discounted at 3 % to the most dominant damage costs due to inhalation, i.e., those of the classical air pollutants, discounted at the same rate (Droste-Franke and Friedrich, 2003), the contribution is marginal. The highest external costs quantified for lead constitute

Table 11-6: Damage factors due to ingestion for a one year pulse emission according to the pan-European emission scenario for 1990 [$€_{2000}$ per $kg_{released}$]

Trace element	Type of effect	Type of monetary value	Discount rate 0 %	3 %
Arsenic	cancer	WTP	25.1	0.0446
		COI[a]	17.1	0.0303
	non-cancer	WTP	533	0.946
		COI	n/a	n/a
Cadmium[b]	non-cancer	WTP	2785	110
		COI	n/a	n/a
Chromium[b]	non-cancer	WTP	0.855	0.00262
		COI	n/a	n/a
Lead	cancer	WTP	4.55	0.0740
		COI[a]	1.52	0.0247
	non-cancer	WTP	1681	27.4
		COI[c]	62	1.01

a.COI for average cancer.
b.Cancer effect information not available.
c.COI for hypertension.

about 0.4 % of those of the classical air pollutants in 1990 of about 230 · 10^9 $€_{2000}$ (value updated, only impacts in EU15 valued, cf. section 11.3). When discounting at 0 %, a different picture is obtained. The total quantifiable external costs due to inhalation of classical air pollutants increase only little to 240 · 10^9 $€_{2000}$ (derived according to Droste-Franke, 2005) whereas those due to ingestion exposure towards the trace elements increase substantially (cf. Table 11-7). As a result, the quantifiable external costs due to lead add about 25 % to those due to the classical air pollutants. Three aspects need to be noted related to this comparison. First, the estimated relative contributions by the trace elements discussed so far and in the following may be overestimated as the external cost assessments by Droste-

Table 11-7: Quantifiable external costs due to ingestion of selected pollutants and in total caused by a one year pulse emission according to the pan-European emission scenario for 1990 [10^6 €$_{2000}$/yr]

Trace element	Type of effect	Type of monetary value	Discount rate 0 %	3 %
Arsenic	cancer	WTP	29.7	0.0528
		COI[a]	20.2	0.0359
	non-cancer	WTP	631	1.12
		COI	n/a	n/a
Cadmium[b]	non-cancer	WTP	1410	55.8
		COI	n/a	n/a
Chromium[b]	non-cancer	WTP	1.91	0.00586
		COI	n/a	n/a
Lead	cancer	WTP	158	2.57
		COI	52.8	0.860
	non-cancer	WTP	58500	952
		COI[c]	2160	35.2
Sum			63000	1050

a.COI for average cancer.
b.Cancer effect information not available.
c.COI for hypertension.

Franke (2005) for the classical air pollutants only consider the damages within the area that is determined by the 15 European Union member countries (EU15; i.e., the countries being member of the European Union as of 1995: Austria, Belgium, Denmark, Finland, France, Germany, Greece, Ireland, Italy, Luxembourg, The Netherlands, Portugal, Spain, Sweden and the United Kingdom). Taking only the damages occurring in these countries into account leads to total quantifiable external costs due to lead exposure that are about half of those reported in Table 11-7. On the other hand, the presented assessment does not contain all exposure pathways so that the damages caused by the investigated contaminants need to be con-

Table 11-8: Total trace element emissions in Europe in 1990 and 2000 estimated according to Droste-Franke et al. (2003) and ESPREME (2004), respectively

Trace element	Emissions [t/yr] in ...		Relation
	1990	2000	[%]
Arsenic	1184	654	55
Cadmium	508	269	53
Chromium	2238	1658	74
Lead	34797	10923	31

sidered lower bound estimates. Further work is needed in order to find out to what extent these incompleteness of both analyses lead to a bias and into which direction. Second, the β_{ED10} slope factor for hyptertension due to lead must be considered particularly uncertain (cf. Table 7-7). Thus, the next highest total quantifiable external costs are those for cadmium adding only 0.59 % or 0.024 % to those of the classical air pollutants when discounting at 0 % and 3 %, respectively. These contributions are reduced by about 60 % when only taking the damages in the EU15 countries into account. Third, when transferring the assessment to more recent years the change in the emission situation needs to be borne in mind. The emissions of contaminants into air have considerably declined since the early 1990s. In the case of the investigated trace elements, this particularly concerns lead (cf. Table 11-8). Assuming the same emission distribution at the reduced level of the year 2000, the total quantifiable ingestion-related external costs from lead, thus, only amount to $19 \cdot 10^9$ €$_{2000}$ (0 % discounting). These can be compared to the external costs assessed for an emission scenario of NO_x, SO_2, NH_3, NMVOC and primary particles for 1998 (Droste-Franke, 2005) which may serve as a proxy for the year 2000. The external costs discounted at a rate of 0 % and updated as described above amount to about $150 \cdot 10^9$ €$_{2000}$. As a result, the contribution by lead to the external costs caused by the emission of classical air pollutants is about 13 %. When using a discount rate of 3 %, again only a very small relation is obtained, i.e., 0.2 %. This emphasizes once more that the exposure towards persistent substances such as the trace elements investigated here involves very long time horizons, substantially lowering their monetised damages when performing non-zero discounting.

Inhalation-related annual external costs due to a one year pulse emission at the level of 1990 have been presented in Table 11-4. These are not only negligible when compared to the classical air pollutants (cf. section 11.3) but also when compared to ingestion exposure of the same trace elements (comparing the totals in Table 11-4 with those in Table 11-7). Discounting the damages following ingestion exposures with up to a discount rate of 3 % does not change this conclusion.

Including substances other than the classical air pollutants in the assessment, thus, leads to an increase in the total quantifiable external costs at most in the order of less than one percent when discounting at 3 % according to the presently available information. A similar picture has been obtained for ingestion exposures to dioxins and dioxin-like substances for selected countries for which the contribution amounts to at most a few percent (Droste-Franke et al., 2003). Assuming that the time preference of society is indifferent towards when a benefit is realized, i.e., when discounting at 0 %, the contribution of the investigated trace elements to the total quantifiable external costs related to human health impacts becomes more substantial. These are assessed to contribute at most 25 % to the total quantifiable external costs caused by the classical air pollutants. Thus, depending on society's time preference, the impact by the investigated trace elements may be substantial.

Some general concluding remarks on the estimated DALYs and external costs for both case studies will be given in sections 12.3.2 and 12.4.

12 Concluding remarks

In the ExternE project series on external costs of energy, exposures and resulting impacts through contaminants present only in air were assessed and valued. In order to perform the external cost assessment in as complete a way as possible, this work has developed and applied an extension of the Impact Pathway Approach (IPA) termed WATSON ('integrated WATer and SOil environmental fate, exposure and impact assessment model of Noxious substances'). WATSON facilitates the coverage of exposures towards hazardous substances released into air, (fresh) water and soil through ingestion of various food items in a spatially-resolved pan-European setting.

12.1 The assessment framework

The approach comprises several special features that shall be recapitulated in the following.

The overall method relies on a coupled set of environmental fate models for air on the one hand and for soil and (fresh) water on the other. While the assessment for air has been adopted from the existing software tool EcoSense (European Commission, 2003d), the contaminants' environmental fate in the terrestrial and aquatic environment is described with the help of a spatially-resolved climatological box model similar to Mackay level III/IV models (Mackay, 1991). Both fate models assume long-term average conditions for the description of the environment. In line with current political concern, the focus is laid on persistent substances such as heavy metals. In particular, the trace elements arsenic, cadmium, chromium and lead are investigated. The methodological development has, therefore, focused on this substance group which had been poorly addressed previously in the realm of multimedia modelling.

Spatial aspects

The geographical coverage and degree of spatial resolution allow for a spatially-dependent assessment of the trace elements as recommended amongst other by Huijbregts (2000) and Huijbregts et al. (2001). This is also in line with for example Potting and Hauschild (1997), Krewitt et al. (2001) and MacLeod et al. (2004) in that a spatially explicit assessment is deemed more credible and informative than an a-spatial or site-generic assessment. This allows the analysis to take account of the spatial variability in landscape characteristics, food production intensities and human population densities. Furthermore, it allows the assessment to be conducted following a bottom-up approach, a main feature of the Impact Pathway Analysis.

Different spatial resolutions are employed for the air compartment (regular grid), the soil and water environment (according to catchment information), and the exposure part (according to administrative units at least at the country level), thereby taking account of the differences in terms of chemical movements in the environment and data availability with respect to exposure based on production data. Also, if trade of food is geographically constrained at all it mostly follows administrative borders. Emissions into air, water and soil are specified at least according to administrative units if not even additionally by emission sector.

Usually multi-zonal multimedia models at most distinguish the terrestrial environment into agricultural/cultivated and non-agricultural/non-cultivated land (Wania et al., 2000; Wania, 2003) whereas the presented approach may differentiate up to six terrestrial compartments (section 5.1.1). In particular the distinction of pastures from arable land appears to influence the overall result when exposure through cattle is important. If in addition the exposure through freshwater fish contributes substantially to ingestion exposures, the separate modelling of sealed surfaces also appears advisable, at least if emissions into air are investigated. According to the way these are described within the model, the impervious surfaces accelerate the transport of substances to freshwater bodies. However, freshwater fish exposure is rather irrelevant for all of the investigated trace elements for the emission scenarios analysed.

Processes and environmental characteristics considered

As regards fish exposures, a distinction between rivers and lakes is made. In particular, a physically meaningful distinction between these two freshwater body types has been introduced in terms of the dynamics of (suspended) particles. The importance of this model development has been demonstrated to increase the exposure through freshwater fish by almost one order of magnitude when spatially differentiating below the catchment level, in contrast to the treatment of all freshwater bodies as lakes as done by state-of-the-art multimedia models. A further need for improvement of the process formulation has been identified.

The terrestrial compartments are distinguished according to different land uses showing rather different susceptibilities especially to the process of water soil erosion. At least when distinguishing arable land, pastures and other soils, the water soil erosion rate has been identified to be very sensitive with respect to the exposure estimates of rather immobile substances. It could be shown for chromium that the variation of the water soil erosion rate influences the overall ingestion exposure situation even more significantly than substance-specific parameters such as the solid-water partitioning coefficient, bioconcentration factors and biotransfer factors. This finding is in contradiction to previous uncertainty and sensitivity analyses conducted with respect to exposure estimates (e.g., Hertwich et al., 1999; Huijbregts et al., 2000a) that found that environmental parameters are rather insensitive. However, their focus was on degradable substances. Recent evidence supporting the importance of the water soil erosion process with respect to exposure estimates is given by Huijbregts et al. (2003). Although the water soil erosion process has been improved towards existing multimedia models in that it is allowed to vary by compartments, further development is needed. A possible approach is suggested in section B.5.3.

In line with the finding of the relevance of the water soil erosion process, it may be worthwhile to consider to include the process of wind soil erosion. Although it has been shown to be rather irrelevant for the environmental fate of selected semi-volatile persistent organic chemicals, i.e., PCDD/Fs, by Suzuki et al. (2000), the wind soil erosion / suspension process may be of importance. Suzuki et al. (2000) did not analyse the influence of this process in a multi-zonal context where spatial variability for example in terms of areas potentially prone to this process and distribution of food production are taken into account. Furthermore, the case may be different especially for non-degrading and rather involatile substances such as most metals (e.g., Guerzoni and Chester, 1996). However, the coupling of the air quality model (WTM) on the one hand and the soil and water environmental fate model (WATSON) on the other requires many subsequent iterative runs of both models in order to consider this process within the presented methodological approach. Furthermore, both models are mostly confined to Europe in terms of their spatial coverage. It is known that even particle-bound trace elements can undergo long-range transport between continents upon resuspension (Church et al., 1990). Thus, further developments need to be done to set up a fully integrated multimedia model with a potentially larger geographical scope that at least covers the northern hemisphere when trying to fully follow the impact pathway of hazardous substances (United States - Environmental Protection Agency, 1997b; Ryaboshapko et al., 1998; Pekar et al., 1999).

The environmental fate model developed is the first one in the realm of multimedia models to include the process of preferential flow. Its influence could clearly be demonstrated, potentially leading to a reduction in food exposures by 50 % when agricultural produce dominates the overall ingestion exposures. A process that also leads to accelerated transport especially of hydrophobic substances to the subsurface has been introduced by McLachlan et al. (2002) which is termed 'sorbed phase transport'. It may be questioned whether the processes such as 'bioturbation', 'cryoturbation' and 'erosion into cracks formed by soil drying' that are held responsible for the sorbed phase transport (McLachlan et al., 2002) are really the main processes driving the downward transport especially of lipophilic substances. Hartmann et al. (2004) have shown that even hydrophobic substances like tributyltin (TBT) reach the zone below the top soils via preferential flow when applied to soils, suggesting that this transport that also affects colloidally bound substances may be another or even the most important candidate for explaining the movement of rather insoluble substances to the subsurface. According to Flury (1996), this process is more the rule than the exception and may have different causes (Wittig et al., 1985; Helling and Gish, 1991; Steenhuis and Parlange, 1991; Schwarz and Kaupenjohann, 2000) including colloidal transport (Jarvis et al., 1999; Noack et al., 2000). It even also applies to atmospheric deposition in forests (Wittig et al., 1985; Chang and Matzner, 2000).

Harvest removal of substances entrained in food items is considered in the environmental fate model. This is in line with Severinsen and Jager (1998) and TRIM.FaTE (United States - Environmental Protection Agency, 2002b) for aboveground plant parts. In the presented approach, additionally harvest removal of belowground produce and 'catch removal' of freshwater fish are included. In particular with respect to plants, the removal is modelled only for the edible portions. The other plant parts are not explicitly addressed. This implicitly leads to the assumption that the non-edible plant parts are added after harvest to those soils on which the produce was grown. The question, however, arises where the trace elements removed from the environment by harvest would re-enter it, for example after being released again from or by the human body. Some portions will reach the subsurface from cemeteries or enter the sewer systems from households. From the sewer system, the substances may reach surface water bodies when entrained in the effluent and/or may be trapped in the sewage sludge and could subsequently be applied to agricultural soils. Not allowing for the harvest removal processes would mean that the trace element amounts present in the respective compartments stay in these compartments and may contribute to exposure in subsequent time steps for which the assessment is conducted. Thereby, the substances may potentially be double-counted at two or more rather close points in time. Thus, the harvest removal processes prevent the double-counting of exposure towards substances for example within a generation while disregarding potential re-exposure of future generations. This may be compensated to some degree by the inclusion of discharges to soil and water if related information was available to the extent necessary. Owing to the substantial contribution of intercepted atmospheric depositions to human exposure, however, the inclusion of harvest removals does not lead to substantial reductions in the human exposure situation when air emissions are analysed, as could be shown in a scenario analysis (section 9.3.3). This exposure pathway may tend to be overestimated because rinsing of aboveground exposed produce as part of a regular kitchen practice is not explicitly taken into account. However, the ingestion exposure assessment only includes one food item of this group of produce, i.e., spinach. Due to the incomplete assessment in terms of other produce that are classified as aboveground exposed produce such as many green salads and fruits, the contribution of this produce group is, therefore, not deemed to be overestimated. It needs to be noted, however, that the exposure at the individual level and maybe even at the national level may, nevertheless, be affected due to differing preferences in terms of 'aboveground exposed produce' consumption by different people.

The inclusion of harvest removals has implications on when exposures and impacts are to be assessed. One may, therefore, consider not including these harvest removals from a Life Cycle Impact Assessment point of view where temporal information especially on emissions usually are not available or when zero-discounting is performed and one tries to cover all potential effects. However, whether the additional exposures would then be assessed in a correct way due to the missing consideration of redirected substances is another open field for discussion.

The environmental fate model takes pH-dependent or organic carbon-dependent partitioning of contaminants into account (section C.1.1). Furthermore, the derivation of the dimensionless Henry's law constant is also modelled in a temperature-dependent way (section C.1.2). A scenario analysis of either letting the solid-water partitioning coefficient depend on a zonally variable pH or one that varies only by compartment has shown that this new element in a multimedia model is influential by increasing the time-integrated effective Intake Fraction due to ingestion of chromium by more than 80 % (cf. section 9.3.4). This influence may even be more significant if solid-water partitioning coefficients became available that are not only given for example for three different pH values as provided by United States - Environmental Protection Agency (1998) but additionally on organic matter or clay content, for example.

Exposure assessment

The proposed methodological framework takes exposures through inhalation and food ingestion into account. The assessment of the latter is more complex due to both the variety of food items to which human beings might be exposed and the spatial distribution of the food production. The estimation of ingestion-related exposures builds on the site-specific risk assessment approach recommended by the US-EPA for hazardous waste combustion facilities (United States - Environmental Protection Agency, 1998), thereby striving for representative rather than for protective estimates. As noted above, the exposure is assessed at the level of administrative units for which food production and population data are usually provided. Unlike other multimedia exposure models, human exposure towards food items is assessed according to nationally variable food supply figures. A correction is included that considers losses not taken into account by this statistical measure.

Unlike most other multimedia exposure models, the food items are assumed to undergo trade within the geographical scope of the assessment framework which can be regarded an extension of the environmental fate of the investigated contaminants. This leads to homogeneous contaminant levels in all traded goods prior to consumption by humans and/or farm animals. By means of this homogenization the actual amounts of food produced at different administrative levels which may be as low as at the municipality level are taken into account in order to weigh the assessed contaminant concentrations. In order not to overestimate exposures towards European residents, the self supply of the respective goods is, furthermore, taken into account also in order to follow the mass conservation principle. However, principally bilateral information between countries is ideally needed in order to more appropriately consider the influence of trade. One such information source is the comprehensive and commercially available United Nations Commodity Trade Statistics Database (UN Comtrade).

The exposure of farm animals via feed and ingestion of soil particles requires very detailed information on the way the animals are kept. In particular the extent to which the animals are kept outdoors will significantly influence their exposure via soil ingestion towards those pollutants that do not directly contaminate the feeding stuff, i.e., that are dispersedly released. For instance, the ingestion of soil particles by cattle may contribute more than 50 % to the human exposure towards chromium stemming from particular areas according to the present assessment.

The originally published concept of the Intake Fraction is principally adopted as the exposure measure and extended in several ways. As is also done by other authors, the Intake Fraction is distinguished according to routes of exposure, i.e., inhalation and ingestion. For ingestion exposures, this measure is further differentiated according to different exposure pathways. Second, the Intake Fraction is confined to effective exposures by only taking into account the chemical form of a contaminant that may cause an adverse effect. Third, the effective Intake Fraction especially for ingestion exposures may be given for different time horizons and not just at steady-state as initially proposed by Bennett et al. (2002). This is particularly desirable when analysing rather persistent contaminants in a policy decision support context in order to give an indication of the time horizons potentially involved. Fourth, this measure may be provided for different nations and/or sub-populations allowing among other for the assessment of imports and exports of contaminants between countries as done by Droste-Franke and Friedrich (2003). As a result, the differentiation of the Intake Fraction allows a better representation of population-based exposure situations in time and space.

Impact assessment

The most limiting information with respect to the complete assessment according to the Impact Pathway Approach is that related to effects following ingestion exposures. Due to the lack of existing epidemiologically derived effect information, use is made of the approach proposed by Crettaz (2000), Crettaz et al. (2002) and Pennington et al. (2002). This derives a linear so-called β_{ED10} slope factor that represents a measure for the population-averaged excess individual risk of an effect per unit daily dose for a lifetime exposure. The linearisation is based on a non-threshold assumption. For consistency reasons, the approach is also applied to inhalation exposures.

Generally, the approach makes use of rather different effect measures in order to derive a β_{ED10} slope factor (cf. section 7.3.1). The related uncertainty in the derived dose-effect model depends amongst other on whether it is derived from dose-response information such as *slope factors* or *unit (lifetime) risks* in US-EPA (United States - Environmental Protection Agency 1996b) or WHO terminology (World Health Organisation, 2000b), respectively, or from threshold effect measures such as NOAEL or LOAEL. This emphasizes the importance of reliable effect information for which a very high need for further research is identified and recommended. More reliable dose-response information such as that based on epidemiological evidence may become available in the near future for the trace elements investigated through ongoing projects such as the EC-funded ESPREME project (Estimation of willingness-to-pay to reduce risks of exposure to heavy metals and cost-benefit analysis for reducing heavy metals occurrence in Europe, contract number: 502527).

In order to arrive at impacts, the approach proposed by Crettaz (2000), Crettaz et al. (2002) and Pennington et al. (2002) employs the Disability Adjusted

Life Year (DALY) concept endorsed by the WHO for considering different severities of the assessed effects. This severity measure is also adopted in the presented methodological framework based on most recent findings (Keller, 2005). It has the advantage of aggregating morbidity and (premature) mortality impacts as equivalents of Years Of Life Lost (YOLLs). This allows the monetary valuation to be performed as commonly done within the ExternE project series. A weak point of the adopted DALY values is the treatment of morbidity which relies on rather uncertain disability weights (cf. section 7.3). Also, the assessment of non-cancer effects which are derived from cancer-related average DALYs is based on a rough classification of these diseases. Consideration may, therefore, be given to look for alternatives with respect to this measure of severity of human health damages and to combine these with the prioritised dose-response information. However, the DALY approach is still deemed a step towards a more differentiated assessment of cancers for whose valuation only one generic monetary value for any type of cancer is used according to the latest ExternE methodology (European Commission, 2004).

Valuation

Due to the very long time horizons involved in the ingestion exposures towards the trace elements investigated, a new discounting scheme is proposed that takes the issue of intergenerational equity into account. It is termed *intergenerationally equal, positive personal discounting*. It combines intergenerational equity by assuming a discount rate of zero between generations with the observation that each individual shows a positive pure time preference. As is argued in section 8.2.4, this discounting scheme yields external costs that are about half of those when constantly discounting at a rate of 0 %.

Implementation

A special feature is also the way in which the methodological approach for the assessment of ingestion exposures and their valuation is implemented. In contrast to the majority of multimedia fate and exposure models which are implemented as spreadsheet models, for instance EUSES (Vermeire et al., 1997), USES-LCA (Huijbregts, 1999), CalTOX (McKone, 1993b) and IMPACT 2000 (Pennington et al., 2005), the software tool WATSON is coded in C++ (MS Visual Studio 6.0) and uses a LINUX-based Oracle database version 8.1.6i. This facilitates a flexible definition of process formulations and combinations as well as the use of different environmental settings allowing the modelling of different substances (e.g., Trapp and Schwartz, 2000). Unlike many existing multimedia models, WATSON's mass balance is based on concentrations (like SimpleBox, Brandes et al., 1996). The software tool also offers the possibility of running in different modes of operation for the investigation for example of continuous and constant emissions over time and at steady-state or of a pulse emission and its consequences in terms of exposure over different time horizons. Storing the data in a database means that the data are kept separately from the simulation code (Robinson, 1999) which facilitates their changeability (Veerkamp and Wolff, 1996) at the expense of computation time however.

12.2 General limitations of the assessment

Although comprising many innovations and providing a reliable exposure and impact assessment approach, the main constraints with respect to the presented methodological framework shall be noted.

The methodology developed is at present limited with respect to substances that are to some extent volatile, i.e., only substances with a low vapour pressure can be assessed.

The assessment of ingestion exposures is incomplete. In particular, no exposure through seafood, drinking water or soil ingestion by humans is at present included in the assessment. Furthermore, several crops classified as aboveground exposed produce are missing. Exposure pathways related to dermal contact, occurring at the working place or through consumer products are also not taken into account due to the assessment being conducted at the regional scale (see next point) and/or for disperse emission sources. This should not be interpreted as implying that transfers from other environmental media through these or other pathways are unimportant.

Exposures occurring in a very localised area or only during short episodes cannot be addressed adequately. The spatial and temporal resolution of the environmental fate model does not allow such localised or temporary exposure assessments to be carried out. This means that an assessment of the exposure of individuals cannot be conducted. This applies especially to those individuals with localised food supply that is produced on contaminated soils/feed (Tennant, 2001).

Due to the use of long-term average data for the description of the environment, computations with time steps that are not full years do not give adequate results in terms of meaningful values for the eventually desired period of time (e.g., seasonal, monthly, daily variations).

Especially with respect to the long time frames involved, until a certain percentage of the steady-state concentration is reached, such long-term analyses face the problem of justifying the assumption of constant long-term environmental and societal conditions (e.g., hydrological cycle, pH, population) which are subject to changes such as climate change, acid rain and shifts in birth and death rates. However, trying to predict these changes is also highly speculative.

As discussed in section 2.3, substances with rather short residence times in the environment require dynamic modelling approaches that do not rely on long-term average conditions. Thus, such substances should be assessed cautiously with the help of the presented approach, if at all.

The quantification of impacts and external costs are related to impacts on human health. These are assessed for the stated contaminants. Thus, impacts of other pollutants and on other receptors such as biodiversity still need to be assessed in order for the analysis to be as comprehensive as desired for a well-informed policy decision-making.

A problem especially related to naturally occurring contaminants is that background levels may need to be taken into account. This is particularly the case if there are non-linear relationships considered either in the environmental fate, exposure or impact assessment which is not the case at present. Not only background levels would be required when there are non-linearities considered but also past and present emission information. Information on present releases of contaminants into water and soil but also of past emissions into all media is incomplete so that for instance local hot-spots due to metal mining and processing, sewage sludge and fertilizer amendments, and local depositions on roadside soils can hardly be included in the assessments, partly owing to the regional spatial resolution. As just indicated, information on releases to soils or waters in particular are identified as not yet existing for the spatial scope required.

Although the present modelling tries to take into account the persistent nature of the trace elements for instance by the distinction of several compartments differing in the rate of advective flows and by the consideration of their pH-dependent partition behaviour and, therefore, comprises a step forward in large scale trace element assessments, it could potentially be improved for example by the inclusion of speciation apart from considering only the effective fractions of the pollutants in food items and air by means of the effective Intake Fraction. However, this is not feasible at the spatial scale needed for national or even pan-European assessments especially due to data availability constraints with respect to transformation rates and concentrations of reaction partners or competing ions in the respective media.

Inactivation processes such as irreversible binding are not explicitly considered but deemed to be part of the solid-water partitioning coefficient that is recommended to be provided for aged samples.

The geographical scope to which the methodology can be applied at present is confined to Europe. However, the model framework exists and 'merely' needs some data acquisition and processing in order to apply it to other parts of the world. This extension of the model may even lead to a globally applicable tool necessitating an air quality model that operates at the same spatial scale (e.g., Leip and Lammel, 2004; Munthe and Palm, 2003).

12.3 Application of the assessment framework

The application of the methodological framework suggests the following conclusions.

12.3.1 Case studies

Different scenarios have been investigated addressing emissions into air from single facilities or for the whole of Europe.

Generally, exposure via staple food items such as cereals and to a lesser extent potatoes contributes substantially to the ingestion exposures of all trace elements analysed. Dairy products are additionally important for chromium and even more so for arsenic. Beef only constitutes a significant share of chromium's Intake Fraction in the long run while freshwater fish and other animal products such as pork, poultry and eggs contribute insignificantly. In line with the findings in European Commission (2000b) for cadmium and arsenic, the inhalation pathway only contributes marginally to the overall human exposure.

The investigation of the development of the human exposure via ingestion towards a one year pulse emission has revealed that not only the total amounts taken in increase slowly over time[33] but also that the food items contributing most to the time-integrated Intake Fraction vary over different time horizons. This variation may even lead to entirely different patterns in terms of the dominating food items at different integration times. For instance, the long-term exposure towards arsenic is dominated by dairy products (about 80 %) while in the short term the composition of the ingestion exposure is shared between cereals, dairy products, potatoes and spinach. Also, the exposure through aboveground exposed produce such as spinach contributes more substantially in the near future after the pulse emissions occurred while its contribution to the effective Intake Fraction may be insubstantial in the long run. The contribution of aboveground exposed produce through interception of atmospheric deposition, thus, appears to be similar to inhalation-related exposures in terms of its intertemporal significance for human exposure towards pulse emissions. Expressed inversely, exposures through the

---

[33] For the trace elements with slower dynamics, i.e., arsenic and chromium, less than 2 % of the fraction that leads to exposure may have reached the human population after 100 years upon a one-year pulse emission according to the present assessment.

media soil and water are most dominant in the intermediate to long term for very persistent substances although for cadmium the contribution of the ingestion pathways to the overall human exposure is already substantial in the short term. Exposures towards very persistent substances through the media soil and water are, therefore, highly relevant with respect to sustainable development especially in terms of intergenerational equity.

The dominance of the ingestion exposures is also reflected in the external costs. Inhalation-related annual external costs according to the investigated emission scenarios are negligible when compared to the related ingestion exposures when discounting at a rate of 0 %. The damage factors due to ingestion are substantially smaller when non-zero discounting is performed, owing to the long-lived nature of these pollutants (cf. Hellweg, 2000; van den Bergh et al., 2000; Huijbregts et al., 2001; de Vries et al., 2004) and associated slow dynamics. Depending on the dynamics of the respective pollutant, the effect is more (e.g., arsenic) or less (e.g., cadmium) pronounced. However, discounting the damages following ingestion exposures with up to a discount rate of 3 % does not change the ranking of the inhalation and ingestion exposures in terms of their contribution to the aggregated impact.

It has been postulated by Spadaro and Rabl (2004) that site-dependency of releases are almost irrelevant for ingestion exposures. However, it could be demonstrated that the variation in terms of damages due to ingestion between sites is similar to the inhalation-caused damages despite the homogenizing effect on food concentrations caused by the present representation of trade. Furthermore, it has been found that the impact of discounting depends on the emission scenario analysed. This can be attributed to different dynamics for the metal to reach the human population from different release sites. This stresses once more that, although trade may lead to homogeneous levels in the food items under consideration, it does not mean that the site of release is almost irrelevant. Thus, employing different discounting schemes may cause comparable damages from different release sites to become distinct. The difference is expected to increase if trade is modelled according to bilateral trade information (see above).

12.3.2 Remarks on the magnitude of the external costs

The damage factors derived in Chapters 10 and 11 have been put into perspective against those for the classical air pollutants and for previously reported trace elements to the extent available. Inhalation-related quantifiable annual external costs are negligible (i.e., four orders of magnitude smaller) according to the pan-European emission scenario for 1990 of the investigated trace elements when compared to an emission scenario for the classical air pollutants of the same year. The consideration of ingestion exposures of these pollutants, however, could lead to an increase in the total quantifiable external costs at most by between 0.4 % and in the order of some 10 % when discounting at a rate of 3 % and 0 %, respectively, according to the presently available information. In this respect, effects due to elevated blood pressure caused by lead are most contributional. A similar finding could also be demonstrated for ingestion exposures to dioxins and dioxin-like substances in selected countries (Droste-Franke et al., 2003), amounting to a few percent when employing a discount rate of 3 %.

The direct use of the damage factors and (annual) external costs as estimated in this study must be performed with caution. As demonstrated in section 9.3, the damage estimates via ingestion exposure may vary by about a factor of two depending on different representations of the environment, particularly when considering the process of preferential flow. Ingestion exposure estimates are still more sensitive towards single parameters such as substance-specific solid-water partitioning coefficients, bioconcentration factors and biotransfer factors, and substance-independent water soil erosion rates. As discussed in section 9.3.1, however, the dose- or rather concentration-response information employed is considered one of the most important component of the analysis in terms of uncertainty emphasizing the importance of reliable effect information. The disregard of chemical speciation constitutes another major source of uncertainty whose impact has not been quantified.

Another problem lies in the incomplete knowledge about the effect-causing characteristic of particulate matter. In general, there is a discussion going on whether the particle size or its composition is (more) responsible for the observed adverse effects. Apparently, "(e)vidence is accumulating that metals may have a role in any toxic response to complex air particles" (Godleski et al., 2000, p. 74). However, also other constituents of particulate matter such as sulphates are considered to be responsible for its toxic effect (Gordon et al., 2000). In any case, care must be taken not to double-count the effects towards particle-associated metals via inhalation. While the effects assessed to occur due to inhalation exposure towards particulate matter are not related to carcinogenesis (cf. e.g. Friedrich and Bickel, 2001a), most of the inhalation-induced effects estimated in the present study are (cf. Tables 7-6 and 7-7). This means that the damage factors derived for the trace elements considered in this study can be added to those for particles due to different effect endpoints. Non-cancer effect information is only used for chromium. However, the quantified, non-cancer related damages via inhalation of hexavalent chromium are rather negligible (Tables 10-6 and 11-3).

12.3.3 Quantitative evaluation of predicted concentrations

A comparison has been conducted of the predicted concentrations according to a 100 year continuous release of the trace elements into air according to the pan-European emission scenario with reported concentrations. It could be demonstrated that the results of the present assessment are almost exclusively within or below the ranges of expected values.

A scenario analysis and a sensitivity analysis of the parameters was conducted in order to evaluate the novel components of the assessment framework such as the compartments distinguished in this work, the pH-dependent partitioning of trace elements, and improved or newly introduced processes (e.g., preferential flow, harvest removals, riverine suspended particle dynamics and compartment-dependent water soil erosion). It could be demonstrated that all of these components are influential on the overall human exposure. These analyses have, furthermore, revealed that the influence of the environmental fate and exposure parameters and/or settings mostly shows in the intermediate to long run. Thus, when analysing one year pulse emission scenarios and performing (regular) non-zero discounting, most of the uncertainties related to these model components become largely irrelevant.

12.4 Applicability of the approach to other contexts

In Chapters 10 and 11, more detailed results have been shown at different levels of the assessment according to the Impact Pathway Approach which may serve different purposes. For instance, the indicator *Intake Fraction* may be used in the context of risk analysis or Life Cycle Impact Assessment (LCIA) as done by Bennett et al. (2002), Bodnar et al. (2002) and Evans et al. (2002) among others. Similarly, the indicator Disability Adjusted Life Years (DALYs) has also been applied in LCIAs in order to characterize a contaminant with respect to an impact indicator ('characterization factor', e.g., Goedkoop et al., 1998; Hofstetter, 1998; Crettaz, 2000; Crettaz et al., 2002; Pennington et al., 2002; Jolliet et al., 2003) although some reservations exist with respect to its use due to the inclusion of value choices (Krewitt et al., 2002, see also section 8.2.3). In many cases, the analysed energy-related emissions lead to the highest impacts within a life cycle study with respect to the toxicity impact category (e.g., Beck et al., 2000; Saouter et al., 2002). Due to the model development undertaken, the presented LCIA-related metrics for trace elements typically released by energy conversion processes constitute a step towards a better assessment of these contaminants within Life Cycle Analyses (LCA). The use of the DALY concept also offers the possibility to compare the assessed impacts to health reports issued by the WHO (e.g., World Health Organisation, 2002) although noting that the DALYs used by the WHO most likely will be derived considering age-weighting and discounting, rendering a direct comparison of the numbers less readily feasible.

The valued impacts may, furthermore, be used in contexts where cost-benefit analyses (CBAs) are conducted. Owing to the monetisation of external effects that are not taken into account when deriving private costs of profit-oriented enterprises, such analyses are typically conducted by public bodies especially at the national or the supranational level. National accounting frameworks that take environmental aspects explicitly into account are one such example (cf. European Commission, 2003d).

12.5 Outlook and closure

Previous prioritisations within the ExternE project series especially of the classical air pollutants, thus, appear justified in the sense that the selected substances have high damage factors and are emitted in rather large quantities. However, the amount of contaminants added by the present work to the list of substances for which external costs can be estimated is small compared to those that remain unaddressed. Their monetised impacts may add up to substantial shares of the so far quantifiable external costs. The main obstacle on the way to a larger substance coverage is seen in the lack of effect information in terms of dose- or exposure-response functions. The appropriate consideration of hydrophobic and (semi-) volatile substances for instance may bring about the need to develop a fully integrated spatially-resolved multimedia model which includes an air compartment and potentially even a plant compartment (Simonich and Hites, 1994; Wagrowski and Hites, 1997; Bennett et al., 1998; McLachlan and Horstmann, 1998; Severinsen and Jager, 1998; Cousins and Mackay, 2001). Furthermore, many substances of public concern are rather long-lived in air and, therefore, require at least hemispheric if not global models for their appropriate assessment (United States - Environmental Protection Agency, 1997b; Ryaboshapko et al., 1998; Pekar et al., 1999). Another issue is that mercury for example is not only long-lived in air but human exposure towards its methylated and most toxic species mostly occurs through fish and especially marine fish (United Nations Environment Programme, 2002). A cost-efficient abatement strategy for this heavy metal which is desirable for setting a strategy on mercury at the EU level[34] for instance would require a link between emissions and exposures that consequently not only comprises the whole medium air but also the marine environment including the organisms relevant in the final human exposure towards mercury. This involves not

---

[34] See e.g. http://europa.eu.int/comm/environment/chemicals/mercury/index.htm as of August 2005

only transport of mercury according to wind or water currents but also entrained in migrating fish and finally trade (United Nations Environment Programme, 2002). Such a global model on fish migration and chemical environmental fate for the marine environment is still to be developed. Thus, further research is needed not only with respect to improving or rather identifying reliable effect information.

The approach taken is a balance between the ambitious goal to be able to address trace element contamination at a continental scale with a regional resolution on the one hand and state-of-the-art in modelling of trace elements on the other. When interpreting the results obtained in decision-making, it is, therefore, important to acknowledge the practical state-of-the-art, the uncertainties and the need for ongoing scientific advances. According to the 'ethos of applied demography' (Essink-Bot, 1998), however, it is better to provide the best possible estimates based on, at times, poor data, than providing no estimates at all. In this sense, the present work constitutes an improvement towards more knowledge about the magnitude of the external costs occurring due to human activities. Before this contribution, hardly any information (if at all) on the external costs for exposure routes other than inhalation had been available. Therefore, the uncertainty is considered acceptable given the model's purpose (Eisenhart, 1968; Scott et al., 2000). Several issues of further development have been named for which hopefully further funding can be obtained.

In supporting the assessment of releases of hazardous substances into air, (fresh) water and soil at the European scale in a spatially-resolved way, the present work is an improvement towards more knowledge about the magnitude of health impacts and external costs occurring due to human activities as hardly any information (if at all) particularly on the external costs for exposure routes other than inhalation had been available prior to this effort.

References

In the following, all references that are mentioned in this work are given regardless of whether these are even personal communications or quotes from other references. In the latter case, it is made explicit in the text that the author has not had access to the respective source. For better traceability purposes of the corresponding information, however, these are also given here.

Aboul-Kassim TAT, Simoneit BRT (2001a) Interaction mechanisms between organic pollutants and solid phase systems. In: Aboul-Kassim TAT and Simoneit BRT (eds) Pollutant-solid phase interactions: mechanisms, chemistry and modeling. Springer, Berlin The handbook of environmental chemistry (Volume 5 Part E), pp 107-167

Aboul-Kassim TAT, Simoneit BRT (2001b) Sorption/desorption of organic pollutants from complex mixtures: modeling, kinetics, experimental techniques and transport parameters. In: Aboul-Kassim TAT and Simoneit BRT (eds) Pollutant-solid phase interactions: mechanisms, chemistry and modeling. Springer, Berlin The handbook of environmental chemistry (Volume 5 Part E), pp 169-242

Addiscott T, Smith J, Bradbury N (1995) Critical evaluation of models and their parameters. Journal of environmental quality 24:803-807

Addiscott TM (1993) Simulation modelling and soil behaviour. Geoderma 60:15-40

Addiscott TM (1998) Modelling concepts and their relation to the scale of the problem. Nutrient Cycling in Agroecosystems 50:239-245

Agency for Toxic Substances and Disease Registry (1999) Toxicological Profile for Lead. U.S. Public Health Service, U.S. Department of Health and Human Services, Atlanta, GA

Agency for Toxic Substances and Disease Registry (2000a) Toxicological Profile for Chromium. U.S. Public Health Service, U.S. Department of Health and Human Services, Atlanta, GA

Agency for Toxic Substances and Disease Registry (2000b) Toxicological Profile for Arsenic. U.S. Public Health Service, U.S. Department of Health and Human Services, Atlanta, GA

Agency for Toxic Substances and Disease Registry (2003) Toxicological Profile Information Sheet. U.S. Public Health Service, U.S. Department of Health and Human Services, Atlanta, GA, available at: http://www.atsdr.cdc.gov/toxpro2.html

Alloway BJ, Steinnes E (1999) Anthropogenic additions of cadmium to soils. In: McLaughlin MJ and Singh BR (eds) Cadmium in soils and plants. Kluwer, Dordrecht Developments in plant and soil sciences, vol 85, pp 97-123

Alloway BJ, Ayres DC, Förstner U (1996) Schadstoffe in der Umwelt: chemische Grundlagen zur Beurteilung von Luft-, Wasser- und Bodenverschmutzungen. Spektrum Akademischer Verlag, Heidelberg

Anonym (2002) ZMP-Marktbilanz: Getreide, Ölsaaten, Futtermittel 2002: Deutschland, Europäische Union, Weltmarkt. Zentrale Markt- und Preisberichtstelle für Erzeugnisse der Land-, Forst- und Ernährungswirtschaft (ZMP), Bonn

Anonym (2003) ZMP-Marktbilanz: Eier und Geflügel 2003: Deutschland, Europäische Union, Weltmarkt. Zentrale Markt- und Preisberichtstelle für Erzeugnisse der Land-, Forst- und Ernährungswirtschaft (ZMP), Bonn

Anonym (2004) Ökomarkt-Jahrbuch: Verkaufspreise im ökologischen Landbau, Jahre 2002/2003. Zentrale Markt- und Preisberichtstelle für Erzeugnisse der Land-, Forst- und Ernährungswirtschaft (ZMP), Bonn

Anonymous (1971) Das Umweltprogramm der Bundesregierung. Bundestags-Drucksache VI/2710

Anonymous (1996) Report on the welfare of pigs kept outdoors. Farm Animal Welfare Council, London

Anonymous (1999a) Understanding variation in partition coefficient, Kd , values - Volume I: The Kd Model, Methods of Measurement, and Application of Chemical Reaction Codes. Office of Radiation and Indoor Air Office of Solid Waste and Emergency Response, U.S. Environmental Protection Agency; Office of Environmental Restoration, U.S. Department of Energy, Herndon, VA, USA

Anonymous (1999b) Understanding variation in partition coefficient, Kd , values - Volume II: Review of Geochemistry and Available Kd Values for Cadmium, Cesium, Chromium, Lead, Plutonium, Radon, Strontium, Thorium, Tritium (3 H), and Uranium. Office of Radiation and Indoor Air Office of Solid Waste and Emergency Response, U.S. Environmental Protection Agency; Office of Environmental Restoration, U.S. Department of Energy, Herndon, VA, USA

Anonymous (2000) Assessment of dietary intake of dioxins and related PCBs by the population of EU - Member States - 7 June 2000. Directorate General for Health and Consumer Protection, Brussels Reports on tasks for scientific cooperation

Anonymous (2002) Contaminants in soil: Collation of toxicological data and intake values for humans. Chromium. Environment Agency, Department for Environment, Food and Rural Affairs and the Environment Agency, Bristol

Anonymous (2004) Poultry egg production in the South East. National Farmers' Union, available at: http://www.nfu.org.uk/stellentdev/groups/public/documents/regional_article/poultry-eggproduc_ia412f4576-1.hcsp

Arnold JG, Allen PM, Bernhardt G (1993) A comprehensive surface-groundwater flow model. Journal of Hydrology 142:47-69

Azar C, Sterner T (1996) Discounting and distributional considerations in the context of global warming. Ecological economics 19:169-184

Bach M, Huber A, Frede H-G (2001) Input pathways and river load of pesticides in Germany - a national scale modeling assessment. Water Science and Technology 43:261-268

Bachmann TM, Droste-Franke B, Friedrich R (2004) Assessing the Sustainability of Heavy Metal Emissions in Europe. In: International Conference on Probabilistic Safety Assessment and Management (PSAM) 7 - European Safety and Reliability Conference (ESREL) '04, Berlin, Germany. Springer, pp 2558-2563

Baker JI, Hites RA (2000) Is Combustion the Major Source of Polychlorinated Dibenzo-p -dioxins and Dibenzofurans to the Environment? A Mass Balance Investigation. Environmental Science & Technology 34:2879-2886

Baker JR, Mihelcic JR, Shea E (2000) Estimating Koc for persistent organic pollutants: limitations of correlations with Kow. Chemosphere 41:813-817

Baker JR, Mihelcic JR, Sabljic A (2001) Reliable QSAR for estimating Koc for persistent organic pollutants: correlation with molecular connectivity indices. Chemosphere 45:213-221

Barbante C, Veysseyre A, Ferrari C, Van De Velde K, Morel C, Capodaglio G, Cescon P, Scarponi G, Boutron C (2001) Greenland Snow Evidence of Large Scale Atmospheric Contamination for Platinum, Palladium, and Rhodium. Environmental Science & Technology 35:835 -839

Barbante C, Schwikowski M, Döring T, Gäggeler HW, Schotterer U, Tobler L, Van de Velde K, Ferrari C, Cozzi G, Turetta A, Rosman K, Bolshov M, Capodaglio G, Cescon P, Boutron C (2004) Historical Record of European Emissions of Heavy Metals to the Atmosphere Since the 1650s from Alpine Snow/Ice Cores Drilled near Monte Rosa. Environmental Science & Technology 38:4085-4090

Barra R, Vighi M, Maffioli G, Di Guardo A, Ferrario P (2000) Coupling SoilFug Model and GIS for Predicting Pesticide Pollution of Surface Water at Watershed Level. Environmental Science & Technology 34:4425 -4433

Bartlett RJ (1999) Characterizing Soil Redox Behaviour. In: Sparks DL (ed) Soil physical chemistry. CRC Press, Boca Raton, Fla., pp 371-397

Batjes NH (1996) Documentation to ISRIC-WISE global data set of derived soil properties on a 1/2° by 1/2° grid (version 1.0). International Soil Reference and Information Centre (ISRIC), Wageningen, The Netherlands, pp 13

Baumgartner A, Liebscher H-J (1990) General hydrology, quantitative hydrology (in German). Gebrüder Borntraeger, Stuttgart

Baxter M, Lewis J (2002) Total and inorganic arsenic concentrations in 1999 UK total diet study. Central Science Laboratory, Sand Hutton, York, pp 24

Beck A, Scheringer M, Hungerbühler K (2000) Fate modelling within LCA - the case of textile chemicals. The International Journal of Life Cycle Assessment 5:335-344

Beck MB, Chen J (2000) Assuring the quality of models designed for predictive tasks. In: Saltelli A, Chan K and Scott EM (eds) Sensitivity analysis. John Wiley & Sons, Chichester Wiley series in probability and statistics, pp 401-420

Becker A (1995) Problems and progress in macroscale hydrological modelling. In: Feddes RA (ed) Space and time scale variability and interdependencies in hydrological processes. Cambridge Univ. Press, Cambridge International hydrology series, pp 135-143

Becker K, Müssig-Zufika M, Hoffmann K, Krause C, Meyer E, Nöllke P, Schulz C, Seiwert M (1997) Umwelt-Survey 1990/92, Band V: Trinkwasser. Umweltbundesamt, Institut für Wasser-, Boden- und Lufthygiene, Berlin

Beitz W, Küttner K-H (1995) Dubbel - Taschenbuch für den Maschinenbau. Springer, Berlin

Bennett DH, McKone TE, Matthies M, Kastenberg WE (1998) General Formulation of Characteristic Travel Distance for Semivolatile Organic Chemicals in a Multimedia Environment. Environmental Science & Technology 32:4023-4030

Bennett DH, Margni MD, McKone TE, Jolliet O (2002) Intake Fraction for Multimedia Pollutants: A Tool for Life Cycle Analysis and Comparative Risk Assessment. Risk Analysis 22:903-916

Berdowski JJM, Baas J, Bloos JPJ, Visschedijk AJH, Zandvend PYJ (1997) The European Atmospheric Emission Inventory of Heavy Metals and Persistent Organic Pollutants for 1990. Umweltbundesamt; TNO Institut für Umwelt, Energie und Verfahrensinnovation, Berlin, Apeldoorn

Berende PLM (1990) Grondopname door melkkoeien. Internal Report No. 312. Institute for Livestock Feeding and Nutrition Research, Lelystad

Bergkvist B, Folkeson L, Berggren D (1989) Fluxes of Cu, Zn, Pb, Cr, and Ni in temperate forest ecosystems. Water, Air, and Soil Pollution 47:217-286

Bernigau W, Becker K, Hoffmann K, Krause C, Friedrich C, Schulz C, Seifert B (2000) Umwelt-Survey 1990/92, Band X: Blei - Zusammenhangsanalyse. Umweltbundesamt, Institut für Wasser-, Boden- und Lufthygiene, Berlin

Berrow MJ, Burridge JC (1991) Uptake, Distribution, and Effects of Metal Compounds on Plants. In: Merian E (ed) Metals and their compounds in the environment: occurrence, analysis, and biological, relevance. VCH, Weinheim, pp 399-410

Beven K (1991) Modeling preferential flow: an uncertain future? In: Gish TJ and Shirmohammadi A (eds) Preferential flow. Proceedings of the national symposium held at Chicago, Illinois 16-17 December 1991. American Society of Agricultural Engineers, St. Joseph, Michigan, pp 1-11

Bey I, Jacob DJ, Yantosca RM, Logan JA, Field BD, Fiore AM, Li Q, Liu HY, Mickley LJ, Schultz MG (2001) Global modeling of tropospheric chemistry with assimilated meteorology: Model description and evaluation. Journal of Geophysical Research 106:23073-23096

Bingham FT, Sposito G, Strong JE (1986) The effect of sulfate on the availability of cadmium. Soil Science 141:172-177

Bintein S, Devillers J (1996a) Evaluating the environmental fate of lindane in France. Chemosphere 32:2427-2440

Bintein S, Devillers J (1996b) Evaluating the environmental fate of atrazine in France. Chemosphere 32:2441-2456

Blanchard PE, Lerch RN (2000) Watershed Vulnerability to Losses of Agricultural Chemicals: Interactions of Chemistry, Hydrology, and Land-Use. Environmental Science & Technology 34:3315-3322

Bleeker I, Fischer AB, Tilkes F, Eikmann T (1999) PCB-Konzentrationen im menschlichen Blut. Umweltmedizin in Forschung und Praxis 4:84-96

Bliefert C (1997) Umweltchemie, 2 edn. Wiley-VCH, Weinheim

Blöschl G (1996) Scale and Scaling in Hydrology Institut für Hydraulik, Gewässerkunde und Wasserwirtschaft. Technische Universität Wien, Wien, pp 346

Bodnar AB, Maddalena RL, McKone TE (2002) The Contribution of Locally Grown Foods in Cumulative Exposure Assessments Journal of Exposure Analysis & Environmental Epidemiology. Environmental Health Sciences, School of Public Health, University of California; Indoor Environment Department, Lawrence Berkeley National Laboratory, Berkeley, CA

Boening DW (2000) Ecological effects, transport, and fate of mercury: a general review. Chemosphere 40:1335-1351

Bogen KT, Spear RC (1987) Integrating uncertainty and interindividual variability in environmental risk assessment. Risk Analysis 7:427-436

Bolt GH, van Riemsdijk WH (1987) Surface chemical processes in soil. In: Stumm W (ed) Aquatic surface chemistry: chemical processes at the particle-water interface. Wiley, New York Environmental science and technology, pp 127-164

Borkovec M, Rusch U, Westall JC (1998) Modeling of competitive ion binding at heterogeneous materials with affinity distributions. In: Jenne EA (ed) Adsorption of metals by geomedia: variables, mechanisms, and model applications. Academic Press, San Diego, pp 467-482

Bowen JE (1987) Physiology of genotyping differences in zinc and copper uptake in rice and tomato. Plant and soil 99:115-125

Brandes LJ, den Hollander H, van de Meent D (1996) SimpleBox 2.0: a nested multimedia fate model for evaluating the environmental fate of chemicals. National Institute of Public Health and the Environment (RIVM), Bilthoven, the Netherlands

Brännvall M-L, Bindler R, Renberg I, Emteryd O, Bartnicki J, Billström K (1999) The Medieval Metal Industry Was the Cradle of Modern Large-Scale Atmospheric Lead Pollution in Northern Europe. Environmental Science & Technology 33:4391-4395

Bredehoeft JD, Konikow LF (1993) Ground-water models: validate or invalidate. groundwater 31:178-179

Breivik K, Wania F (2003) Expanding the Applicability of Multimedia Fate Models to Polar Organic Chemicals. Environmental Science & Technology 37:4934-4943

Briggs GG, Bromilow RH, Evans AA (1982) Relationships Between Lipophilicity and Root Uptake and Translocation of Non-ionized Chemicals by Barley. Pesticide science 13:495-504

Brode RW, Wang J (1992) Users's Guide for the Industrial Source Complex (ISC2) Dispersion Models (Volumes I-III). U.S. Environmental Protection Agency, Research Triangle Park, NC

Bromilow RH, Chamberlain K (1995) Principles governing uptake and transport of chemicals. In: Trapp S and Mc Farlane JC (eds) Plant contamination: modeling and simulation of organic chemical processes. Lewis, Boca Raton, pp 37-68

Brown SK, Sim MR, Abramson MJ, Gray CN (1994) Concentrations of Volatile Organic Compounds in Indoor Air - A Review. Indoor Air 4:123-134

Büchert A, Cederberg T, Dyke P, Fiedler H, Fürst P, Hanberg A, Hosseinpour J, Hutzinger O, Kuenen JG, Malisch R, Needham LL, Olie K (2001) Dioxin Contamination in Food. Environmental Science & Pollution Research 8:84-88

Buckley-Golder DH, Coleman P, Davies M, King K, Petersen A, Watterson J, Woodfield M, Fiedler H, Hanberg A (1999) Compilation of EU Dioxin Exposure and Health Data. AEA Technology plc, Abingdon, UK

Burke TA, Doull J, McKone T, Paustenbach D, Scheuplein R, Udo de Haes HA, Young JS (1996) Human health impact assessment In life cycle assessment: Analysis by an expert panel. International Life Sciences Institute (ILSI), Health and Environmental Sciences Institute, Life Cycle Assessment Technical Committee, Washington, DC

Burmaster DE, Anderson PD (1994) Principles of good practice for the use of Monte Carlo techniques in human health and ecological risk assessments. Risk Analysis 14:477-481

Buse A, Norris D, Harmens H, Büker P, Ashenden T, Mills G (2003) Heavy metals in European mosses: 2000/2001 survey. Centre for Ecology & Hydrology and The United Nations Economic Commission for Europe International Cooperative Programme on effects of Air Pollution on Natural Vegetation and Crops (UNECE ICP Vegetation), Bangor, pp 45

Campolongo F, Kleijnen J, Andres T (2000a) Screening methods. In: Saltelli A, Chan K and Scott EM (eds) Sensitivity analysis. John Wiley & Sons, Chichester Wiley series in probability and statistics, pp 65-80

Campolongo F, Saltelli A, Sørensen T, Tarantola S (2000b) Hitchhiker's guide to sensitivity analysis. In: Saltelli A, Chan K and Scott EM (eds) Sensitivity analysis. John Wiley & Sons, Chichester Wiley series in probability and statistics, pp 15-47

Caswell H (1976) The validation problem. In: Patten BC (ed) Systems Analysis and Simulation in Ecology. Academic, New York, vol IV, pp 313-325

Cataldo DA, Garland TR, E WR (1983) Cadmium uptake kinetics in intact soybean plants. Plant physiology 73:844-848

Central Intelligence Agency (CIA) (2003) The World Factbook. Central Intelligence Agency, available at: http://www.odci.gov/cia/publications/factbook/index.html

Chaney RL, Ryan JA (1994) Risk based standards for arsenic, lead, and cadmium in urban soils: summary of information and methods developed to estimate standards for Cd, Pb, and As in urban soils. DECHEMA, Frankfurt am Main

Chaney RL, Ryan JA, Li Y-M, Brown SL (1999) Soil cadmium as a threat to human health. In: McLaughlin MJ and Singh BR (eds) Cadmium in soils and plants. Kluwer, Dordrecht Developments in plant and soil sciences, vol 85, pp 219-256

Chang AC, Page AL, Warneke JE (1987) Long-term sludge application on cadmium and zinc accumulation in Swiss chard and radish. Journal of environmental quality 16:217-221

Chang S-C, Matzner E (2000) The effect of beech stemflow on spatial patterns of soil solution chemistry and seepage fluxes in a mixed beech/oak stand. Hydrological Processes 14:135-144

Chapman PM (2001) How toxic is toxic? (Editorial). Marine Pollution Bulletin 42:1279-1280

Charles R, Jolliet O (2003) Processes governing fate of pesticides in plant. unpublished manuscript

Chiou CT, McGroddy SE, Kile DE (1998) Partition Characteristics of Polycyclic Aromatic Hydrocarbons on Soils and Sediments. Environmental Science & Technology 32:264-269

Choudhury H, Cogliano J, Hertzberg R, Mukerjee D, Rice G, Teuschler L, Doyle E, Woo Y, Schoeny R (2000) Supplementary Guidance for Conducting Health Risk Assessment of Chemical Mixtures. Risk Assessment Forum, Washington, DC

Chung N, Alexander M (1998) Differences in Sequestration and Bioavailability of Organic Compounds Aged in Dissimilar Soils. Environmental Science & Technology 32:855 -860

Church TM, Véron A, Patterson CC, Settle D, Erel Y, Maring HR, Flegal AR (1990) Trace elements in the north atlantic troposphere: shipboard results of precipitation and aerosols. Global biogeochemical cycles 4:431-443

Cleveland WA, et al. (1984) Britannica Atlas. Encyclopaedia Britannica, Chicago

Colman SM (1981) Rock-weathering rates as a function of time. Quaternary research 15:250-264

Councell TB, Duckenfield KU, Landa ER, Callender E (2004) Tire-Wear Particles as a Source of Zinc to the Environment. Environmental Science & Technology

Council of the European Union (1996a) Council Directive 96/61/EC of 24 September 1996 concerning integrated pollution prevention and control. Official Journal of the European Communities L 257:0026-0040

Council of the European Union (1996b) Council Directive 96/62/EC of 27 September 1996 on ambient air quality assessment and management. Official Journal of the European Communities L 296:0055-0063

Cousins IT, Mackay D (2001) Strategies for including vegetation compartments in multimedia models. Chemosphere 44:643-654

Cowan CE, Versteeg DJ, Larson RJ, Kloepper-Sams PJ (1995a) Integrated approach for environmental assessment of new and existing chemicals. Regulatory Toxicology and Pharamacology 21:3-31

Cowan CE, Mackay D, Feijtel TCJ, van de Meent D, di Guardo A, Davies J, Mackay N (1995b) The multi-media fate model: a vital tool for predicting the fate of chemicals. In: workshop organized by the Society of Environmental Toxicology and Chemistry (SETAC), Leuven, Belgium and Denver, Colorado. SETAC press, pp 78

Cox DC, Baybutt P (1981) Methods for uncertainty analysis: a comparative survey. Risk Analysis 1:251-258

Crettaz P (2000) From toxic releases to damages on human health: a method for life cycle impact assessment, with a case study on domestic rainwater use Laboratory of Ecosystem Management. Ecole Polytechnique Fédérale de Lausanne (EPFL), Switzerland, Lausanne

Crettaz P, Pennington DW, Rhomberg L, Brand K, Jolliet O (2002) Assessing Human Health in Life Cycle Assessment using ED10 s and DALYs: Part 1 - Cancer effects. Risk Analysis 22:931-946

Crump KS (1995) Calculation of benchmark doses from continuous data. Risk Analysis 15:79-89

Crump KS (1998) Investigation of the potential impact of benchmark dose and pharmacokinetic modeling in noncancer risk assessment. II. Investigaton of impact on MRLs for methylmercury, manganese, cadmium, perchloroethylene, chloroform, and metallic mercury vapor. Agency for Toxic Substances and Disease Registry (ATSDR)

Cutler JM, Rains DW (1974) Characterization of cadmium uptake by plant tissue. Plant physiology 54:67-71

Daly GL, Wania F (2004) Simulating the Influence of Snow on the Fate of Organic Compounds. Environmental Science & Technology

Daly HE, Cobb JB (1989) For the common good: Redirecting the economy toward community, the environment, and a sustainable future. Beacon Press, Boston

Davies T (1998) The Pollution Control System is Broken. Risk Analysis 18:365-366

de Roo APJ (1993) Modelling surface runoff and soil erosion in catchments using geographical information systems: validity and applicability of the "ANSWERS" model in two catchments in the loess area of South Limburg (The Netherlands) and one in Devon (UK) Faculteit Ruimtelijke Wetenschappen. Rijksuniversiteit Utrecht, Utrecht, pp 295

de Vries W (1999) Approaches and Criteria to Calculate Critical Loads of Heavy Metals for Soils and Surface Waters. In: Gregor H-D, Mohaupt-Jahr B and

Hönerbach F (eds) Workshop on Effects-based Approaches for Heavy Metals, Schwerin, 12. bis 15. Oktober 1999. Proceedings, in UBA-Texte 87/99. Umweltbundesamt, Berlin, pp 33-41

de Vries W, Bakker DJ (1998) Manual for calculating critical loads of heavy metals for terrestrial ecosystems. Guidelines for critical limits, calculation methods and input data. DLO Winand Staring Centre, Wageningen, The Netherlands

de Vries W, Bakker DJ, Sverdrup HU (1998a) Manual for calculating critical loads of heavy metals for aquatic ecosystems. Guidelines for critical limits, calculation methods and input data. DLO Winand Staring Centre, Wageningen, The Netherlands

de Vries W, Bakker DJ, Sverdrup HU, Paces T, Tipping E (1998b) Effect-based approaches to assess the risk of heavy metal inputs to soils - overview methods and models. In: UN-ECE CLRTAP TF Mapping (ed) Proceedings of the Workshop on Critical Limits and Effect Based Approaches for Heavy Metals and Persistent Organic Pollutants. Federal Environmental Agency, Berlin Texte 98,5, pp I-125-I-224

de Vries W, Schütze G, Lofts S, Tipping E, Meili M, Römkens PFAM, Groenenberg JE (2004) Calculation of critical loads for cadmium, lead and mercury: Background document to a Mapping Manual on Critical Loads of cadmium, lead and mercury. Alterra, Wageningen

del Re AAM, Trevisan M (1995) Selection criteria of xenobiotic leaching models in soil. European Journal of Agronomy 4:465-472

Derwent RG, Nodop K (1986) Long-range Transport and Deposition of Acidic Nitrogen Species in North-west Europe. Nature 324:356-358

Derwent RG, Dollard GJ, Metcalfe SE (1988) On the Nitrogen Budget for the United Kingdom and North-west Europe. Q.J.R. Meteorol. Soc. 114:1127-1152

Desmet PJJ, Govers G (1996) A GIS procedure for automatically calculating the USLE LS factor on topographically complex landscape units. Journal of soil and water conservation 51:427-433

Deutsche Gesellschaft für Ernährung e.V. (2000) Ernährungsbericht. hrsg. von der Deutschen Gesellschaft für Ernährung im Auftrag des Bundesministers für Jugend, Familie und Gesundheit und des Bundesministeriums für Ernährung, Landwirtschaft und Forsten, Frankfurt, M, pp 394

Deutscher Verband Tiernahrung (2003) Rohstoffverbrauch zur Mischfutterherstellung. Deutscher Verband Tiernahrung e.V. (DVT), found at: http://www.dvtiernahrung.de/

Deutsches Nationalkomitee für das internationale Hydrologische Programm (IHP) der UNESCO und das Operationelle Hydrologische Programm

(OHP) der WMO (1998) International Glossary of Hydrology: Version: Englisch/Deutsch IHP/OHP-Berichte. Bundesanstalt für Gewässerkunde - IHP/OHP-Sekretariat, Koblenz, vol 12, pp 243

Devillers J, Bintein S, Karcher W (1995) CHEMFRANCE: a regional level III fugacity model applied to France. Chemosphere 30:457-476

Di Guardo A, Calamari D, Zanin G, Consalter A, Mackay D (1994) A fugacity model of pesticide runoff to surface water: development and validation. Chemosphere 28:511-531

Diamond M, Mackay D, Welbourn PM (1992) Models of multimedia partitioning of multi-species chemicals: The fugacity/aquivalence approach. Chemosphere 25:1907-1921

Diamond ML, Priemer DA, Law NL (2001) Developing a multimedia model of chemical dynamics in an urban area. Chemosphere 44:1655-1667

DIN EN ISO (14042:2000) Umweltmanagement - Ökobilanz - Wirkungsabschätzung

Döll P, Lehner B (2002) Validation of a new global 30-min drainage direction map. Journal of Hydrology 258:214-231

Döll P, Lehner B, Kaspar F (2002) Global modeling of groundwater recharge. In: Schmitz GH (ed) Proceedings of Third International Conference on Water Resources and the Environment Research, Technical University of Dresden, Germany, vol I, pp 27-31

Döll P, Kaspar F, Lehner B (2003) A global hydrological model for deriving water availability indicators: model tuning and validation. Journal of Hydrology 270:105-134

Draper NR, Smith H (1966) Applied regression analysis. Wiley, New York

Drever JI (1997a) Weathering processes. In: Saether OM and de Caritat P (eds) Geochemical processes, weathering and groundwater recharge in catchments. Balkema, Rotterdam, pp 3-19

Drever JI (1997b) Catchment mass balance. In: Saether OM and de Caritat P (eds) Geochemical processes, weathering and groundwater recharge in catchments. Balkema, Rotterdam, pp 241-261

Drever JI, Clow DW (1995) Weathering rates in catchments. In: White AF and Brantley SL (eds) Chemical weathering rates of silicate minerals. Mineralogical Society of America, Washington, DC Reviews in mineralogy, vol 31, pp 463-484

Droppo IG, Walling DE, Ongley ED (1998) Suspended sediment structure: implications for sediment and contaminant transport modelling. In: Summer W, Klaghofer E and Zhang W (eds) Modelling Soil Erosion, Sediment Transport and Closely Related Hydrological Processes. IAHS Press, Wallingford, UK Proceedings and Reports (Red books), vol 249, pp 437-444

Droste-Franke B (2005) Quantifizierung von Umweltschäden als Beitrag zu Umweltökonomischen Gesamtrechnungen. Institut für Energiewirtschaft und Rationelle Energieanwendung. Stuttgart, Universität Stuttgart, Stuttgart pp. 232; available at: http://elib.uni-stuttgart.de/opus/volltexte/2005/2204/

Droste-Franke B, Friedrich R (2003) Air pollution. In: European Commission (ed) An applied integrated environmental impact assessment framework for the European Union (GREENSENSE). European Commission, DG Research, EESD, Brussels

Droste-Franke B, Bachmann TM, Friedrich R (2003) Toxic substances. In: European Commission (ed) An applied integrated environmental impact assessment framework for the European Union (GREENSENSE). European Commission, DG Research, EESD, Brussels

Edwards S (2004) Personal communication on free-range keeping of pigs. University of Newcastle, School of Agriculture, Food and Rural Development, Newcastle upon Tyne

Efroymson RA, Will ME, Suter II GW, Wooten AC (1997) Toxicological Benchmarks for Screening Contaminants of Potential Concern for Effects on Terrestrial Plants: 1997 Revision. U.S. Department of Energy

Eggleston JR, Rojstaczer SA (2000) Can We Predict Subsurface Mass Transport? Environmental Science & Technology 34:4010-4017

Eisenhart C (1968) Expression of the uncertainties of final results: clear statements of the uncertainties of reported values are needed for their critical evaluation. Science 160:1201-1204

Eitzer BD, Hites RA (1989) Polychlorinated dibenzo-p-dioxins and dibenzofurans in the ambient atmosphere of Bloomington, Indiana. Environmental Science & Technology 23:1389-1395

EROS Data Center (1996) HYDRO1k geographic database developed from the USGS' 30 arc-second digital elevation model (DEM) of the world (GTOPO30). U.S. Geological Survey (USGS) in cooperation with UNEP/GRID Sioux Falls,
available at: http://edcdaac.usgs.gov/gtopo30/hydro/

EROS Data Center, University of Nebraska-Lincoln, Joint Research Centre of the European Commission (2000) Global land cover characteristics data base (version 2.0). U.S. Geological Survey (USGS) in cooperation with UNEP/GRID Sioux Falls,
available at: http://lpdaac.usgs.gov/glcc/glcc.asp

Eschenbach A, Wienberg R, Mahro B (1998) Fate and Stability of Nonextractable Residues of [14 C]PAH in Contaminated Soils under Environmental Stress Conditions. Environmental Science & Technology 32:2585 -2590

Escher BI, Hermens JLM (2002) Modes of Action in Ecotoxicology: Their Role in Body Burdens, Species Sensitivity, QSARs, and Mixture Effects. Environmental Science & Technology 36:4201 -4217

ESPREME (2004) Personal communication within the EC-funded ESPREME project on total air emissions in Europe in 2000

Essink-Bot M-L (1998) DALYs in Europe. In: Joint ECE-WHO Meeting on Health Statistics, Rome, Italy. World Health Organization, Office for Europe

Euromonitor (1992) European Marketing Data and Statistics 1992. Euromonitor Plc.

European Centre for Ecotoxicology and Toxicology of Chemicals (1994) Assessment of Non-Occupational Exposure to Chemicals. ECETOC, Brussels

European Centre for Ecotoxicology and Toxicology of Chemicals (1999) GREAT-ER 1.0. ECETOC, Brussels

European Commission (1995) Externalities of Fuel Cycles - ExternE Project. European Commission DG XII, Science Research and Development, JOULE, Brussels - Luxembourg

European Commission (1996a) EUSES, the European Union System for the Evaluation of Substances. National Institute of Public Health and the Environment (RIVM), the Netherlands. Available from the European Chemicals Bureau (EC/JRC), Ispra, Italy, Ispra, Italy

European Commission (1996b) Technical guidance document in support of Commission directive 93/67/EEC on risk assessment for new notified substances and Commission regulation (EC) no 1488/94 on risk assessment for existing substances (Part I). Office for Official Publications of the European Communities, Luxembourg

European Commission (1998) The European Soil Data Base (Version 1.0). Joint Research Center, European Soil Bureau, Ispra

European Commission (1999a) Externalities of Fuel Cycles - ExternE Project. Vol. 7 - Methodology (2nd edition). European Commission DG XII, Science Research and Development, JOULE, Brussels - Luxembourg

European Commission (1999b) Externalities of Fuel Cycles - ExternE Project. Vol. 10 - National Implementation. European Commission DG XII, Science Research and Development, JOULE, Brussels - Luxembourg

European Commission (2000a) Communication from the Commission on the precautionary principle. In: European Commission (ed). Commission of the European Communities, Brussels

European Commission (2000b) Ambient air pollution by As, Cd and Ni compounds - Position Paper. Office for Official Publications of the European Communities, Luxembourg, pp 361

European Commission (2001a) Strategy for a future chemicals policy - white paper. Commission of the european communities, Brussels

European Commission (2001b) Fact Sheet on dioxin in feed and food. European Commission, Brussels

European Commission (2002) Communication from the Commission on impact asessment. In: European Commission (ed). Commission of the European Communities, Brussels

European Commission (2003a) Technical guidance document in support of Commission directive 93/67/EEC on risk assessment for new notified substances and Commission regulation (EC) no 1488/94 on risk assessment for existing substances and Directive 98/8/EC of the European Parliament and of the Council concerning the placing of biocidal products on the market (Part I), 2 edn. European Chemicals Bureau (ECB), Joint Research Centre (JRC), Ispra (VA), Italy

European Commission (2003b) Technical guidance document in support of Commission directive 93/67/EEC on risk assessment for new notified substances and Commission regulation (EC) no 1488/94 on risk assessment for existing substances and Directive 98/8/EC of the European Parliament and of the Council concerning the placing of biocidal products on the market (Part II), 2 edn. European Chemicals Bureau (ECB), Joint Research Centre (JRC), Ispra (VA), Italy

European Commission (2003c) Technical guidance document in support of Commission directive 93/67/EEC on risk assessment for new notified substances and Commission regulation (EC) no 1488/94 on risk assessment for existing substances and Directive 98/8/EC of the European Parliament and of the Council concerning the placing of biocidal products on the market, 2 edn. European Chemicals Bureau (ECB), Joint Research Centre (JRC), Ispra (VA), Italy

European Commission (2003d) An applied integrated environmental impact assessment framework for the European Union (GREENSENSE). European Commission, DG Research, EESD, Brussels

European Commission (2003e) Eurostat - NewCronos - Theme 1 (General Statistics) - European Regional Statistics. Office for Official Publications of the European Communities, Luxembourg, CD-ROM

European Commission (2003f) Communication from the Commission to the Council, the European Parliament and the European Economic and Social Committee - A European Environment and Health Strategy. Commission of the European Communities, Brussels

European Commission (2003g) Communication from the Commission to the Council, the European Parliament, the Economic and Social Committee and the Committee of the Regions - Towards a Thematic Strategy for Soil Protection. In: European Commission (ed). Commission of the European Communities, Brussels

European Commission (2004) New Elements for the Assessment of External Costs from Energy Technologies (NewExt). European Commission, DG Research, Technological Development and Demonstration (RTD), Brussels

European Environment Agency (2000) CORINE land cover database

European Environment Agency Data Service (1998) European rivers and catchments database (ERICA). European Environment Agency Data Service, available at: http://dataservice.eea.eu.int/dataservice/metadetails.asp?id=235

Evans JS, Wolff SK, Phonboon K, Levy JI, Smith KR (2002) Exposure efficiency: an idea whose time has come? Chemosphere 49:1075-1091

Ewers U, Schlipköter H-W (1991) Intake, distribution, and excretion of metals and metal compounds in humans and animals. In: Merian E (ed) Metals and their compounds in the environment: occurrence, analysis, and biological, relevance. VCH, Weinheim, pp 571-583

Ewers U, Wilhelm M (1995) Metalle/Cadmium. In: Wichmann H-E, Schlipköter H-W and Fülgraff G (eds) Handbuch der Umweltmedizin. ecomed, Landsberg/Lech, vol 18. Erg. Lfg. 3/2000, pp 25

Fekete BM, Vörösmarty CJ, Lammers RB (2001) Scaling gridded networks for macro-scale hydrology: Development and analysis and control of error. Water resources research 37:1955-1967

Fenner K, Scheringer M, Hungerbühler K (2000) Persistence of Parent Compounds and Transformation Products in a Level IV Multimedia Model. Environmental Science & Technology 34:3809-3817

Ferrario JB, Byrne CJ, Cleverly DH (2000) 2,3,7,8-Dibenzo-p -dioxins in Mined Clay Products from the United States: Evidence for Possible Natural Origin. Environmental Science & Technology 34:4524-4532

Fiedler H (2003) Dioxins and Furans (PCDD/PCDF). In: Fiedler H (ed) The handbook of environmental chemistry Vol 3: Anthropogenic Compounds Part O: Persistent organic pollutants. Springer, Berlin, pp 123-201

Fiedler H, Hutzinger O, Welsch-Pausch K, Schmiedinger A (2000) Evaluation of the Occurrence of PCDD/PCDF and POPs in Wastes and Their Potential to Enter the Foodchain. Final Report. University of Bayreuth (Ecological Chemistry and Geochemistry) and European Commission, Bayreuth, pp 121

Finkel AM (1990) Confronting uncertainty in risk management: a guide for decision-makers. Center for Risk Management, Resources for the Future, Washington, DC, pp 68

Finlayson BL, McMahon TA (1995) Understanding river hydrology. In: Singh VP (ed) Environmental hydrology. Kluwer Academic Publishers, Dordrecht Water Science and Technology Library, vol 15, pp 107-135

Finley B, Paustenbach D (1994) The benefits of probabilistic exposure assessment: three case studies involving contaminated air, water, and soil. Risk Analysis 14:53-73

Fitzgerald WF (1994) Global Biogeochemical Cycling of Mercury. Presented at the DOE/FDA/EPA Workshop on Methylmercury and Human Health, Bethesda, MD

Flury M (1996) Experimental evidence of transport of pesticides through field soils - a review. Journal of environmental quality 25:25-45

Food and Agriculture Organization of the United Nations - Statistics Division (2002a) Food Balance Sheets, available at: http://apps.fao.org/

Food and Agriculture Organization of the United Nations - Statistics Division (2002b) Agriculture Data: Livestock Primary, available at: http://faostat.fao.org/faostat/collections?subset=agriculture

Food and Agriculture Organization of the United Nations - Statistics Division (2003) Agriculture Data: Crops Primary, available at: http://faostat.fao.org/faostat/collections?subset=agriculture

French CL, Maxwell WH, Peters WD, Rice GE, Bullock OR, Vasu AB, Hetes R, Colli A, Nelson C, Lyons BF (1998) Study of Hazardous Air Pollutant Emissions from Electric Utility Steam Generating Units - Final Report to Congress. U.S. Environmental Protection Agency: Emission Standards Division/Air Quality Strategies and Standards Division; Office of Air Quality Planning and Standards

Friedrich R, Bickel P (2001a) Environmental External Costs of Transport. Springer-Verlag, Berlin Heidelberg New York, pp 326

Friedrich R, Bickel P (2001b) Estimation of External Costs Using the Impact-Pathway-Approach. Results from the ExternE project series. TA-Datenbank-Nachrichten 10:74-82

Gauglhofer J, Bianchi V (1991) Chromium. In: Merian E (ed) Metals and their compounds in the environment: occurrence, analysis, and biological, relevance. VCH, Weinheim, pp 853-878

Gawel JE, Trick CG, Morel FMM (2001) Phytochelatins Are Bioindicators of Atmospheric Metal Exposure via Direct Foliar Uptake in Trees near Sudbury, Ontario, Canada. Environmental Science & Technology 35:2108-2113

Gebel T (1999) Metalle/Arsen. In: Wichmann H-E, Schlipköter H-W and Fülgraff G (eds) Handbuch der Umweltmedizin. ecomed, Landsberg/Lech, vol 22. Erg. Lfg. 7/2001, pp 26

Georgopoulos PG, Walia A, Roy A, Lioy PJ (1997) Integrated Exposure and Dose Modeling and Analysis System. 1. Formulation and Testing of Microenvironmental and Pharmacokinetic Components. Environmental Science & Technology 31:17 -27

Geßl (2004) Personal communication on free-range keeping of farm animals. Freiland, Vienna

Gish TJ, Shirmohammadi A (1991) Preferential flow. Proceedings of the national symposium held at Chicago, Illinois 16-17 December 1991. American Society of Agricultural Engineers, St. Joseph, Michigan

Gisi U (1990) Bodenökologie. Thieme, Stuttgart

Godleski JJ, Verrier RL, Koutrakis P, Catalano P (2000) Mechanisms of Morbidity and Mortality from Exposure to Ambient Air Particles. Health Effects Institute, Cambridge MA, pp 105

Goedkoop M, Hofstetter P, Müller-Wenk R, Spriemsma R (1998) The Eco-Indicator 98 Explained. The International Journal of Life Cycle Assessment 3:352-360

Gold LS, Zeiger E (1997) Handbook of carcinogenic potency and genotoxicity databases. CRC press, Boca Raton, pp 754

Golubev GN (1982) Soil erosion and agriculture in the world: an assessment and hydrological implications. In: Walling DE (ed) Recent developments in the explanation and prediction of erosion and sediment yield : proceedings of a symposium held during the First Scientific General Assembly of the International Association of Hydrological Sciences (IAHS) at Exeter, UK, 19-30 July 1982. International Association of Hydrological Sciences, Washington, DC IAHS-AISH publication, vol 137, pp 261-268

Gordon T, Nadziejko C, Chen LC, Schlesinger R (2000) Effects of Concentrated Ambient Particles in Rats and Hamsters: An Exploratory Study. Health Effects Institute, Cambridge MA, pp 43

Green ML, DePinto JV, Sweet C, Hornbuckle KC (2000) Regional Spatial and Temporal Interpolation of Atmospheric PCBs: Interpretation of Lake Michigan Mass Balance Data. Environmental Science & Technology 34:1833-1841

Greger M (1999) Metal Availability and Bioconcentration in Plants. In: Prasad MNV and Hagemeyer J (eds) Heavy metal stress in plants: from molecules to ecosystems. Springer, Berlin, Heidelberg, pp 1-27

Gressmann A, Bickel P (1997) Der Wert eines verlorenen Lebensjahres. In: Friedrich R and Krewitt W (eds) Umwelt- und Gesundheitsschäden durch die Stromerzeugung. Springer, Berlin, pp 55-60

Guerzoni S, Chester R (1996) The impact of desert dust across the Mediterranean Environmental science and technology library - no 11. Kluwer Academic, Dordrecht, pp 389

Guinée J, Heijungs R, van Oers L, van de Meent D, Vermeire T, Rikken M (1996) LCA impact assessment of toxic releases: generic modelling of fate, exposure and effect for ecosystems and human beings with data for about 100 chemicals. Ministerie van Volkshuisvesting, Ruimtelijke Ordening en Milieubeheer, Centrale Directie Voorlichting en Externe Betrekkingen, Den Haag

Gustafsson Ö, Haghseta F, Chan C, MacFarlane J, Gschwend PM (1997) Quantification of the Dilute Sedimentary Soot Phase: Implications for PAH Speciation and Bioavailability. Environmental Science & Technology 31:203 -209

Haab TC, McConnell KE (2002) Valuing Environmental and Natural Resources - The Econometrics of Non-Market Valuation. Edward Elgar, Cheltenham, UK

Håkanson L (1984) Aquatic contamination and ecological risk: an attempt to a conceptual framework. Water Research 18:1107-1118

Hamby DM (1994) A review of techniques for parameter sensitivity analysis of environmental models. Environmental monitoring and assessment 32:135-154

Hammitt JK (2000) Valuing Mortality Risk: Theory and Practice. Environmental Science & Technology 34:1396-1400

Hansen M, DeFries R, Townshend JRG, Sohlberg R (1998) 1 km Land Cover Classification Derived from AVHRR. The Global Land Cover Facility, University of Maryland, College Park, Maryland, available at: http://glcf.umiacs.umd.edu/data/landcover/data.shtml

Harrison SN (2001a) Inorganic contaminants in food. In: Watson DH (ed) Food chemical safety 1: Contaminants. CRC Press, Boca Raton, pp 148-168

Harrison SN (2001b) Environmental organic contaminants in food. In: Watson DH (ed) Food chemical safety 1: Contaminants. CRC Press, Boca Raton, pp 169-192

Hartmann E, Bischoff W-A, Kaupenjohann M (2004) Untersuchung von Klärschlamm auf ausgewählte Schadstoffe und ihr Verhalten bei der landwirtschaftlichen Klärschlammverwertung. Umweltbundesamt, Berlin

Harvey C (1994) The reasonableness of non-constant discounting. Journal of Public Economics 53:31-51

Hasselrot B, Grennfelt P (1987) Deposition of air pollutants in a wind exposed forest edge. Water, Air, and Soil Pollution 34:135-143

Hattemer-Frey HA, Travis CC, Land ML (1990) Benzene: Environmental partitioning and human exposure. Advances in Environmental Research 53:221-232

Hauschild M, Potting J (2003) Spatial differentiation in life cycle impact assessment - the EDIP2000 methodology. Department of Manufacturing Engineering and Management, Technical University of Denmark, Lyngby

Heijungs R (1995) Harmonization of methods for impact assessment. Environmental Science & Pollution Research 2:217-224

Heijungs R (2000) Dynabox : A dynamic multi-media fate model with applications to heavy metals. In: van der Voet E, Guinée JB and Udo de Haes HA (eds) Heavy metals: a problem solved? - Methods and models to evaluate policy strategies for heavy metals. Kluwer Acad. Publ., Dordrecht, pp 65-76

Heijungs R, Suh S (2002) The computational structure of Life Cycle Assessment. Kluwer, Dordrecht

Helling CS, Gish TJ (1991) Physical and chemical processes affecting preferential flow. In: Gish TJ and Shirmohammadi A (eds) Preferential flow. Proceedings of the national symposium held at Chicago, Illinois 16-17 December 1991. American Society of Agricultural Engineers, St. Joseph, Michigan, pp 77-86

Hellweg S (2000) Time- and Site-Dependent Life Cycle-Assessment of Thermal Waste Treatment Processes Chemical Engineering Department. ETH Zürich, Zürich

Hellweg S, Hofstetter T, Hungerbühler K (2003) Discounting and the Environment - Should Current Impacts be Weighted Differently than Impacts Harming Future Generations? The International Journal of Life Cycle Assessment 8:8-18

Helmke PA (1999) Chemistry of cadmium in soil solution. In: McLaughlin MJ and Singh BR (eds) Cadmium in soils and plants. Kluwer, Dordrecht Developments in plant and soil sciences, vol 85, pp 39-64

Hennings V (1994) Methodendokumentation Bodenkunde. E. Schweizerbart'sche Verlagsbuchhandlung, Stuttgart

Henrion M, Fischhoff B (1986) Assessing uncertainty in physical constants. Am. J. Phis. 54:791-798

Hering JG, Morel FMM (1990) The kinetics of trace metal complexation: implications for metal reactivity in natural waters. In: Stumm W (ed) Aquatic chemical kinetics: reaction rates of processes in natural waters. Wiley, New York, pp 145-171

Hertl M, Merk HF (1999) Metalle/Chrom. In: Wichmann H-E, Schlipköter H-W and Fülgraff G (eds) Handbuch der Umweltmedizin. ecomed, Landsberg/Lech, vol 3. Erg. Lfg. 1/1994, pp 8

Hertwich EG (1999) Toxic Equivalency: Addressing Human Health Effects in Life Cycle Impact Assessment Energy and Resources Group. University of California, Berkeley

Hertwich EG (2001) Intermittent Rainfall in Dynamic Multimedia Fate Modeling. Environmental Science & Technology 35:936-940

Hertwich EG, McKone TE, Pease W (1999) Parameter Uncertainty and Variability In Evaluative Fate and Exposure Models. Risk Analysis 19:1193-1204

Hertwich EG, McKone TE, Pease WS (2000) A systematic uncertainty analysis of an evaluative fate and exposure model. Risk Analysis 20:439-454

Hertwich EG, Mateles SF, Pease WS, McKone TE (2001) Human Toxicity Potentials for Life-Cycle-Assessment and Toxics: Release inventory risk screening. Environmental toxicology and chemistry 20:928-939

Hertwich EG, Jolliet O, Pennington DW, Hauschild M, Schulze C, Krewitt W, Huijbregts MAJ (2002) Fate and exposure assessment in the Life Cycle Impact Assessment of Toxic Chemicals. In: Udo de Haes HA, Finnveden G, Goedkoop M, Hauschild M, Hertwich EG, Hofstetter P, Jolliet O, Klöpffer W, Krewitt W, Lindeijer E, Müller-Wenk R, Olsen SI, Pennigton DW, Potting J and Steen B (eds) Life-cycle impact assessment: striving towards best practice. Society of Environmental Toxicology and Chemistry (SETAC), Pensacola, Florida, pp 101-122

Hettelingh J-P, Slootweg J, Posch M, Dutchak S, I.Ilyin (2002) Preliminary Modelling and Mapping of Critical Loads for Cadmium and Lead. Corrdination Center for Effects (CCE) at the National Institute of Public Health and the Environment (RIVM) and EMEP-Meteorological Synthesizing Centre - East, Bilthoven, the Netherlands

Hoffman FO, Hammonds JS (1994) Propagation of uncertainty in risk assessments: the need to distinguish between uncertainty due to lack of knowledge and uncertainty due to variability. Risk Analysis 14:707-712

Hofstetter P (1998) Perspectives in life cycle impact assessment: a structured approach to combine models of the technosphere, ecosphere, and valuesphere. Kluwer Academic Publishers, Boston

Hofstetter P, Hammitt JK (2001) Human Health Metrics for Environmental Decision Support Tools: Lessons from Health Economics and Decision Analysis. U.S.Environmental Protection Agency, Office of Research and Development, National Risk Management Research Laboratory, Cincinnati, Ohio, pp 59

Hohl R (1985) Die Entwickungsgeschichte der Erde. Verlag für Kunst und Wissenschaft, Leipzig, pp 703

Hoosbeek MR, Bryant RB (1992) Towards the quantitative modeling of pedogenesis - a review. Geoderma 55:183-210

Hopke PK, Borak TB, Doull J, Cleaver JE, Eckerman KF, Gundersen LCS, Harley NH, Hess CT, Kinner NE, Kopecky KJ, McKone TE, Sextro RG, Simon SL (2000) Health Risks Due to Radon in Drinking Water. Environmental Science & Technology 34:921-926

Horstmann M, McLachlan MS (1998) Atmospheric deposition of semivolatile organic compounds to two forest canopies. Atmospheric environment 32:1799-1809

Huijbregts MAJ (1999) Priority Assessment of Toxic Substances in the frame of LCA - Development and application of the multi-media fate, exposure and effect model USES-LCA. Interfaculty Department of Environmental Science, Faculty of Environmental Sciences, University of Amsterdam, Amsterdam

Huijbregts MAJ (2000) Priority Assessment of Toxic Substances in the frame of LCA - Time horizon dependency in toxicity potentials calculated with the multi-media fate, exposure and effects model USES-LCA. Institute of Biodiversity and Ecosystem Dynamics, University of Amsterdam, Amsterdam

Huijbregts MAJ, Thissen U, Jager T, van de Meent D, Ragas AMJ (2000a) Priority assessment of toxic substances in life cycle assessment. Part II: assessing parameter uncertainty and human variability in the calculation of toxicity potentials. Chemosphere 41:575-588

Huijbregts MAJ, Thissen U, Guinée JB, Jager T, Kalf D, van de Meent D, Ragas AMJ, Wegener Sleeswijk A, Reijnders L (2000b) Priority assessment of toxic substances in life cycle assessment. Part I: Calculation of toxicity potentials for 181 substances with the nested multi-media fate, exposure and effects model USES-LCA. Chemosphere 41:541-573

Huijbregts MAJ, Guinée JB, Reijnders L (2001) Priority assessment of toxic substances in life cycle assessment. Part III: Export of potential impact over time and space. Chemosphere 44:59-65

Huijbregts MAJ, Lundi S, McKone TE, van de Meent D (2003) Geographical scenario uncertainty in generic fate and exposure factors of toxic pollutants for life-cycle impact assessment. Chemosphere 51:501-508

Hunsaker CT, Graham RL, Glenn WSI, O'Neill RV, Barnthouse LW, Gardner RH (1990) Assessing ecological risk on a regional scale. Environmental management 14:325-332

Hunt A (2001) Monetary valuation of noise effects. Draft Final Report prepared for the EC UNITE Project, subcontracted to IER, Germany. Metroeconomica Ltd., Bath (UK), pp 27

Hunt A, Markandya A (2001) Chapter 8 - Economic valuation, sustainability indicators and alternative assessment techniques. In: Friedrich R and Bickel P (eds) Environmental External Costs of Transport. Springer-Verlag, Berlin Heidelberg New York, pp 87-120

Hurley F, Miller B (2001) Chapter 5 - Health Effects: Exposure-Response Functions. In: Friedrich R and Bickel P (eds) Environmental External Costs of Transport. Springer-Verlag, Berlin Heidelberg New York, pp 35-58

Hurley F, Miller B (2004) Life tables for different discount rates: Summary description of Methods and Results (Draft). Institute for Occupational Medicine (IOM), Edinburgh, pp 6

Ilyin I, Ryaboshapko A, Afinogenova O, Berg T, Hjellbrekke A-G (2001) Evaluation of transboundary transport of heavy metals in 1999. Trend analysis. Meteorological Synthesizing Centre - East, Chemical Co-ordinating Centre, Moscow, Russia

International Atomic Energy Agency (1989) Evaluating the reliability of predictions using environmental transfer models. International Atomic Energy Agency (IAEA), Vienna

International Atomic Energy Agency (2001) Generic models for use in assessing the impact of discharges of radioactive substances to the environment. International Atomic Energy Agency (IAEA), Vienna

International Council of Chemical Associations (1998) Position on Persistent Organic Pollutants (POPs)

International Programme on Chemical Safety (1999) Principles for the Assessment of Risks to Human Health from Exposure to Chemicals. Environmental Health Criteria 210

Irwin RJ, van Mouwerik M, Stevens L, Seese MD, Basham W (1998) Environmental Contaminants Encyclopedia: Chromium VI (hexavalent chromium) entry. National Park Service, Water Resources Division, Fort Collins, Colorado, pp 43

Ivens W, Tank AK, Kauppi P, Alcamo J (1989) Atmospheric deposition of sulphur, nitrogen and basic cations onto European forests: observations and model calculations. In: Kämäri J, Brakke DF, Jenkins A, Norton SA and Wright RF (eds) Regional Acidification Models. Springer, Berlin, pp 103-111

Jaenicke R (1998) Atmospheric aerosol size distribution. In: Harrison RM and van Grieken R (eds) Atmospheric particles. John Wiley & Sons, Chichester IUPAC series on analytical and physical chemistry of environmental systems, vol 5, pp 1-28

Jarvis NJ, Villholth KG, Ulén B (1999) Modelling particle mobilization and leaching in macroporous soil. European Journal of Soil Science 50:621-632

Jenne EA (1998a) Adsorption of metals by geomedia: data analysis, modeling, controlling factors, and related issues. In: Jenne EA (ed) Adsorption of metals by geomedia: variables, mechanisms, and model applications. Academic Press, San Diego, pp 1-73

Jenne EA (1998b) Adsorption of metals by geomedia: variables, mechanisms, and model applications. Academic Press, San Diego, pp 583

Joint Research Centre of the European Commission (2003) Integrated Pollution Prevention and Control (IPPC): Draft Reference Document on Best Available Techniques for Large Combustion Plants. Institute for Prospective Technological Studies, Joint Research Centre of the European Commission, Seville, Spain, pp 539

Jolliet O, Margni M, Charles R, Humbert S, Payet J, Rebitzer G, Rosenbaum R (2003) IMPACT 2002+: A New Life Cycle Impact Assessment Methodology. The International Journal of Life Cycle Assessment 8:324-330

Jonas R, Heinemann K (1985) Studies on the dry deposition of aerosol particles on vegetation and plane surfaces. Journal of Aerosol Science 16:463-471

Jørgensen SE, Bendoricchio G (2001) Fundamentals of Ecological Modelling. Elsevier, Amsterdam

Jury WA, Russo D, Streile G, El Abd H (1990) Evaluation of volatilization by organic chemicals residing below the soil surface. Water resources research 26:13-20

Kabata-Pendias A, Pendias H (1992) Trace elements in soils and plants, 2 edn. CRC Pr., Boca Raton

Kabata-Pendias A, Pendias H (2001) Trace elements in soils and plants, 3 edn. CRC Pr., Boca Raton

Karimi-Lotfabad S, Pickard MA, Gray MR (1998) Fate and Stability of Nonextractable Residues of [14 C]PAH in Contaminated Soils under Environmental Stress Conditions. Environmental Science & Technology 30:1145 -1151

Kaupp H, Towara J, McLachlan MS (1994) Distribution of polychlorinated dibenzo-p -dioxins and dibenzofurans in atmospheric particulate matter with respect to particle size. Atmospheric environment 28:585-593

Keller S-P (2005) Assessing Human Effect Factors for Cancer in Life Cycle Impact Assessment (LCIA). Diploma thesis. Laboratory of Ecosystem Management. Ecole Polytechnique Fédérale de Lausanne (EPFL), Switzerland, Lausanne, pp 30

Kirkby MJ, Imeson AC, Bergkamp G, Cammeraat LH (1996) Scaling up processes and models from the field plot to the watershed and regional areas. Journal of soil and water conservation 51:391-396

Kleeberg H-B (1992) Diskussionsergebnisse. In: Kleeberg H-B (ed) Regionalisierung in der Hydrologie. VCH, Weinheim Mitteilung der Senatskommission für Wasserforschung, pp 419-429

Klepper O, den Hollander HA (1999) A comparison of spatially explicit and box models for the fate of chemicals in water, air and soil in Europe. Ecological Modelling 116:183-202

Korte F (1992) Lehrbuch der Ökologischen Chemie - Grundlagen und Konzepte für die ökologische Beurteilung von Chemikalien. Georg-Thieme, Stuttgart

Korzun VI, Sokolov AA, Bodyko MI (1974) Atlas of the world water balance (in Russian). Gidrometeorologiceskoe izdatel stvo, Moscow, Leningrad

Krewitt W, Mayerhofer P, Trukenmüller A, Friedrich R (1998) Application of the Impact Pathway Analysis in the Context of LCA. The International Journal of Life Cycle Assessment 3:86-94

Krewitt W, Trukenmüller A, Bachmann TM, Heck T (2001) Country-specific Damage Factors for Air Pollutants: A Step Towards Site Dependent Life Cycle Impact Assessment. The International Journal of Life Cycle Assessment 6:199-210

Krewitt W, Pennington DW, Olsen SI, Crettaz P, Jolliet O (2002) Indicators for human toxicity in Life-Cycle Impact Assessment. In: Udo de Haes HA, Finnveden G, Goedkoop M, Hauschild M, Hertwich EG, Hofstetter P, Jolliet O, Klöpffer W, Krewitt W, Lindeijer E, Müller-Wenk R, Olsen SI, Pennigton DW, Potting J and Steen B (eds) Life-cycle impact assessment: striving towards best practice. Society of Environmental Toxicology and Chemistry (SETAC), Pensacola, Florida, pp 123-148

Kroes R (1996) Toxicity testing and human health. In: van Leeuwen CJ and Hermens JLM (eds) Risk Assessment of Chemicals: An Introduction. Kluwer Acad. Publ., Dordrecht, pp 147-174

Länderarbeitsgemeinschaft Wasser (LAWA) (1993) Richtlinie für die Gebietsbezeichnung und die Verschlüsselung von Fließgewässern

Lasaga AC (1995) Fundamental approaches in describing mineral dissolution and precipitation rates. In: White AF and Brantley SL (eds) Chemical weathering rates of silicate minerals. Mineralogical Society of America, Washington, DC Reviews in mineralogy, vol 31, pp 12-86

Lee DS (2003) Personal communication on parameters for heavy metals and organics. Manchester Metropolitan University, Manchester

Lehner B, Döll P (2001) A global wetlands, lakes and reservoirs data set. Center for Environmental Systems Research, University of Kassel, Germany, Kassel

Leip A, Lammel G (2004) Indicators for persistence and long-range transport potential as derived from multicompartment chemistry-transport modelling. Environmental Pollution 128:205-221

Léonhard A (1991) Arsenic. In: Merian E (ed) Metals and their compounds in the environment: occurrence, analysis, and biological, relevance. VCH, Weinheim, pp 751-774

Lick W, McNeil J (2001) Effects of sediment bulk properties on erosion rates. The Science of the Total Environment 266:41-48

Lide DR (2002) CRC handbook of chemistry and physics: a ready-reference book of chemical and physical data, 83 edn. CRC Press, Boca Raton

Linares Llamas P (2003) Biodiversity. In: European Commission (ed) An applied integrated environmental impact assessment framework for the European Union (GREENSENSE). European Commission, DG Research, EESD, Brussels

Lindberg SE (1989) Behavior of Cd, Mn, and Pb in forest-canopy throughfall. In: Pacyna JM and Ottar B (eds) Control and fate of atmospheric trace metals. Proceedings of the NATO Advanced Research Workshop on Fate and Control of Toxic Metals in the Atmosphere 12-16 September 1988. Kluwer, Dordrecht NATO advanced study institutes series: C, vol 268, pp 233-257

Lindqvist O, Rodhe H (1985) Atmospheric Mercury - a review. Tellus 37B:136-159

Lopez AD, Salomon JA, Ahmad OB, Murray CJL, Mafat D (2001a) Life Tables for 191 Countries: Data, Methods, Results. World Health Organization

Lopez AD, Ahmad OB, Guillot M, Inoue M, Ferguson BD, Salomon JA (2001b) Life Tables for 191 Countries for 2000: Data, Methods, Results. Harvard Burden of Disease Unit, Cambrigde

Lovett GM, Reiners WA, Olson RK (1982) Cloud Droplet Deposition in Subalpine Balsam Fir Forests: Hydrological and Chemical Inputs. SCIENCE 218:1303-1304

Lumsdon DG, Evans LJ (1995) Predicting chemical speciation and computer simulation. In: Ure AM and Davidson CM (eds) Chemical speciation in the environment. Blackie Academic & Professional, London, pp 86-134

Luthy RG, Aiken GR, Brusseau ML, Cunningham SD, Gschwend PM, Pignatello JJ, Reinhard M, Traina SJ, Weber (Jr.) WJ, Westall JC (1997) Sequestration of Hydrophobic Organic Contaminants by Geosorbents. Environmental Science & Technology 31:3341-3347

Luxmoore RJ (1991) On preferential flow and its measurement. In: Gish TJ and Shirmohammadi A (eds) Preferential flow. Proceedings of the national symposium held at Chicago, Illinois 16-17 December 1991. American Society of Agricultural Engineers, St. Joseph, Michigan, pp 113-121

Mackay D (1979) Finding fugacity feasible. Environmental Science & Technolology 13:1218-1223

Mackay D (1985) Air/water exchange coefficients. In: Neely WB and Blau GE (eds) Environmental exposure from chemicals. Volume I. CRC Press, Boca Raton, Florida, pp 91-108

Mackay D (1991) Multimedia Environmental Models: The Fugacity Approach. Lewis Publishers, Chelsea, Michigan

Mackay D (2001) Multimedia Environmental Models: The Fugacity Approach, 2 edn. Lewis Publishers, Boca Raton

Mackay D, Diamond M (1989) Application of the QWASI (quantitative water air sediment interaction) fugacity model to the dynamics of organic and inorganic chemicals in lakes. Chemosphere 18:1343-1365

Mackay D, Southwood JM (1992) Modelling the Fate of Organochlorine Chemicals in Pulp Mill Effluents. Water Pollution Research Journal of Canada 27:509-537

Mackay D, Hickie B (2000) Mass balance model of source apportionment, transport and fate of PAHs in Lac Saint Louis, Quebec. Chemosphere 41:681-692

Mackay D, Paterson S, Shiu WY (1992) Generic Models for Evaluating the Regional Fate of Chemicals. Chemosphere 24:695-717

Mackay D, di Guardo A, Paterson S, Cowan E (1996a) Evaluating the environmental fate of a variety of types of chemicals using the EQC model. Environmental toxicology and chemistry 15:1627-1637

Mackay D, di Guardo A, Paterson S, Kicsi G, Cowan E (1996b) Assessing the Fate of New and Exisiting Chemicals: A Five-stage Process. Environmental toxicology and chemistry 15:1618-1626

MacLeod M (2002) Personal communication on the BETR North-America model. Lawrence Berkeley National Laboratory, Berkeley

MacLeod M, Woodfine DG, Mackay D, McKone TE, Bennett DH, Maddalena R (2001) BETR North America: A regionally segmented multimedia contaminant fate model for North America. Environmental Science & Pollution Research 8:156-163

MacLeod M, Bennett DH, Perem M, Maddalena RL, McKone TE, Mackay D (2004) Dependence of intake fraction on release location in a multi-media framework: A case study of four contaminants in North America. Journal of Industrial Ecology 8:89-102

Maddalena R, Bennett DH, McKone TE, Lyon BF, Efroymson RA, Jones DS, Eyth A, Lee M, McVey ME, Burch D, Cleland J, Jones B (2002) Evaluation of TRIM.FaTE. Volume I: Approach and Initial Findings. Office of Air Quality, Planning and Standards, Research Triangle Park, NC

Margni M (2002) Personal communication on feedback fractions. École Polytechnique Fédéral de Lausanne, Lausanne

Margni M (2003) Source to Intake Modeling in Life Cycle Impact Assessment Section Science et Ingénierie de l'Environnement. Swiss Federal Institute of Technology (EPFL), Lausanne, pp. 138 p

Margni M, Pennington DW, Bennett DH, Jolliet O (2004) Cyclic Exchanges and Level of Coupling between Environmental Media: Intermedia Feedback in Multimedia Fate Models. Environmental Science & Technology 38:5450 - 5457

Markandya A, Hunt A, Ortiz RA, Desaigues B, Bounmy K, Ami D, Masson S, Rabl A, Santoni L, Salomon M-A, Alberini A, Scarpa R, Krupnick A (2004) Mortality Risk Valuation. Draft final report prepared for the EC NewExt Project. University of Bath and others, Bath and others, pp 101

Märker B, Urhahn T, Ballschmiter K (2000) Regionale Verteilungsmodelle für Chemikalien im Vergleich. Akademie für Technikfolgenabschätzung in Baden-Württemberg, Stuttgart, pp 118

Markert B (1998) Distribution and biogeochemistry of inorganic chemicals in the environment. In: Schüürmann G and Markert B (eds) Ecotoxicology: ecological fundamentals, chemical exposure, and biological effects. Wiley, New York, NY Environmental science and technology, pp 165-222

Martínez García MJ, Moreno-Grau S, Martínez García JJ, Moreno J, Bayo J, Guillén Pérez JJ, Moreno-Clavel J (1999) Distribution of the Metals Lead, Cadmium, Copper, and Zinc in the Top Soil of Cartagena, Spain. Water, Air, and Soil Pollution 131:329-347

Mason P (2002) Personal communication on the meaning of 'contingent' in 'contingent valuation'. University of Bath, Bath

McBride MB (1994) Environmental chemistry of soils. Oxford University Press, New York

McColl S, Hicks J, Craig L, Shortreed J (2000) Environmental health risk managment: a primer for Canadians. Institute for Risk Research, University of Waterloo, Waterloo, Ontario, Canada

McCutcheon SC, Martin JL, Barnwell (Jr.) TO (1993) Water quality. In: Maidment DR (ed) Handbook of hydrology. McGraw-Hill, New York, NY, pp 11.1-11.73

McKone TE (1993a) CalTOX, A Multimedia Total-Exposure Model for Hazardous-Wastes Sites, Part I: Executive Summary. Lawrence Livermore National Laboratory, Livermore, CA

McKone TE (1993b) CalTOX, A Multimedia Total-Exposure Model for Hazardous-Wastes Sites, Part II: The Dynamic Multimedia Transport and Transformation Model. Lawrence Livermore National Laboratory, Livermore, CA

McKone TE (2003) Personal communication on CalTOX scientific documentation. Lawrence Berkeley National Laboratory, Berkeley

McKone TE, Ryan PB (1989) Human exposures to chemicals through the food chains: an uncertainty analysis. Environmental Science & Technology 23:1154-1163

McKone TE, Hertwich EG (2001) The Human Toxicity Potential and a Strategy for Evaluating Model Performance in Life Cycle Impact Assessment. The International Journal of Life Cycle Assessment 6:106-109

McKone TE, Enoch KG (2002) CalTOX, A Multimedia Total-Exposure Model Spreadsheet User's Guide Version 4.0 (Beta). Ernest Orlando Lawrence Berkeley National Laboratory, Berkeley, CA

McKone TE, Bennett DH (2003) Chemical-Specific Representation of Air-Soil Exchange and Soil Penetration in Regional Multimedia Models. Environmental Science & Technology 37:3123-3132

McLachlan MS (1994) Model of the fate of hydrophobic contaminants in cows. Environmental Science & Technology 28:2407-2414

McLachlan MS (1996) Bioaccumulation of hydrophobic chemicals in agricultural food chains. Environmental Science & Technology 30:252-259

McLachlan MS (1997) A simple model to predict accumulation of PCDD/Fs in an agricultural food chain. Chemosphere 34:1263-1276

McLachlan MS, Horstmann M (1998) Forests as Filters of Airborne Organic Pollutants: A Model. Environmental Science & Technology 32:413-420

McLachlan MS, Horstmann M, Hinkel M (1996) Polychlorinated dibenzo-p -dioxins and dibenzofurans in sewage sludge: sources and fate following sludge application to land. The Science of the Total Environment 185:109-123

McLachlan MS, Czub G, Wania F (2002) The Influence of Vertical Sorbed Phase Transport on the Fate of Organic Chemicals in Surface Soils. Environmental Science & Technology 36:4860-4867

Mehra RK, Tripathi RD (2000) Phytochelatins and Metal Tolerance. In: Agrawal SB and Agrawal M (eds) Environmental Pollution and Plant Responses. Lewis Publ., Boca Raton, Fla., pp 367-382

Mekel OCL, Fehr R (2000) Probabilistische Expositionsabschätzung (Teil III): Berücksichtigung von Variabilität und Unsicherheit in quantitativen Risikoabschätzungen (QRA). Umweltwissenschaften und Schadstoff - Forschung 12:42-50

Menz (2004) Personal communication on the composition of fodder in Germany. Zentrale Markt- und Preisberichtstelle für Erzeugnisse der Land-, Forst- und Ernährungswirtschaft (ZMP), Bonn

Mersch-Sundermann V (1996) Wirkungen von Kohlenwasserstoffen in Säugetieren - zwischen Spekulation und Erkenntnis. In: Straub H-P (ed) Belastung von Säugetieren mit Umweltschadstoffen: Analytik, Ergebnisse und Konsequenzen. Landesanstalt für Umweltschutz Baden-Württemberg, Karlsruhe Ökologisches Wirkungskataster Baden-Württemberg 1, pp 65-78

Mileson B, Faustman E, Olin S, Ryan PB, Ferenc S, Burke T (1999) A Framework for Cumulative Risk Assessment. In: Cumulative Risk Assessment workshop. International Life Sciences Institute, pp 55

Miller BG (2001) Annex 1 - Life-table methods for predicting and quantifying long-term impacts on mortality. In: World Health Organization (ed) Quantification of the Health Effects of Exposure to Air Pollution. Report of a WHO Working Group (meeting at Bilthoven, Netherlands the 20-22 November 2000). WHO Regional Office for Europe, Copenhagen, pp 20-28

Milliman JD, Meade RH (1983) World-wide delivery of river sediment to the oceans. The Journal of Geology 91:1-21

Milliman JD, Syvitski JPM (1992) Geomorphic/tectonic control of sediment discharge to the ocean: the importance of small mountainous rivers. The Journal of Geology 100:525-54

Moore ID, Turner AK, Wilson JP, Jenson SK, Band LE (1993) GIS and land-surface-subsurface process modeling. In: Goodchild MF, Parks BO and Steyaert LT (eds) Environmental modeling with GIS. Oxford University Press, New York, pp 196-230

Morel FMM, Hering JG (1993) Principles and applications of aquatic chemistry. Wiley, New York

Morgan JJ, Stumm W (1991) Chemical Processes in the Environment, Relevance of Chemical Speciation. In: Merian E (ed) Metals and their compounds in the environment: occurrence, analysis, and biological, relevance. VCH, Weinheim, pp 67-103

Morgan MG, Henrion M (1990) Uncertainty: a guide to dealing with uncertainty in quantitative risk and policy analysis. Cambridge Univ. Press, Cambridge

Morgan RPC (1999) Soil erosion and conservation (German translation). Enke, Stuttgart

Mosbaek H, Tjell JC, Hovmand MF (1989) Atmospheric lead input to agricultural crops in Denmark. Chemosphere 19:1787-1799

Mosley MP, McKerchar AI (1993) Streamflow. In: Maidment DR (ed) Handbook of hydrology. McGraw-Hill, New York, NY, pp 8.1-8.39

Mücke W (6/1995) Chemische Stoffe in der Umwelt - Praktische Anwendung toxikologischer Erkenntnisse im Umwelthygienerecht. In: Vogl J (ed) Handbuch des Umweltschutzes. Ecomed, Landsberg am Lech

Mulkey LA, Donigian (Jr.) AS, Allison TL, Raju CS (1993) Evaluation of Source Term Initial Conditions for Modeling Leachate Migration from Landfills. U.S. Environmental Protection Agency, Environmental Research Laboratory, Athens, Georgia

Müller-Wenk R, Hofstetter P (2003) Monetarisierung verkehrslärmbedingter Gesundheitsschäden. Bundesamt für Umwelt, Wald und Landschaft, Bern, pp 93

Muñoz O, Vélez D, Montoro R (1999) Optimization of the solubilization, extraction and determination of inorganic arsenic [As(III) + As(V)] in seafood products by acid digestion, solvent extraction and hydride generation atomic absorption spectrometry. The Analyst 124:601-607

Munthe J, Palm A (2003) MEPOP - Atmospheric Cycling of Mercury and Persistent Organic Pollutants. EUROTRAC-2 Subproject Final Report. International Scientific Secretariat (ISS), GSF - National Research Center for Environment and Health, Munich, Germany, pp 102

Murray CJL (1994) Quantifying the burden of disease: the technical basis for disability-adjusted life years. Bulletin of the World Health Organization 72:429-445

Murray CJL, Lopez AD (1996a) The global burden of disease: a comprehensive assessment of mortality and disability from diseases, injuries, and risk factors in 1990 and projected to 2020. World Health Organization, Harvard School of Public Health, Cambridge, Massachusettes

Murray CJL, Lopez AD (1996b) Global health statistics: a compendium of incidence, prevalence, and mortality estimates for over 200 conditions. Harvard University on behalf of the World Health Organization and the World Bank, Cambridge, Massachusettes

Murray CJL, Lopez AD, Jamison DT (1994) The global burden of disease in 1990: summary results, sensitivity analysis and future directions. Bulletin of the World Health Organization 72:495-509

Neal C, Robson AJ, Christophersen N (1997) Towards coupling hydrological, soil and weathering processes within a modelling perspective. In: Saether OM and de Caritat P (eds) Geochemical processes, weathering and groundwater recharge in catchments. Balkema, Rotterdam, pp 329-380

New M, Hulme M, Jones P (1999) Representing Twentieth-Century Space-Time Climate Variability. Part I: Development of a 1961-90 Mean Monthly Terrestrial Climatology. Journal of Climate 12:829-856

Nicholas AP, Walling DE (1996) The significance of particle aggregation in the overbank deposition of suspended sediment on river floodplains. Journal of Hydrology 186:275-293

Nichols P, Hauschild M, Potting J, White P (1996) Part V: Impact assessment of non toxic pollution in life cycle assessment. In: Udo de Haes HA (ed) Towards a methodology for life cycle impact assessment. Society of Environmental Toxicology and Chemistry - Europe, Brussels, pp 63-73

Nigge K-M (2000) Life Cycle Assessment of natural gas vehicles - Development and application of site-dependent impact indicators. Springer, Berlin

Nigge K-M (2001) Generic Spatial Classes for Human Health Impacts. Part I: Methodology. The International Journal of Life Cycle Assessment 6:257-264

Noack AG, Grant CD, Chittleborough DJ (2000) Colloid Movement through Stable Soils of Low Cation-Exchange Capacity. Environmental Science & Technology 34:2490-2497

Nord E (2002) My goodness - and yours: a history, and some possible futures, of DALY meanings and valuation procedures. In: Murray CJL, Salomon JA, Mathers CD and Lopez AD (eds) Summary measures of population health: concepts, ethics, measurement and applications. World Health Organisation, Geneva, pp 139-146

Norgaard RB, Howarth RB (1991) Sustainability and discounting the future. In: Costanza R (ed) Ecological economics: the science and management of sustainability. Columbia University Press, New York, pp 88-101

North Atlantic Treaty Organization/Committee on the Challenges of Modern Society (1988) International toxicity equivalency factors (I-TEF) method of risk assessment for complex mixtures of dioxins and related compounds. North Atlantic Treaty Organization, Brussels

Nriagu JO (1978) Lead in soils, sediments and major rock types. In: Nriagu JO (ed) The biogeochemistry of lead in the environment. Elsevier/North-Holland Biomedical Press, Amsterdam, Netherlands Topis in environmental health, vol 1A, pp 15-72

Nriagu JO (1989) A global assessment of natural sources of atmospheric trace metals. Nature 338:47-49

Oh J-E, Choi J-S, Chang Y-S (2001) Gas/particle partitioning of polychlorinated dibenzo-p -dioxins and dibenzofurans in atmosphere; evaluation of predicting models. Atmospheric environment 35:4125-4134

Olivie-Lauquet G, Gruau G, Dia A, Riou C, Jaffrezic A, Henin O (2001) Release of Trace Elements in Wetlands: Role of Seasonal Variability. Water Research 35:943-952

Olsen SI, Møller Christensen F, Hauschild M, Pedersen F, Larsen HF, Tørsløv J (2001) Life cycle impact assessment and risk assessment of chemicals - a methodological comparison. Environmental Impact Assessment Review 21:385-404

Olson BH, Panigrahi AK (1991) Bacteria, fungi, and blue-green algae. In: Merian E (ed) Metals and their compounds in the environment: occurrence, analysis, and biological, relevance. VCH, Weinheim, pp 419-448

Oreskes N, Shrader-Frechette K, Belitz K (1994) Verification, Validation, and Confirmation of Numerical Models in the Earth Sciences. Science 263

Organisation for Economic Co-operation and Development (1999) Environmental Exposure Assessment Strategies for Existing Industrial Chemicals in OECD Memeber Countries. Environment Directorate of the OECD, Paris

Otto WH, Carper WR, Larive CK (2001) Measurement of Cadmium(II) and Calcium(II) Complexation by Fulvic Acids Using ^{113}Cd NMR. Environmental Science & Technology 35:1463-1468

Owens JW (1997a) Life-Cycle Assessment: Constraints on Moving from Inventory to Impact Assessment. Journal of Industrial Ecology 1:37-49

Owens JW (1997b) Life-Cycle assessment in relation to risk assessment: an evolving perspective. Risk analysis 17:359-365

Owens JW (2001) Chemical toxicity indicators for human health: Case study for classification of chronic non-cancer chemical hazards in life cycle assessment. Environmental toxicology and chemistry 21:207-225

Pacyna JM (1987) Atmospheric emissions of arsenic, cadmium, lead and mercury from high temperature processes in power generation and industry. In: Hutchinson TC and Meema KM (eds) Lead, mercury, cadmium and arsenic in the environment. Wiley, Chichester SCOPE 31, pp 69-87

Parliament and Council of the European Union (2000) Directive 2000/60/EC of the European Parliament and of the Council of 23 October 2000 establishing a framework for Community action in the field of water policy. Official Journal of the European Communities L 327:0001-0073

Paterson S, Mackay D, Mc Farlane C (1994) A Model of Organic Chemical Uptake by Plants from Soil and the Atmosphere. Environmental Science & Technolology 28:2259-2266

Pearce DW, Turner RK (1990) Economics of natural resources and the environment. The Johns Hopkins University Press, Baltimore

Pearce DW, Moran D (2001) The value of biological diversity. Organisation for Economic Co-operation and Development, Paris

Pekar M, Pavlova N, Gusev A, Shatalov V, Vulikh N, Ioannisian D, Dutchak S, Berg T, Hjellbrekke A-G (1999) Long-Range Transport of Selected Persistent Organic Pollutants - Development of Transport Models for Polychlorinated Biphenyls, Benzo[a]pyrene, Dioxins/Furans and Lindane. Meteorological Synthesizing Centre - East, Moscow, Russia

Pelichet T (2003) Development of a spatial multimedia chemical fate and human exposure model for Europe, with a focus on air advection Laboratory of Ecosystem Management. Ecole Polytechnique Fédérale de Lausanne (EPFL), Switzerland, Lausanne, pp 75

Pennington DW, Crettaz P, Tauxe A, Rhomberg L, Brand K, Jolliet O (2002) Assessing Human Health in Life Cycle Assessment using ED10 s and DALYs: Part 2 - Noncancer effects. Risk Analysis 22:947-963

Pennington DW, Margni M, Ammann C, Jolliet O (2005) Multimedia Fate and Human Intake Modeling: Spatial versus Nonspatial Insights for Chemical Emissions in Western Europe. Environmental Science and Technology 39:1119-1128

Peterson PJ, Alloway BJ (1979) Cadmium in soils and vegetation. In: Webb M (ed) The chemistry, biochemistry, and biology of cadmium. Elsevier/ North-Holland Biomedical Press, Amsterdam, Netherlands Topis in environmental health, vol 2, pp 45-92

Pope CA, Thun MJ, Namboodri MM, et al. (1995) Particulate air pollution as a predictor of mortality in a prospective study of US adults. Am. J. Resp. Critical Care Med. 151:669-674

Popper KR (1968) The logic of scientific discovery, 4 edn. Hutchinson, London

Potting J, Hauschild M (1997) Predicted Environmental Impact and Expected Occurence of Actual Environmental Impact - Part II: Spatial Differentiation in Life-Cycle Assessment via the Site-Dependent Characterisation of Environmental Impact from Emissions. The International Journal of Life Cycle Assessment 2:209-216

Potting J, Schöpp W, Blok K, Hauschild M (1998) Site-dependent life-cycle impact assessment of acidification. Journal of Industrial Ecology 2:63-87

Powell JC, Pearce DW, Craighill AL (1997) Approaches to valuation in LCA impact assessment. The International Journal of Life Cycle Assessment 2:11-15

Prevedouros K, MacLeod M, Jones KC, Sweetman AJ (2004) Modelling the fate of persistent organic pollutants in Europe: parameterisation of a gridded distribution model. Environmental Pollution 128:251-261

Price PS, Shu SH, Harringto JR, Keenan RE (1996) Uncertainty and Variation in Indirect Exposure assessments: An Analysis of Exposure to Tetrachlorodibenzo-*p*-dioxin from a Beef Consumption Pathway. Risk Analysis 16:263-277

Purohit V, Basu AK (2000) Mutagenicity of Nitroaromatic Compounds. Chemical Research in Toxicology 13

Puxbaum H (1991) Metal compounds in the atmosphere. In: Merian E (ed) Metals and their compounds in the environment: occurrence, analysis, and biological, relevance. VCH, Weinheim, pp 257-286

Rabl A (1996) Discounting of Long Term Costs: What Would Future Generations Prefer Us to Do? Ecological Economics 17:137-145

Rabl A, Spadaro JV (1999) Damages and costs of air pollution: an analysis of uncertainties. Environment International 25:29-46

Rabl A, Spadaro JV, McGavran PD (1998) Health risks of air pollution from incinerators: a perspective. Waste Management & Research 16:365-388

Ragas AMJ, Etienne RS, Willemsen FH, van de Meent D (1999) Assessing model uncertainty for environmental decision making: a case study of the coherence of independently derived environmental quality objectives for air and water. Environmental toxicology and chemistry 18:186-1867

Rantio T, Paasivirta J (1996) Modelled and observed fate of chlorocymenes. Chemosphere 33:453-466

Rat von Sachverständigen für Umweltfragen (2004) Sondergutachten "Meeresumweltschutz für Nord- und Ostsee". Rat von Sachverständigen für Umweltfragen (SRU), Berlin, pp 462

Rawls WJ, Ahuja LR, Brakensiek DL, Shirmohammadi A (1993) Infiltration and soil water movement. In: Maidment DR (ed) Handbook of hydrology. McGraw-Hill, New York, NY, pp 5.1-5.51

Rea AW, Lindberg SE, Keeler GJ (2001) Dry deposition and foliar leaching of mercury and selected trace elements in deciduous forest throughfall. Atmospheric environment 35:3453-3462

Reimann C, de Caritat P (1998) Chemical elements in the environment: factsheets for the geochemist and environmental scientist. Springer-Verlag, Berlin

Reimann C, Siewers U, Tarvainen T, Bityukova L, Eriksson J, Gilucis A, Gregorauskiene V, Lukashev V, Matinian NN, Pasieczna A (2000) Baltic soil survey: total concentrations of major and selected trace elements in arable soils from ten countries around the Baltic Sea. The Science of the Total Environment 257:155-170

Reimann C, Siewers U, Tarvainen T, Bityukova L, Eriksson J, Gilucis A, Gregorauskiene V, Lukashev VK, Matinian NN, Pasieczna A (2003) Agricultural soils in Northern Europe: a geochemical atlas. Schweizerbart, Stuttgart

Reinds GJ, Bril J, de Vries W, Groenenberg JE, Breeuwsma A (1995) Critical loads and excess loads of cadmium, copper and lead for European forest soils. DLO Winand Staring Centre & Haren (Gr.) DLO Institute for Agrobiological and Soil Fertility Research, Wageningen, The Netherlands, pp 91

Renard KG, Foster GR, Weesies GA, McCool DK, Yoder DC (1997) Predicting soil erosion by water: a guide to conservation planning with the revised universal soil loss equation (RUSLE). Agricultural Research Service, Washington, D. C.

Rennings K (1994) Indikatoren für eine dauerhaft-umweltgerechte Entwicklung. Metzler-Poeschel, Stuttgart

Rennings K (1997) Ökonomische Bewertung von externen Effekten der Stromerzeugung. In: Friedrich R and Krewitt W (eds) Umwelt- und Gesundheitsschäden durch die Stromerzeugung. Springer, Berlin, pp 37-67

Rentz O, Martel C (1998) Analyse der Schwermetallströme in Steinkohlefeuerungen - Einfluß der Kohlesorte und des Lastzustandes. Deutsch-Französisches Institut für Umweltforschung (DFIU) der Universität Karlsruhe (TH), Karlsruhe, pp 254

Richards D, Rowe WD (1999) Decision-making with heterogeneous sources of information. Risk Analysis 19:69-81

Richter O, Diekkrüger B, Nörtersheuser P (1996) Environmental Fate Modelling of Pesticides. VCH, Weinheim

Rickard DT, Nriagu JO (1978) Aqueous environmental chemistry of lead. In: Nriagu JO (ed) The biogeochemistry of lead in the environment. Elsevier/ North-Holland Biomedical Press, Amsterdam, Netherlands Topis in environmental health, vol 1A, pp 219-284

Riederer M (1995) Partitioning and transport of organic chemicals between the atmospheric environment and leaves. In: Trapp S and Mc Farlane JC (eds) Plant contamination: modeling and simulation of organic chemical processes. Lewis, Boca Raton, pp 153-190

Ritchie GSP, Sposito G (1995) Speciation in soils. In: Ure AM and Davidson CM (eds) Chemical speciation in the environment. Blackie Academic & Professional, London, pp 201-233

Robarge WP (1999) Precipitation/Dissolution Reactions in Soils. In: Sparks DL (ed) Soil physical chemistry. CRC Press, Boca Raton, Fla., pp 193-238

Robinson S (1999) Simulation Verification, Validation and Confidence: A Tutorial. TRANSACTIONS of the Society for Computer Simulation International 16:63-69

Rodhe A, Killingtveit Å (1997) Catchment hydrology. In: Saether OM and de Caritat P (eds) Geochemical processes, weathering and groundwater recharge in catchments. Balkema, Rotterdam, pp 77-107

Römbke J, Moltmann JF (1996) Applied ecotoxicology. Lewis Publ., Boca Raton

Rossetti di Valdalbero D (2004) Quantification and tentative internalisation of energy external costs in the European Union. In: International Conference on Probabilistic Safety Assessment and Management (PSAM) 7 - European Safety and Reliability Conference (ESREL) '04, Berlin, Germany. Springer, pp 2301-2307

Rowe WD (1994) Understanding uncertainty. Risk Analysis 14:743-750

Ryaboshapko A, Ilyin I, Gusev A, Afinogenova O (1998) Mercury in the atmosphere of Europe: concentrations, deposition patterns, transboundary fluxes. Meteorological Synthesizing Centre - East, Moscow, Russia

Rykiel (Jr.) EJ (1996) Testing ecological models: the meaning of validation. Ecological Modelling 90:229-244

Saltelli A (2000) What is sensitivity analysis? In: Saltelli A, Chan K and Scott EM (eds) Sensitivity analysis. John Wiley & Sons, Chichester Wiley series in probability and statistics, pp 3-13

Samara C, Voutsa D (2005) Size distribution of airborne particulate matter and associated heavy metals in the roadside environment. Chemosphere 59:1197-1206

Saouter E, van Hoof G, Feijtel TCJ, Owens JW (2002) The Effect of Compact Formulations on the Environmental Profile of Northern European Granular Laundry Detergents. Part II: Life Cycle Assessment. The International Journal of Life Cycle Assessment 7:27-38

Sargent RG (1984) Simulation model validation. In: Ören TI, Zeigler BP and Elzas MS (eds) Simulation and model based methodologies: an integrative view. Proceedings of the NATO Advanced Study Institute on Simulation and Model-Based Methodologies; an Integrative View, held at Ottawa, Ontario/Canada, July 26 - August 6, 1982. Springer, Berlin NATO ASI series: Series F, Computer and systems sciences; Vol 10

Sauerbeck D (1989) Der Transfer von Schwermetallen in die Pflanze. In: Behrens D and Wiesner J (eds) Beurteilung von Schwermetallkontaminationen im Boden. Dechema, Frankfurt, pp 281-316

Sauerbeck D, Lübben S (1991) Auswirkungen von Siedlungsabfällen auf Böden, Bodenorganismen und Pflanzen: BMFT Forschungsvorhaben 0339059 Berichte aus der ökologischen Forschung. Forschungszentrum Jülich - Zentralbibliothek, Jülich, vol 6, pp 416

Sauvé S (2002) Speciation of metals in soils. In: Allen HE (ed) Bioavailability of Metals in Terrestrial Ecosystems: Importance of Partitioning for Bioavailability to Invertebrates, Microbes and Plants. Society for Environmental Toxicology and Chemistry, Pensacola, Fla., pp 7-37

Sauvé S, Hendershot W, Allen HE (2000) Solid-Solution Partitioning of Metals in Contaminated Soils: Dependence on pH, Total Metal Burden, and Organic Matter. Environmental Science & Technology 34:1125-1131

Scheffer F, Schachtschabel P (1989) Textbook of soil science (in German), 12 edn. Enke, Stuttgart

Scheidleder A, Grath J, Winkler G, Stärk U, Koreimann C, Gmeiner C, Nixon S, Casillas J, Gravese P, Leonard J, Elvira M (1999) Groundwater quality and quantity in Europe. European Environment Agency, Copenhagen, pp 123

Schelling TC (2000) Intergenerational and international discounting. Risk Analysis 20:771-778

Scheringer M, Wania F (2003) Multimedia Models of Global Transport and Fate of Persistent Organic Pollutants. In: Fiedler H (ed) The handbook of environmental chemistry Vol 3: Anthropogenic Compounds Part O: Persistent organic pollutants. Springer, Berlin, pp 237-269

Scheringer M, Halder D, Hungerbühler K (2000a) Comparing the environmental performance of fluorescent whitening agents with peroxide bleaching of mechanical pulp. Journal of Industrial Ecology 3:77-95

Scheringer M, Wegmann F, Fenner K, Hungerbühler K (2000b) Investigation of the Cold Condensation of Persistent Organic Pollutants with a Global Multimedia Fate Model. Environmental Science & Technology 34:1842-1850

Schmid-Grob I, Thöni L, Hertz J (1993) Bestimmung der Deposition von Luftschadstoffen in der Schweiz mit Moosanalysen. Bundesamt für Umwelt, Wald und Landschaft, Bern, pp 173

Schmitt HW, Sticher H (1991) Heavy Metal Compounds in the Soil. In: Merian E (ed) Metals and their compounds in the environment: occurrence, analysis, and biological, relevance. VCH, Weinheim, pp 311-331

Schnitzer M (1978) Humic Substances: Chemistry and Reactions. In: Schnitzer M and Khan SU (eds) Soil organic matter. Elsevier Scientific Publ. Co., Amsterdam Developments in soil science, vol 8, pp 1-64

Schnoor JL (1996) Environmental Modeling: Fate and Transport of Pollutants in Water, Air, and Soil. John Wiley &Sons, Inc., New York

Schultz R (1987) Vergleichende Betrachtung des Schwermetallhaushalts verschiedener Waldökosysteme Norddeutschlands Forschungszentrum Waldökosysteme-Waldsterben. Kassel, Gesamthochschule, Göttingen Berichte des Forschungszentrums Waldökosysteme, Waldsterben Reihe A (32), pp 217

Schulz (2004) Personal communication on pig keeping. Zentralverband der Deutschen Schweineproduktion e.V. (ZDS), Bonn

Schumm SA (1977) The fluvial system. Wiley, New York

Schütte (2003) Personal communication on tillage practices and homogenized soil depth. University of Hohenheim, Stuttgart

Schütze G (1999) Critical Loads für terrestrische Ökosysteme - Critical Loads für Schwermetalle und persistente organische Verbindungen. In: Nagel H-D and Gregor H-D (eds) Ökologische Belastungsgrenzen: Critical Loads & Levels - Ein internationales Konzept für die Luftreinhaltepolitik. Springer Verlag, Berlin, pp 110-124

Schütze G, Nagel H-D (1998) Kriterien für die Erarbeitung von Immissionsminderungszielen zum Schutz der Böden und Abschätzung der langfristigen räumlichen Auswirkungen anthropogener Stoffeinträge auf die Bodenfunktionen. Umweltbundesamt, Berlin, pp 251

Schwartz S (2000) Quality Assurance of Exposure Models for Environmental Risk Assessment of Substances Department of Mathematics and Computer Science. University of Osnabrück, Osnabrück, pp 186

Schwartz S, Berding V, Trapp S, Matthies M (1998) EU Risk Assessment Guidelines Part I: Quality Criteria for Environmental Risk Assessment Software - Using the Example of EUSES. Environmental Science & Pollution Research 5:217-222

Schwarz A, Kaupenjohann M (2000) Grundwasserbelastungen durch in Böden eingetragene Schadstoffe unter besonderer Berücksichtigung des schnellen Flusses in bevorzugten Fließbahnen - Abschlussbericht des Arbeitskreises

"Schneller Stofftransport in Böden" im Fachausschuss "Bodenschutz, Boden- und Grundwasserverunreinigungen" des ATV-DVWK. Institut für Bodenkunde und Standortlehre, Universität Hohenheim, Hohenheim

Schwarzenbach RP, Gschwend PM, Imboden DM (1993) Environmental organic chemistry. Wiley, New York

Schwarzinger M, Stouthard ME, Burström K, Nord E (2003) Cross-national agreement on disability weights: the European Disability Weights Project. Population Health Metrics 1

Scott EM, Saltelli A, Sørensen T (2000) Practical experience in applying sensitivity and uncertainty analysis. In: Saltelli A, Chan K and Scott EM (eds) Sensitivity analysis. John Wiley & Sons, Chichester Wiley series in probability and statistics, pp 267-274

Scudlark JR, Rice KC, Conko KM, Bricker OP, Church TM (2005) Transmission of Atmospherically Derived Trace Elements Through an Undeveloped, Forested Maryland Watershed. Water, Air, and Soil Pollution 163:53-79

Searl A (2002) List of recommended dose respose functions and threshold values for toxic substances. Institute for Occupational Medicine (IOM), Internal paper for the GreenSense project, Edinburgh

Searl A (2004) Personal communication on latency times. Institute for Occupational Medicine (IOM), Edinbourgh

Seinfeld JH (1986) Atmospheric chemistry and physics of air pollution. John Wiley & Sons, New York

Seiwert M, Becker K, Friedrich C, Helm D, Hoffmann K, Krause C, Nöllke P, Schulz C, Seifert B (1999) Umwelt-Survey 1990/92, Band VIII: Arsen - Zusammenhangsanalyse. Umweltbundesamt, Institut für Wasser-, Boden- und Lufthygiene, Berlin

Selim HM, Amacher MC (2001) Sorption and release of heavy metals in soils: nonlinear kinetics. In: Selim HM and Sparks DL (eds) Heavy metals release in soils. Lewis publishers, Boca Raton, pp 1-29

Seth R, Mackay D, Muncke J (1999) Estimating the Organic Carbon Partition Coefficient and Its Variability for Hydrophobic Chemicals. Environmental Science & Technology 33:2390-2394

Severinsen M, Jager T (1998) Modelling the influence of terrestrial vegetation on the environmental fate of xenobiotics. Chemosphere 37:41-62

Severinsen M, Andersen MB, Chen F, Nyholm N (1996) A Regional Chemical Fate and Exposure Model Suitable for Denmark and its coastal Sea. Chemosphere 32:2159-2175

Sharpe S, Mackay D (2000) A Framework for Evaluating Bioaccumulation in Food Webs. Environmental Science & Technology 34:2373-2379

Shen HW, Julien PY (1993) Erosion and sediment transport. In: Maidment DR (ed) Handbook of hydrology. McGraw-Hill, New York, NY, pp 12.1-12.61

Shrader-Frechette K (2000) Duties to future generations, proxy consent, intra- and intergenerational equity: the case of nuclear waste. Risk Analysis 20:833-837

Shuttleworth WJ (1993) Evaporation. In: Maidment DR (ed) Handbook of hydrology. McGraw-Hill, New York, NY, pp 4.1-4.53

Simonich SL, Hites RA (1994) Importance of vegetation in removing polycyclic aromatic hydrocarbons from the atmosphere. Nature 370:49-51

Simpson D, Eliassen A (1997) Control strategies for ozone and acid deposition - an iterative approach. Norwegian Meteorological Institute, EMEP

Simpson D, Olendrzynski K, Semb A, Støren E, Unger S (1997) Photochemical oxidant modelling in Europe: multi-annual modelling and source-receptor relationships. Norwegian Meteorological Institute, EMEP MSC-W

Smedley PL, Kinniburgh DG (2002) A review of the source, behaviour and distribution of arsenic in natural waters. Applied Geochemistry 17:517-568

Smedley PL, Kinniburgh DG (2003) Source and behaviour of arsenic in natural waters. In: World Health Organisation (ed) United Nations Synthesis Report on Arsenic in Drinking Water - draft

Spadaro JV, Rabl A (1999) Estimates of real damage from air pollution: site dependence and simple impact indices for LCA. The International Journal of Life Cycle Assessment 4:229-243

Spadaro JV, Rabl A (2004) Pathway Analysis for Population-Total Health Impacts of Toxic Metal Emissions. Risk Analysis

Speir TW, August JA, C.W. F (1992) Assessment of the feasibility of using CCA treated sawdust as soil amendments. I. Plant growth and element uptake. Plant and soil 142:235-248

Stagnitti F, Parlange J-Y, Steenhuis TS, Boll J, Pivetz B, Barry DA (1995) Transport of moisture and solutes in the unsaturated zone by preferential flow. In: Singh VP (ed) Environmental hydrology. Kluwer Academic Publishers, Dordrecht Water Science and Technology Library, vol 15, pp 193-224

Stanners D, Bourdeau P (1995) Europe's Environment - The Dobris Assessment. European Environment Agency, Copenhagen

Statistisches Bundesamt (various volumes) Länderbericht Statistik des Auslandes. Metzler-Poeschel, Stuttgart

Steenhuis TS, Parlange J-Y (1991) Preferential flow in structured and sandy soils. In: Gish TJ and Shirmohammadi A (eds) Preferential flow. Proceedings of the national symposium held at Chicago, Illinois 16-17 December 1991. American Society of Agricultural Engineers, St. Joseph, Michigan, pp 12-21

Steinberg C, Brüggemann R, Hartmann A, Heller W, Kirchner M, Lienert D, Müller K, Pestlin G, Scheunert I, Seiler K-P, Ernst D, Spieser OH, Klein J (6/1995) Ökotoxikologische Testverfahren. In: Vogl J (ed) Handbuch des Umweltschutzes. Ecomed, Landsberg am Lech

Stern R, Thomsen E, Furst A (1984) Cr(VI) and other metallic mutagens in fly ash and welding fumes. Toxicological and Environmental Chemistry 8:95-108

Stoeppler M (1991) Cadmium. In: Merian E (ed) Metals and their compounds in the environment: occurrence, analysis, and biological, relevance. VCH, Weinheim, pp 803-851

Stoeppler M (1992) Cadmium. In: Stoeppler M (ed) Hazardous metals in the environment. Elsevier, Amsterdam Techniques and instrumentation in analytical chemistry, vol 12, pp 177-230

Strasburger E (1991) Lehrbuch der Botanik für Hochschulen (Textbook of botany for academy). Gustav Fischer, Stuttgart, pp 1030

Stumm W, Morgan JJ (1996) Aquatic Chemistry, 3 edn. Wiley-Interscience, New York

Suzuki N, Yasuda M, Sakurai T, Nakanishi J (2000) Simulation of long-term environmental dynamics of polychlorinated dibenzo-p -dioxins and polychlorinated dibenzofurans using the dynamic multimedia environmental fate model and its implication to the time trend analysis of dioxins. Chemosphere 40:969-976

Temm (2004) Personal communication on swine keeping. Pig Improvement Company (PIC), Germany, Schleswig

Tennant DR (2001) Risk analysis. In: Watson DH (ed) Food chemical safety 1: Contaminants. CRC Press, Boca Raton, pp 15-36

Tidblad J, Kucera V, Mikhailov AA (1998) Statistical analysis of 8 year materials exposure and acceptable deterioration and pollution levels. Swedish Corrosion Institute, Stockholm, Sweden

Tolle DA, Hesse DJ, Chadwell GB, Cooper JS, Evers DP (2001) Comparison of Two Equivalency Factor Approaches with Simplified Risk Assessment for LCIA of Toxicity Impact Potential. The International Journal of Life Cycle Assessment 6:96-105

Tolls J, McLachlan MS (1994) Partitioning of semivolatile organic compounds between air and Lolium multiflorum (Welsh Ray Grass). Environmental Science & Technology 28:159-166

Tompson AFB (1993) Numerical simulation of chemical migration in physically and chemically heterogeneous porous media. Water resources research 29:3709-3726

Traina SJ (1999) The environmental chemistry of cadmium. In: McLaughlin MJ and Singh BR (eds) Cadmium in soils and plants. Kluwer, Dordrecht Developments in plant and soil sciences, vol 85, pp 11-37

Trapp S (1995) Model for uptake of xenobiotics into plants. In: Trapp S and Mc Farlane JC (eds) Plant contamination: modeling and simulation of organic chemical processes. Lewis, Boca Raton, pp 107-151

Trapp S (2002) Dynamic root uptake model for neutral lipophilic organics. Environmental toxicology and chemistry 21:203-206

Trapp S, Matthies M (1995) Generic one-compartment model for uptake of organic chemicals by foliar vegetation. Environmental Science & Technology 29:2333-2338

Trapp S, Matthies M (1998) Chemodynamics and Environmental Modeling - an introduction. Springer, Berlin

Trapp S, Schwartz S (2000) Proposals to overcome limitations in the EU chemical risk assessment scheme. Chemosphere 41:965-971

Trapp S, Rantio T, Paasivirta J (1994) Fate of Pulp mill effluent compounds in a Finnish watercourse. Environmental Science & Pollution Research 1:246-252

Travis CC, Arms AD (1988) Bioconcentration of organics in beef, milk, and vegetation. Environmental Science & Technology 22:271-274

Trudgill ST (2000) Weathering overview - measurement and modelling. In: Viles HA (ed) Recent advances in field and laboratory studies of rock weathering. Borntraeger, Berlin Zeitschrift für Geomorphologie: Supplementband, vol 120, pp 187-193

Trukenmüller A (1998) Using WMI - Implementing atmospheric trajectory models with the Wind rose Model Interpreter. Institute of Energy Economics and the Rational Use of Energy, University of Stuttgart, Stuttgart, pp 59

Trukenmüller A, Friedrich R (1995) Die Abbildung der großräumigen Verteilung, chemischen Umwandlung und Deposition von Luftschadstoffen mit dem Trajektorienmodell WTM. In: Arbeitsgruppe Luftreinhaltung der Universität Stuttgart (ed) Jahresbericht 1995 "Ausbreitung von Luftverunreinigungen". Schwäbische Druckerei, Stuttgart, pp 93-108

Tsang C-F (1991) The modeling process and model validation. groundwater 29:825-831

Tsiros IX (2001) A screening model-based study of transport fluxes and fate of airborne mercury deposited onto catchment areas. Chemosphere 44:99-107

Turner DR (1995) Problems in trace metal speciation modeling. In: Tessier A and Turner DR (eds) Metal speciation and bioavailability in aquatic systems. Wiley, Chichester IUPAC series on analytical and physical chemistry of environmental systems, vol 3, pp 149-203

Udo de Haes HA (1996) Part I: Discussion of general principles and guidelines for practical use. In: Udo de Haes HA (ed) Towards a methodology for life cycle impact assessment. Society of Environmental Toxicology and Chemistry - Europe, Brussels, pp 7-30

Udo de Haes HA, Jolliet O, Finnveden G, Hauschild M, Krewitt W, Müller-Wenk R (1999) Best Available Practice Regarding Impact Categories and Category Indicators in Life Cycle Impact Assessment - Part I. The International Journal of Life Cycle Assessment 4:66-74

Ulrich B (1991) Deposition of Acids and Metal Compounds. In: Merian E (ed) Metals and their compounds in the environment: occurrence, analysis, and biological, relevance. VCH, Weinheim, pp 369-378

Umweltbundesamt (1999) Nährstoffbilanzierung der Flußgebiete Deutschlands. Institut für Gewässerökologie und Binnenfischerei im Forschungsverbund Berlin e.V., Berlin, pp 288

Umweltbundesamt (2000) Emissionsinventar Wasser für die Bundesrepublik Deutschland. Fraunhofer-Institut für Systemtechnik und Innovationsforschung (ISI), Berlin, pp 130

United Nations - Economic Commission for Europe (1998) Proceedings of the workshop on Critical Limits and Effect Based Approaches for Heavy Metals and Persistent Organic Pollutants, Bad Harzburg, Germany. Federal Environmental Agency

United Nations - Economic Commission for Europe, Co-operative programme for monitoring and evaluation of long range transmission of air pollutants in Europe (2002) UNECE/EMEP emission database. UNECE/EMEP, available at: http://webdab.emep.int/index.html

United Nations Environment Programme (2002) Global mercury assessment. Inter-Organization Programme for the sound management of chemicals, Geneva, Switzerland, pp 258

United States - Environmental Protection Agency (1992) Guidelines for Exposure Assessment. U.S. Environmental Protection Agency, Risk Assessment Forum, Washington, DC

United States - Environmental Protection Agency (1994) Methods for Derivation of Inhalation Reference Concentrations and Application of Inhalation Dosimetry. U.S. Environmental Protection Agency Office of Research and Development, Washington, DC

United States - Environmental Protection Agency (1995) Use of the Benchmark Dose Approach in Health Risk Assessment. U.S. Environmental Protection Agency Office of Research and Development, Washington, DC

United States - Environmental Protection Agency (1996a) Soil Screening Guidance: Technical Background Document and User's Guide (2nd edition).

U.S. Environmental Protection Agency Office of Solid Waste and Emergency Response, Washington, DC

United States - Environmental Protection Agency (1996b) Proposed Guidelines for Carcinogen Risk Assessment-Availability. U.S. Environmental Protection Agency Office of Solid Waste and Emergency Response, Washington, DC

United States - Environmental Protection Agency (1997a) Exposure Factors Handbook (Volume 3) - Draft. U.S. Environmental Protection Agency, Office of Research and Development, Washington, DC

United States - Environmental Protection Agency (1997b) Mercury Study Report to Congress. Volume III: Fate and transport of mercury in the environment. U.S. Environmental Protection Agency Office of Air Quality Planning and Standards and Office of Research and Development

United States - Environmental Protection Agency (1997c) Exposure Factors Handbook (Volume 1): General Factors. U.S. Environmental Protection Agency, Office of Research and Development, Washington, DC

United States - Environmental Protection Agency (1997d) Guiding Principles for Monte Carlo Analysis. U.S. Environmental Protection Agency, Risk Assessment Forum, Washington, DC, pp 35

United States - Environmental Protection Agency (1998) Human Health Risk Assessment Protocol for Hazardous Waste Combustion Facilities (Peer review draft). U.S. Environmental Protection Agency Region 6 U.S. EPA Multimedia Planning and Permitting Division Office of Solid Waste, Center for Combustion Science and Engineering

United States - Environmental Protection Agency (1999a) Total Risk Integrated Methodology. Office of Air Quality, Planning and Standards, Research Triangle Park, NC

United States - Environmental Protection Agency (1999b) TRIM - Total Risk Integrated Methodology - Status Report. United States - Environmental Protection Agency, Office of Air and Radiation, Office of Air Quality, Planning and Standards, Research Triangle Park, NC

United States - Environmental Protection Agency (2001) Dioxin: Scientific Highlights from Draft Reassessment (2000): 2001 Update information sheet 2. US Environmental Protection Agency - Office of Research and Development, Washington, DC, pp 7

United States - Environmental Protection Agency (2002a) TRIM.FaTE Technical support document Volume I: Description of Module. Office of Air Quality, Planning and Standards, Research Triangle Park, NC

United States - Environmental Protection Agency (2002b) TRIM.FaTE Technical support document Volume II: Description of Chemical Transport and

Transformation Algorithms. Office of Air Quality, Planning and Standards, Research Triangle Park, NC

United States - Environmental Protection Agency (2005) Integrated Risk Information System (IRIS) (accessed via internet on 21 April 2005)

Ure AM, Davidson CM (1995) Chemical speciation in the environment. Blackie Academic & Professional, London, pp 1-5

Ursínyová M, Hladíová V (2000a) Cadmium in the environment of Central Europe. In: Markert B and Friese K (eds) Trace elements - their distribution and effects in the environment. Elsevier, Amsterdam Trace metals in the environment, vol 4, pp 87-107

Ursínyová M, Hladíová V (2000b) Lead in the environment of Central Europe. In: Markert B and Friese K (eds) Trace elements - their distribution and effects in the environment. Elsevier, Amsterdam Trace metals in the environment, vol 4, pp 109-134

van de Meent D, de Bruijn JHM, de Leeuw FAAM, de Nijs ACM, Jager DT, Vermeire TG (1996) Exposure Modelling. In: van Leeuwen CJ and Hermens JLM (eds) Risk Assessment of Chemicals: An Introduction. Kluwer Acad. Publ., Dordrecht, pp 103-145

van den Berg M, Birnbaum L, Bosveld ATC, Brunström B, Cook P, Feeley M, Giesy JP, Hanberg A, Hasegawa R, Kennedy SW, Kubiak T, Larsen JC, Rolaf van Leeuwen FX, Liem AKD, Nolt C, Peterson RE, Poellinger L, Safe S, Schrank D, Tillitt D, Tysklind M, Younes M, Waern F, Zacharewski T (1998) Toxic Equivalency Factors (TEFs) for PCBs, PCDDs, PCDFs for Humans and Wildlife. Environmental Health Perspectives 106:775-792

van den Bergh JCJM, Boelens J, Bouman MN, Guinée JB, Heijungs R, Huppes G, Kandelaars PPAAH, Lexmond TM, Moolenaar SW, van Oers L, Olsthoorn X, Udo de Haes HA, Verkuijlen E, van der Voet E (2000) Summary, conclusions and recommendations. In: van der Voet E, Guinée JB and Udo de Haes HA (eds) Heavy metals: a problem solved? - Methods and models to evaluate policy strategies for heavy metals. Kluwer Acad. Publ., Dordrecht, pp 211-230

van der Knijff JM, Jones RJA, Montanarella L (2000) Soil Erosion Risk - Assessment in Europe. European Soil Bureau (ESB) and Space Applications Institute (SAI) at the Joint Research Centre (JRC) of European Commission, Ispra, Italy, pp 34

van Eijkeren, J. (2002). Personal communication on the dynamic solution implemented in SimpleBox 2.0. Bilthoven, the Netherlands, National Institute of Public Health and the Environment (RIVM)

van Jaarsveld JA (1990) An operational atmospheric transport model for Priority Substances; specification and instructions for use. National Institute of

Public Health and the Environment (RIVM), Bilthoven, the Netherlands, pp 101

van Pul WAJ, de Leeuw FAAM, van Jaarsveld JA, van der Gaag MA, Sliggers CJ (1998) The potential for long-range transboundary atmospheric transport. Chemosphere 37:113-141

Veerkamp W, Wolff C (1996) Fate and Exposure Models in Relation to Risk Assessment: Developments and Validation Criteria. Environmental Science & Pollution Research 3:91-95

Verdin KL (1997) A System for Topologically Coding Global Drainage Basins and Stream Networks. In: 17th Annual ESRI Users Conference, Environmental Systems Research Institute, San Diego, CA

Vermeire TG, Jager DT, Bussian B, Devillers J, den Haan K, Hansen B, Lundberg I, Niessen H, Robertson S, Tyle H, van der Zandt PTJ (1997) European Union System for the Evaluation of Substances (EUSES). Principles and Structure. Chemosphere 34:1823-1836

Versteegh JFM, van Gaalen FW, Rietveld LC, Evers EG, Aldenberg TA, Cleij P (2001) TAPWAT: Definition, structure and applications for modelling drinking-water treatment. National Institute of Public Health and the Environment (RIVM), Bilthoven, the Netherlands

Vink RJ, Peters S (2003) Modelling point and diffuse heavy metal emissions and loads in the Elbe basin. Hydrological Processes 17:1307- 1328

Vörösmarty CJ, Federer CA, Schloss A (1998) Potential evaporation functions compared on US watersheds: possible implications for global-scale water balance and terrestrial ecosystem modeling. Journal of Hydrology 207:147-169

Vossiniotis G, Arabatzis G, Assimacopoulos D (1996) Dispersion modelling on a local scale in the ExternE Transport Project : A description of ROADPOL. National Technical University of Athens, Laboratory of Industry and Energy Economics, Athens

Vuceta J, Morgan JJ (1978) Chemical modeling of trace metals in fresh waters: role of complexation and adsorption. Environmental Science & Technology 12:1302-1309

Vulava VM, Kretzschmar R, Rusch U, Grolimund D, Westall JC, Borkovec M (2000) Cation Competition in a Natural Subsurface Material: Modeling of Sorption Equilibria. Environmental Science & Technology 34:2149-2155

Wagenet RJ (1998) Scale issues in agroecological research chains. Nutrient Cycling in Agroecosystems 50:23-34

Wagrowski DM, Hites RA (1997) Polycyclic Aromatic Hydrocarbon Accumulation in Urban, Suburban, and Rural Vegetation. Environmental Science & Technology 31:279-282

Walker CH, Hopkin SP, Sibly RM, Peakall DB (2001) Principles of Ecotoxicology, 2 edn. Bell & Bain Ltd, Glasgow

Walling DE (1983) The sediment delivery problem. Journal of Hydrology 65:209-37

Walling DE, Webb BW (1983) Patterns of sediment yield. In: Gregory KJ (ed) Background to Palaeohydrology. John Wiley, Chichester International geological correlation programme, vol Project 158, pp 69-100

Wania F (1996) Spatial Variability in Compartmental Fate Modelling - Linking Fugacity Models and GIS. Environmental Science & Pollution Research 3:39-46

Wania F (2003) Assessing the Potential of Persistent Organic Chemicals for Long-Range Transport and Accumulation in Polar Regions. Environmental Science & Technology 37:1344-1351

Wania F, Mackay D (1993a) Modelling the global distribution of toxaphene: a discussion of feasibility and desirability. Chemosphere 27:2079-2094

Wania F, Mackay D (1993b) Global fractionation and cold condensation of low volatility organochlorine compounds in polar regions. Ambio 22:10-18

Wania F, Mackay D (1995) A global distribution model for persistent organic chemicals. The Science of the Total Environment 160/161:211-232

Wania F, Mackay D (1999) The evolution of mass balance models of persistent organic pollutant fate in the environment. Environmental Pollution 100:223-240

Wania F, McLachlan MS (2001) Estimating the Influence of Forests on the Overall Fate of Semivolatile Organic Compounds Using a Multimedia Fate Model. Environmental Science & Technology 35:582-590

Wania F, Persson J, Di Guardo A, McLachlan MS (2000) The POPCYCLING-Baltic Model - A Non-Steady State Multicompartment Mass Balance Model of the Fate of Persistent Organic Pollutants in the Baltic Sea Environment. Norwegian Institute for Air Research, NILU, Kjeller

Watson D (2001) Introduction. In: Watson DH (ed) Food chemical safety 1: Contaminants. CRC Press, Boca Raton, pp 1-12

Weaver RW, Melton JR, Wang D, Duble RL (1984) Uptake of arsenic and mercury from soil by bermudagrass Cynodon dactylon . Environmental pollution (Series A) 33:133-142

Wedepohl KH (1991) The composition of the upper earth's crust and the natural cycles of selected metals. Metals in natural raw materials. Natural sources. In: Merian E (ed) Metals and their compounds in the environment: occurrence, analysis, and biological, relevance. VCH, Weinheim, pp 3-17

Wedepohl KH (1995) The composition of the continental crust. Geochimica et Cosmochimica Acta 59:1217-1232

Wegener Sleeswijk A (2005) Doctoral thesis (in preparation). Leiden University, Leiden, The Netherlands

Weigert P (1991) Metal Loads of Food of Vegetable Origin Including Mushrooms. In: Merian E (ed) Metals and their compounds in the environment: occurrence, analysis, and biological, relevance. VCH, Weinheim, pp 449-468

Weitzmann ML (1999) "Just keep discounting, but ..." In: Portney PR and Weyant JP (eds) Discounting and intergenerational equity. Resources for the Future, Washington, DC, pp 23-29

Welch RM, Norvell WA (1999) Mechanisms of cadmium uptake, translocation and deposition in plants. In: McLaughlin MJ and Singh BR (eds) Cadmium in soils and plants. Kluwer, Dordrecht Developments in plant and soil sciences, vol 85, pp 125-150

Welsch-Pausch K, McLachlan MS, Umlauf G (1995) Determination of the principal pathways of polychlorinated dibenzo-p -dioxins and dibenzofurans to Lolium multiflorum (Welsh Ray Grass). Environmental Science & Technology 29:1090-1098

Whelan G, Buck JW, Strenge DL, Droppo (Jr) JG, Hoopes BL (1992) Overview of the Multimedia Environmental Pollutant Assessment System (MEPAS). Hazardous Waste & Hazardous Materials 9:191-208

Whelan G, Castleton KJ, Buck JW, Hoopes BL, Pelton MA, Strenge DL, Gelston GM, Kickert RN (1997) Concepts of a Framework for Risk Analysis In Multimedia Environmental Systems (FRAMES). Pacific Northwest National Laboratory, Richland, Washington, pp 121

White AF, Brantley SL (1995) Chemical weathering rates of silicate minerals: an overview. In: White AF and Brantley SL (eds) Chemical weathering rates of silicate minerals. Mineralogical Society of America, Washington, DC Reviews in mineralogy, vol 31, pp 1-22

Wickenkamp V, Duttmann R, Mosimann T (2000) A Multiscale Approach to Predicting Soil Erosion on Cropland Using Empirical and Physically Based Soil Erosion Models in a Geographic Information System. In: Schmidt J (ed) Soil erosion: application of physically based models. Springer, Berlin Environmental science, pp 109-134

Wilhelm M, Ewers U (1999) Metalle/Blei. In: Wichmann H-E, Schlipköter H-W and Fülgraff G (eds) Handbuch der Umweltmedizin. ecomed, Landsberg/Lech, vol 18. Erg. Lfg. 3/2000, pp 25

Wischmeier WH, Smith DD (1978) Predicting rainfall erosion losses - a guide to conservation planning. U.S. Gov. Print. Off., Washington

Wittig R, Ballach H-J, Brandt CJ (1985) Increase of number of acid indicators in the herb layer of the millet grass-beech forest of the Westphalian bight. Angewandte Botanik 59:219-232

Wolt JD (1994) Soil solution chemistry: applications to environmental science and agriculture. John Wiley & Sons, New York

Woodfine D, MacLeod M, Mackay D (2002) A regionally segmented national scale multimedia contaminant fate model for Canada with GIS data input and display. Environmental Pollution 119:341-355

Woodfine DG, MacLeod M, Mackay D, Brimacombe JR (2001) Development of continental scale multimedia contaminant fate models: Integrating GIS. Environmental Science & Pollution Research 8:164-172

World Health Organisation (1992a) Cadmium: environmental aspects. World Health Organization, Geneva

World Health Organisation (1992b) Cadmium. World Health Organization, Geneva

World Health Organisation (2000a) Hazardous chemicals in human and environmental health. Produced under the joint sponsorship of the United Nations Environment Programme, the International Labour Organisation and the World Health Organization, and within the framework of the Inter-Organization Programme for the Sound Management of Chemicals, Geneva, Switzerland

World Health Organisation (2000b) Air quality guidelines for Europe (2nd edition). World Health Organization, Regional Office for Europe, Copenhagen, pp 273

World Health Organisation (2002) The European health report 2002. WHO Regional Office for Europe, Copenhagen

Zachara JM, Westall JC (1999) Chemical Modeling of the Soil Solution. In: Sparks DL (ed) Soil physical chemistry. CRC Press, Boca Raton, Fla., pp 47-95

Zaslavsky MN (1979) Erozia Pochv (Soil erosion). Mysl Publishing House, Moscow

Zayed A, Lytle CM, Qian J-H, Terry N (1998) Chromium accumulation, translocation and chemical speciation in vegetable crops. Planta 206:293-299

Zhang Q, Crittenden JC, Shonnard D, Mihelcic JR (2003) Development and evaluation of an environmental multimedia fate model CHEMGL for the Great Lakes region. Chemosphere 50:1377-1397

Zimdahl RL, Koeppe DE (1979) Uptake by plants. In: Boggess WR and Wixson BG (eds) Lead in the environment. Castle House Publ, London, pp 99-104

Zöttl HW (1985) Heavy metal levels and cycling in forest ecosystems. Experientia 41:1104-1113

Zoumis T, Schmidt A, Grigorova L, Calmano W (2001) Contaminants in sediments: remobilisation and demobilisation. The Science of the Total Environment 266:195-202

Appendix A Model formulation

In this Appendix, the calculations within the different modules of the Impact Pathway Approach as implemented in the WATSON model are described. First, the mathematical formulation of the environmental fate model is presented including the different types of temporal modes of operations (section A.1). Secondly, the processes constituting either the matrix or perturbation vector elements are formulated (section A.3 through A.6). In section A.7, the equations used in the exposure assessment are given. The equations used during the impact assessment and the monetary valuation are given to the extent not yet documented in the main text in sections A.8 and A.9, respectively.

A.1 Overall modelling approach of the environmental fate model

The water and soil environmental fate model is formulated as an inhomogeneous system of ordinary linear first order differential equations. It is 'inhomogeneous' because there is a 'perturbation' term in the differential equations that neither contains the dependent variable (here: concentration) nor its derivative(s) and that is not zero. This perturbation term describes the exogenous inputs from outside the model's scope (i.e., emissions from technosphere, depositions from air, possibly also import via advection from outside the model's scope). The differential equations are called 'first order ordinary' since they only have the first derivative in one variable (here: time).[35] The differential equations are 'linear' as they are linear combinations of the dependent variable and its derivatives.

Note that in the following symbols will be employed that are only used in this section (i.e., A.1 including sub-sections) and are not given in Appendix D.

Assuming that the perturbation term is independent of time one can write the ordinary differential equation (ODE) system in matrix notation as follows:

---

[35] If there were different derivatives with respect to more than one variable (e.g., time t and space x, y and/or z) one would have to deal with partial differential equations.

$$\vec{v} \cdot \frac{d\vec{c}}{dt} = A \times \vec{c} + \vec{b} \tag{A-1}$$

where

A : coefficient matrix of dimension n x n [m^3/s]

$\vec{b}$: perturbation vector of dimension n with exogenous inputs like atmospheric deposition or direct emissions to the compartments [kg/s]

$\vec{c}$: concentration vector of dimension n [kg/m^3]

t : time [s]

$\vec{v}$: volume vector of dimension n [m^3].

There are two solutions of this ODE system implemented: steady-state and dynamic. For computational efficiency reasons, WATSON in both cases tries to subdivide the overall environmental fate matrix in linearly independent sub-matrices before further solving the set of differential equations. In case no air compartment and no marine environment are considered, the different river catchments will constitute linearly independent sets of differential equations that are treated one after the other.

Note that the volume vector only occurs on the left hand side of equation (A-1). For the steady-state solution, it is irrelevant (see below). For the dynamic solution, however, all volumes need to be known in order to solve for the concentration vector. Within WATSON, the matrix A as well as the perturbation vector b are, therefore, divided by the respective volume vector in any case.

A.1.1 Steady-state solution

In particular for sustainability questions, one may want to know what environmental concentrations will occur if a society (or national economy) proceeds at a certain emission level. For this, the steady-state solution can be computed. Steady-state means that there is no concentration change in time (any more), given a constant and continuous emission into the modelled system. Eq. (A-1) hence becomes:

$$\vec{v} \cdot \frac{d\vec{c}}{dt} = 0 = A \times \vec{c} + \vec{b} \Rightarrow \vec{c} = A^{-1} \times -\vec{b}\,. \tag{A-2}$$

Overall the matrix of a spatially-resolved environmental fate model is rather sparse, i.e., contains many zero-elements. This is because not all compartments are interconnected. Thus, only routines based on sparse linear algebra are implemented for the matrix inversion. These make use of the coordinate storage scheme. The routines for sparse matrix inversion are taken from the NAG C library (mark 6). These routines are iterative methods trying to determine the solution through a sequence of approximations until some user-specified termination criterion is met or until some pre-defined maximum number of iterations has been carried out. In order to decrease the number of iterations required for convergence, a preconditioner is often used that is mandatory for the inversion routines as used here. Preconditioning matrices are based on incomplete factorization, in this case incomplete Lower-Upper (LU) factorization. In order to increase the accuracy indicated by the number of pivot modifications, the preconditioning matrices are allowed to become less sparse by increasing the level of fill successively. For details, refer to the NAG C library (mark 6) documentation. Due to the fact that the NAG C library (mark 6) does not contain a routine to invert a sparse matrix as a whole in one step (so-called matrix-matrix operations or Level-3 Basic Linear Algebra Subprograms (BLAS)), each row is successively inverted in a matrix-vector operation (Level-2 BLAS). Due to the fact that one iterative method for the inversion of nonsymmetric linear systems cannot cope with any matrix equally well, different methods and options are implemented that are tried successively if the former try did not result (e.g., an infinite value or an internal error occurred). Without explaining these methods, it shall be stated here that the following methods are tried one after the other while also varying between the inversion of the sparse matrix itself and its transpose for one method: the stabilized bi-conjugate gradient method, the restarted generalized minimum residual method, and the conjugate gradient squared method. The interested reader is referred to the NAG C library (mark 6) documentation and the references given therein.

In some cases, the numerical stability of these methods is not assured if the matrix is ill-conditioned. One way to address this issue is to rescale the matrix (cf. Heijungs and Suh, 2002). Thus, before trying to invert the matrix the minimum and maximum values per row are defined in absolute terms from which the geometric mean is built. The different matrix elements of each row are then divided by the respective resulting value prior to inverting this rescaled matrix. Before the elements of the inverse are stored, the values are back transformed accordingly.

It depends on the removal rates from the system when a substance will reach the steady-state situation. With very persistent substances like heavy metals, the steady-state situation will only be reached after some hundred or even thousands and more years given the potentially very long residence times of these contaminants, for example, in soils (Alloway et al., 1996). Principally, possible removal rates are degradation or ultimately mineralization, radioactive decay and export to beyond the model's scope.

For pulse emission situations (like in LCA), the steady-state solution may also serve for assessing time-integrated exposures as shown by Heijungs (1995). This, however, depends on the time after which the following key assumption/condition becomes true:

$$\lim_{t \to \infty} e^{t \cdot A} = 0\,. \tag{A-3}$$

If it is really only after millennia or longer that this condition becomes true (e.g of very persistent substances) it is questionable to what extent the calculated time-integrated exposures and consequently impacts are valuable for decision-making purposes.

A.1.2 Dynamic solution

There are principally two ways to arrive at a dynamic solution: analytic and numeric. As was demonstrated for multimedia models (Brandes et al., 1996; Heijungs, 2000; van Eijkeren, 2002), there is an analytical solution to Eq. (A-1) containing a matrix exponential.

$$\vec{c} = e^{t \cdot A'} \times \vec{c}_0 + -A'^{-1} \times (I - e^{t \cdot A'}) \times \vec{b}' \tag{A-4}$$

where

A' : coefficient matrix A multiplied by the inverse of the volume vector v, dimension n x n [1/s]

$\vec{b}'$: perturbation vector b multiplied by the inverse of the volume vector v, dimension n [$kg/m^3/s$]

$\vec{c}$: vector containing the concentrations at a certain time *t* [kg/m^3]

$\vec{c}_0$: vector containing the initial concentrations [kg/m^3]

I : identity matrix of dimension n x n; diagonal elements are 1, off-diagonal elements are zero

t : time for which concentrations are computed [s].

In order to solve this matrix exponential, one would need to find the value to which it converges for the following series:

$$e^{A'} = \sum_{n=0}^{\infty} \frac{1}{n!} \cdot A'^{n} \approx \sum_{n=0}^{m_{\text{convergence}}} \frac{1}{n!} \cdot A'^{n} . \tag{A-5}$$

This might be very resource-intensive for systems where the matrix A has a dimension of several hundred or even thousands. Matrix A can be rewritten as the product of its eigenvector matrix (P) times the diagonal matrix with eigenvalues λ_i (D) times the inverse of the eigenvector matrix (P^{-1}):

$$A' = P \times D \times P^{-1} . \tag{A-6}$$

The matrix exponential hence becomes:

$$\begin{aligned} e^{t \cdot A'} &= \sum_{n=0}^{\infty} \frac{1}{n!} \cdot t^{n} \cdot A'^{n} = \sum_{n=0}^{\infty} \frac{1}{n!} \times P \times t^{n} \times D^{n} \times P^{-1} \\ &= P \times \left(\sum_{n=0}^{\infty} \frac{1}{n!} \cdot t^{n} \cdot D^{n} \right) \times P^{-1} = P \times e^{t \cdot D} \times P^{-1} \end{aligned} \tag{A-7}$$

and, thus, the overall analytical solution can be written as:

$$\vec{c} = P \times e^{t \cdot D} \times P^{-1} \times \vec{c}_0 - P \times D^{-1} \times (I - e^{t \cdot D}) \times P^{-1} \times \vec{b}' . \tag{A-8}$$

The solution of the matrix exponential consequently simplifies to computing the eigenvalues and eigenvectors (and its inverse matrix) as well as the matrix exponential of the diagonal matrix of the eigenvalues. The latter can be facilitated according to:

$$e^{t \cdot D} = \begin{bmatrix} e^{t \cdot \lambda_1} & 0 & \dots \\ 0 & e^{t \cdot \lambda_2} & \dots \\ \dots & \dots & \dots \end{bmatrix} . \tag{A-9}$$

However, there might be two drawbacks to the analytic solution of the ODE system. First it needs to be ensured that the matrix is 'well conditioned' so that it is diagonalisable[36] which might not always be the case. Second - and more importantly - it should be made sure that the eigenvalues for the analytic solution are calculated with a high degree of accuracy (i.e., preferably analytically as opposed to by means of numeric methods). Rounding and the tolerance allowed in the numeric derivation of the eigenvalues may produce small but significant inaccuracies in the eigenvalues which might have a major influence on the concentration computations.

In order to find out whether the accuracy of the analytic solution is sufficient, the analytic solution of a two-compartment system was compared to the solution given by a numeric method (Adams method, see below) with the highest tolerance for which a computation could have been successfully performed. The results were identical. Due to computation time reasons, the analytic solution is preferred. For the case that the eigenvalues of the matrix are complex, however, the numeric solution is also implemented. The way how the numeric solution is implemented is described in the following.

When numerically solving an ODE system, one must be aware that these systems could be 'stiff'. If a system is stiff and one wants to be computationally efficient, one needs to adjust the step length to that process ruling 'at the moment'/working point. A system is stiff if the processes involved have substantially different dynamics with respect to the different process rates. An indicator for this is if the eigenvalues have very different negative real parts. In order to decide whether an ODE system is stiff, the following stiffness measure is used:

$$S = \frac{\max\limits_j (|\Re\lambda_j|)}{\min\limits_j (|\Re\lambda_j|)} . \tag{A-10}$$

This stiffness measure can obtain values as big as 10^6. There are different perceptions of what is the threshold for stiff systems. As a default a value of 500 is assumed here. This value can be changed by the user.

Depending on the stiffness of the ODE system, two different numeric solution methods[37] are implemented (NAG C library, mark 6):

---

[36] A matrix of dimension n is 'well conditioned' if the n eigenvectors are linearly independent. Distinct eigenvalues will ensure linear independence of eigenvectors, but there are cases when degenerate (repeated) eigenvalues give rise to linearly independent eigenvectors.

- for stiff systems: variable-order, variable-step method implementing the Backward Differentiation Formulae (BDF) provided with the Jacobian of the system which is identical to the coefficient matrix, and
- for non-stiff systems: variable-order, variable-step Adams method.

In the NAG documentation of the two numeric methods, it is highly recommended to vary the tolerance before accepting a result. Therefore, if the user has specified to automatically adjust the tolerance for the methods then the computation is started with the default tolerance value (or the tolerance value of a former computation for the scenario-pollutant computation if existent). If a solution was successfully computed, the tolerance is tightened by one order of magnitude and the computation is done again. This is done until an error condition occurs (errors: "the tolerance value is too small for the function to take an initial step" or "the tolerance value is too small for the function to make any further progress across the integration range"). Without giving notice of this error to the user, the results of the last run that was successfully completed are then saved. If the first tolerance value is already too strict, it is loosened by four orders of magnitude and tightened consecutively as described above.

Both methods also require to set the type of (local) error and hence step size control. There are three types to choose from:

1. relative: error requirement is in terms of the number of correct significant digits,
2. absolute: error requirement is in terms of the number of correct decimal places, or
3. mixed: error requirement is a mixture of the two types stated above.

The NAG C library recommends the relative option for the BDF whereas it strongly suggests to use the mixed option for the Adams method. However, in a comparison of the two methods for a system of two equations both methods only yielded similar results when using the same type of step size control. Hence, it was chosen to use the mixed option for both methods.

A.1.3 Dynamic solution until a certain fraction of the steady-state solution

Some substances persist a very long time span in the environment. As was stated above, the steady-state solution might serve as an indicator of whether a certain emission level is sustainable. If such a condition will only occur in many thou-

[37] For more details on the respective methods please refer to numeric method maths books.

sands of years or more, however, the steady-state solution - even if used for time-integrated exposures - may not be as meaningful any more at least in the context of policy decision-making. Therefore, WATSON allows the user to calculate the time span until a certain percentage of the steady-state solution is reached. This feature is implemented for the analytic as well as for the numeric solution.

One main distinction between the analytic and the numeric solution approaches is that the analytic solution is done in discrete steps. If the required percentage of the steady-state solution is reached or exceeded, the time is assessed by linearly interpolating between the results of the latest and the previous time step. This might lead to overestimations especially for the concentrations computed for the first time step if initial values are equal to zero. The time steps are different for the time span for which the dynamic solution is calculated and for the time afterwards until the maximum time limit. For the first interval the time steps are equal to the time steps specified by the user. For the second interval the time steps are set according to the constraints set by the user ('default settings'): The remaining time is divided into a number of time steps of between two (user-changeable) default minimum and maximum values also taking a 'threshold time step' into account. If the remaining time divided by the minimum time step yields a larger value than the 'threshold time step' the time step is adjusted to have at most the maximum allowed amount of time steps at a time span close to the 'threshold time step' if possible.

In contrast to the analytic solution, the numeric methods implemented (see section A.1.2) compute results continuously. Therefore, no interpolation between results is necessary. With both numeric methods, apart from specifying the end of the integration interval, the user can supply a function for setting another cut-off criterion. This is used when computing the 'time to steady-state' (or a fraction of it) by checking whether the concentrations in all compartments have reached the specified fraction (> 0-100 %) of the steady-state solution or whether the specified time limit has been reached.

If the time limit is reached for both the analytic and the numeric approach, the percentage of the steady-state solution reached until this moment is saved alongside with the time limit.

A.2 Partitioning of substances and equilibrium distribution coefficients

The Mackay-type multimedia models rely to a rather large extent on the equilibrium partitioning of substances between different phases (Mackay, 1979, 1991). In these box models, the world is separated into homogeneous compartments on which the mass balance is based. A substance in either of the distinguished compartments is assumed to be in equilibrium between the different phases present, i.e., the solid phase which may consist of lipophilic (i.e., living or non-living organic matter) and non-lipophilic phases, the aqueous phase and potentially a gas phase. Several processes will only involve one of these phases. In order to allow processes only to involve a substance's amount present in just one of these phases within a compartment, the concept of the *equilibrium distribution coefficient* between the bulk compartment and the respective single phase may be used (Brandes et al., 1996) which builds on the substance-dependent partitioning coefficients (cf. section C.1).

In order to define the equilibrium distribution coefficient, the rule is followed here to relate the concentration of a substance in the bulk compartment to its concentration in the minority phases. Such minority phases are for example for soils the aqueous and gas phases, and for water compartments the suspended matter phase. For sediments in particular, the definition of a minority phase is difficult due to the high vertical variability in the prevalence of its constituents. At present, water is still the dominant phase according to the 'volume fraction that is solid phase' used (cf. section B.5.4). Nevertheless, sediments are treated in the same way as soils.

Note that in this document the term 'water' is normally used for the water compartment whereas 'aqueous' is used for the water phase in a compartment. Notable exceptions are the established names of parameters such as air-water partitioning coefficient K_{aw}, octanol-water partitioning coefficient K_{ow}, or the solid-water partitioning coefficient K_{sw}.

A.2.1 Bulk compartment-aqueous phase or solid phase equilibrium distribution coefficients

Following the rule as stated above, the equilibrium distribution coefficients for the compartments with a significant solid phase relate the bulk phase concentration to the aqueous phase or potentially gas phase concentration according to:

(A-11)

$$\begin{aligned} ED_{\text{bulk/aqueous,p}} &= \frac{C\_w/v_{\text{bulk}}}{C\_w/v_{\text{aqueous phase}}} \\ &= (fr\_V_{\text{aqueous phase}} \cdot C\_w/v_{\text{aqueous phase}} \\ &\quad + fr\_V_{\text{solid phase/bulk}} \cdot C\_w/v_{\text{solid phase}} \\ &\quad + fr\_V_{\text{gas phase/bulk}} \cdot C\_w/v_{\text{gas phase}}]/C\_w/v_{\text{aqueous phase}} \end{aligned}$$

where

C_w/v : concentration in the bulk compartment or in one of its phases [kg per m^3]

ED : equilibrium distribution coefficient relating the bulk compartment concentration to that of the aqueous phase [-]

fr_V : volume fraction of soil that is solid or gas phase [m^3_{phase} per $m^3_{bulk\ compartment}$].

Note that in the following the volume fraction of aqueous phase is expressed as the complement of the sum of those of the solid and gas phase.

For surface compartments with a substantial gas phase, i.e., soils, the bulk compartment-water phase equilibrium distribution coefficient, thus, becomes:

$$ED_{bulk/aqueous,p} = (1 - fr\_V_{solid\ phase/bulk} - fr\_V_{gas\ phase/bulk}) + fr\_V_{solid\ phase/bulk} \cdot K_{sw,p} \cdot \rho_{solid\ phase} + fr\_V_{gas\ phase/bulk} \cdot K_{aw,p} \tag{A-12}$$

where

ED : equilibrium distribution coefficient relating the bulk compartment concentration to that of the aqueous phase [-]

fr_V : volume fraction of soil that is solid or gas phase [m^3_{phase} per $m^3_{bulk\ compartment}$]

K_{aw} : air-water partitioning coefficient or dimensionless Henry's law constant of substance p [-] (defined by Eq. (C-3))

K_{sw} : solid-water partitioning coefficient of substance p that may depend on pH or the organic carbon content of the respective compartment [kg/kg$_{solid\ phase}$ per kg/m^3_{water}] (defined in section C.1.1)

ρ : density of the solid phase [kg$_{solid\ phase}$ per $m^3_{solid\ phase}$].

For sediment and ground water (if distinguished), principally only the volume fraction of the gas phase becomes zero. Eq. (A-12) thus reduces to:

$$ED_{bulk/aqueous,p} = (1 - fr\_V_{solid\ phase/bulk}) + fr\_V_{solid\ phase/bulk} \cdot K_{sw,p} \cdot \rho_{solid\ phase} \quad . \tag{A-13}$$

The respective bulk-solid phase equilibrium distribution coefficient of sediments and ground water can be derived based on the corresponding bulk-aqueous phase equilibrium distribution coefficient:

$$ED_{\text{bulk/solid,p}} = \frac{(1 - fr\_V_{\text{solid phase/bulk}})}{K_{\text{sw,p}} \cdot \rho_{\text{solid phase}}} + fr\_V_{\text{solid phase/bulk}} = \frac{ED_{\text{bulk/aqueous,p}}}{K_{\text{sw,p}} \cdot \rho_{\text{solid phase}}} \quad \text{(A-14)}$$

The parameter $\rho_{\text{solid phase}}$ may be chosen by the user to differ for the land uses arable soil, pasture, semi-natural ecosystems, non-vegetated land and sediment based on data derived from a GIS dataset (Batjes, 1996) and the differentiation into streams and large lakes (cf. Eq. (B-10)).

A.2.2 Bulk water-suspended matter or aqueous phase equilibrium distribution coefficients

As discussed in section 6.1, the freshwater compartment only consists of water and suspended solids. The concentration in the bulk water compartment is defined accordingly:

$$C\_w/v_{\text{bulk water,p}} = C\_w/v_{\text{solid phase,p}} \cdot fr\_V_{\text{solid phase/bulk}} + C\_w/v_{\text{aqueous phase,p}} \cdot (1 - fr\_V_{\text{solid phase/bulk}}) \quad \text{(A-15)}$$

where

C_w/v : concentration in the bulk compartment or in one of its phases [kg per m^3]

ED : equilibrium distribution coefficient relating the bulk compartment concentration to that of the aqueous phase [-]

fr_V : volume fraction of soil that is solid phase [$m^3_{\text{solid phase}}$ per $m^3_{\text{bulk compartment}}$] (defined in section 5.1.3).

Relating the bulk concentration to the solid phase concentration yields the respective equilibrium distribution coefficient:

$$ED_{\text{bulk/solid,p}} = \frac{C\_w/v_{\text{bulk water,p}}}{C\_w/v_{\text{solid phase,p}}} \quad \text{(A-16)}$$

$$= fr\_V_{\text{solid phase/bulk}} + \frac{C\_w/v_{\text{aqueous phase,p}} \cdot (1 - fr\_V_{\text{solid phase/bulk}})}{C\_w/v_{\text{solid phase,p}}}$$

$$= fr\_V_{\text{solid phase/bulk}} + \frac{(1 - fr\_V_{\text{solid phase/bulk}})}{K_{\text{sw,p}} \cdot \rho_{\text{suspended matter}}}$$

$$= \frac{1}{ED_{\text{suspended matter/bulk water,p}}}$$

where

ED : equilibrium distribution coefficient relating the bulk compartment concentration to that of the solid phase (or relating the suspended matter phase to the bulk water compartment concentration) [-]

fr_V : volume fraction of freshwater that is solid phase [$m^3_{\text{solid phase}}$ per $m^3_{\text{bulk compartment}}$] (computed according to Eq. (A-17))

K_{sw} : solid-water partitioning coefficient of substance *p* [kg/$kg_{\text{solid phase}}$ per kg/m^3_{water}]

ρ : density of the solid phase [$kg_{\text{solid phase}}$ per $m^3_{\text{solid phase}}$].

$$fr\_V_{\text{solid phase/bulk}} = \frac{C\_w/v_{\text{suspended matter}}}{\rho_{\text{suspended matter}}} \quad \text{(A-17)}$$

The bulk water-aqueous phase equilibrium distribution coefficient (for diffusive intermedia exchange between water compartment and sediment compartment) can be computed analogously. Here, it is defined based on the bulk water-solid phase equilibrium distribution coefficient according to:

$$ED_{\text{bulk/aqueous,p}} = ED_{\text{bulk/solid,p}} \cdot K_{\text{sw,p}} \cdot \rho_{\text{suspended matter}} \, . \quad \text{(A-18)}$$

A.3 Environmental fate process formulations

In the following, the different environmental fate processes are described for which formulae are provided by WATSON. These can be combined in different ways as a so-called *process set* (cf. section 5.1).

A.3.1 Degradation

Degradation or rather chemical transformation may occur principally via biotic or abiotic processes (e.g., Schnoor, 1996; European Commission, 2003b). Such processes comprise hydrolysis, photolysis, biodegradation and co-metabolism.

A better notion for 'degradation' which might imply that a substance has been fully mineralised and does not pose any harm any longer could be 'chemical transformation' or 'inactivation'. In particular the latter notion might well be suited to comprise all processes that keep toxic substances from becoming effective (again).

Except for photolysis at the interface between air and the ground, degradation in the terrestrial and aquatic environment is assumed to occur in all compartments with liquid water, i.e., freshwater body (*i*: w), freshwater sediment (*i*: ws), impervious surface (*i*: u), non-vegetated land (*i*: b), (semi-)natural ecosystems (*i*: n), pasture/grassland (*i*: p) and arable land (*i*: ag), and is formulated according to:

$$k_{i,\,\mathrm{deg}}(p, i, z) = A(z) \cdot fr\_A(i, z) \cdot d(i, z) \cdot \frac{\ln(2)}{t_{1/2}(p, i)} \qquad \text{(A-19)}$$

where

A	:	area of zone z [m^2] (defined in section B.2)
d	:	depth of the compartment i in zone z [m] (defined in sections 5.1 and B.4.3)
fr_A	:	area fraction of compartment i in zone z [-] (defined in section B.3)
k	:	process rate for degradation [m^3 per s]
$t_{1/2}$	:	degradation half-life of substance p in compartment i [s^{-1}].

Note that the degradation half-life aggregates the different chemical transformation processes occurring simultaneously in one compartment.

A.3.2 Radioactive decay

Another process which leads to the disappearance of a modelled substance may be radioactive decay. In this case, single isotopes are addressed since the radioactive decay may indeed lead to a change in the nuclear composition of an atom but the number of protons might stay the same.

Radioactive decay is formulated equivalently to degradation but is not confined to compartments in which liquid water occurs, thus, *i* may correspond to any compartment distinguished:

$$k_{i,\,\mathrm{decay}}(p, i, z) = A(z) \cdot fr\_\mathrm{A}(i, z) \cdot d(i, z) \cdot \frac{\ln(2)}{t_{1/2}(p, i)} \tag{A-20}$$

where

A	:	area of zone z [m^2] (defined in section B.2)
d	:	depth of the compartment i in zone z [m] (defined in sections 5.1 and B.4.3)
fr_A	:	area fraction of compartment i in zone z [-] (defined in section B.3)
k	:	process rate for radioactive decay [m^3 per s]
$t_{1/2}$	:	decay half-life of radionuclide p in compartment i [s^{-1}].

A.3.3 Water soil erosion

Generally, erosion may be defined as "wearing away and transport of the soil by running water, glaciers, wind or waves" (Deutsches Nationalkomitee für das internationale Hydrologische Programm (IHP) der UNESCO und das Operationelle Hydrologische Programm (OHP) der WMO, 1998, p. 54). Here, only the erosion by water is modelled which is in line with all of the reviewed multimedia models (cf. sections 3.1 and 4.2.2).

Principally one needs to distinguish between different types of water soil erosion (e.g., sheet, rill, inter-rill, gully erosion, Shen and Julien, 1993; Morgan, 1999). However, models usually only try to estimate one to few types of erosion. For instance, the empirical Universal Soil Loss Equation (USLE, Wischmeier and Smith, 1978) or its revised version (RUSLE, Renard et al., 1997) have experienced a wide range of applications because of their simplicity (least data demanding, van der Knijff et al., 2000). They are used for on-site soil losses and have been developed for sheet and rill erosion (Wischmeier and Smith, 1978). Most erosion models are usually developed only for being applied to a certain site so that absolute values of these models at the regional scale are not reliable (van der Knijff et al., 2000). Erosion models for the regional scale itself that provide quantitative data are, however, lacking (Wickenkamp et al., 2000; Bach et al., 2001). Even simple models that only predict potential erosion rates require at least information on soil texture (Hennings, 1994), a soil property for which hardly any information is available in publicly available GIS datasets that would support regionally differentiated erosion assessments.

As indicated above, when assessing soil erosion from a soil or agricultural science perspective, usually only the loss at a given site is of interest which leads especially to a reduced soil fertility or production capacity (Morgan, 1999). As a consequence, very few of the erosion models predict how much of the soil arrives at adjacent areas or compartments. Attempts have been made to relate the results of the RUSLE to inputs into streams for example by means of the sediment delivery ratio concept (Umweltbundesamt, 1999). However, the RUSLE is still too data demanding at the regional scale and the sediment delivery ratio concept is highly questioned (Walling, 1983).

No transport of eroded soil from one terrestrial compartment to another is considered in WATSON for two reasons: (a) the compartments distinguished are assumed to be homogeneous implying that re-distribution of eroded soil within one compartment is irrelevant and (b) there is a lack of information about the situation of one compartment relative to another (cf. section 4.2.2). Rather, only the transport from the terrestrial environment into surface freshwater bodies is assessed. Zaslavsky (1979) quoted by Golubev (1982) estimated that only 10 % of the gross erosion is transported to the larger rivers, the remainder mostly being only re-distributed in the terrestrial environment (e.g., deposited on the lower parts of slopes). Walling (1983) estimates that only about 0.1 % to 38 % of the gross soil loss reach the rivers' outlets and are represented in the so-called sediment yield (see section B.5.3).

Although noting that the erosion process is selective with respect to particles of different size (e.g., Walling, 1983), it is assumed here to affect the bulk soil even including pore waters. One may argue that the process overland flow is responsible for the transport of pore waters. However, overland flow is perceived here to entrain that amount of a substance contained in soils that is in equilibrium with water that flows at the surface or near the surface ('interflow') as described in section A.3.4.

Due to the potentially low erosion rate on permanently vegetated areas like pastures/grassland and semi-natural ecosystems, water soil erosion is substantially reduced for these compartments (cf. section B.5.3). It is clear that this assumption is not appropriate in any situation. It is considered a justified first approximation, however, as this distinction is in line with both the considerably lower crop management factor of the Universal Soil Loss Equation (USLE) for forest and pasture soils (e.g., Golubev, 1982; Morgan, 1999; Umweltbundesamt, 1999) as well as with existing forest soil models (e.g., Reinds et al., 1995). Allowing the water soil erosion rate only to vary by compartments is, furthermore, supported by the present paucity or rather absence of regional erosion estimates or modelling capabilities at the regional scale (Bach et al., 2001) for the whole of Europe.

The process of water soil erosion which is allowed to occur on arable land (i: ag), pastures (i: p), semi-natural ecosystems (i: n) and non-vegetated land (i: b) is calculated according to:

$$k_{i\text{-}w,\,\text{erosion}}(z,i) = A(z)\cdot fr\_A(i,z)\cdot v_{\text{erosion}}(i) \tag{A-21}$$

where

A : area of zone z [m^2] (defined in section B.2)

fr_A : area fraction of compartment i in zone z [-] (defined in section B.3)

k : process rate for water soil erosion [m^3 per s]

v : erosion velocity of compartment i [m per s] (defined in Table 5-7).

A.3.4 Overland flow

Overland flow or rather saturated overland flow (Mosley and McKerchar, 1993) may be defined as "(f)low of water over the ground before it enters a definite channel" (Deutsches Nationalkomitee für das internationale Hydrologische Programm (IHP) der UNESCO und das Operationelle Hydrologische Programm (OHP) der WMO, 1998, p. 109). This process is contained in many multimedia models (cf. Table 5-4).

There are different causes why water does not penetrate the ground but flows over it instead (Rawls et al., 1993). The probably most important example is the so-called Hortonian overland flow (Rodhe and Killingtveit, 1997) which occurs when the infiltration capacity of a soil is exceeded by the rain intensity.

From a runoff formation point of view, i.e., the formation of that "part of the precipitation that appears as streamflow" (Deutsches Nationalkomitee für das internationale Hydrologische Programm (IHP) der UNESCO und das Operationelle Hydrologische Programm (OHP) der WMO, 1998, p. 109), one may want to distinguish between the three components (a) saturated overland flow, (b) interflow and (c) baseflow or return flow from ground water (Mosley and McKerchar, 1993). While vertical percolation of water through a soil column is mostly responsible for ground water recharge and, thus, contributes or sustains the baseflow, interflow passes through the subsurface similar to the baseflow but is quicker resembling more the dynamics of the saturated overland flow. This is also why interflow together with saturated overland flow are also referred to as 'quickflow' (Mosley and McKerchar, 1993).

The data available for the water balance within WATSON allow the distinction of ground water recharge from the overall runoff (cf. section B.5.2). As a result, the process of overland flow is extended to comprise the whole water undergoing 'quickflow', i.e., including interflow. Although interflow water may pass the subsurface at depth below 30 cm (corresponding to the default soil compartment depth; cf. section 5.1.2), it is assumed here that it does not leave the topsoil towards the deeper subsurface.

One may argue that the extended overland flow process is responsible for the transport of pore waters. However, overland flow is perceived here to lead to an equilibration of substances contained in soils with water flowing at the surface or near the surface ('interflow') whereas the process of water soil erosion is responsible for soil pore water displacements (cf. section A.3.3). Due to the fact that the compartments are rather large in this regional scale environmental fate modelling approach, the contact time of the waters undergoing quickflow is assumed to be sufficiently long for the substances to reach equilibrium, noting that this will not be the case for any substance.

The extended overland flow process for the pervious compartments, i.e., arable land (*i*: ag), pastures (*i*: p), semi-natural ecosystems (*i*: n) and non-vegetated land (*i*: b), is defined as:

$$k_{i\text{-}w,\,\text{overland flow},\,pH|\text{C}_{\text{org}}}(p,i,z) = \text{A}(z)\cdot fr\_A(i,z)\cdot \frac{v_{\text{runoff}}(z)\cdot fr\_\text{v}_{\text{quick flow/runoff}}(z)}{ED_{\text{bulk/aqueous}\,,\,pH|\text{C}_{\text{org}}}(p,i,z)} \tag{A-22}$$

where

A : area of zone z [m^2] (defined in section B.2)

ED : equilibrium distribution coefficient of a substance p of the respective compartment i of zone z that may depend on a compartment's pH or organic carbon content [-] (defined in section A.2)

fr_A : area fraction of compartment i in zone z [-] (defined in section B.3)

fr_V : fraction of runoff being quickflow in zone z [-] (defined in section B.5.2)

k : process rate for the extended overland flow [m^3 per s]

v : runoff in zone z [m per s] (defined in section B.5.2).

For the impervious terrestrial compartments, one has to further distinguish between glaciers and sealed areas. Whereas precipitation to glaciers is assumed to be solid ('snow') which only start to flow substantially upon melting (cf. section A.3.5), saturated overland flow (in its strict sense) is modelled for impervious surfaces according to:

$$k_{u-w,\text{ overland flow, pH}|\,C_{org}}(p, u, z) = A(z) \cdot fr\_A(u, z) \cdot \frac{v_{runoff}(z)}{ED_{\text{bulk/aqueous, pH}|C_{org}}(p, u, z)} \qquad \text{(A-23)}$$

where

A : area of zone z [m^2] (defined in section B.2)

ED : equilibrium distribution coefficient of a substance p of the respective compartment i of zone z that may depend on a compartment's pH or organic carbon content [-] (defined in section A.2)

fr_A : area fraction of compartment i in zone z [-] (defined in section B.3)

k : process rate for overland flow from impervious surfaces [m^3 per s]

v : runoff in zone z [m per s] (defined in section B.5.2).

A.3.5 Ice melt

As with soils, the assumption of homogeneity is unlikely to be true for glaciers (Baumgartner and Liebscher, 1990). As it seems that so far nobody has ever addressed the influence of glaciers on the overall fate of persistent pollutants in a multimedia context, a simple formulation has been adopted to start with. For the reasoning why glaciers are distinguished at all, refer to section 5.1.11.

The process ice melt leads to the release of flowing water by glaciers and consequently of substances contained in the ice which are delivered to the freshwater compartment:

$$k_{gl\text{-}w,\text{ ice melt}}(z, gl) = A(z) \cdot fr\_A(gl, z) \cdot \frac{d(gl, z)}{t_{residence}(gl)} \qquad \text{(A-24)}$$

where

A : area of zone z [m^2] (defined in section B.2)

d : depth of glaciers gl [m] (defined in section 5.1.11)

fr_A : area fraction of compartment i in zone z [-] (defined in section B.3) k : process rate for ice melt [m^3 per s]

$t_{residence}$: residence time of water in glaciers *gl* [s].

The rate by which this process takes place is defined according to the residence time. The residence of water in Alpine glaciers amounts to 100 years according to Table 9.1 in Baumgartner and Liebscher (1990) which is adopted here and which is assumed to be also valid for the other glaciers occurring in the modelled area.

A.3.6 Matrix leaching

The process matrix leaching transports substances dissolved (at equilibrium) in soil pore water flowing towards the subsurface. This flowing water constitutes the ground water recharge and finally the baseflow in the runoff formation process (Mosley and McKerchar, 1993, cf. section A.3.4). The matrix leaching process is defined for pervious soils, i.e., arable land (*i*: ag), pastures (*i*: p), semi-natural ecosystems (*i*: n) and non-vegetated land (*i*: b):

$$k_{i\text{-}gw,\ \mathrm{leaching},\ \mathrm{pH}|C_{\mathrm{org}}}(z, i, p) = A(z) \cdot fr\_\mathrm{A}(i, z) \cdot \frac{(1 - fr\_v_{\mathrm{quick\ flow/runoff}}(z)) \cdot v_{\mathrm{runoff}}(z)}{ED_{\mathrm{bulk/aqueous},\ \mathrm{pH}|C_{\mathrm{org}}}(p, i, z)} \tag{A-25}$$

where

A : area of zone *z* [m^2] (defined in section B.2)

ED : equilibrium distribution coefficient of a substance *p* of the respective compartment *i* of zone *z* that may depend on a compartment's pH or organic carbon content [-] (defined in section A.2)

fr_A : area fraction of compartment *i* in zone *z* [-] (defined in section B.3)

fr_V : fraction of runoff being quickflow in zone *z* [-] (defined in section B.5.2)

k : process rate for matrix leaching [m^3 per s]

v : runoff in zone *z* [m per s] (defined in section B.5.2).

An example of water percolating through soil that is not at equilibrium with the soil matrix is presented in section A.3.7.

If a ground water compartment was distinguished, the process 'ground water exfiltration with sorption' would be formulated correspondingly connecting the ground water compartment to the surface freshwater compartment of the same zone.

A.3.7 Considering vertical substance transport in soils due to stochastic processes

Many soil parameters are conceived as the realization of a random spatial field (e.g., Richter et al., 1996) which is due to the rather stochastic soil behaviour with respect to water and substance transport. A prominent example for a stochastic transport process within soils is preferential flow (Gish and Shirmohammadi, 1991). This is a non-equilibrium process in terms of both water flow (Beven, 1991; 'preferential flow' strictly speaking) and solutes entrained therein (Helling and Gish, 1991; Luxmoore, 1991; Stagnitti et al., 1995; Schwarz and Kaupenjohann, 2000; 'preferential transport'). This process is more the rule than the exception (Flury, 1996) and may have different causes (Wittig et al., 1985; Helling and Gish, 1991; Steenhuis and Parlange, 1991; Schwarz and Kaupenjohann, 2000). It even also applies to atmospheric deposition to forests (Wittig et al., 1985; Chang and Matzner, 2000).

As stated in Steenhuis and Parlange (1991), the amount of water percolating through the top soil layer may be distinguished into preferential and matrix flow which is adopted here.

Another stochastic process is colloidal transport (Jarvis et al., 1999; Noack et al., 2000) which can be considered to be part of the process 'preferential transport' defined by Eq. (A-27). This is also relevant especially for those trace elements which bind to organic matter such as lead and cadmium (Bergkvist et al., 1989).

Reduced matrix leaching due to preferential flow

This process is introduced in order to take into account that a portion of the wet atmospheric deposition is directly transferred to the subsurface soil layers for permeable terrestrial land uses (cf. section A.6.4). The amount of water undergoing this process does not have the time to fully equilibrate with the soil matrix ('non-equilibrium transport', Schwarz and Kaupenjohann, 2000) allowing to distinguish the rain water from the soil pore water in equilibrium with the soil matrix (Luxmoore, 1991). As a consequence, it is assumed here that the preferential flow portion of the wet precipitation is not available to matrix leaching. The equation is, therefore, introduced to subtract the amount of water undergoing preferential flow.

The reduced matrix leaching process is defined for pervious compartments, i.e., arable land (*i*: ag), pastures (*i*: p), semi-natural ecosystems (*i*: n) and non-vegetated land (*i*: b), as follows:

$$k_{i\text{-}gw,\ \mathrm{pref\ flow,\ pH|C_{org}}}(z,i,p) = -A(z)\cdot fr\_\mathrm{A}(i,z)\cdot\frac{v_{\mathrm{rain}}(z)\cdot fr\_v_{\mathrm{pref\ flow/rain}}(z)}{ED_{\mathrm{bulk/aqueous,\ pH|C_{org}}}(p,i,z)} \tag{A-26}$$

where

A	:	area of zone z [m^2] (defined in section B.2)
ED	:	equilibrium distribution coefficient of a substance p of the respective compartment i of zone z that may depend on a compartment's pH or organic carbon content [-] (defined in section A.2)
fr_A	:	area fraction of compartment i in zone z [-] (defined in section B.3)
fr_V	:	fraction of precipitation undergoing preferential flow in zone z [-] (defined in section B.5.2)
k	:	process rate for reduced matrix leaching [m^3 per s]
v	:	precipitation in zone z [m per s] (defined in section B.5.2).

Assuming that preferential flow does not lead to an accelerated movement of a substance already contained in a soil to the subsurface is rather conservative in the sense that preferential flow will carry away some of the dissolved ('displacement of matrix water', cf. Helling and Gish, 1991) and adsorbed phases of substances in soils. Therefore, another process is introduced which is described next.

Preferential transport

Preferential flow may displace part of matrix water (cf. Helling and Gish, 1991). Thus, only subtracting the amount of rainwater immediately undergoing preferential flow may not be sufficient to account for this process (cf. equation (A-26)) as parts of the substance contained in the soil will also be affected. For instance, the amounts of pesticides lost due to this process normally lie in the range of smaller than 0.1 % and 1 % and may reach up to 5 % under worst case conditions (Flury, 1996). When also including colloidal transport, a value for the amount to bypass the top soil layers of 0.1 %, thus, appears to be a reasonable first (conservative) estimate. In order to convert this overall mass balance into a rate, the 0.1 %

are assumed to apply to an annual mass balance meaning that 0.1 % of the annual amount of substances present in the soil reaches the subsurface by preferential transport. The respective rate is, thus, 0.001 per year. One has to note, however, that this rate may be substantially higher for non-degrading substances such as trace elements. However, different volatilisation and adsorption behaviours, for instance, play a role here so that the value is adopted for the time being for any substance until more specific information becomes available.

The preferential transport process is defined for pervious compartments, i.e., arable land (*i*: ag), pastures (*i*: p), semi-natural ecosystems (*i*: n) and non-vegetated land (*i*: b), as follows:

$$k_{i\text{-}gw,\ \text{preferential transport}}(z, i, p) = A(z) \cdot fr\_\mathrm{A}(i, z) \cdot r_{\text{preferential transport}}(p, i) \qquad \text{(A-27)}$$

where

A : area of zone *z* [m^2] (defined in section B.2)

fr_A : area fraction of compartment *i* in zone *z* [-] (defined in section B.3)

k : process rate for the extended overland flow [m^3 per s]

r : rate of preferential transport of substance *p* in compartment *i* [s^{-1}] (defined in the text above).

A.3.8 Uptake by biota and removal

As described in section 5.2 on plants and 6.2 on freshwater fish, living organisms do not constitute separate compartments in the environmental fate model. In regulatory risk assessments when following rather conservative assessment principles, removal of substances from the environment due to intake by organisms and subsequent consumption by (other) animals or humans is often not considered (e.g., European Commission, 1996a). This causes the environmental media concentrations to be larger due to lower removal rates. In spite of not distinguishing biotic compartments in the environmental fate modelling, a substance's removal across the model's boundary due to uptake by biota followed by harvest or catches, respectively, may still be considered.

The harvest and catch rates are set equivalent to the amounts produced per year. This is because the root uptake by plants as well as bioconcentration by fish are assumed to be in equilibrium with the medium on which the organisms thrive. When assessing the amount removed due to intercepting a part of the atmospheric deposition, the actual time the produce is exposed is also considered (see section A.6.5).

Root uptake by and harvest of belowground produce

As argued in section 5.2, belowground produce can be considered in equilibrium with soil for both organic substances and metals while receiving negligible amounts from aboveground plant parts. In order not to distinguish a separate belowground plant compartment for computational efficiency reasons but still allow for removal of the amount of substances that is contained in the harvested plant parts, a combined process is, thus, formulated here.

Based on the bioconcentration factor for root produce relating bulk dry weight root concentration to bulk dry weight soil concentration (equation 5-20B from United States - Environmental Protection Agency (1998), modified) and the production rate of the root produce, the root uptake by and harvest of belowground produce can be described. Additionally converting the bulk soil (volumetric) concentration into a dry soil (mass-based) concentration the combined process can be written as:

$$k_{\text{i, uptake+harvest root crops}} = \frac{1}{fr\_V_{\text{solid phase/bulk}}(i) \cdot \rho_{\text{solid phase}}(i, z)} \cdot emp_{\text{BCF, root crops}}(p, r, e) \cdot fr\_w_{\text{solid phase/bulk}}(r, e) \cdot BCF\_dw/dw_{\text{root/soil}}(p, r, e) \cdot P(r, n) \quad \text{(A-28)}$$

where

BCF_dw/dw: bioconcentration factor of substance *p* due to root crop *r* uptake from soil [kg_{soil} DW per kg_{plant} DW] (defined in section C.2)

emp : empirical correction factor for equilibrium uptake of substance *p* by belowground produce *r* dependent on the substance's octanol-water partitioning coefficient (K_{ow}) [-]

fr_V : volume fraction of soil that is solid phase [$m^3_{\text{solid phase}}$ per $m^3_{\text{bulk compartment}}$] (defined in section 5.1.3)

fr_w : mass fraction of food (*r*) dry matter [kg DW per kg FW] (defined in Table B-22)

k : process rate of root uptake by and harvest of root crops with respect to compartment *i* [m^3 per s]

P : production rate of crop *r* in administrative unit *n* [kg FW per s] (defined as described in section B.6.1)[38]

ρ : density of the solid phase [$kg_{solid\ phase}$ per $m^3_{solid\ phase}$] (defined by Eq. (B-10)).

The empirical correction factor assumes values between 1 and 0.01. According to the recommendations given by United States - Environmental Protection Agency (1998), a value of 1 should be used if log K_{ow} is less than 4 and 0.01 otherwise. As argued in section 5.2.2, an intermediate value of 0.1 for log K_{ow} range from 2 to 4 could additionally be introduced based on the findings by Riederer (1995) and Trapp (2002).

Note that the k-value is representative only for one type of root crop. If there are different types of root crops produced on one agricultural soil compartment and if any of the parameters 'production rate', 'mass fraction of food dry matter', or 'BCF' differs, a sum over the respectively resulting k-values needs to be computed according to (for the explanation of the symbols refer to the equation above):

$$k_{i,\ uptake+harvest\ root\ crops} = \frac{1}{fr\_V_{solid\ phase/bulk}(i) \cdot \rho_{solid\ phase}(i, z)} \cdot emp_{BCF,\ root\ crops}(p, r, e) \cdot \sum_{x = r_1, r_2, \ldots} [fr\_w_{solid\ phase/bulk}(x, e) \cdot BCF\_dw/dw_{root/soil}(p, x, e) \cdot P(x, n)] \quad \text{(A-29)}$$

Note that the empirical factor at present does not distinguish between different belowground crops and is, therefore, not contained in the sum. Further note that the production rate needs to be distributed from administrative units (denoted by *n* here) to zones. This is done on an area-weighted basis.

Root uptake by and harvest of aboveground produce for non-volatile substances

As phloem flow for non-essential heavy metals can be disregarded, the concentrations found in aboveground protected produce solely depend on soil concentrations and corresponding uptake. For aboveground exposed produce, the

[38] The removal will be underestimated based on the amounts produced per year provided by the Food Balance Sheets (FBSs, Food and Agriculture Organization of the United Nations - Statistics Division, 2002a). This is because losses for example between the harvest and the sale are not included in the production data.

contribution by atmospheric deposition needs to be considered additionally (see section A.6.5).[39] Its exposure via root uptake is formulated in the same way as for aboveground protected produce. Note that this process is not formulated for forage taken in for example by cattle. This is mainly because there is no statistical production data available in the FAO statistical database presumably due to the fact that forage is not traded across national borders.

Based on the bioconcentration factor for aboveground produce relating bulk dry weight aboveground protected produce concentration to bulk dry weight soil concentration (equation 5-20B United States - Environmental Protection Agency (1998), modified) and the production rate, the root uptake by and harvest of aboveground produce can be described. Additionally converting the bulk soil (volumetric) concentration into a dry soil (mass-based) concentration, the combined process can be written as:

$$k_{i,\ \text{uptake+harvest aboveground crops}} = \frac{1}{fr\_V_{\text{solid phase/bulk}}(i) \cdot \rho_{\text{solid phase}}(i, z)} \cdot fr\_w_{\text{solid phase/bulk}}(r, e) \cdot BCF\_dw/dw_{\text{plant/soil}}(p, r, e) \cdot P(r, n) \tag{A-30}$$

where

BCF_dw/dw: bioconcentration factor of substance p due to aboveground produce r uptake from soil [kg_{soil} DW per kg_{plant} DW] (defined in section C.2)

fr_V : volume fraction of soil that is solid phase [$m^3_{\text{solid phase}}$ per $m^3_{\text{bulk compartment}}$] (defined in section 5.1.3)

fr_w : mass fraction of food (r) dry matter [kg DW per kg FW] (defined in Table B-22)

k : process rate of root uptake by and harvest of aboveground crops with respect to compartment i [m^3 per s]

P : production rate of crop r in administrative unit n [kg FW per s] (defined as described in section B.6.1)

---

[39] In the case of (semi-) volatile substances, diffusive air-plant exchanges may need to be included for exposed produce. In order to consider this process, it is preferred to follow an approach that allows for kinetic, i.e., non-equilibrium transfer at the plant surface. This would make it necessary that a plant compartment is introduced in the environmental fate model.

ρ : density of the solid phase [$kg_{solid\ phase}$ per $m^3_{solid\ phase}$] (defined by Eq. (B-10)).

Again note that the k-value is representative only for one type of aboveground produce. If there are different types of aboveground produce produced on one agricultural soil compartment and if any of the parameters 'production rate', 'mass fraction of food dry matter', or 'BCF' differs, a sum over the respectively resulting k-values needs to be computed according to (for the explanation of the symbols refer to the equation above):

$$k_{i,\ uptake+harvest\ aboveground\ crops} = \frac{1}{fr\_V_{solid\ phase/bulk}(i) \cdot \rho_{solid\ phase}(i, z)} \cdot \sum_{x = r_1, r_2, \ldots} [BCF\_dw/dw_{plant/soil}(p, x, e) \cdot fr\_w_{solid\ phase/bulk}(x, e) \cdot P(x, n)] \quad \text{(A-31)}$$

Note that r stands for protected and exposed aboveground produce equally. Further note that the production rate needs to be distributed from administrative units (denoted by n here) to zones. This is done on an area-weighted basis.

Uptake by and catch of freshwater fish for non-volatile substances

Similar to the removal by plant harvest, a removal by fish catches is proposed. Based on the bioconcentration factor for fish relating bulk fish concentration to aqueous phase water concentration (equation 5-48, United States - Environmental Protection Agency, 1998) and the production rate, the uptake by and catch of freshwater fish can be described. Additionally converting the bulk water concentration into the aqueous phase concentration of the water compartment, the combined process can be written as:

$$k_{w,\ uptake+catch\ fish} = \frac{1}{Ksw \cdot ED_{bulk/solid} \cdot \rho_{suspendend\ matter}(w, z)} \cdot BCF\_V/fw_{fish/water}(p, r, e) \cdot P(r, n) \quad \text{(A-32)}$$

where

BCF_V/fw : bioconcentration factor of substance p due to fish r uptake from water [$m^3_{aqueous\ phase}$ per kg_{fish} FW] (defined in section C.2)

ED : bulk water compartment-suspended matter phase equilibrium distribution coefficient [$m^3_{\text{bulk compartment}}$ per $m^3_{\text{solid phase}}$] (defined in section A.2)

k : process rate of uptake by and catch of fish in freshwater *w* [m^3 per s]

K_{sw} : solid-water partitioning coefficient [$m^3_{\text{aqueous phase}}$ per $kg_{\text{solid phase}}$] (defined in section C.2)

P : production rate of freshwater fish *r* in administrative unit *n* [kg FW per s] (defined as described in section B.6.1)

ρ : density of the solid phase in the freshwater compartment of zone *z* [$kg_{\text{solid phase}}$ per $m^3_{\text{solid phase}}$] (defined as described in section B.5.4).

The k-value is representative only for one type of freshwater fish. If there are different types of freshwater fish caught in one freshwater compartment and if any of the parameters 'production rate' or 'BCF' differs, a sum over the respectively resulting k-values needs to be computed according to (for the explanation of the symbols refer to the equation above):

$$k_{\text{w, uptake+catch fish}} = \frac{1}{Ksw \cdot ED_{\text{bulk/solid}} \cdot \rho_{\text{suspendend matter}}(w, z)} \cdot \sum_{x = r_1, r_2, \ldots} \{BCF\_V/fw_{\text{fish/water}}(p, r, e) \cdot P(r, n)\} \qquad \text{(A-33)}$$

Note that the production rate needs to be distributed from administrative units (denoted by *n* here) to zones. This is done on an area-weighted basis.

A.3.9 Discharge

Discharge or rate of flow is defined as "volume of water flowing through a river (or channel) cross section in unit time" (Deutsches Nationalkomitee für das internationale Hydrologische Programm (IHP) der UNESCO und das Operationelle Hydrologische Programm (OHP) der WMO, 1998, p. 45). It is simply modelled by employing the value for discharge:

$$k_{w, z1 - z2, \text{discharge}}(z) = Q_{\text{discharge}}(z) \qquad \text{(A-34)}$$

where

k : process rate for discharge [m^3 per s]

Q : discharge occurring in zone z [m^3 per s] (defined in section B.5.2).

A.3.10 Water circulation in large lakes

In section B.2.1, reasons are given why some larger lakes are distinguished as separate zones. Following the Pfafstetter code system (section 4.3), only cascade-like downstream orientated flows can be determined. Due to the rather unnatural herringbone-like differentiation of larger lakes (cf. Fig. 6-2), the additional process 'water circulation in large lakes' has been introduced in order to also allow for an 'upstream' flow between zones of larger lakes. It is formulated analogously to the downstream flow process 'discharge' (section A.3.9) while adding the factor fr_Q:

$$k_{w,\, z_{\text{down}} - z_{\text{up,i}},\, \text{lake ciculation}}(z, w) = Q_{\text{discharge}}(z_{\text{down}}, w) \cdot fr\_Q_{\text{lake circulation}}(w) \qquad \text{(A-35)}$$

where

k : process rate for water circulation in large lakes [m^3 per s]

fr_Q : fraction of the discharge flowing out of zone z_{down} that is allowed to undergo 'upstream' flow into zone $z_{\text{up,i}}$ where the count of i may range from 0 to 2 depending on how many 'upstream' lake zones exist [-]; set to unity

Q : discharge occurring in zone z_{down} [m^3 per s] (defined in section B.5.2).

In order for the water mass balance to result, the same amount of water is set to flow from the potentially two upstream lake zones $z_{\text{up,i}}$ into the one downstream z_{down} according to:

$$k_{w,\, z_{\text{up,i}} - z_{\text{down}},\, \text{lake ciculation}}(z, w) = Q_{\text{discharge}}(z_{\text{down}}, w) \cdot fr\_Q_{\text{lake circulation}}(w)\,. \qquad \text{(A-36)}$$

A.3.11 Sedimentation (or sediment deposition) in freshwater compartments

Sedimentation is defined as the "(p)rocess of settling and depositing by gravity of suspended matter in water" (Deutsches Nationalkomitee für das internationale Hydrologische Programm (IHP) der UNESCO und das Operationelle Hydrologische Programm (OHP) der WMO, 1998, p. 133). It is, thus, a process involved in the particle mass turn-over in an aquatic ecosystem.

As discussed in sections 6.1, B.4 and B.5.4, the behaviour of streams is treated differently from that of large lakes. The overall process of sediment deposition is calculated according to:

$$k_{w\text{-}ws,\ \text{sedimentation, pH|pH inv|C}_{\text{org}}}(p, w, z) = \tag{A-37}$$

$$\frac{\mathrm{A}(z) \cdot fr\_A(w, z)}{ED_{\text{bulk/aqueous, pH|pH inv|C}_{\text{org}}}(p, w, z)} \cdot$$
$$[v_{\text{sedimentation, lake}}(w) \cdot fr\_\mathrm{V}_{\text{stagnant}}(w, z) +$$
$$v_{\text{sedimentation, stream}}(w) \cdot (1 - fr\_\mathrm{V}_{\text{stagnant}}(w, z))]$$

where

A	:	area of zone z [m^2] (defined in section B.2)
ED	:	equilibrium distribution coefficient of a substance p of the respective compartment i of zone z that may depend on a compartment's pH or organic carbon content [-] (defined in section A.2)
fr_A	:	area fraction of the freshwater compartment in zone z [-] (defined in section B.3)
fr_V	:	volume fraction of the freshwater compartment in zone z that is stagnant water [-] (defined in section B.5.4)
k	:	process rate for sedimentation [m^3 per s]
v	:	suspended matter deposition velocity in stagnant or flowing waters [m per s] (defined in section B.5.4).

For evaluative purposes, an additional formulation is implemented in WATSON which is in line with state-of-the-art multimedia models and does not take into account the weighting by the stagnant water volume. Instead an overall sedimentation rate is assumed for all water bodies. The rate corresponds to the pure lake condition as given in Table 6-4.

A.3.12 Resuspension of bottom sediment matter

Resuspension may be defined as the process that causes solids in the bottom sediment of a water body to become suspended again in the water column. Thus, resuspension is a process involved in the particle mass turn-over in an aquatic ecosystem. It is, therefore, mostly concerned with the translocation of particles. In most of the multimedia models which focus on the fate of lipophilic organic compounds which are hardly encountered in solution, it is reasonable to concentrate on the fraction of the substances that are bound to particles. However, particles are set into motion by eddies or currents in the water which will also entrain the surrounding aqueous phase of the sediments. This is especially important for more hydrophilic compounds like several metals and their compounds. As a result, the process 'resuspension' is considered here to not only set a part of the sediment compartment into motion so that the sediment particles become suspended again but also to drag along the sediment pore water formerly surrounding those re-suspended particles. The rate is assumed to be the same for both of these phases. Thus, no equilibrium distribution coefficient is considered in Eq. (A-38) describing this process.

As discussed in sections 6.1, B.4 and B.5.4, the behaviour of streams is treated differently from that of large lakes. The overall process of resuspension is calculated according to:

$$k_{ws\text{-w, resuspension}}(ws, z) = A(z) \cdot fr\_A(w, z) \cdot [v_{\text{resuspension, lake}}(ws) \cdot fr\_A_{\text{stagnant water}}(ws, z) + v_{\text{resuspension, stream}}(ws) \cdot (1 - fr\_A_{\text{stagnant water}}(ws, z))] \quad \text{(A-38)}$$

where

A : area of zone z [m^2] (defined in section B.2)

fr_A : fr_A: area fraction of the freshwater compartment in zone z [-] (defined in section B.3)

$fr\_A_{stagnant}$: area fraction of the freshwater sediment compartment in zone z that is located below stagnant water [-] (defined in section B.5.4)

k : process rate for resuspension [m^3 per s]

v : resuspension velocity in stagnant or flowing waters [m per s] (defined in section B.5.4).

For evaluative purposes, an additional formulation is implemented in WATSON which is in line with state-of-the-art multimedia models. It reads for pH-dependent partitioning:

$$k_{ws\text{-}w,\ \mathrm{resuspension,\ pH}}(ws, z) = \frac{\mathrm{A}(z) \cdot fr\_A(w, z) \cdot v_{\mathrm{sedimentation}}(w) \cdot fr\_v_{\mathrm{resuspended/sedimentation}}(ws) \cdot Ksw(p, pH(z, ws)) \cdot \rho_{\mathrm{solid\ phase}}(ws, z)}{ED_{\mathrm{bulk/aqueous,\ pH}}(p, ws, z)} \qquad \text{(A-39)}$$

and for organic carbon-dependent partitioning:

$$k_{ws\text{-}w,\ \mathrm{resuspension,\ Corg}}(ws, z) = \frac{\mathrm{A}(z) \cdot fr\_A(w, z) \cdot v_{\mathrm{sedimentation}}(w) \cdot fr\_v_{\mathrm{resuspended/sedimentation}}(ws) \cdot Ksw_{C_{org}}(p, ws, z) \cdot \rho_{\mathrm{solid\ phase}}(ws, z)}{ED_{\mathrm{bulk/aqueous,}\ C_{org}}(p, ws, z)} \qquad \text{(A-40)}$$

where

A	:	area of zone z [m^2] (defined in section B.2)
ED	:	equilibrium distribution coefficient of a substance p of the sediment compartment of zone z relating the bulk concentration to the aqueous phase concentration [-] (defined in section A.2)
fr_A	:	area fraction of the freshwater compartment in zone z [-] (defined in section B.3)
fr_v	:	fraction of sedimentation rate being resuspended [-] (defined as described in Table 6-4 for pure lake conditions)
K_{sw}	:	solid-water partitioning coefficient of substance p that may depend on organic carbon or pH [$\mathrm{m^3}_{\mathrm{aqueous\ phase}}$ per $\mathrm{kg}_{\mathrm{solid\ phase}}$] (defined in section C.1.1)
k	:	process rate for resuspension [m^3 per s]
ρ	:	density of the solid phase [$\mathrm{kg}_{\mathrm{solid\ phase}}$ per $\mathrm{m^3}_{\mathrm{solid\ phase}}$] (defined as described in section B.5.4)
v	:	sedimentation velocity [m per s] (defined as described in Table 6-4 for pure lake conditions).

A.3.13 Sediment burial

Burial refers to the rate at which contaminants move from the active to the inactive sediment layer. In contrast to resuspension in which both the solid and the aqueous phase are involved, only the particles are assumed to undergo this process. This is because the volume fraction of water decreases substantially with sediment depth so that the water is thought to 'stay' whereas the solids settle and become compacted.

As discussed in sections 6.1, B.4 and B.5.4, the behaviour of streams is treated differently from that of large lakes. The overall process of sediment burial for substances whose partitioning behaviour is dependent on the sediment's pH is calculated according to:

$$k_{ws,\,\text{burial, pH|pH}_{\text{inv}}}(p, ws, z) = \mathrm{A}(z) \cdot fr\_A(w, z) \cdot \frac{\rho_{\text{solid phase}}(ws, z) \cdot Ksw(p, pH(ws, z))}{ED_{\text{bulk/aqueous, pH|pH}_{\text{inv}}}(p, ws, z)} \cdot [v_{\text{burial, lake}}(ws) \cdot fr\_\mathrm{A}_{\text{stagnant water}}(ws, z) + v_{\text{burial, stream}}(ws) \cdot (1 - fr\_\mathrm{A}_{\text{stagnant water}}(ws, z))] \qquad \text{(A-41)}$$

For partitioning dependent on the sediment's organic carbon content, the calculation reads:

$$k_{ws,\,\text{burial, C}_{\text{org}}}(p, ws, z) = \mathrm{A}(z) \cdot fr\_A(w, z) \cdot \frac{\rho_{\text{solid phase}}(ws, z) \cdot Ksw_{\text{C}_{\text{org}}}(p, ws, z)}{ED_{\text{bulk/aqueous, C}_{\text{org}}}(p, ws, z)} \cdot [v_{\text{burial, lake}}(ws) \cdot fr\_\mathrm{A}_{\text{stagnant water}}(ws, z) + v_{\text{burial, stream}}(ws) \cdot (1 - fr\_\mathrm{A}_{\text{stagnant water}}(ws, z))] \qquad \text{(A-42)}$$

where

A : area of zone *z* [m^2] (defined in section B.2)

ED : equilibrium distribution coefficient of a substance *p* of the respective compartment *i* of zone *z* relating the bulk concentration to the aqueous phase concentration [-] (defined in section A.2)

fr_A : fr_A: area fraction of the freshwater compartment in zone *z* [-] (defined in section B.3)

$fr\_A_{stagnant}$: area fraction of the freshwater sediment compartment in zone z that is located below stagnant water [-] (defined in section B.5.4)

K_{sw} : solid-water partitioning coefficient of substance p that may depend on organic carbon or pH [$m^3_{aqueous\ phase}$ per $kg_{solid\ phase}$] (defined in section C.1.1)

k : process rate for sediment burial [m^3 per s]

ρ : density of the solid phase [$kg_{solid\ phase}$ per $m^3_{solid\ phase}$] (defined as described in section B.5.4)

v : sediment burial velocity in stagnant or flowing waters [m per s] (defined in section B.5.4).

For evaluative purposes, an additional formulation is implemented in WATSON which is in line with state-of-the-art multimedia models. It reads for pH-dependent partitioning:

$$k_{ws,\ burial,\ pH}(p, ws, z) = \frac{A(z) \cdot fr\_A(w, z) \cdot v_{sedimentation}(w) \cdot fr\_v_{burial/sedimentation}(ws) \cdot Ksw(p, pH(z, ws)) \cdot \rho_{solid\ phase}(ws, z)}{ED_{bulk/aqueous,\ pH}(p, ws, z)} \tag{A-43}$$

and for organic carbon-dependent partitioning:

$$k_{ws,\ burial,\ C_{org}}(p, ws, z) = \frac{A(z) \cdot fr\_A(w, z) \cdot v_{sedimentation}(w) \cdot fr\_v_{burial/sedimentation}(ws) \cdot Ksw_{C_{org}}(p, ws, z) \cdot \rho_{solid\ phase}(ws, z)}{ED_{bulk/aqueous,\ C_{org}}(p, ws, z)} \tag{A-44}$$

where

A : area of zone z [m^2] (defined in section B.2)

ED : equilibrium distribution coefficient of a substance p of the respective compartment i of zone z relating the bulk concentration to the aqueous phase concentration [-] (defined in section A.2) fr_A : area fraction of the freshwater compartment in zone *z* [-] (defined in section B.3)

fr_v : fraction of sedimentation rate finally buried [-] (defined as described in Table 6-4 for pure lake conditions)

K_{sw} : solid-water partitioning coefficient of substance *p* that may depend on organic carbon or pH [$m^3_{aqueous\ phase}$ per $kg_{solid\ phase}$] (defined in section C.1.1)

k : process rate for resuspension [m^3 per s]

ρ : density of the solid phase [$kg_{solid\ phase}$ per $m^3_{solid\ phase}$] (defined as described in section B.5.4)

v : sedimentation velocity [m per s] (defined as described in Table 6-4 for pure lake conditions).

A.3.14 Diffusion from water body to sediment

Apart from advective processes, substances may also migrate from one compartment into another due to diffusion. This migration is usually described based on the stagnant two-film model or two-resistance theory (Mackay, 1985; Schwarzenbach et al., 1993; Cowan et al., 1995b; Brandes et al., 1996; Wania et al., 2000). The inverse of the mass transfer coefficients or velocities can be interpreted as a transfer resistance. This also applies to diffusion taking place at the sediment-water interface. In contrast to the soil-air interface, there are only two resistances which are connected in series. The overall mass transfer coefficients $v_{diffusion}$ results accordingly:

$$\frac{1}{v_{diffusion}} = \frac{1}{v_{diffusion,\ sediment\text{-}side}} + \frac{1}{v_{diffusion,\ water\text{-}side}} \quad \text{(A-45)}$$

$$\Rightarrow v_{diffusion} = \frac{v_{diffusion,\ sediment\text{-}side} + v_{diffusion,\ water\text{-}side}}{v_{diffusion,\ sediment\text{-}side} \cdot v_{diffusion,\ water\text{-}side}}.$$

The respective sediment-side and water-side partial mass transfer coefficients can generally be computed by dividing the respective effective diffusivities by their corresponding diffusion path lengths (Schwarzenbach et al., 1993). However, a generic value for the overall mass transfer coefficient will be employed here (see section B.4.4).

The overall process of diffusion from water body into sediment for substances whose partitioning behaviour is dependent on the sediment's pH is calculated according to:

$$k_{w-ws,\,\text{diffusion},\,\text{pH}|\text{pH}_{\text{inv}}}(p, w, z) = (A(z) \cdot fr\_A(w, z) \cdot v_{\text{diffusion}}(w)) / [ED_{\text{bulk/solid},\,\text{pH}|\text{pH}_{\text{inv}}}(p, w, z) \cdot Ksw(p, pH(w, z)|pH(w)) \cdot \rho_{\text{suspended matter}}(w, z)] \quad \text{(A-46)}$$

For partitioning dependent on the sediment's organic carbon content, the calculation reads:

$$k_{w-ws,\,\text{diffusion},\,C_{\text{org}}}(p, w, z) = (A(z) \cdot fr\_A(w, z) \cdot v_{\text{diffusion}}(w)) / [ED_{\text{bulk/solid},\,C_{\text{org}}}(p, w, z) \cdot Ksw_{C_{\text{org}}}(p, w, z) \cdot \rho_{\text{suspended matter}}(w, z)] \quad \text{(A-47)}$$

where

A : area of zone z [m^2] (defined in section B.2)

ED : equilibrium distribution coefficient of a substance p of the respective compartment i of zone z relating the bulk concentration to the solid phase concentration [-] (defined in section A.2)

fr_A : area fraction of the freshwater compartment in zone z [-] (defined in section B.3)

K_{sw} : solid-water partitioning coefficient of substance p that may depend on organic carbon or pH [$m^3_{\text{aqueous phase}}$ per $kg_{\text{solid phase}}$] (defined in section C.1.1)

k : process rate for diffusion from water body into sediment [m^3 per s]

ρ : density of the solid phase in the freshwater compartment of zone z [$kg_{\text{solid phase}}$ per $m^3_{\text{solid phase}}$] (defined as described in section B.5.4)

v : overall mass transfer coefficient for diffusion at the sediment-water interface [m per s] (defined in section B.4.4).

Note that the denominator corresponds to the equilibrium distribution coefficient that relates the bulk concentration to the aqueous phase concentration in the water compartment (cf. Eq. (A-18)).

A.3.15 Diffusion from sediment to water body

The process 'diffusion from sediment to water body' is described in analogy to that of the reverse process presented in section A.3.14 where also a discussion on the overall mass transfer coefficient is provided:

$$k_{ws\text{-}w,\ \mathrm{diffusion,\ pH|pH\ inv|C_{org}}}(p, ws, z) = \mathrm{A}(z) \cdot fr\_A(w, z) \cdot \frac{v_{\mathrm{diffusion}}(ws)}{ED_{\mathrm{bulk/aqueous,\ pH|pH\ inv|C_{org}}}(p, ws, z)} \tag{A-48}$$

where

A : area of zone z [m^2] (defined in section B.2)

ED : equilibrium distribution coefficient of a substance p of the respective compartment i of zone z relating the bulk concentration to the aqueous phase concentration [-] (defined in section A.2)

fr_A : area fraction of the freshwater compartment in zone z [-] (defined in section B.3)

k : process rate for diffusion from water body into sediment [m^3 per s]

v : overall mass transfer coefficient for diffusion at the sediment-water interface [m per s] (defined in section B.4.4).

A.4 Volume calculations

In order to compute the dynamic solution (cf. section A.1), it is necessary to know the volumes of each of the compartments. Three different equations are employed taking account of the different ways the volumes are determined:

1. terrestrial compartments other than impervious surfaces are assumed to have an invariant depth throughout the entire model's scope (cf. section 5.1.2),
2. impervious surfaces such as pavements are by definition impervious and do, thus, not have a real depth. On the other hand, they are not expected to constitute compartments that show long retention times. Therefore, their volume is set to the total annual amount of precipitation occurring at a given site (cf. section 5.1.10), and
3. the freshwater compartments have variable volumes depending on whether large lakes are present in a zone and also depending on the location within a

larger catchment (freshwater volume increases towards the river mouth, cf. section B.4). The volumes are at present determined externally and are directly provided. The same applies to freshwater sediments although having a constant depth.

The determination of the volumes is described in the following.

A.4.1 Volume calculation: non-urban terrestrial compartments

Volumes of terrestrial compartments with constant depths, i.e., arable land (*i*: ag), pastures (*i*: p), semi-natural ecosystems (*i*: n), non-vegetated land (*i*: b), glaciers (*i*: gl), are calculated according to:

$$V(i, z) = \mathrm{A}(z) \cdot fr\_A(i, z) \cdot d(i) \qquad \text{(A-49)}$$

where

A	: area of zone z [m^2] (defined in section B.2)
fr_A	: area fraction of compartment i in zone z [-] (defined in section B.3)
d	: depth of compartment i [m] (defined in section 5.1)
V	: volume of compartment i in zone z [m^3].

A.4.2 Volume calculation: urban/built-up area

The depth of the impervious compartment varies between zones (cf. section 5.1.10). The volume is calculated according to:

$$V(u, z) = \mathrm{A}(z) \cdot fr\_A(u, z) \cdot d(u, z) \qquad \text{(A-50)}$$

where

A	: area of zone z [m^2] (defined in section B.2)
fr_A	: area fraction of the impervious land compartment in zone z [-] (defined in section B.3)
d	: depth of the impervious land compartment [m] (defined in section 5.1.10)
V	: volume of the impervious land compartment in zone z [m^3].

A.4.3 Volume calculation: water and sediment

The volumes of the freshwater (i: w) and sediment compartments (i: ws) are calculated externally and provided in the database. The volume calculation simplifies to:

$$V(i, z) = V(i, z) \tag{A-51}$$

where
V : volume of compartment i in zone z [m^3].

A.5 Background concentration calculation

When calculating dynamically in the followed mathematical approach (cf. Eq. (A-1)), an initial concentration needs to be specified. If a 'pristine' environment is assumed, these background concentrations are set to zero. However, if emission takes places into an environment in which appreciable substance amounts are already present, it can be set to non-zero values for any compartment i distinguished:

$$\begin{aligned} bg_{\text{zero}}(i, z) &= 0 && \text{when no background is assumed} \\ bg_{\text{non-zero}}(p, i, z) &= C\_w/v_{\text{background}}(p, i) && \text{when background is considered} \end{aligned} \tag{A-52}$$

where
bg : background concentration of substance p in compartment i of zone z [kg per m^3]

C_w/v : background concentration of substance p in compartment i [kg per m^3].

Note that the non-zero background concentrations are at present only allowed to vary by compartments and not by zones.

A.6 Exogenous input formulations

Any model that is confined to a part of a system that is not entirely closed needs to set boundary conditions. According to the followed mathematical approach, the boundary conditions consist of the perturbation vector ($\vec{b}$ in Eq. (A-1)) that defines exogenous inputs into the modelled system. Results from air quality models or releases directly into the media soil or water may constitute such exogenous inputs. The way these are formulated is described in the following sections.

A.6.1 Direct emissions into soil or water

Direct emissions may principally occur into any compartment distinguished although substantial releases of substances directly into sediments or glaciers are rather unlikely to occur. At present only releases into arable land (*i*: ag) and freshwater (*i*: w) are distinguished which may be due to soil amendments or sewer effluents for instance (note that similar to the exposure assessment the specification of direct releases into water and soil is according to administrative units, cf. Fig. B-4):

$$S_{j,\text{ direct input}}(s, p, i, z) = S(s, p, i, z) \qquad \text{(A-53)}$$

where

S : source strength of substance p into compartment i of zone z according to scenario s due to direct releases [kg per s].

A.6.2 Atmospheric deposition - wet

Atmospheric deposition is usually distinguished into wet and dry (e.g., Seinfeld, 1986). During wet atmospheric deposition, substances in air are absorbed by droplets which in turn are removed from the atmosphere by precipitation. Any compartment in contact with the atmosphere, i.e., arable land (*i*: ag), pastures (*i*: p), semi-natural ecosystems (*i*: n), non-vegetated land (*i*: b), glaciers (*i*: gl), impervious surfaces (*i*: u) and freshwater (*i*: w), may receive inputs by this process:

$$S_{a\text{-}i,\text{ wet atmospheric deposition}}(z, s, p, i) = A(z) \cdot fr\_\mathrm{A}(i, z) \cdot ATMDEP_{\text{wet}}(s, p, z) \qquad \text{(A-54)}$$

where

A : area of zone z [m^2] (defined in section B.2)

ATMDEP : wet atmospheric deposition of substance p in zone z for scenario s [kg per m^2 per s][40]

fr_A : area fraction of compartment i in zone z [-] (defined in section B.3)

---

[40] Note that the atmospheric deposition may stem from different sources. These may be reported depositions or those estimated by means of air quality models. Presently, the results from the Windrose Trajectory Model (WTM) as described in section 4.1 are used.

S : source strength of substance p into compartment i of zone z according to scenario s due to wet atmospheric deposition [kg per s].

A.6.3 Atmospheric deposition - dry

Atmospheric deposition is usually distinguished into wet and dry (e.g., Seinfeld, 1986). During dry atmospheric deposition, substances in air are taken up by the earth's surface which may constitute of soil, water, or vegetation. Any compartment in contact with the atmosphere, i.e., arable land (i: ag), pastures (i: p), semi-natural ecosystems (i: n), non-vegetated land (i: b), glaciers (i: gl), impervious surfaces (i: u) and freshwater (i: w), may receive inputs by this process:

$$S_{a\text{-}i,\,\text{dry atmospheric deposition}}(z,s,p,i) = A(z)\cdot fr\_\text{A}(i,z)\cdot ATMDEP_{\text{dry}}(s,p,z) \qquad \text{(A-55)}$$

where

A : area of zone z [m^2] (defined in section B.2)

ATMDEP : dry atmospheric deposition of substance p in zone z for scenario s [kg per m^2 per s][40]

fr_A : area fraction of compartment i in zone z [-] (defined in section B.3)

S : source strength of substance p into compartment i of zone z according to scenario s due to dry atmospheric deposition [kg per s].

A.6.4 Wet atmospheric deposition considering preferential flow/leaching

When considering preferential flow which is discussed in section A.3.7, the wet atmospheric deposition needs to be treated differently from what was presented in section A.6.2. In general, one needs to distinguish permeable from impermeable surfaces. This is because the process formulation for impermeable compartments follows that of the 'ordinary' case.

Wet atmospheric deposition to permeable soils (preferential flow distinguished)

When allowing preferential flow to be active (cf. section A.3.7), it is assumed that a certain fraction of the precipitation instantly passes the top soil which is represented by the soil compartment (cf. section 5.1.2). Thus, this portion of the precipitation and the corresponding substances contained therein are directly moved to below the top soil. As a result, this portion of the wet atmospheric deposition needs to be disregarded in terms of input to the top soil. The process affects any compartment that may receive inputs from the atmosphere and is permeable, i.e., arable land (i: ag), pastures (i: p), semi-natural ecosystems (i: n) and non-vegetated land (i: b):

$$S_{a\text{-}i,\ \text{wet atmospheric deposition/pref flow}}(z, s, p, i) = A(z) \cdot fr\_A(i, z) \cdot ATMDEP_{\text{wet}}(s, p, z) \cdot (1 - fr\_v_{\text{pref flow/rain}}(z)) \qquad \text{(A-56)}$$

where

A	:	area of zone z [m^2] (defined in section B.2)
ATMDEP	:	wet atmospheric deposition of substance p in zone z for scenario s [kg per m^2 per s][40]
fr_A	:	area fraction of compartment i in zone z [-] (defined in section B.3)
fr_V	:	fraction of precipitation undergoing preferential flow in zone z [-] (defined in section B.5.2)
S	:	source strength of substance p into compartment i of zone z according to scenario s due to wet atmospheric deposition allowing for preferential flow [kg per s].

Wet atmospheric deposition to compartments other than permeable soils (preferential flow distinguished)

The process formulation for impermeable compartments including freshwater follows that as presented in section A.6.2. The only difference that exists concerns the compartments to which it applies. These are freshwater (i: w), glacier (i: gl) and urban/built-up area/impervious surface (i: u).

Wet atmospheric deposition to the subsurface through preferential flow/leaching

If the subsurface of the top soil was distinguished (e.g., ground water), the direct input from the atmosphere to this part of the environment via preferential flow would need to be described explicitly. Preferential flow can of course only occur if the ground that receives atmospheric inputs is permeable at all, i.e., covered by the compartments arable land (*i*: ag), pastures (*i*: p), semi-natural ecosystems (*i*: n) and non-vegetated land (*i*: b). In order to define the permeable share of the zonal area, the area shares of freshwater (*i*: w), glacier (*i*: gl) and urban/built-up area/ impervious surface (*i*: u) are subtracted from the total area share of 100 % if these compartments exist:

$$S_{a\text{-}j,\text{ wet atmospheric deposition}}(z,s,p) = A(z) \cdot fr\_v_{\text{pref flow/rain}}(z) \cdot (1 - fr\_A(w,z) - fr\_A(gl,z) - fr\_A(u,z)) \cdot ATMDEP_{\text{wet}}(s,p,z) \tag{A-57}$$

where

A : area of zone *z* [m^2] (defined in section B.2)

ATMDEP : wet atmospheric deposition of substance *p* in zone *z* for scenario *s* [kg per m^2 per s][40]

fr_A : area fraction of the compartments freshwater (*i*: w), glacier (*i*: gl) and/or urban/built-up area/impervious surface (*i*: u) in zone *z* [-] (defined in section B.3)

fr_V : fraction of precipitation undergoing preferential flow in zone *z* [-] (defined in section B.5.2)

S : source strength of substance *p* into compartment *j* of zone *z* according to scenario *s* due to preferential flow [kg per s].

A.6.5 Removal of atmospheric deposition due to harvest of exposed aboveground produce

In general, aboveground plant parts intercept a portion of the dry and wet atmospheric deposition. In the case of exposed aboveground produce, i.e., produce that is in direct contact with the atmosphere, the intercepted portion of the substance may contribute directly or indirectly to human exposure. In order to allow for removal of substances which are intercepted due to harvest, two process formulations are suggested here.

Table A-1: Parameter needs for the assessment of particle deposition to aboveground produce that are neither related to substance nor to plant characteristics (like plant biomass, time until harvest)

Reference	Parameter required	Remarks
TRIM.FaTE (United States - Environmental Protection Agency, 2002b)	Interception fraction for dry deposition [-]	used in equations TF 7-1 and TF 7-2 (ibid.); can be derived if vegetation attenuation factor [m^2/kg], wet aboveground non-woody vegetation biomass inventory per unit area [kg/m^2] and water content of leaves [-] are known
	Interception fraction for wet deposition [-]	used in equations TF 7-3 and TF 7-4a (ibid.); can be derived by the LAI [-], vegetation-dependent leaf-wetting factor [m] and amount of rainfall of a rainfall event [m] are known or use the default value of 0.2
Equation 5-13 in (United States - Environmental Protection Agency, 1998)	Fraction of wet deposition that adheres to plant surfaces [-]	recommended value (Table B-2-7, ibid.): 0.2 for anions 0.6 for cations and organics and insoluble particles
	Interception fraction of the edible portion of plant tissue [-]	can either be derived with the help of an empirical constant and the standing crop biomass [kg/m^2] or a recommended value can be used which is 0.39 (see section 5.3.1.1, ibid.)
	Plant surface loss coefficient [$time^{-1}$]	recommended value (section 5.3.1.2, ibid.): 18 [$year^{-1}$] ~ 0.05 [day^{-1}]; the parameter allows for wind removal, water removal and growth dilution and is stated to be conservative as it does not include degradation

There are only two models given in Table 5-8 describing particulate deposition to plant surfaces (United States - Environmental Protection Agency, 1998, 2002b). Both methods are fairly data-intensive, requiring data for the parameters described in Table A-1 that are neither related to substance nor to plant characteristics (like plant biomass, time until harvest).

A closer look at the definition of the parameters in Table A-1 reveals that the parameter 'Interception fraction of the edible portion of plant tissue' and 'Interception fraction for dry deposition' are identical (defined by the same formula of the same reference). The recommended value for 'Interception fraction of the edible portion of plant tissue' in United States - Environmental Protection Agency (1998) could, thus, also be used as a default value for 'Interception fraction for dry deposition' used by TRIM.FaTE (United States - Environmental Protection Agency, 2002b).

It appears that there are two options for the inclusion of the particulate deposition process for non-volatile substances:

1. relying on net adsorption rates as provided by United States - Environmental Protection Agency (1998) which can be combined with a harvest rate without distinguishing a separate 'particles on plant/leaves' compartment or
2. modelling deposition and additionally removal either due to blow off or wash off in the environmental fate model according to TRIM.FaTE (United States - Environmental Protection Agency, 2002b) by introducing a separate 'particles on plant/leaves' compartment.

In either case, the use of quite a few default values seems to be necessary. Also it must be taken account of the fact that the soil below the vegetation compartment receives less input directly from air.

The net adsorption approach under number 1) is adopted for the following reasons. In TRIM.FaTE the processes wash off and blow off of particles from leaves only occur when there is or there is no rain, respectively. This would bring about the need to distinguish between rain and non-rain episodes being accomplished by a meteorological (on/off) toggle in TRIM.FaTE which is not available in the air quality model WTM (described in section 4.1) based on which the present environmental fate and exposure assessment is performed. A second reason is that it is tried here not to introduce too many compartments into the environmental fate model. A third reason might be that the formulation of exchange processes with the plant interior poses difficulties (Riederer, 1995; and note in Maddalena et al., 2002) although these are not so much relevant for non-volatile metals for which the question whether these penetrate the plant cuticle or not is unresolved (see section 5.2.1).

United States - Environmental Protection Agency (1998) recommends equation 5-14 (given therein) for the assessment of concentrations in exposed aboveground produce. This equation relates emissions to plant concentrations. However, interception concerns depositions of particles or droplets which is why equation 5-13 (ibid.) relating depositions to plant concentrations is made use of here. This also complies to the mathematical formulation of multimedia models in general and WATSON specifically.

The Leaf Area Index (LAI) is implicitly taken into account by the two correction factors for the adhering fraction of wet deposition and the interception fraction of edible parts. In the '1 minus exponent' term the time duration of the actual exposure of the edible parts needs to be specified. Unlike for leafy produce, the exposure time of fruits that only appear after impregnation of the blossom will be shorter than the full growing season of the respective plant. Fruits are not explicitly mentioned here but can be treated equivalently.

Removal processes need to be formulated for dry and wet atmospheric deposition separately in order to allow for subtraction from the respective 'pure' atmospheric deposition process. Note that this process is not formulated for forage taken in for example by cattle. This is mainly because there is no statistical production data available in the FAO statistical database presumably due to the fact that forage is not traded (across national borders).

Removal from dry atmospheric deposition due to harvest of exposed aboveground produce

The removal from the dry atmospheric deposition is formulated as:

$$S_{\text{a-ag, dry deposition+harvest exposed crops}} = -ATMDEP_{\text{dry}}(s, p, z) \cdot emp_{\text{plant surface loss}}(r, e) \cdot fr\_w_{\text{intercept/deposition}}(r, e) \cdot \frac{P(r, n)}{Y\_fw(r, n, e)} \qquad \text{(A-58)}$$

where

ATMDEP : dry atmospheric deposition of substance p in zone z for scenario s [kg per m^2 per s][40]

emp : empirical correction factor for physical surface loss from plant r [s] (defined below)

fr_w : mass fraction of a substance that is intercepted by aboveground exposed produce r during atmospheric deposition [kg per kg]; 0.39 (United States - Environmental Protection Agency, 1998, p. 5-28)

P : annual production rate of crop r in administrative unit n [kg FW per s] (defined as described in section B.6.1)

S : source of substances [kg per s]; note that this is negative here as this part of the atmospheric deposition is directly redirected into the exposure assessment

Y_fw : yield of aboveground exposed produce r in administrative unit n [kg FW per m^2] (defined as described in section B.6.1).

The empirical correction factor is pre-calculated according to:

$$emp_{\text{plant surface loss}}(r, e) = \frac{1 - 10^{-(r_{\text{plant surface loss}}(r, e) \cdot t_{\text{exposure duration}}(r, e))}}{r_{\text{plant surface loss}}(r, e)} \qquad \text{(A-59)}$$

where

emp : Empirical correction factor for physical surface loss from plant r [s]

r : Physical surface loss rate for plant r [per s]; $5.7 \cdot 10^{-7}$ (United States - Environmental Protection Agency, 1998, p. 5-29)

t : Exposure duration of exposed produce r [s]; 5184000 (United States - Environmental Protection Agency, 1998, p. 5-30).

The S-value is representative only for one type of crop. If there are different types of aboveground exposed crops produced on one agricultural soil compartment and if any of the parameters 'production rate', 'yield of aboveground exposed produce', 'mass fraction of a substance that is intercepted', or 'empirical correction factor' differs, a sum over the respectively resulting S-values needs to be computed according to (for the explanation of the symbols refer to Eq. (A-58)):

$$S_{\text{a, dry deposition+harvest exposed crops}} = -ATMDEP_{\text{dry}}(s, p, z) \cdot emp_{\text{plant surface loss}}(r, e) \cdot \sum_{x = r_1, r_2, \ldots} \left[fr\_w_{\text{intercept/deposition}}(x, e) \cdot \frac{P(x, n)}{Y\_fw(x, n, e)} \right] \qquad \text{(A-60)}$$

Note that the empirical factor at present does not distinguish between different aboveground exposed crops and is, therefore, not contained in the sum. Further note that the production rate needs to be distributed from administrative units to zones, denoted by n and z respectively (cf. sections B.6 and B.2 on the respective spatial differentiation). This is done on an area-weighted basis.

Removal from wet atmospheric deposition due to harvest of exposed aboveground produce

The removal from wet atmospheric deposition due to harvest of exposed above-ground produce is formulated as:

$$S_{\text{a-ag, wet deposition+harvest exposed crops}} = -ATMDEP_{\text{wet}}(s, p, z) \cdot fr\_w_{\text{adhere/wet deposition}}(p, r, e) \cdot emp_{\text{plant surface loss}}(r, e) \cdot fr\_w_{\text{intercept/deposition}}(r, e) \cdot \frac{P(r, n)}{Y\_fw(r, n, e)} \tag{A-61}$$

where

ATMDEP : dry atmospheric deposition of substance *p* in zone *z* for scenario *s* [kg per m^2 per s][40]

emp : empirical correction factor for physical surface loss from plant *r* [s] (for its computation see above)

fr_w : $fr\_w_{\text{adhere/wet deposition}}$: mass fraction of a substance's *p* wet deposition that adheres to aboveground exposed produce *r* [kg per kg] (defined in Table C-7)

$fr\_w_{\text{intercept/deposition}}$: mass fraction of a substance that is intercepted by aboveground exposed produce *r* during atmospheric deposition [kg per kg]; 0.39 (United States - Environmental Protection Agency, 1998, p. 5-28)

P : annual production rate of crop *r* in administrative unit *n* [kg FW per s] (defined as described in section B.6.1)

S : source of substances [kg per s]; note that this is negative here as this part of the atmospheric deposition is directly redirected into the exposure assessment

Y_fw : yield of aboveground exposed produce *r* in administrative unit *n* [kg FW per m^2] (defined as described in section B.6.1).

The S-value is representative only for one type of crop. If there are different types of aboveground exposed crops produced on one agricultural soil compartment and if any of the parameters 'production rate', 'yield of aboveground exposed produce', 'mass fraction of a substance that is intercepted', 'mass fraction of a substance's wet deposition that adheres to aboveground exposed produce', or 'empirical correction factor' differs a sum over the respectively resulting S-values needs to be computed according to (for the explanation of the symbols refer to the equation above):

$$S_{\text{a, wet deposition+harvest exposed crops}} = -ATMDEP_{\text{wet}}(s, p, z) \cdot emp_{\text{plant surface loss}}(r, e) \cdot \sum_{x = r_1, r_2, \ldots} \left[\frac{P(x, n)}{Y\_fw(x, n, e)} \cdot fr\_w_{\text{intercept/deposition}}(x, e) \cdot fr\_w_{\text{adhere/wet deposition}}(p, x, e) \right] \quad \text{(A-62)}$$

Note that the empirical factor at present does not distinguish between different aboveground exposed crops and is, therefore, not contained in the sum. Further note that the production rate needs to be distributed from administrative units to zones, denoted by *n* and *z* respectively (cf. sections B.6 and B.2 on the respective spatial differentiation). This is done on an area-weighted basis.

Remaining atmospheric deposition to agricultural soil

The combined root uptake and harvest process can be regarded as an additional removal process. In the case of atmospheric deposition and harvest, however, one takes out a portion of processes that connects two compartments (air and soil), i.e., wet and dry atmospheric deposition. In order not to violate the mass conservation principle by taking out portions of the atmospheric wet and dry deposition due to harvest of aboveground exposed plant parts, the remaining input from air to soil due to atmospheric deposition needs to be defined. It shall, furthermore, be challenged whether it could possibly assume non-realistic values, i.e., become negative. The amount of atmospheric dry deposition that reaches the soil $S_{\text{a-j,effective dry atmospheric deposition}}$ is given according to Eq. (A-63). The respective amount of atmospheric wet deposition that reaches the soil $S_{\text{a-j,effective wet atmospheric deposition}}$ is defined accordingly (Eq. (A-64)). For the meaning of the symbols, refer to the previous sections.

$$S_{a\text{-}j,\ \text{effective dry atmospheric deposition}} = S_{a\text{-}j,\ \text{dry atmospheric deposition}} + S_{\text{a, dry deposition+harvest exposed crops}} = ATMDEP_{\text{dry}}(s,p,z)\cdot \left\{ A(z)\cdot fr\_A(i,z) - emp_{\text{plant surface loss}}(r,e)\cdot \sum_x \left[\frac{fr\_w_{\text{intercept/deposition}}(x,e)\cdot P(x,n)}{Y\_fw(x,n,e)}\right]\right\} \tag{A-63}$$

$$S_{a\text{-}j,\ \text{effective wet atmospheric deposition}} = S_{a\text{-}j,\ \text{wet atmospheric deposition}} + S_{\text{a, wet deposition+harvest exposed crops}} = ATMDEP_{\text{wet}}(s,p,z) \left\{ A(z)\cdot fr\_A(i,z) - emp_{\text{plant surface loss}}(r,e)\cdot \sum_x \left[\frac{P(x,n)}{Y\_fw(x,n,e)}\cdot fr\_w_{\text{intercept/deposition}}(x,e)\cdot fr\_w_{\text{adhere/wet deposition}}(p,x,e)\right]\right\} \tag{A-64}$$

The mass conservation principle would be violated if the term in braces became smaller than zero. This situation would occur if the area of the compartment was smaller than the product of the empirical plant surface loss factor and the sum in the equations above, i.e.:

$$A(z)\cdot fr\_A(i,z) < emp_{\text{plant surface loss}}(r,e)\cdot \sum_x \left[\frac{fr\_w_{\text{intercept/deposition}}(x,e)\cdot P(x,n)}{Y\_fw(x,n,e)}\right] \tag{A-65}$$

$$A(z)\cdot fr\_A(i,z) < emp_{\text{plant surface loss}}(r,e)\cdot \sum_x \left[\frac{P(x,n)}{Y\_fw(x,n,e)}\cdot fr\_w_{\text{intercept/deposition}}(x,e)\cdot fr\_w_{\text{adhere/wet deposition}}(p,x,e)\right] \tag{A-66}$$

It shall be explored when this would be the case by a worst case approach in which the right hand side assumes values as large as possible. The parameters 'mass fraction of a substance that is intercepted' and 'mass fraction of a substance's wet deposition that adheres to aboveground exposed produce' can at most become equal to one and are, hence, disregarded in this discussion. Both inequations become identical in this case. The following equation, therefore, needs to be fulfilled in order to obey the mass conservation principle:

$$A(z) \cdot fr\_A(i, z) > emp_{\text{plant surface loss}}(r, e) \cdot \sum_x \frac{P(x, n)}{Y\_fw(x, n, e)} \tag{A-67}$$

$$\frac{A(z) \cdot fr\_A(i, z)}{\sum_x \frac{P(x, n)}{Y\_fw(x, n, e)}} > emp_{\text{plant surface loss}}(r, e) = \frac{1 - 10^{-(r_{\text{plant surface loss}}(r, e) \cdot t_{\text{exposure duration}}(r, e))}}{r_{\text{plant surface loss}}(r, e)} \tag{A-68}$$

If the exposure duration was zero, the numerator of the empirical factor would become zero which would not constitute a problem. The other extreme would be that the numerator assumes a value close to one. In order to guarantee that in any case not more of a substance is removed than is actually deposited on the crops, this upper boundary limit of the numerator is considered:

$$\frac{A(z) \cdot fr\_A(i, z)}{\sum_x \frac{P(x, n)}{Y\_fw(x, n, e)}} > \frac{1}{r_{\text{plant surface loss}}(r, e)}. \tag{A-69}$$

The parameters 'annual production rate', 'cropland area' and 'yield of aboveground exposed produce' are interlinked in that only a certain cropland area ($A \cdot fr\_A$) can sustain an annual production rate (P) given the crop and location-specific yield (Y). A side-condition is that a crop is only once produced on a given area within the balancing period. If this was not the case the yield would need to be increased to obtain a yield integrated over a one year period. The annual production rate and the yield can be rewritten as:

$$P = M_{\text{crop x}} \cdot t_{\text{balance}}$$
$$Y\_fw = \frac{M_{\text{crop x}}}{A_{\text{crop x}}} \quad (A\text{-}70)$$

Assuming that only aboveground exposed produce was grown on the available agricultural area (i.e., $A(z) \cdot fr\_A(i,z) = A_{\text{crop x}}$) which is again an upper bound estimate, rarely the case at municipal levels or higher for which the production data are given (cf. section B.6.1), the left hand side assumes its smallest value which corresponds to the time over which the production balance is performed, i.e., the duration of one year:

$$t_{\text{balance}} > \frac{1}{r_{\text{plant surface loss}}(r, e)}$$
$$r_{\text{plant surface loss}}(r, e) > \frac{1}{t_{\text{balance}}} = \frac{1}{1 \text{ year}} = \frac{1}{31536000 \text{ seconds}} \quad (A\text{-}71)$$

Thus, as long as the plant surface loss rate is larger than the inverse of a one year period (here: in seconds), the removal of parts of the atmospheric deposition can be formulated in the way presented without violating the mass conservation principle. United States - Environmental Protection Agency (1998) suggests to use a value of 18 per year which fulfils this condition.

A.7 Exposure assessment

Two exposure assessment frameworks are presently implemented in WATSON. One is from the health physics (radionuclides) context (International Atomic Energy Agency, 2001) and the other concerned with hazardous air contaminants (United States - Environmental Protection Agency, 1998). Equations for both exposure assessment frameworks are given below as far as they are implemented. Some parameter values may depend on the exposure assessment employed which is denoted by an *e* in the brackets after the parameter's symbol in the equations to come.

Different exposure pathways are considered. Here, *exposure pathway* (or *food chain*) means any combination of (a) an environmental medium concentration as predicted by the fate model (e.g., agricultural soil concentration) based on which (b) different interrelated intermediate food concentrations are derived (e.g., wheat consumed by cow, milk) finally being (c) taken in by humans. This brings about that human exposure for example to milk is composed of the exposure pathways based on the ingestion of soil particles, forage, silage and grains by milk cattle. Each of the linkages or steps of an exposure pathway is termed an *exposure transfer*, i.e., a transfer from one medium, substrate, or receptor to another.

The calculation of the different exposure pathways principally may start with a unit conversion of the environmental fate results (section A.7.1). The different steps or exposure transfers of each of the exposure pathways are not shown separately below. Rather, these are aggregated into an overall equation that relates the concentration in the media as assessed by the environmental fate model to those in the different food items for each of the exposure pathways considered (section A.7.4 and following). These concentrations in the different food items are converted by a human consumption rate into the effective personal intake rate (section A.7.14) after taking trade of the respective food or potentially feed items into account (section A.7.13).

Note that when calculating dynamically, the initialization of the environmental fate concentrations needs special treatment which is presented in section A.7.3.

Further note that the intake rates provided in the following sections need to be multiplied by the population at the respective administrative unit in order to yield the overall mass taken up which is used for the computation of the (effective) Intake Fraction (cf. Eq. (7-3)).

A.7.1 Concentration conversion

The environmental fate model results in bulk concentrations that are given in weight of a substance per volume of a medium (kg per m^3). However, many of the equations in the exposure assessment of terrestrial food chains are based on concentrations that are given in weight of a substance per (dry or fresh) weight of the medium (kg per kg FW or kg per kg DW) according to United States - Environmental Protection Agency (1998). The food chains in the aquatic environment, in contrast, are based on the dissolved fraction of the substance. Consequently, different unit conversions need to be performed.

Conversion bulk soil to solid phase concentration

In the terrestrial environment, especially the transfer from soils into aboveground plant parts but also the ingestion of soil particles is based on bulk solid phase concentrations of the dried soil. The conversion from bulk concentrations (kg per m^3) into dry weight concentrations (kg per kg DW) for the compartments arable land (*i*: ag) and pastures (*i*: p) is performed according to:

$$C\_w/dw(i,z) = \frac{1}{fr\_V_{\text{solid phase/bulk}}(i) \cdot \rho_{\text{solid phase}}(i,z)} \cdot C\_w/v(i,z) \tag{A-72}$$

where

C_w/dw : concentration of a substance in compartment *i* of zone *z* [$kg_{chemical}$ per $kg_{solid\ phase}$ DW]

C_w/v : volumetric concentration of a substance in compartment *i* of zone *z* [$kg_{chemical}$ per $m^3_{bulk\ compartment}$] (result from the environmental fate model)

fr_V : volume fraction of compartment *i* that is solid phase [$m^3_{bulk\ compartment}$ per $m^3_{solid\ phase}$] (defined in section 5.1.3)

ρ : density of the solid phase in compartment *i* of zone *z* [kg_{solid} per m^3_{solid}] (defined by Eq. (B-10)).

Conversion bulk soil to solid phase concentration divided by solid-water partitioning coefficient

In the terrestrial environment, the transfer from soils into belowground produce is modelled based on the Root Concentration Factor (RCF). It relates the concentration of a substance in roots to its concentration in soil pore water. In order to use the concept of the RCF for substances that are not metals, the bulk concentration needs to be converted into the dissolved phase concentration according to United States - Environmental Protection Agency (1998) (cf. section A3.4.1). Note that for metals the so-called 'Plant-Soil Bioconcentration Factor in Root Vegetables' is used and consequently requires a different concentration conversion (see above). The conversion from bulk concentrations (kg per m^3) into aqueous phase weight concentrations (kg per kg of aqueous phase) for non-metals present in the compartments arable land (*i*: ag) and pastures (*i*: p) is, thus, performed according to:

$$C\_w/w_{i,\text{aqueous}} = \frac{1}{fr\_V_{\text{solid phase/bulk}}(c) \cdot \rho_{\text{solid phase}}(c,z) \cdot K_{sw,p} \cdot \rho_{\text{water}}(c)} \cdot C\_w/v_i \tag{A-73}$$

where

C_w/dw : concentration of a substance in compartment *i* of zone *z* [$kg_{chemical}$ per $kg_{solid\ phase}$ DW]

C_w/v	:	volumetric concentration of a substance in compartment *i* of zone *z* [$kg_{chemical}$ per $m^3_{bulk\ compartment}$] (result from the environmental fate model)
fr_V	:	volume fraction of compartment *i* that is solid phase [$m^3_{bulk\ compartment}$ per $m^3_{solid\ phase}$] (defined in section 5.1.3)
K_{SW}	:	solid-water partitioning coefficient of substance *p* that may depend on pH or the organic carbon content of the respective compartment [$kg/kg_{solid\ phase}$ per kg/m^3_{water}] (defined in section C.1.1)
ρ	:	density of the solid phase in compartment *i* of zone *z* [kg_{solid} per m^3_{solid}] (defined by Eq. (B-10)).

Conversion bulk water to dissolved phase concentrations

Transfer of substances from water into freshwater fish depends exclusively on the dissolved fraction of the substance according to the equations 5-48 and 5-49 given in United States - Environmental Protection Agency (1998). The conversion from bulk concentrations (kg per m^3 of bulk compartment) into concentrations in the dissolved phase (kg per m^3 of aqueous phase of the compartment) for non-metals in freshwater bodies is, thus, performed according to:

$$C\_w/v_{w,\text{aqueous}} = \frac{1}{K_{sw,p} \cdot ED_{\text{bulk/solid}} \cdot \rho_{\text{suspendend matter}}(w)} \cdot C\_w/v_{w,\text{bulk}} \qquad \text{(A-74)}$$

where

C_w/v	:	$C\_w/v_{aqueous}$: concentration of a substance in the aqueous phase of compartment *i* in zone *z* [$kg_{chemical}$ per $m^3_{aqueous\ phase\ of\ compartment}$] C_w/v_{bulk}: concentration of a substance in compartment *i* of zone *z* [$kg_{chemical}$ per $m^3_{bulk\ compartment}$] (result from the environmental fate model)
ED	:	equilibrium distribution coefficient of a substance *p* of the respective compartment *i* of zone *z* that may depend on a compartment's pH or organic carbon content [-] (defined in section A.2)

K_{sw} : solid-water partitioning coefficient of substance *p* that may depend on pH or the organic carbon content of the respective compartment [$kg/kg_{solid\ phase}$ per kg/m^3_{water}] (defined in section C.1.1)

fr_V : volume fraction of compartment *i* that is solid phase [$m^3_{bulk\ compartment}$ per $m^3_{solid\ phase}$] (defined in section 5.1.3)

ρ : density of suspended matter [kg_{solid} per m^3_{solid}] (defined in section B.5.4).

A.7.2 Assessment of inhalation exposures

Unlike ingestion, inhalation exposures are assessed with the help of the EcoSense model (European Commission, 1999a). In the case of trace elements, the relevant results are the concentrations in air that are given in microgram per cubic metre which need to be converted into kilogram per cubic metre. These concentrations are multiplied by the affected population in order to yield the accumulated inhalation exposure.

In order to apply the cancer and non-cancer slope factors as given in Tables 7-6 and 7-7, respectively, one needs to convert the accumulated inhalation exposure into an amount taken up. For this, the inhalation rate of the affected people is needed which principally depends on age, gender and body weight (United States - Environmental Protection Agency, 1997c, 1998). Values given in the literature range from 4.5 (United States - Environmental Protection Agency, 1997c) to 23 cubic metres per day (value quoted in Table 9.5 in European Commission, 1999a) for babies and male adults, respectively. Average rates of 20 and 20.6 cubic metres of inhaled air per day are used by United States - Environmental Protection Agency (1998) and Spadaro and Rabl (2004), respectively. The value of 20 cubic metres per day is adopted here although noting that average personal inhalation rates from about 14 to 23 cubic metres per day may be obtained for instance when following the approach taken in section 9.3.2 of European Commission (1999a) and using either the values provided therein or those by United States - Environmental Protection Agency (1997c).

The accumulated exposure as provided by the EcoSense tool is translated into the (effective) Intake Fraction due to inhalation at steady-state by taking the effective portion of the trace element into account according to:

$$IF_{\text{inhalation}} = \frac{fr\_w_{\text{effective/total}}(p) \cdot \frac{INH}{1000^3} \cdot \sum_n C\_w/v_{a,\text{n,bulk}} \cdot Population_n}{S} \tag{A-75}$$

where:

1000^3	:	conversion factor [µg per kg]
C_w/v	:	concentration of a substance in the air compartment of administrative unit n [$\mu g_{chemical}$ per m^3]
fr_w	:	mass fraction of substance *p* in air leading to an effect [kg per kg] (defined in Table C-2)
IF	:	(effective) Intake Fraction of a substance due to inhalation [$kg_{effective\ exposure}$ per $kg_{released}$]
INH	:	inhalation rate [m^3 per capita and s]; $2.32 \cdot 10^{-4} \sim 20$ m^3 per capita and day according to United States - Environmental Protection Agency (1998)
Population	:	population at administrative unit *n* [capita]
S	:	source strength of a substance [kg per s].

Note that the accumulated exposure yielded by the sum in the above equation is calculated with the help of the EcoSense software tool.

As for ingestion exposures, the Intake Fraction for inhalation in the dynamic case at time *t* (in full years) is given as:

$$IF_{\text{inhalation,t}} = \frac{fr\_w_{\text{effective/total}}(p) \cdot \dfrac{INH}{1000^3} \cdot \sum_n \sum_t C\_w/v_{a,\text{n,bulk,t}} \cdot Population_n}{\sum_t S_t}. \qquad \text{(A-76)}$$

A.7.3 Performing dynamic exposure assessment when removal due to harvest is included in the environmental fate model

In previous sections, processes leading to exposure were described that remove a substance at a certain rate from the environmental fate model. At steady-state and when the removal only affects the exogenous input (cf. sections A.6.5 and A.7.4 related to atmospheric interception), the exposure assessment can be based on the predicted environmental concentrations since the continuous release of a substance to the environment is balanced by all removals. When computing dynamically while considering harvest removals, in contrast, one needs to know how much of a substance has been removed in order to know the 'original' concentration without removal for example by plants. This is because 'original' concentration without removal is actually the concentration to which the process rate applied leading to the (reduced) predicted environmental concentration.

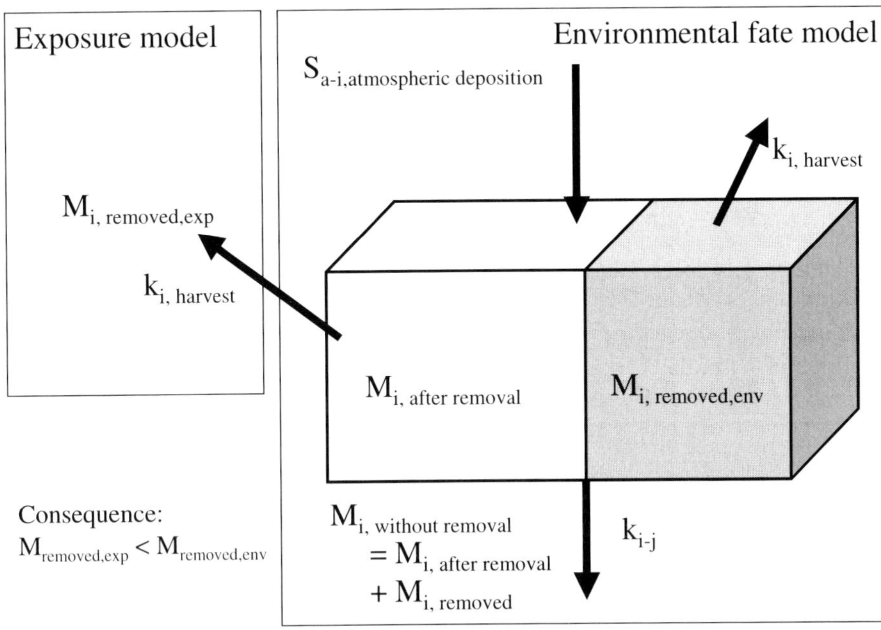

Fig. A-1: Masses with respect to removal due to harvest resulting in the environmental fate and exposure model in the dynamic case

Thus, in order not to assume a transfer rate based on a lower concentration when performing the exposure assessment, one needs to correct the depleted concentrations by the respective removal according to the following equation (cf. Fig. A-1):

$$\begin{aligned} M_{i,\text{ without removal}} &= M_{i,\text{ after removal}} + M_{\text{removed}} \\ C\_w/v_{i,\text{ without removal}} \cdot V_i &= C\_w/v_{i,\text{ after removal}} \cdot V_i + M_{\text{removed}} \end{aligned} \tag{A-77}$$

where

C_w/v : $C\_w/v_{i,\text{ without removal}}$: concentration that would have occurred in compartment *i* if no removal due to harvest of food had taken place [kg per m^3]

		$C\_w/v_{i,\text{ after removal}}$: concentration that was predicted by the environmental fate model in compartment *i* [kg per m^3]
M	:	M_{removed}: mass of substance removed [kg]
		$M_{i,\text{ after removal}}$: mass that was predicted by the environmental fate model in compartment *i* [kg]
		$M_{i,\text{ without removal}}$: mass that would have been contained in compartment *i* if no removal due to harvest of food had taken place [kg]
V_i	:	volume of compartment *i* [m^3] (defined in section A.4).

The 'mass of substance removed' can be calculated according to:

$$M_{\text{removed}} = C\_w/v_{i,\text{ without removal}} \cdot k_{\text{i, harvest}} \cdot \Delta t \tag{A-78}$$

where

C_w/v	:	concentration that would have occurred in compartment *i* if no removal due to harvest of food had taken place [kg per m^3]
k	:	process rate of combined uptake by and harvest of the organism [m^3 per s]
M_{removed}	:	mass of substance removed [kg]
Δt	:	time step of the iteration [s].

The concentration without removal can, thus, be computed as:

$$C\_w/v_{i,\text{ without removal}} = C\_w/v_{i,\text{ after removal}} + C\_w/v_{i,\text{ without removal}} \cdot \frac{k_{\text{i, harvest}} \cdot \Delta t}{V_i} \tag{A-79}$$

$$\Rightarrow C\_w/v_{i,\text{ without removal}} = \frac{C\_w/v_{i,\text{ after removal}}}{1 - \frac{k_{\text{i, harvest}} \cdot \Delta t}{V_i}}$$

The computation of the k-values differs for root uptake by belowground and aboveground produce as well as for bioconcentration by freshwater fish (cf. section A.3.8).

Note that the denominator might become zero or negative especially if the volume of the compartment is rather small. WATSON, therefore, checks internally whether the compartment's area share of the respective zone is smaller than the internally set cut-off criterion of 0.5 %. If so, the volume is considered almost negligible and the denominator is set to 0.5 by default.

A.7.4 Food concentration for the exposure pathway 'atmospheric deposition - aboveground exposed produce - humans' for the example of spinach

Although there is little evidence that the amount of substance deposited onto aboveground exposed produce contributes substantially to the overall load contained in a plant (e.g., World Health Organisation, 1992a; Gebel, 1999), this does not mean that exposure due to anthropogenically released substances is not significant via this exposure route. In fact, in EUSES this exposure pathway is not included, at the same time it is noted that "this route may be important for some chemicals" (European Commission, 1996a, p. II-44).

When selecting a crop for an exemplary food chain of this kind, it needs to be borne in mind that

- the produce is grown on open-land and not in a greenhouse (e.g., tomatoes to some extent),
- agricultural practice allows for significant exposure (e.g., cauliflower is protected for a certain amount of time in order not to change its colour to yellow), and
- most of the aboveground plant parts that are eaten are exposed; this is not the case for instance for lettuces and round cabbage.

Spinach appears to comply with all these aspects and has, therefore, been included in the assessment.

The removal from atmospheric deposition builds on the equations presented in section A.6.5 and can be formulated for one type of aboveground exposed produce such as spinach as:

$$C\_w/fw(r, n, p, e) = -[S_{\text{a, dry deposition+harvest exposed crops}} + S_{\text{a, wet deposition+harvest exposed crops}}] \cdot \frac{1}{P(r, n)} = \frac{emp_{\text{plant surface loss}}(r, e) \cdot fr\_w_{\text{intercept/deposition}}(r, e)}{Y\_fw(r, n, e)} \cdot [ATMDEP_{\text{dry}}(s, p, z) + ATMDEP_{\text{wet}}(s, p, z) \cdot fr\_w_{\text{adhere/wet deposition}}(p, r, e)] \quad \text{(A-80)}$$

where:

ATMDEP : dry or wet atmospheric deposition of substance p in zone z for scenario s [kg per m^2 per s][41]

emp : empirical correction factor for physical surface loss from plant r [s]

C_w/fw : concentration of substance p in food item r at the administrative unit n [kg_{chemical} per kg_{food} FW]

fr_w : $fr\_w_{\text{adhere/wet deposition}}$: mass fraction of a substance's p wet deposition that adheres to aboveground exposed produce r [kg per kg]

$fr\_w_{\text{intercept/deposition}}$: mass fraction of substance p that is intercepted by aboveground exposed produce r during atmospheric deposition [kg per kg]

P : production rate of crop r in administrative unit n [kg FW per s] (defined as described in section B.6.1)

S : removal of parts of the source of substances (i.e., dry or wet atmospheric deposition) due harvest of exposed aboveground crops [kg per s]; note that the values are negative indicating removal and need, therefore, be subtracted here

Y_fw : yield of aboveground exposed produce r in administrative unit n [kg FW per m^2] (defined as described in section B.6.1).

In contrast to many other exposure pathways, there is no need to convert units of concentrations. However, when calculating dynamically, interception might only occur in specific time periods. In any case, at time zero no emission

[41] See footnote 40 on page 421.

has as yet occurred. Therefore, the atmospheric deposition is set to zero. When assessing a pulse emission, the atmospheric deposition will cease after the pulse emission has terminated plus the length of the residence time of the respective substance in air. As a consequence, the atmospheric deposition after this time period also needs to be set to zero. The trace elements considered here occur in the atmosphere usually attached to particles. Particles of intermediate size show the longest residence times that are typically in the order of days (Jaenicke, 1998). Thus, the residence times in air can be neglected as pulse emissions of a one year period are usually considered (cf. Chapters 10 and 11).

A.7.5 Food concentration for the exposure pathway 'atmospheric deposition - forage/silage - cattle - humans'

Potentially, forage and silage like any other exposed aboveground produce may be exposed due to atmospheric deposition as well. However, the exposure pathways related to silage and/or forage exposure followed by transfer into dairy milk and beef/veal are not included into the assessment. This is due to the fact that (spatially-resolved) information especially on production data are not readily available for silage and forage which is necessary to compute this exposure pathway (cf. section A.7.4).

A.7.6 Food concentration for the exposure pathway 'arable land - aboveground protected produce - humans' for the example of cereals

The exposure pathway 'arable land - aboveground protected produce - humans' is based on the unit-converted concentration in the arable land compartment. At present only the cereals wheat, barley, rye and oats are considered. The related equation when following the exposure assessment provided by United States - Environmental Protection Agency (1998) reads:

$$C\_w/fw(r, n, p, e) = BCF\_dw/dw_{\text{plant/soil}}(p, r, e) \cdot fr\_w_{\text{solid phase/bulk}}(r, e) \cdot C\_w/dw_{\text{ag,solid}} \tag{A-81}$$

and the one according to International Atomic Energy Agency (2001) is:

$$C\_w/fw(r, n, p, e) = BCF\_dw/fw_{\text{plant/soil}}(p, r, e) \cdot C\_w/dw_{\text{ag,solid}} \tag{A-82}$$

where

BCF_dw/dw: bioconcentration factor of substance p due to crop r uptake from soil [kg_{soil} DW per kg_{plant} DW] (defined in section C.2)

BCF_dw/fw: bioconcentration factor of substance p due to crop r uptake from soil [kg_{soil} DW per kg_{plant} FW] (defined in section C.2)

C_w/fw : concentration of substance p in food item r at the administrative unit n [$kg_{chemical}$ per kg_{food} FW]

C_w/dw : concentration of substance p in arable land ag of zone z [$kg_{chemical}$ per $kg_{solid\ phase}$ DW] (unit-converted result of the environmental fate model)

fr_w : mass fraction of dry weight per fresh weight of food item r [kg_{food} DW per kg_{food} FW] (defined in Table B-22).

A.7.7 Food concentration for the exposure pathway 'arable land - aboveground exposed produce - humans'

As stated in section A.7.4, the only aboveground exposed produce considered is spinach. The assessment of root uptake follows that for aboveground protected produce given by Eq. (A-81).

A.7.8 Food concentration for the exposure pathway 'arable land - belowground produce - humans' for the example of potato

The exposure pathway 'arable land - belowground produce - humans' is based on the unit-converted concentration in the arable land compartment. Presently only potatoes are considered. The related equation when following the exposure assessment for metals provided by United States - Environmental Protection Agency (1998) reads:

$$C\_w/fw(r, n, p, e) = emp_{\text{BCF, root crops}}(p, r, e) \cdot BCF\_dw/dw_{\text{root/soil}}(p, r, e) \cdot fr\_w_{\text{solid phase/bulk}}(r, e) \cdot C\_w/dw_{\text{ag, solid}} \tag{A-83}$$

and the one according to International Atomic Energy Agency (2001):

$$C\_w/fw(r, n, p, e) = BCF\_dw/fw_{\text{plant/soil}}(p, r, e) \cdot C\_w/dw_{\text{ag, solid}} \tag{A-84}$$

where

BCF_dw/dw: bioconcentration factor of substance p due to crop r uptake from soil [kg_{soil} DW per kg_{plant} DW] (defined in section C.2)

BCF_dw/fw: bioconcentration factor of substance p due to crop r uptake from soil [kg_{soil} DW per kg_{plant} FW] (defined in section C.2)

C_w/dw : concentration of substance p in arable land ag of zone z [$kg_{chemical}$ per $kg_{solid\ phase}$ DW] (unit-converted result of the environmental fate model)

C_w/fw : concentration of substance p in food item r at the administrative unit n [$kg_{chemical}$ per kg_{food} FW]

fr_w : mass fraction of dry weight per fresh weight of food item r [kg_{food} DW per kg_{food} FW] (defined in Table B-22)

emp : empirical correction factor for equilibrium uptake of substance p by belowground produce r dependent on the substance's octanol-water partitioning coefficient (K_{ow}) [-] (defined in Table C-6).

A.7.9 Food concentration for the exposure pathways 'pasture/arable land - feed - milk cattle - humans'

The exposure pathways 'pasture/arable land - feed - milk cattle - humans' are based on the unit-converted concentration in the pasture and arable land compartment, respectively. To be more specific, 'feed' could mean forage, silage, or grains. These either grow on pastures (forage) or on arable land (silage and grains).

When following the exposure assessment provided by United States - Environmental Protection Agency (1998), the related equation for silage and forage reads:

$$C\_w/fw(r, n, p, e) = \{ING_{feed}(r_{animal}, e) \cdot BTF\_t/w_{milk/feed}(p, r_{animal}, e)\} \cdot BCF\_dw/dw_{plant/soil}(p, r_{plant}, e) \cdot C\_w/dw_{p|ag,solid} \quad \text{(A-85)}$$

The one for grains for which only wheat is presently considered is formulated as:

$$C\_w/fw(r, n, p, e) = fr\_w_{\text{wheat/total grain}}(r_{\text{animal}}, e) \cdot \{ING_{\text{feed}}(r_{\text{animal}}, e) \cdot BTF\_t/w_{\text{milk/feed}}(p, r_{\text{animal}}, e)\} \cdot BCF\_dw/dw_{\text{plant/soil}}(p, r_{\text{plant}}, e) \cdot C\_w/dw_{\text{ag,solid}} \tag{A-86}$$

Note that the 'soil bioavailability factor' and the 'metabolism factor' are not considered in Eqs. (A-85) and (A-86) as the recommended values are 1 (ibid., sections 5.4.4.6 and 5.4.4.7).

Only the exposure pathway 'pasture - forage - milk cattle - humans' is presently implemented for the IAEA exposure assessment (International Atomic Energy Agency, 2001):

$$C\_w/fw(r, n, p, e) = \frac{BTF\_t/v_{\text{milk/feed}}(p, r_{\text{animal}}, e) \cdot ING_{\text{forage}}(r_{\text{animal}}, e)}{\rho_{\text{food}}(r, e)} \cdot BCF\_dw/dw_{\text{plant/soil}}(p, r_{\text{plant}}, e) \cdot C\_w/dw_{\text{p, solid}} \tag{A-87}$$

where

BCF_dw/dw: bioconcentration factor of substance p due to crop r uptake from soil [kg_{soil} DW per kg_{plant} DW] (defined in section C.2)

BTF_t/v : biotransfer factor relating the amount of substance p contained the feed's volume taken in by animal r [s · capita per m^3] (defined in section C.2)

BTF_t/w : biotransfer factor relating the amount of substance p contained the feed's mass taken in by animal r [s · capita per kg FW] (defined in section C.2)

C_w/dw : concentration of substance p in arable land ag of zone z [$kg_{chemical}$ per $kg_{solid\ phase}$ DW] (unit-converted result of the environmental fate model)

C_w/fw : concentration of substance p in food item r at the administrative unit n [$kg_{chemical}$ per kg_{food} FW]

fr_w : mass fraction of grains fed to farm animals r consisting of wheat [-] (defined in Table B-23)

ING : ingestion rate of feed taken in by animal r [kg DW/capita/s] (defined in section B.6.3)

ρ : density of food (milk) [kg per m^3]; here: 1030.

Unlike the other exposure pathways, trade may not only be considered for the animal product that is finally consumed by the human population. Rather, also feed may be traded prior to consumption by the farm animals. This is especially the case for grains. Trade of grains is considered analogously to the trade of food items (cf. section A.7.13).

A.7.10 Food concentration for the exposure pathways 'pasture/arable land - feed - beef and veal cattle - humans'

The exposure pathways 'pasture/arable land - feed - beef cattle - humans' are computed analogously to the equations given in section A.7.9. The only adaptation that needs to be made is to choose the adequate BCF, BTF and feed ingestion values for beef cattle instead of milk cattle.

A.7.11 Food concentration for the different exposure pathways 'pasture (soil particles) - animal products - humans'

The exposure pathways 'pasture (soil particle) - animal products - humans' are based on the unit-converted concentration in the pasture compartment. To be more specific, 'animal products' could mean cattle milk, beef and veal, poultry meat, eggs from laying hens as well as pork.

The related equation when following the exposure assessment provided by United States - Environmental Protection Agency (1998) reads:

$$C\_w/fw(r, n, p, e) = fr\_w_{\text{free-range/total}}(r, n, e) \cdot C\_w/dw_{\text{p, solid}} \cdot [BTF\_t/w_{\text{animal product/feed}}(p, r, e) \cdot ING_{\text{soil}}(r, e)] \tag{A-88}$$

where

C_w/dw : concentration of substance p in arable land ag of zone z [kg_{chemical} per $kg_{\text{solid phase}}$ DW] (unit-converted result of the environmental fate model)

BTF_t/w : biotransfer factor relating the amount of substance p entrained by soil particles (or any other mass like feed) taken in by animal r [s · capita per kg FW] (defined in Table C-5 of section C.2)

fr_w : mass fraction of produce stemming from animals r kept in the free-range at administrative unit n [kg per kg] (defined in section 7.1.1)

ING : ingestion of soil by the animal r [kg DW/capita/s] (defined in section B.6.3).

Note that the 'soil bioavailability factor' and the 'metabolism factor' are not considered in Eq. (A-88) as the recommended values are 1 (ibid., sections 5.4.4.6 and 5.4.4.7).

A.7.12 Food concentration for the exposure pathway 'freshwater - fish - humans'

The exposure pathway 'freshwater - fish - humans' is based on the unit-converted concentration in the arable land compartment.

The related equation when following the exposure assessment provided by United States - Environmental Protection Agency (1998) reads:

$$C\_w/fw(r, n, p, e) = BCF\_V/fw_{\text{fish/water}}(p, r, e) \cdot C\_w/v_{w,\text{aqueous}} \tag{A-89}$$

where

C_w/fw : concentration of substance p in food item r at the administrative unit n [kg_{chemical} per kg_{food} FW]

C_w/v : concentration of a substance in the aqueous phase of compartment i in zone z [kg_{chemical} per $m^3_{\text{aqueous phase of compartment}}$] (unit-converted result of the environmental fate model)

BCF_V/fw : bioconcentration factor of substance p due to fish r uptake from water [$m^3_{\text{aqueous phase}}$ per kg_{fish} fresh weight] (defined in section C.2).

For non-lipophilic substances, only uptake from the water body into freshwater fish is relevant according to United States - Environmental Protection Agency (1998) (cf. section 5.7.5.3). The fish concentration of metals other than mercury consequently only results from the transfer from the dissolved phase of the substance in the water body.

A.7.13 Consideration of trade

From trade statistics (Food and Agriculture Organization of the United Nations - Statistics Division, 2002a), it is obvious that the net trade of certain food products differs between countries. This may lead on the one hand to higher exposures even at the society level if the food items produced in a country show a higher contaminant load while at the same being exported to a small extent. On the other hand, rather active trade relationships between countries will lead to exposures of people that may live at quite some distance from the contaminated environment in case of more localised sources.

In order to consider trade in an exposure pathway, it may be specified for each of the respective exposure transfers whether it involves trade. At present, trade is assumed to lead to homogeneous concentrations in food in general and also in certain types of feed across the geographical scope of WATSON. This 'homogenisation' may occur even more than once for an exposure pathway (e.g., both the wheat and the milk from the exposure pathway 'arable land - wheat - cattle milk - humans' is allowed to be traded). In future developments, a more detailed approach may be realized in which the amounts that are eaten nationally are distinguished from those transported across national borders. An aggregation at least at the national level is suggested as food consumption/supply data are only provided at this level within WATSON (see below and section B.6.2). There may be produces, however, that are not produced in one country but may as well be eaten in the respective country. This is the case for spinach for example. One cannot do without trade between countries in such instances unless one takes the risk to underestimate the overall exposure. The consideration of trade is, therefore, strongly recommended albeit its present initial status of consideration.

The transfer from an environmental compartment into an organism and from organism to organism is based on an equilibrium approach according to United States - Environmental Protection Agency (1998). When trade is assumed to occur, the predicted concentrations in the different food items are first multiplied by the production (or stock) occurring in the respective region. This production may be zero which is why the concentration predicted to this end is termed 'theoretical'. Then, the resulting substance masses given for the different administrative units are added and divided by the production of the reference area. This reference area could possibly be a country, but is at present the entire area covered by WATSON as given in Fig. B-1. Eq. (A-90) shows the involved calculation when trade is considered:

$$C\_w/fw(r, Europe, p, e)_{\text{average}} = \frac{t_{\text{year}} \cdot \sum_n C\_w/fw(r, n, p, e)_{\text{theoretical}} \cdot P(r, n)}{t_{\text{year}} \cdot \sum_n P(r, n)} \qquad \text{(A-90)}$$

where

C_w/fw : C_w/fw_{average}: average concentration of substance p in food item r in the geographical scope of the assessment ('Europe') as a result of considering production data [$kg_{chemical}$ per kg_{food} FW]

$C\_w/fw_{theoretical}$: concentration of substance p in food item r at the administrative unit n which is theoretical as this concentration may be assessed to occur in an administrative unit in which no respective food item is produced [$kg_{chemical}$ per kg_{food} FW] (defined in sections A.7.4 through A.7.12)

P : production rate of crop r in administrative unit n [kg FW per s] (defined as described in section B.6.1)

t : time for which the production rate is given [s], i.e., corresponding to one year.

This production-based weighting scheme leads to homogeneous concentrations of the food and feed items across the reference area. The human consumption of the respective food items is calculated according to nationally provided consumption data (cf. section B.6.2).

A.7.14 Computation of the effective personal intake rate from food concentrations

In order to arrive at the effective personal intake rate related to a respective exposure pathway, the corresponding fresh weight concentration in a food item is multiplied by the human consumption rate. As is discussed in more detail in sections 7.2 and B.6.2, furthermore, the amount of the food supply not consumed, the degree of the European food self-supply, and the portion of the substance potentially leading to an effect are taken account of:

$$\begin{aligned} IR\_p(r, n, p, e) = \; & fr\_w_{\text{effective/total}}(p, r, e) \cdot ING_{\text{human supply}}(r, n) \cdot \\ & fr\_w_{\text{self-supply}}(r, e) \cdot (1 - fr\_w_{\text{not consumed/food supply}}(r, e)) \cdot \\ & C\_w/fw(r, n, p, e) \end{aligned} \tag{A-91}$$

where

C_w/fw : concentration of substance p in food item r at the administrative unit n [$kg_{chemical}$ per kg_{food} FW] (defined in sections A.7.4 through A.7.12, note the comments in section A.7.13) fr_w : $fr\_w_{effective/total}$: mass fraction of substance *p* contained in food *r* leading to an effect [kg per kg] (defined in Table C-2)

$fr\_w_{self\text{-}supply}$: mass fraction of produce *r* produced in the geographical scope of the assessment [kg per kg] (defined in section B.6.2)

$fr\_w_{not\ consumed/food\ supply}$: mass fraction of (fresh) food that is produced and traded but not consumed [kg per kg] (defined in section B.6.2)

ING : ingestion of food item *r* by humans according to food supply information for the administrative unit *n* [kg FW/capita/s]

IR_p : effective personal intake rate of substance *p* contained in food item *r* by humans at the administrative unit *n* [kg/capita/s].

Trade is considered by averaging the food concentration across Europe prior to consumption according to the produced amounts of foods in the different countries, states, districts and/or municipalities (cf. section A.7.13).

It shall be noted that when the impact assessment is performed in a risk group-specific way (i.e., the dose-response function is given for only a sensitive portion of the population such as asthmatics, children, elderly people) particularly the respective food consumption behaviours also need to be given accordingly (for the explanation of most of the symbols refer to the equation above):

$$\begin{aligned} IR\_p_{\text{risk group}}(r(i), n, p, e) = \; & ING_{\text{human supply}}(r(i), n) \cdot \\ & fr\_r_{\text{risk group/population}}(r(i), n) \cdot fr\_w_{\text{self-supply}}(r, e) \cdot \\ & (1 - fr\_w_{\text{not consumed/food supply}}(r, e)) \cdot \\ & fr\_w_{\text{effective/total}}(p, r, e) \cdot C\_w/fw(r, n, p, e) \end{aligned} \tag{A-92}$$

where

fr_r : fraction of the population *r* that belongs to a certain risk group *i* in country *n* [-].

In order to compute the effective Intake Fraction, the sum of the effective personal intake rates of all risk groups need to be performed:

$$IR\_p(r, n, p, e) = \sum_i IR\_p_{\text{risk group}}(r(i), n, p, e). \tag{A-93}$$

A.8 Impact assessment

The equations used for the impact assessment are already fully contained in the main text. The reader is referred to Eqs. (7-16) through (7-19) in section 7.3.

A.9 Monetary valuation

The equations used for the monetary valuation have already been fully described in the main text. The reader is referred to Chapter 8.

Appendix B Substance-independent data

In this Appendix, the derivation of the spatially-resolved information necessary for the methodological framework is described. The focus is on the spatial information necessary to run the environmental fate model for soil and water, i.e., the spatial differentiation of the continental areas into zones or compartments and the derivation of parameter values varying spatially. However, section B.6 is also dedicated to the exposure as well as to the impact assessment. These follow a spatial differentiation based on administrative units mostly according to the Nomenclature of Territorial Units for Statistics (Nomenclature des Unités Territoriales Statistiques, NUTS) used by the Statistical Office of the European Communities (EUROSTAT).

In the following, first the geographical scope of the external cost assessment methodology is defined (section B.1). Secondly, the spatial differentiation of the 'continental environment' comprising the non-marine environment into zones is presented (section B.2). After the zones have been defined, their constituents namely the compartment entities need to be defined. This will be done separately for the soils and/or land uses on the one hand (section B.3) and freshwater bodies on the other hand (section B.4). In these sections, the dimensions of the different compartments will be defined. What remains to describe are the ways how the other environmental properties including fluxes of water are derived.

Generally, one may distinguish four different kinds of parameters in the spatially-resolved environmental fate model:

1. those that are invariant: such as universal or molar gas constant; a default ambient air temperature
2. those that vary by compartment (and not by zone): erosion rate; fraction of runoff being quick/direct flow; fraction of rain rate being preferential flow; depth (of soils, glaciers and sediment); sedimentation velocity lake; sedimentation velocity stream; sediment resuspension rate lake; sediment resuspension rate stream; net sediment burial rate; sediment burial rate lake;

sediment burial rate stream; volume fraction of sediment, ground water or soil that is solid phase; volume fraction of soil that is gas phase; density of the solid phase (default value); overall mass transfer coefficient diffusion at sediment-water interface; fraction of discharge in lake circulation; density of the organic solid phase; density of the mineral solid phase; density of water; mass fraction of organic carbon (Corg) in organic matter; pH (default values); volume fraction of freshwater that is stagnant water; volume fraction of freshwater that is stagnant water at large river mouth; fraction of sedimentation rate being resuspended; fraction of sedimentation rate finally buried

3. those that vary by region: most hydrology-related data fall into this category such as discharge, runoff, precipitation rate, evapotranspiration rate, temperature, fraction of runoff being quick/direct flow, and fraction of rain rate being preferential flow; furthermore: area of the different zones, area fraction of permeable soils, temperature
4. those that vary by region and compartment: depth (of freshwater bodies and impervious areas), volume (depending on the area of a compartment as the product of the zone, the corresponding compartment's area fraction and the depth), area fraction of a compartment, flow rate of lake water circulation, area fraction of total freshwater sediment lying below stagnant waters, volume fraction of freshwater that is stagnant water; parameters only varying for the different types of soils are density of the solid phase (depending on the organic carbon content), pH and Corg; density of suspended matter; concentration of suspended matter in freshwater bodies.

In section B.5, the spatially variable data of category 3 and 4 for the terrestrial environment as well as the hydrological cycle will be presented.

B.1 Defining the geographical scope of the model

The EcoSense model for stationary sources for Europe (European Commission, 1995; Krewitt et al., 2001) covers most of Europe and small parts of Asia (parts of Turkey) and Africa (parts of Morocco, Algeria, Tunisia and Libya; see Fig. B-1). For consistency reasons, the same geographical coverage is selected.

B.2 Spatial differentiation into zones

In site-dependent modelling, the whole area covered by the model needs to be distinguished into sub-areas. These sub-areas will be called 'zones' in this text.

For the definition of the zones, one has principally to distinguish between two environments: the terrestrial domain and the marine domain.

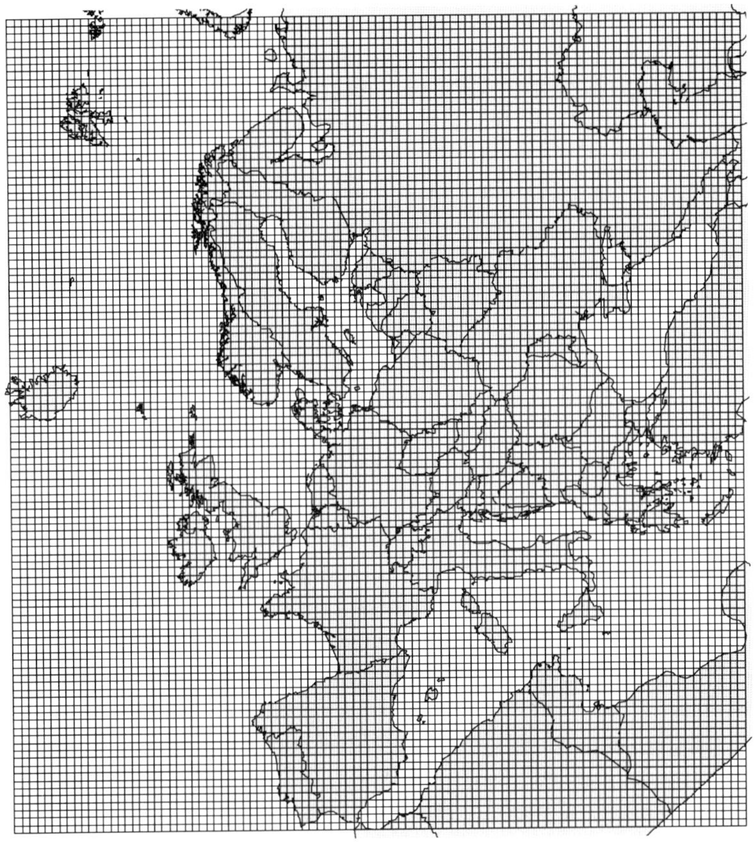

Fig. B-1: Area for which concentrations and depositions are calculated on the EMEP 50 km grid within the single and multi source EcoSense Europe version (European Commission, 1999a; Friedrich and Bickel, 2001a)

For the terrestrial regions to which also rivers, lakes and swamps are counted, the different zones are distinguished according to the drainage basins to which they contribute. These drainage basins were taken from the HYDRO1k geographic database developed at the EROS Data Center (1996). The European basin dataset as well as parts of the Asian and African basin datasets after conversion of their coordinate systems have been used.

The HYDRO1k database consists of topographically derived datasets, including streams, drainage basins and ancillary layers based on the USGS' 30 arc-second digital elevation model of the world (GTOPO30). Within this dataset, the drainage basins are organized following the Pfafstetter code (cf. Verdin, 1997).

This code allows to identify whether and where a zone is situated within a drainage basin. According to this code, each drainage basin of larger rivers is subdivided into nine sub-basins if at least four larger tributaries can be identified. These are coded with even numbers from downstream to upstream. The drainage areas between these basins (called interbasins) assume the respective odd numbers and constitute the main stem of the subdivided river. This procedure can be repeated for each basin and interbasin if again at least four tributaries can be identified. The Pfafstetter code can also be applied starting at the continental level. For Europe, the Rhine catchment, for instance, is identified at the third subdivision level by the code '914' (cf. Fig. 4-4). A further subdivision is also possible at least at the fourth level (as indicated in Fig. 4-4), and for some (inter)basins even below. As a result, the Pfafstetter code allows to identify the connectivities of zones by water currents as provided by the HYDRO1k dataset (EROS Data Center, 1996).[42]

Although a resolution of 1 km^2 is fairly high in a continent-wide analysis, this abstraction might lead to wrong descriptions of the real watersheds (cf. Fekete et al., 2001) and, thus, to the imprecise assessment of the environmental fate of pollutants. Therefore, a qualitative comparison of the drainage basins of the HYDRO1k dataset with the European rivers and catchments database (ERICA Version 1998, European Environment Agency Data Service, 1998) was performed. This database at scale 1:1,000,000 contains over 1500 catchments to river confluences for the largest rivers in the European Environment Agency (EEA) member states. These are located in western Europe (from Portugal through to Germany), Sweden, Greece, parts of Finland, Norway, Italy, England, Ireland and Iceland.

Another comparison was conducted between the HYDRO1k dataset and the Britannica Atlas (Cleveland et al., 1984). In the first place, this was undertaken in order to assign names to the different zones.

The comparison between the HYDRO1k dataset and the other two data sources showed generally good agreement. However, a few significant deviations became obvious which were taken into account (see Table B-1). From these deviations, the assignment of large lakes (with long residence times) to wrong drainage basins was deemed particularly severe. This is especially the case for the Lake Geneva area. However, also further differentiation possibilities have taken into account. Particularly these adaptations may not always result in a subdivision of a (sub-) catchment into 5 interbasins and 4 basins following the Pfafstetter code.

---

42 The Pfafstetter code is to some degree similar to the official German codification of drainage basins which has been in use for some decades already (Länderarbeitsgemeinschaft Wasser (LAWA), 1993).

Table B-1: Adjusted representation of catchments as given by the HYDRO1k dataset (EROS Data Center, 1996)

Drainage basin (identification code)	Country or region	Description[a] / tributary	Original code	Adjusted code[b]
Area between Ljusnan (95576) and Indalselven (9556)	Sweden, river mouth near Sundsvall	Upper part of river identified by '95572' is assigned to Indalselven	955660	955723
			955720	955721
Area between Tana-Elv and Muonioelv	Norway, Finland	Correct northern Scandinavian coastal area	957367	357359
			957368	957359
			957369[c]	957359
			957369[c]	954400
Axios/Vardas (91116)	Serbia, Macedonia	Head waters of the southern Morava (tributary to the Danube) falsely assigned to the upper part of the Vardas (tributary to Axios); parts of the (White) Drin falsely assigned to Vardas	911166[c]	838800
			911166[c]	911166
			911169[c]	911169
			911169[c]	911180
Bann (913774)	Ireland, United Kingdom	Adjusting the proper outflow of the Bann river to the sea	913773[c]	913773
			913773[c]	913774
Caspian Sea (02)	Kazakhstan	The lowest region with Pfaffsteter code '021000' falsely located within the Caspian Sea	021000	020300
	Turkey	Tuz gölü lake	355010	355020
			355070	355020
			355080	355020
			355090	355020

Table B-1: Adjusted representation of catchments as given by the HYDRO1k dataset (EROS Data Center, 1996)

Drainage basin (identification code)	Country or region	Description[a] / tributary	Original code	Adjusted code[b]
Caspian Sea (02) (continued)	Turkey (continued)	Eber Gü	355040	355060
			355050	355060
		Beysehir Gölü	355061	355040
			355062	355040
			355063	355040
			355064	355040
			355065	355040
			355066	355040
			355067	355040
			355068	355040
			355069	355040
Danube (8)	Germany	Parts of the Danube river falsely assigned to the Neckar river (west) or Main river (north, both tributaries to the Rhine)	914698[c]	899500
			914699[c]	899500
			914760[c]	899900
Dolelv (9558)	Sweden	The main two tributaries which after their confluence build the Dolelv are not well represented	955820	955830
			955830	955820
			955840	955820
			955850	955850
			955860	955850
			955870	955850
			955880	955850
			955890	955850

Table B-1: Adjusted representation of catchments as given by the HYDRO1k dataset (EROS Data Center, 1996)

Drainage basin (identification code)	Country or region	Description[a] / tributary	Original code	Adjusted code[b]
Douro/Duero (9118)	Portugal	Parts have not been correctly assigned	911790[c]	911790
			911790[c]	911813
	Spain	Parts were not correctly assigned	911880[c]	911858
			911880[c]	911880
Duna (936)	Russia, Belarus	Subdivision into uppermost tributary and headwaters could not be identified; most of the headwater area (936900) actually belongs to the Dnjepr (see below)	936800	936900
Duna (936), Dnjepr (6)	Russia, Belarus	Most of the headwater area (936900) belongs to the Dnjepr	936900[c]	936900
			936900[c]	662400
Glomma, Glåma (9572)	(mostly) Norway	Upper parts of Glomma river could not be identified to follow disaggregation given by HYDRO1k dataset	957240	957290
			957250	957290
			957260	957290
			957270	957290
			957280	957290
			957290	957250
Guadalquivir (91174)	Spain	Part of the river mouth area falsely assigned to adjacent zone	911739[c]	911739
			911739[c]	911741
Guadiana (91176)	Portugal, Spain	River mouth area is not complete	911750[c]	911741
			911750[c]	911750

Table B-1: Adjusted representation of catchments as given by the HYDRO1k dataset (EROS Data Center, 1996)

Drainage basin (identification code)	Country or region	Description[a] / tributary	Original code	Adjusted code[b]
Guadiana (91176) (continued)	Portugal, Spain (continued)	River mouth area is not complete (continued)	911750[c]	911761
			911770[c]	911761
			911770[c]	911770
Kalixälven (95512)	Sweden (border to Finland)	Upper part of the Kalixälven falsely assigned to the Torneälv	954600	955123
			955120	955121
Kemijoki (9538)	Sweden, Finland, Norway	Upper part of the Ounaskjoki (tributary of the Kemijoki) is assigned to the Torneelv	954200[c]	954200
			954200[c]	953810
			954400[c]	953810
			954400[c]	954400
Loire (912)	France	The following tributaries to the Loire had not been distinguished prior to the adjustment: Mayenne and Loie to Sarthe; Creuse to Vienne; Indre	912200[d]	912210
			912200[d]	912220
			912200[d]	912230
			912200[d]	912240
			912200[d]	912250
			912400[d]	912410
			912400[d]	912420
			912400[d]	912430
			912500[d]	912510
			912500[d]	912520
			912500[d]	912530

Table B-1: Adjusted representation of catchments as given by the HYDRO1k dataset (EROS Data Center, 1996)

Drainage basin (identification code)	Country or region	Description[a] / tributary	Original code	Adjusted code[b]
Minho/Miño (91192)	Spain, Portugal	Subdivision into one tributary 'Sil' and two interbasins introduced	911920[d]	911921
			911920[d]	911922
			911920[d]	911923
Neva (94), Vuoksi (942)	Finland, Russia	According to HYDRO1k, the Vuoksi river (942) and, hence, the Ladoga lake are not fed by Saimaa lake catchment (952); instead the latter area is supposed to be completely drained by the Saimaa canal to the Gulf of Finland; it is assumed here that hardly any water flow occurs via the Saimaa canal and most of the water from the Saimaa lake catchment flows through the Ladoga lake	942400	942411
			952100	942413
			952210	942421
			952220	942422
			952230	942423
			952240	942423
			952250	942423
			952260	942423
			952270	942423
			952280	942423
			952290	942423
			952300	942430
			952400	942440
			952500	942450
			952600	942460
			952700	942470
			952800	942480
			952900	942490

Table B-1: Adjusted representation of catchments as given by the HYDRO1k dataset (EROS Data Center, 1996)

Drainage basin (identification code)	Country or region	Description[a] / tributary	Original code	Adjusted code[b]
Oulujoki (95374)	Finland	Upper part of Oulo river including Oulu-järvi lake falsely placed in another zone	953600	953743
			953740	953741
Pasvikelv (95738)	Norway, Finland, Russia	Lower parts including river mouth of Pas-vikelv are falsely set to be further east; these areas are assigned to the area in between the new Pas-vikelv's lower parts and the Tana-Elv	957384	957383
			957392	957381
			957381	957370
			957382	957370
			957383	957370
Rhine (914)	Germany, France	Moselle, Saar adjust-ments River mouth of Saar represented by new code: 914421 Saar + Blies + Schwarzbach repre-sented by new code: 914423 Seille represented by new code: 911460	914420	914421
			914460[c]	914423
			914460[c]	914460
	Germany	Lahn is a tributary to the Rhine, there is no closed basin in central Germany	915000	914500
	Nether-lands, Ger-many	Only part of the area belongs to the Vechte	915200[c]	914310
			915200[c]	915200

Table B-1: Adjusted representation of catchments as given by the HYDRO1k dataset (EROS Data Center, 1996)

Drainage basin (identification code)	Country or region	Description[a] / tributary	Original code	Adjusted code[b]
Rhine/Meuse (914)	France, Belgium	Parts of the upper Meuse river are assigned to the Oise river, a tributary to the Seine; the Meuse river confluences with the Rhine river (Meuse represented by leading code: 9142)	913245	914293
			913246	914294
			913247	914295
			913248	914296
			913249	914297
			914100	914210
			914290	914291
Rhone (9114)	France, Switzerland	Area around lake Geneve region is falsly assigned to the Rhine catchment	914980	911473
			914990	911475
	France	River mouth is shifted to West Durance (tributary to the Rhone river) is partly assigned to the Côte d'Azur coastal area	911396[c]	911396
			911396[c]	911420
			911398[c]	911398
			911398[c]	911420
			911399[c]	911399
			911399[c]	911410
			911399[c]	911420
			911399[c]	911510
			911410[c]	911410
			911410[c]	911510

Table B-1: Adjusted representation of catchments as given by the HYDRO1k dataset (EROS Data Center, 1996)

Drainage basin (identification code)	Country or region	Description[a] / tributary	Original code	Adjusted code[b]
Rhone (9114) (continued)	France (continued)	Rearrangement of first order sub-basins Ain represented by new code: 911471; in this zone also the main stem of the Rhone river (at least in terms of the name) is situated Saone represented by new code: 911461	911460	911471
			911470	911461
			911480	911462
			911491	911463
			911492	911463
			911493	911463
			911494	911464
			911495	911465
			911496	911466
			911497	911467
			911498	911468
			911499	911469
Scheldt (9134)	Belgium, Nether-lands, France	Joining two zones into one	913500	913400
Segre (91162)	Espana	Subdivision into uppermost tributary and headwaters could not be identified	911628	911629
Seine (9132)	France, Belgium	Oise	913242[c]	913243
		Sambre	913242[c]	914270
	France	Joining two zones to identify the Aisne and to distinguish the Oise	913243	913242
			913244	913242

Table B-1: Adjusted representation of catchments as given by the HYDRO1k dataset (EROS Data Center, 1996)

Drainage basin (identification code)	Country or region	Description[a] / tributary	Original code	Adjusted code[b]
Skellefteelv (95518)	Sweden	Upper parts of the Skelleftelv including the Uddjaur lake is falsely assigned to the Vindelelv	955180	955181
			955240	955183
Weser (9158)	Germany	Parts of the Elbe river belong to the Weser	916300[c]	915840
			916440[c]	915840
			916490[c]	915860

a. Note: The way how the Pfafstetter code is employed did not allow a further subdivision of catchments within the HYDRO1k dataset in some cases. Therefore, the HYDRO1k basins should not be considered as incorrect in those cases in which further, partly 'incomplete' subdivisions are introduced in this work (see also footnote b).
b. Note that the adaptations made may not always result in a subdivision of a (sub-) catchment into 5 interbasins and 4 basins following the Pfafstetter code.
c. The zone has only in parts been newly allocated.
d. The whole zone has been further sub-divided.

Two identified irregularities could not be adjusted. One is the Adige river in northern Italy which confluences with the Po river according to the GIS dataset although discharging into the Adriatic Sea in parallel channels. The second is the Kokemäenjoki in southern Finland which partly drains to the Gulf of Finland according to the HYDRO1k dataset.

The areas of the zones were determined from the respective GIS dataset resulting after correction and joining the European, Asian, African and a lake GIS datasets. The derivation of this latter lake dataset is described in the following section.

B.2.1 Definition of large lakes

The lake coverage mentioned above was yielded by taking the geo-datasets on land uses into account presented in section B.3. These were updated by the WELAREM dataset (Lehner and Döll, 2001) where information on the so-called global lakes exist. From this geo-dataset, all water bodies were extracted that are larger than 100 km^2. As mentioned in section B.4.1, these lakes are assumed to have a depth of 74 m.

Some corrections have been made in order for some resulting lakes not to be considered as such. This is because these either do not constitute pure freshwater bodies or do not have a depth as large as 74 m. These are

- the Elbe estuary,
- the bay at the Rügen island,
- the river mouth of the Odra river,
- wetland in southern Finland,
- wetland in northern Denmark and Ringkoebing fjord,
- part of the Mediterranean northwest of Cyprus,
- bay in Tunisia,
- bay in southern France (however keeping the Camarque as wetland with a smaller depth),
- river mouth of the Rhine, and
- bay in northern Ireland.

Some of these larger lakes are fully contained within the zones identified by the HYDRO1k basin dataset (EROS Data Center, 1996; cf. Fig. 6-2). These are only considered in terms of a larger depth. However, many of these lakes spread over different zones. All of these lake portions which are connected by the downstream flow of water constitute separate zones in the proposed methodology (cf. the example of lake Vänern in Fig. 6-2).

B.3 Distinction of different compartments

For the definition of different terrestrial compartments, three sources have been used:

1. one GIS dataset covering some of the EU countries (European Environment Agency, 2000) with a resolution of 250 m and distinguishing 44 land use classes as given in Table B-2 (base year 1990),
2. one GIS dataset covering the whole globe (EROS Data Center et al., 2000) with a resolution of 1 km and distinguishing 24 land use classes as given in Table B-3 (base year April 1992-March 1993),
3. one GIS dataset covering the whole globe (Hansen et al., 1998) from the University of Maryland with a resolution of 1 km (base years 1981-1994, average values used); this is basically used for the definition of the arable land compartment outside the CORINE land cover dataset termed 'cropland' which is why the full set of 14 distinguished land use classes are not shown here.

Additionally, a GIS dataset on lakes, reservoirs and wetlands (Lehner and Döll, 2001) has been used for a better definition of lakes.

Note that these datasets contain information on the different land covers existing in the respective areas. Although land use and land cover are different concepts (e.g., grasslands can or cannot be used as pastures; cf. Moore et al., 1993), these two terms are mostly used synonymously in the present work.

The usage of three datasets was necessary as the one by the EEA has a higher spatial resolution and - more importantly - a more comprehensive set of land uses distinguished than the one by the USGS and GLCF (44 towards 24 and 14, respectively). The distinction of different agricultural land uses with the EEA dataset is a major advantage of this dataset over the other two especially when dealing with human exposures via food. While the USGS dataset has the advantage to be more detailed in terms of land uses distinguished, it does not provide explicit information on crop lands. Due to this shortcoming, the third dataset by the GLCF was used to identify those and 'update' the USGS dataset. The translation of the originally distinguished land covers by the EEA and USGS datasets into the different compartments distinguished by WATSON (cf. sections 5.1.1 and B.3) is given in Tables B-2 and B-3 (see also section B.4 for the treatment of water bodies). The area shares of all compartments present in a zone have been extracted from the resulting GIS dataset.

B.3.1 Considerations with respect to depths of terrestrial compartments

Above, the areas of the different compartments have been defined. In order to arrive at volumes, also the depths need to be known (cf. section A.4). These are defined in the main text for the terrestrial compartments (cf. section 5.1) and are not repeated here.

B.3.2 Considerations with respect to soil depths of volatile substances

Potentially different from exposure models, pure environmental fate models try to capture as much of a substance as possible. This has bearings on the subdivision of these models in terms of compartments as is discussed in the following.

Table B-2: Translation of CORINE land uses (European Environment Agency, 2000) into WATSON land uses

CORINE land use class	Land use type	Assigned compartment type
1.1 Urban fabric	Continuous urban fabric	urban areas
	Discontinuous urban fabric	urban areas
1.2 Industrial, commercial and transport units	Industrial or commercial units	urban areas
	Road and rail networks and associated land	urban areas
	port areas	urban areas
	Airports	urban areas
1.3 Mine, dump and construction sites	Mineral extraction sites	non vegetated land
	Dump sites	non vegetated land
	Construction sites	non vegetated land
1.4 Artificial non-agricultural vegetated areas	Green urban areas	semi natural ecosystems
	Sport and leisure facilities	semi natural ecosystems
2.1 Arable land	Non-irrigated arable land	arable land
	Permanently irrigated land	arable land
	Rice fields	arable land
2.2 Permanent crops	Vineyards	arable land
	Fruit trees and berry plantations	arable land
	Olive groves	arable land
2.3 Pastures	Pastures	pasture
2.4 Heterogeneous agricultural areas	Annual crops associated with permanent crops	arable land
	Complex cultivation patterns	arable land
	Land principally occupied by agriculture	arable land
	Agro-forestry areas	semi natural ecosystems

Table B-2: Translation of CORINE land uses (European Environment Agency, 2000) into WATSON land uses

CORINE land use class	Land use type	Assigned compartment type
3.1 Forests	Broad-leaved forest	semi natural ecosystems
	Coniferous forest	semi natural ecosystems
	Mixed forest	semi natural ecosystems
3.2 Shrubs and/or herbaceous vegetation associations	Natural grassland	semi natural ecosystems
	Moors and heathland	semi natural ecosystems
	Sclerophyllous vegetation	semi natural ecosystems
	Transitional woodland-shrub	semi natural ecosystems
3.3 Open spaces with little or no vegetation	Beaches	non vegetated land
	Bare rocks	non vegetated land
	Sparsely vegetated areas	non vegetated land
	Burnt areas	non vegetated land
	Glaciers and perpetual snow	glacier snow
4.1 Inland wetlands	Inland marshes	semi natural ecosystems
	Peat bogs	semi natural ecosystems
4.2 Coastal wetland	Salt-marshes	semi natural ecosystems
	Salines	non vegetated land
	Intertidal flats	non vegetated land
5.1 Inland waters (cf. footnote 43)	Water courses	water course
	Water bodies	water
5.2 Marine waters	Coastal lagoons	(nothing assigned)
	Estuaries	water
	Sea and ocean	(nothing assigned)
	no information (terrestrial)	(nothing assigned)
	no information (aquatic)	(nothing assigned)

Table B-3: Translation of USGS land uses (EROS Data Center et al., 2000) into WATSON land uses

Land use type	Assigned compartment type
Urban and Built-Up Land	urban areas
Dryland Cropland and Pasture	arable land / pasture
Irrigated Cropland and Pasture	arable land / pasture
Mixed Dryland/Irrigated Cropland and Pasture	arable land / pasture
Cropland/Grassland Mosaic	arable land / pasture
Cropland/Woodland Mosaic	semi natural ecosystems
Grassland	semi natural ecosystems
Shrubland	semi natural ecosystems
Mixed Shrubland/Grassland	semi natural ecosystems
Savanna	semi natural ecosystems
Deciduous Broadleaf Forest	semi natural ecosystems
Deciduous Needleleaf Forest	semi natural ecosystems
Evergreen Broadleaf Forest	semi natural ecosystems
Evergreen Needleleaf Forest	semi natural ecosystems
Mixed Forest	semi natural ecosystems
Water Bodies	water
Herbaceous Wetland	semi natural ecosystems
Wooded Wetland	semi natural ecosystems
Barren or Sparsely Vegetated	non-vegetated land
Herbaceous Tundra	semi natural ecosystems
Wooded Tundra	semi natural ecosystems
Mixed Tundra	semi natural ecosystems
Bare Ground Tundra	non-vegetated land

Table B-3: Translation of USGS land uses (EROS Data Center et al., 2000) into WATSON land uses

Land use type	Assigned compartment type
Snow or Ice	glacier / snow
no data	(not assigned)
Interrupted areas (global Goodes homolosine projection)	(not assigned)

With respect to soils, Mackay (1991) found out that a single soil layer may underestimate volatilisation of those substances for which this process is relevant. There exist different recommendations in order to cope with this underestimation (Cowan et al., 1995b) of which a substance-dependent soil compartment depth (e.g., Brandes et al., 1996) as well as distinguishing at least two soil layers are most often used (e.g., McKone, 1993a). In a recent work, McKone and Bennett (2003) give the recommendation based on theoretical considerations to represent the soil compartment at least as two layers one of which consisting of a thin surface layer in order to properly account for the air-soil mass transfer coefficient of (semi-) volatile compounds. The layer below this should be adjusted to the chemical-specific penetration depth (derived by means of the so-called Damkoehler number). One shortcoming of this adjusted compartment depth, however, is that it may range from 0.1 to several metres (see Table 4 in McKone and Bennett, 2003). When implementing a variable soil depth in a model which is not parameterised for a specific site, this may lead to erroneous assumptions with regard to the structure of the subsurface (e.g., unweathered solid rock, ground water) where penetration is unlikely or at least substantially reduced. This is why in SimpleBox 2.0 the maximally allowed soil depth is set to 1 m (Brandes et al., 1996). The implementation of the effective penetration depth would also have implications on the data needs if one was to represent this part of the terrestrial environment appropriately. This is because the two soil layers would have different characteristics depending on the chemical's effective penetration depth. This shall be illustrated with a rough example. Consider a soil that has a humus rich surface horizon ('layer') of 20 cm followed by 1 m of unconsolidated sand layer which in turn is followed by a consolidated rock layer (e.g., shale). It is assumed here that the surface soil layer is always 2 cm deep and the soil layer below is referred to as 'rooting layer'. If the effective penetration depth was 20 cm the soil layers in the multimedia model could be delimited at 2 cm and 20 cm soil depth having the same properties. However, if the effective penetration depth was

40 cm the rooting layer would have mixed properties of the humus rich soil horizon and the underlying sand rock. This would especially concern the organic carbon content in the case of lipophilic compounds. The situation would be even worse if the effective penetration depths was larger than 1.2 m extending into the shale.

When deriving a Damkoehler number-based effective penetration depth of organic compounds, one has to bear in mind that chemical transformation ('degradation') in soils is mostly dependent on the activity of microorganisms although abiotic transformation processes may also be of importance (McBride, 1994; Alloway et al., 1996), especially photodegradation at the soil surface. Degradation is, thus, mostly confined to areas of biological activity in soils. Correspondingly, it is deemed reasonable principally not to assume Damkoehler number-derived penetration depths larger than 1 m which conforms with SimpleBox 2.0 (Brandes et al., 1996).

In general, however, there are two aspects that suggest not to include a variable soil depth. First, in the context of a spatially-resolved model of continental scope such detailed information on all relevant soil properties (such as partitioning influencing key parameters like organic carbon content for organics and pH for dissociating substances, impermeable subsurface layers) for several decimetres or even metres is not available. Second, if these information became available the averaging of the properties would need to be done for each substance to be modelled separately requiring additional algorithms and a longer computation time. The distinction of several soil layers, thus, touches upon implementation constraints. These are storage of information as well as the dimension of the set of linear differential equations to be handled and, thus, computation time.

Another aspect is to what degree terrestrial vegetation can compensate for the underestimation of volatilisation of a single layer soil compartment. Bennett et al. (1998) used a multimedia model whose soil compartment is two-layered and has an 'effective soil depth' in order to investigate the vegetation influence. They found for TCDD that vegetation is more important on the regional fate of this compound than the soil compartment: the Characteristic Travel Distance (CTD) decreased by an order of magnitude when introducing a vegetation compartment. However, it cannot be assessed what CTD would have resulted if the soil had been represented to consist only of one layer. Nevertheless, vegetation significantly enhances a substance's retention (also supported by findings of Wania and McLachlan, 2001) possibly exerting even a higher effect than does a single soil layer multimedia model. This could mean that the underestimation of the volatilisation from soil may no longer be effective.

Overall, the recommendations with respect to layers and also to variable penetration depths apply to (semi-) volatile organic compounds and are neither feasible (in terms of environmental data acquisition) nor scientifically defendable in terms of potentially allowing unrealistically deep soil compartments in a non-site-specific multi-zonal model of a rather large geographical scope. One also has to keep in mind that even more sophisticated models seem to fail to model more than one zone appropriately (del Re and Trevisan, 1995).

B.4 Dimensions and spatially invariant properties of freshwater compartments

Surface water bodies containing freshwater can roughly be classified into lakes and streams. These show particularly differences in terms of their morphology (depth and width) and flow velocity. Whereas the land use and lake geo-datasets described in a previous section allow for the distinction of larger lakes, reaches (stream extents) are usually too narrow to be represented in such large scale mapping exercises.[43] Nevertheless, one needs to define water volumes for the compartments in order to perform a mass balance based on concentrations. The volumes of unregulated water bodies vary according to the meteorological conditions. In WATSON, however, climatological data are used. Therefore, one needs to base the water volume calculations on long-term averages that are assumed to be constant in time.

As hydrologists usually are more interested for example in flood prevention or drinking/irrigation water supply assessments there is no need to determine such static (long-term) volumes of water bodies from their point of view. Also concentration calculations are usually performed by building the quotient of a mass emission rate (e.g., in kg/s) and the discharge of a stream (e.g., in m^3/s). This may serve as an explanation why no data source on water volumes has been found. The only source found that deals with average volumes is Korzun et al. (1974) cited in Baumgartner and Liebscher (1990) on a global scale.

B.4.1 Dimensions of lakes

According to Korzun et al. (1974) cited in Baumgartner and Liebscher (1990), freshwater lakes globally cover $1.24 \cdot 10^6$ km^2 while containing 91 000 km^3 of water. This means lakes are on average 74 m deep. This value is used as a default depth unless other values are provided.

This depth, however, will only be reached by rather large lakes. For the definition of large lakes, a cut-off value of 100 km^2 was used based on a GIS dataset

---

[43] Note that in Table B-2 water courses are distinguished from other water bodies; this is because the resulting geo-dataset is also used to determine lake zones.

on lakes which was specifically created for the purpose of this work (cf. section B.5.2).

B.4.2 Dimensions of streams

Korzun et al. (1974) cited in Baumgartner and Liebscher (1990) also estimated the freshwater volume contained in streams. It amounts to 2 120 km^3. As they did not estimate the land area covered by streams and due to lack of such data, it is necessary to estimate the stream water volume as well as its area for the catchments within the geographical scope of the model. Data on area (section B.2) as well as on runoff and discharge (section B.5.2) are readily available on a per zone basis. In order to make a valid water mass balance, however, information on either the residence times of the water or the flow velocities are necessary. These are difficult to obtain.

In order to distribute the global stream freshwater volume, a more pragmatic estimation method is, thus, followed by deriving a continent- and area-specific water volume. The global stream freshwater volume is distributed to the different continents weighted by the total discharge from each continent divided by the global discharge from land (discharge weights in Table B-4). The area-specific stream water volume (per continent) is yielded by dividing this value by the continental area. It is assumed that within one catchment the total stream freshwater volume is given as the product of the total drainage area of the catchment and the area-specific stream water volume:

$$V_{\text{total freshwater volume of catchment c}} = A_{\text{area of catchment c}} \cdot emp_{\text{stream freshwater volume per area}} \cdot \qquad \text{(B-1)}$$

If the catchment consists of more than one zone, the water volume is, furthermore, distributed to the different zones as a function of the total contributing catchment area per zone according to the general observation for rivers in humid areas (Finlayson and McMahon, 1995). As the zones may vary considerably in terms of their spatial extent, the total contributing drainage area per zone is further weighted by the area share of the zone with respect to the total catchment area. The total weight for the water volume distribution within catchment c is, hence, given for zone i according to Eq. (B-2).

Table B-4: Deriving stream freshwater volumes per catchment area depending on the continent (drainage areas and discharges in the peripheral and central regions of the world taken from Baumgartner and Liebscher, 1990)

Continent	Area $[10^6\ km^2]$		Discharge $[10^3\ km^3/yr]$		Discharge weights	Discharge-weighted stream freshwater volume	Stream freshwater volume per area
	peripheral	central	peripheral	central	[%]	$[km^3]$	$[m^3/m^2]$
Europe	8.3	1.7	2.5	0.3	6.3	133	0.013
Asia	31.4	12.7	12.5	-0.3	31.4	666	0.015
Africa	17.6	12.2	3.4	n/a	8.5	181	0.0061
Australia	4.7	4.2	2.4	n/a	6.0	128	0.014
North America	23.2	0.9	5.9	n/a	14.8	314	0.013
South America	16.4	1.5	11.1	n/a	27.9	591	0.033
Antarctica	14.1	n/a	2.0	n/a	5.0	107	0.0076
Sum	115.7	33.2	39.8	0.0	n/a	n/a	n/a

$$Weight_{\text{volume of zone i in catchment c}} = \frac{A_{\text{drainage area of zone i}} \cdot \dfrac{A_{\text{area of zone i}}}{A_{\text{area of catchment c}}}}{\sum_{n}^{\text{zones of catchment c}} A_{\text{drainage area of zone n}} \cdot \dfrac{A_{\text{area of zone n}}}{A_{\text{area of catchment c}}}} \qquad \text{(B-2)}$$

One sees that the total catchment area cancels down. The freshwater volume of streams in each zone is computed accordingly as:

$$V_{\text{water compartment in zone i}} = Weight_{\text{volume of zone i in catchment c}} \cdot V_{\text{total freshwater volume of catchment c}} \qquad \text{(B-3)}$$

Furthermore, one needs to define the area of the water compartments as it constitutes the interface between the atmosphere and the water bodies (e.g., for atmospheric deposition). Assuming that the total area of river water bodies constitutes 0.5 % of the total land areas showing discharge would yield an average depth of 2.7 m for Europe according to the world water balance given in Table B-1. A value of 0.5 % of a zone's area is, therefore, assumed as a default. In small zones through which a large river flows, however, the water compartment's depth might become unrealistically large following this rule. A further rule is, therefore, set into place: If the stream water's depth is larger than the sum of the incoming streams' depths, a larger zone area share of between 0.5 % and up to 100 % is adopted assuming at least a depth that is as big as the mentioned sum of the incoming streams' depths.

B.4.3 Dimensions of the freshwater compartment

In the water volume derivation for streams in the previous section, the volumes and areas given for lakes (section B.4.1) are not considered. These are finally added if applicable to yield the ultimate values for the freshwater compartment. Their average depth is yielded by dividing the volume by the respective area covered. Note that this way it is assumed that all of the water entering a zone flows through all lakes contained therein.

B.4.4 Mass transfer coefficient at the water-sediment interface

In order to define the diffusion from water body to sediment and vice versa, the overall mass transfer coefficient needs to be known (cf. sections A.3.14 and

Table B-5: Organic carbon content and pH values for compartments other than permeable soils as used by WATSON

Compartment	pH	Organic carbon content $[kg_{Corg} / kg_{solid}]$
Glaciers	not applicable	not applicable
Impervious surfaces	5.5[a]	0.1[b]
Freshwater bodies	7.0[c]	variable[d]
Freshwater sediment	7.0[e]	variable[d]

a. pH of 'pristine' rain water at 25°C (Stumm and Morgan, 1996, p. 161) adjusted to 0.5 pH units.
b. Analogy assumption to freshwater bodies.
c. Huijbregts (1999).
d. Refer to Table B-11.
e. According to Huijbregts (1999) and Devillers et al. (1995) noting that the pH value may be higher than in freshwater due to less oxidizing conditions.

A.3.15). Reported values range from about $2.8 \cdot 10^{-8}$ (Mackay et al., 1992; 1996a; Wania and Mackay, 1995; Brandes et al., 1996; Severinsen et al., 1996) to $2 \cdot 10^{-6}$ metres per second at the shore line of a lake (Wania, 1996). The values tend to be smaller for (the deeper parts of) lakes (Mackay and Diamond, 1989; Wania, 1996) than for generic freshwater bodies. This tendency may be explained by the on average lower temperatures and, thus, slower Brownian motion (Schwarzenbach et al., 1993) in deep water environments. In any case, it is not plausible to assume a quicker transport of substances in rivers with a lot of water currents and eddies due to diffusive processes than due to water advection or resuspension (cf. section 6.1). Thus, an overall applicable value of $2.8 \cdot 10^{-8}$ metres per second is adopted.

B.5 Computation of spatially-resolved compartment properties and process rates

There is only little information on variable soil and water properties readily available in a GIS format without substantial payments. An example for a relatively expensive data source for soils is the European Soil Data Base (European Commission, 1998).[44] Nevertheless, information on soil pH and organic carbon content (C_{org}) could be found from the International Soil Reference and Information Centre (ISRIC, Batjes, 1996) which are given on a half-degree grid. These datasets only provide information on the respective properties of those soils that are classified as pervious in this study. For the other compartments, the default pH and C_{org} values are given in Table B-5.

Spatially-resolved data on the hydrological cycle were also found. Their description and processing are presented in section B.5.2.

In contrast to these environmental parameters, there are other parameters whose values are not allowed to vary between zones and which were adopted from the literature. These are given in the sections which describe the respective processes or in the following sub-sections.

B.5.1 Spatially variable properties of soils

Values for pH and organic carbon content have been assigned to the different soil compartments after intersecting the land use coverage (cf. section B.3) with the respective geo-datasets. The ISRIC datasets distinguish classes of pH and organic carbon reservoir values that are not assigned single numbers but span ranges (cf. Fig. B-2). Single values have been assigned to the given ranges according to Table B-6 and Table B-7.

Calculation of soil-related pH values

The pH of a permeable soil compartment has generally been derived from the original data (Batjes, 1996) according to the following formula:

$$pH_{\text{compartment}} = -\log \frac{\Sigma(A_{\text{compartment with same pH}} \cdot 10^{-pH})}{A_{\text{compartment total}}} \tag{B-4}$$

where

A : area of the compartment [m]

pH : soil reaction, i.e., pH value [-].

The values have been rounded according to 0.5 pH units.

For arable land and pastures, however, the minimally allowed (and default) pH values have been set to 6.0 and 5.5, respectively, due to land management practices taking place ('optimal pH'). If no data had been available for certain zones, the default values of 6.5 and 6.0 have been used for semi-natural ecosystems and non-vegetated land, respectively.

---

[44] Note that an aggregated version has become publicly available via the internet only recently.

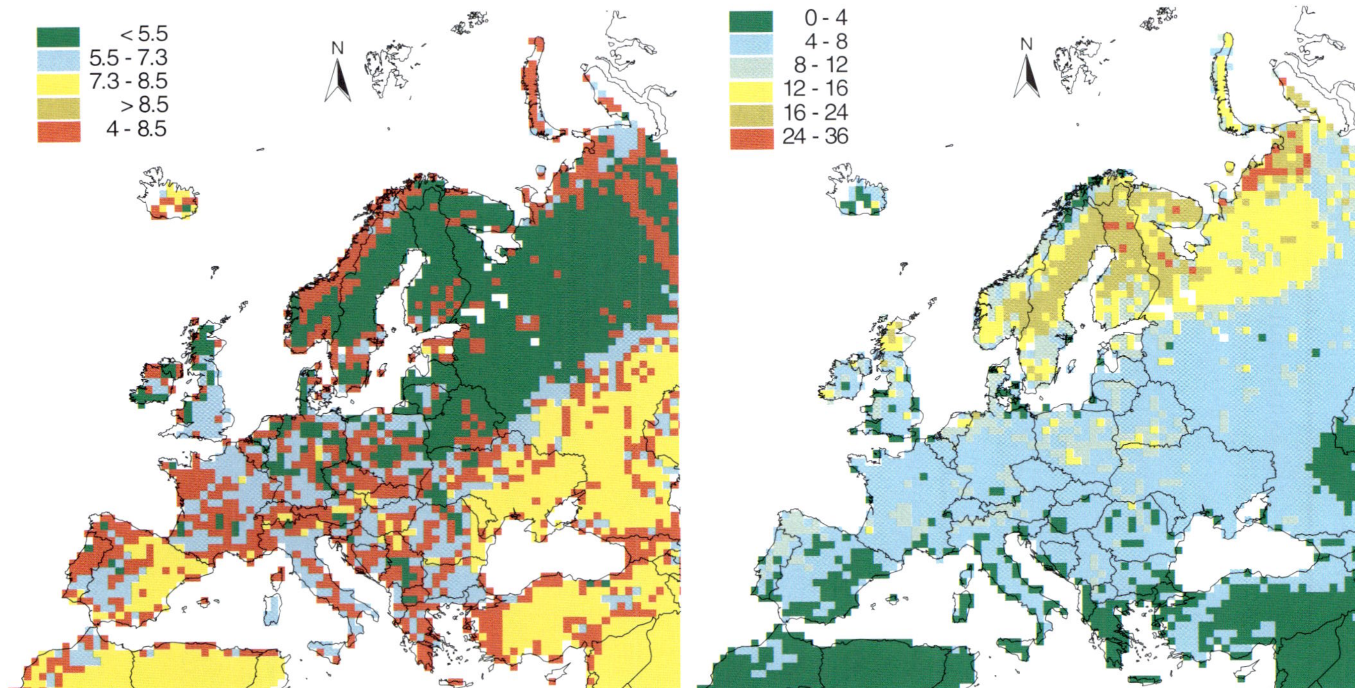

Fig. B-2: Properties of top soil in terms of soil reaction (pH, left) and organic carbon reservoir (right, [kg_{carbon}/m^2]; taken from Batjes, 1996)

Table B-6: Classes of pH values as given by Batjes (1996) and assigned representative single pH values

Range class	Assigned pH value
$pH \leq 5.5$	5.0
$5.5 < pH \leq 7.3$	6.5
$7.3 < pH \leq 8.5$	8.0
$8.5 < pH$	9.0 [a]
$4.0 < pH \leq 8.5$ (complex unit)	6.0

a.Soil types rich in soda can have pH values up to 11.

Table B-7: Organic carbon classes as given by Batjes (1996) and assigned organic carbon reservoir values [kg_{carbon}/m^2]

Range class	Assigned value
0-4	2.0
4-8[a]	6.0
8-12	10.0
12-16	14.0
16-24	20.0
24-36	30.0
36-48	42.0
>48	60.0 [b]

a.Mode value in the area covered.

b.Explanation: bogs have up to 200 kg_{carbon}/m^2 in the first metre which is exactly 60 kg_{carbon}/m^2 in the first 0.3 m (Gisi, 1990).

Calculation of soil-related organic carbon content values

The organic carbon contents of soils are given in mass per square metres for a given soil depth, i.e., 0-30 and 30-100 cm (Batjes, 1996). In order to arrive at the organic carbon concentration for a given compartment in one zone, the original data are multiplied by the area to which they apply. These are then summed over all patches of the same compartment and finally divided by the overall respective compartment area in a respective zone. Division by the appropriate depth yields the organic carbon concentration according to:

$$C\_w/v_{\mathrm{Corg}}(i, z) = \frac{1}{d} \cdot \frac{\Sigma(A_{i,\ \mathrm{with\ same\ Corg\ content}}(z) \cdot Corg)}{A_i(z)} \tag{B-5}$$

where

A	:	area of the compartment i in zone z; either as total or for which the same organic carbon content is given [m^2]
C_w/v	:	concentration of organic carbon in the bulk volume of compartment i in zone z [kg C_{org} per m^3]
C_{org}	:	reservoir or inventory of organic carbon in soil [kg C_{org} per m^2] according to Batjes (1996)
d	:	depth for which the reservoir data are provided [m]; here: 0.3 m.

The mass fraction of organic carbon related to total solid matter in permeable soils, i.e., arable land (i: ag), pastures (i: p), semi-natural ecosystems (i: n) and non-vegetated land (i: b), is computed according to:

$$fr\_w_{\mathrm{organic\ carbon/solid\ phase}}(i, z) = \frac{M_{\mathrm{Corg}}(i, z)}{M_{\mathrm{total\ solids}}(i, z)} = \frac{M_{\mathrm{Corg}}(i, z)}{M_{\mathrm{OM}}(i, z) + M_{\mathrm{MM}}(i, z)} \tag{B-6}$$

where

fr_w	:	mass fraction of organic carbon in overall solid matter of compartment i in zone z [kg C_{org} per kg_{solid}]
M_{Corg}	:	mass of organic carbon of compartment i in zone z [kg C_{org}]
M_{MM}	:	mass of mineral matter (MM) of compartment i in zone z [kg_{MM}]
M_{OM}	:	mass of organic matter (OM) of compartment i in zone z [kg_{OM}].

In the following, the computation of the different parameters on the right hand side of Eq. (B-6) will be presented. Note that the dependency on the compartment and the zone will not be denoted although existing.

The organic carbon mass is simply calculated by multiplying the organic carbon concentration by the total volume:

$$M_{\mathrm{Corg}} = C\_w/v_{\mathrm{Corg,\,c}} \cdot V_{\mathrm{compartment\ total}} \tag{B-7}$$

where

C_w/v : concentration of organic carbon in the bulk volume of a compartment [kg C_{org} per m^3]

M_{Corg} : mass of organic carbon [kg C_{org}]

V : volume of the bulk compartment [m^3].

The organic matter mass (M_{OM}) consists of compounds containing carbon as well as other elements. Thus:

$$\begin{aligned} M_{\mathrm{OM}} &= M_{\mathrm{Corg}} + M_{\mathrm{non\text{-}Corg}} \\ &= \frac{M_{\mathrm{Corg}}}{fr\_w_{\mathrm{Corg\ mass\ fraction\ of\ total\ organic\ solids}}} \end{aligned} \tag{B-8}$$

where

fr_w : mass fraction of organic carbon in organic matter [kg C_{org} per kg_{OM}]

M_{Corg} : mass of organic carbon [kg C_{org}]

$M_{non\text{-}Corg}$: mass in organic matter not consisting of organic carbon [kg non-C_{org} elements]

M_{OM} : mass of organic matter [kg_{OM}].

The mass fraction of organic carbon in organic matter generally assumes values of 0.5 according to 'model' humic and fulvic acids as given by Schnitzer (1978). For impervious land uses, the value is set to 0.7 based on the consideration that the organic matter on roads mostly consists of soot which is richer in organic carbon (e.g., Gustafsson et al., 1997).

The mineral matter mass (M_{MM}) is yielded by subtracting the organic matter volume from the overall (constant) solid matter volume and multiplying this difference by the mineral matter density:

$$\begin{aligned} M_{MM} &= \rho_{MM} \cdot V_{MM} \\ &= \rho_{MM} \cdot (V_{solids} - V_{OM}) \\ &= \rho_{MM} \cdot \left(fr\_V_{solids} \cdot V_{bulk} - \frac{M_{OM}}{\rho_{OM}}\right) \end{aligned} \tag{B-9}$$

where

fr_V : volume fraction of solids in bulk compartment [$m^3{}_{solids}$ per $m^3{}_{bulk}$]; defined as described in section 5.1.3

M_{MM} : mass of mineral matter [kg_{MM}]

M_{OM} : mass of organic matter [kg_{OM}]

ρ_{MM} : density of mineral matter [kg_{MM} per $m^3{}_{MM}$]

ρ_{OM} : density of organic matter [kg_{OM} per $m^3{}_{OM}$]

V : volume of mineral matter (MM), organic matter (OM), solids, or the bulk compartment [m^3].

The density of mineral and organic matter is not allowed to vary in space and set to 2650 and 1400 kg/m^3 (Scheffer and Schachtschabel, 1989), respectively. Note that the mineral matter density was set equal to that of quartz which makes up the most part of the mineral phase. The volume fraction of soils consisting of solids is invariantly set to 0.5 according to Mackay et al. (1992) and McKone and Bennett (2003) corresponding to a loamy soil, i.e., a soil that is neither rather sandy nor rather clayey.

In the case that the mass of mineral matter (M_{MM}) would become negative, i.e., the term in parenthesis of Eq. (B-9) is negative due to the fact that the soil is very rich in organic carbon, M_{OM} is adjusted so that the total solid matter in a compartment consists of 10 vol.-% mineral solids as a default. Exceptions to this default value apply to freshwater bodies with a value for suspended matter of 5 vol.-% and to the solids in the urban environment and in aquifers (ground water compartment if distinguished) with 10 vol.-% and 50 vol.-%, respectively.

The solid phase density is computed according to:

$$\rho_{solids} = \frac{M_{OM} + M_{MM}}{fr\_V_{solids} \cdot V_{bulk}} \tag{B-10}$$

where

fr_V : volume fraction of solids in bulk compartment [m^3_{solids} per m^3_{bulk}]; defined as described in section 5.1.3

M_{MM} : mass of mineral matter [kg_{MM}]

M_{OM} : mass of organic matter [kg_{OM}]

ρ_{solids} : density of solid matter [kg_{solids} per m^3_{solids}]

V : volume of the bulk compartment [m^3].

In case no organic carbon contents could be assigned to a compartment, default values have been assumed. Arable land, pastures and semi-natural ecosystems were assigned to the category containing 4-8 kg C_{org}/m^2 and non-vegetated land to category with 0-4 kg C_{org}/m^2 corresponding to the mode value and the lowest value in the area covered, respectively (cf. Table B-7).

B.5.2 Hydrological data

In search of a consistent dataset on all components of the hydrological cycle, i.e., at least two of the list of precipitation, evaporation and runoff when disregarding storage changes, the dataset by the Center for Environmental Systems Research at Kassel university, Germany could be found (Döll and Lehner, 2002; Döll et al., 2002, 2003) which builds on precipitation data by New et al. (1999). These provide consolidated 30 year (1961-90) long-term average estimates on precipitation, runoff and ground water recharge. In addition to these data, global GIS data on lakes, wetlands and reservoirs have also been made available (Lehner and Döll, 2001) which have been used for the derivation of a GIS dataset on lakes (cf. section B.2.1).

One problem has occurred when computing the derived figures described below. There are cases in which precipitation is smaller than runoff. This problem had already been identified and reported in Döll et al. (2003). It is due to a calibration exercise performed on measured runoff data which overrules the information on precipitation that are considered to be too small also in parts of Europe. This calibration is owing to the generally recognised fact in hydrology that runoff measurements provide more reliable data than those of precipitation (e.g., Shuttleworth, 1993). The respective values for evapotranspiration have been set to zero in the present study although not fulfilling the water mass balance. However, the measure evapotranspiration is presently not used in the assessment.

Consideration of evaporation

In the geo-datasets used, evaporation is considered to occur from canopies, soils and so-called global lakes and wetlands (Döll et al., 2003). While the evaporation from canopies and soils is included in the runoff values employed, those for lakes and wetlands could not be considered. In order to account for lake water evaporation, the watershed-based distinction of zones in WATSON would need to be allocated to the respective lakes. This, however, has not been possible due to the way how a lake's water balance is considered in the global hydrological model. It is only the most downstream grid cell in which the whole water balance of the global lakes and wetlands is performed. This may even be a grid cell in which two lake water balances happen to be computed. The same problem exists for the consideration of the consumptive use of water by man. Although information on both lake evaporation and water abstraction are principally provided by the hydrological data sources, these have not been considered partly leading to an overestimation of runoff and, thus, discharge.

Computation of runoff and groundwater recharge

Runoff is defined as "(t)hat part of precipitation that appears as streamflow" (Deutsches Nationalkomitee für das internationale Hydrologische Programm (IHP) der UNESCO und das Operationelle Hydrologische Programm (OHP) der WMO, 1998, p. 130). The information provided by Döll and co-workers (Döll et al., 2002, 2003) is given on a grid cell base (cf. Fig. B-3). The environmental fate model of WATSON, in turn, is spatially differentiated according to catchment delineations (see section B.2). In order to transform the original data to match catchments, these are intersected using the GIS tool ArcInfo 7.0. The runoff of a particular zone in WATSON is then computed by multiplying the specified runoff by the area for which it is applicable first. These are summed for all areas contained in a zone. Finally, the resulting value is divided by the overall area. Unfortunately not all grid cells contain valid runoff data. Therefore, also the area by which it is divided is equal to that area for which valid entries are given.

Groundwater recharge, recharge, or accretion is defined as the "process by which water is added from outside to the zone of saturation of an aquifer, either directly into a formation, or indirectly by way of another formation" (Deutsches Nationalkomitee für das internationale Hydrologische Programm (IHP) der UNESCO und das Operationelle Hydrologische Programm (OHP) der WMO, 1998, p. 123). The same computational procedure as for runoff applies to ground water recharge. Groundwater recharge is not used within WATSON as such. Rather the share of the precipitation that reaches the rivers via the so-called quickflow is computed. This is done by first computing the baseflow or base runoff

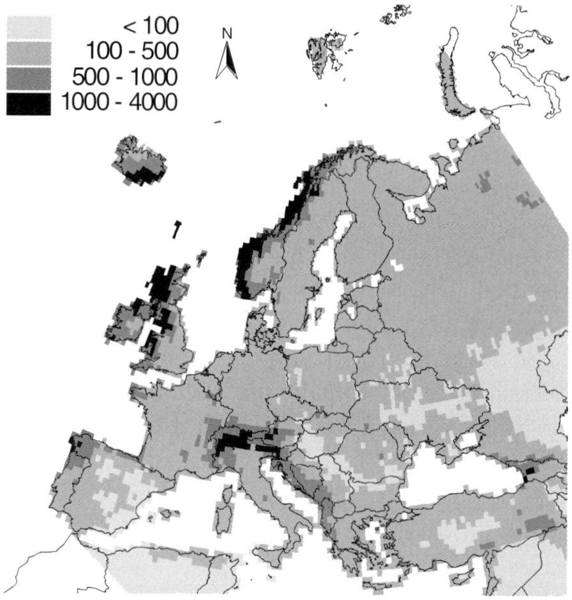

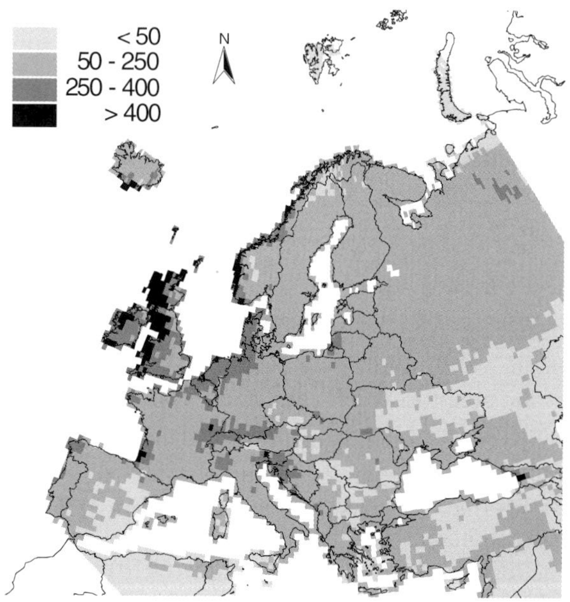

Fig. B-3: Long-term values for runoff from land (top) and ground water recharge (bottom) in the area of interest according to Döll and co-workers (Döll and Lehner, 2002; Döll et al., 2002, 2003) [mm/yr]

which is defined as "part of the discharge which enters a stream channel mainly from groundwater, but also from lakes and glaciers during long periods when no precipitation or snowmelt occurs" (ibid., p. 18) relating the groundwater recharge to the runoff. The complement is considered the share of quickflow.

Computation of discharge

Discharge or rate of flow is defined as the "volume of water flowing through a river (or channel) cross section in unit time" (Deutsches Nationalkomitee für das internationale Hydrologische Programm (IHP) der UNESCO und das Operationelle Hydrologische Programm (OHP) der WMO, 1998, p. 45). Based on the runoff information (see above), discharge is simply computed by multiplying the runoff (in metre per second) and the area of a zone (in square metres). In case there are several interconnected zones distinguished in a catchment, the discharge of an upstream zone adds to all downstream zones. Note that evaporation and anthropogenic water abstraction from larger water body surfaces such as lakes is not taken into account in WATSON at present (see above).

Preferential flow

Preferential flow is a non-equilibrium process in soils that rapidly transfers waters and substances entrained towards the subsurface (cf. section A.3.7). It may, therefore, constitute an important removal process of substances from the modelled system unless the subsurface and/or groundwater is considered.

In order to account for this process, it must be known which portion of the vertical water balance, i.e., runoff equals precipitation minus evaporation plus/minus storage (Becker, 1995; Döll et al., 2003), undergoes this rapid flow through the soil. Since preferential flow is known to also occur in arid climates with little to no runoff formation, the amount of water preferentially flowing through soils is assessed based on precipitation rather than on runoff.

Preferential flow was chosen to be 1 % of the rain rate. When applying this value it occurred at times that this amount of the rain rate exceeded the total groundwater recharge. In such instances, it has, therefore, been assumed that 50 % of groundwater recharge happens as preferential flow if there is groundwater recharge at all. If a zone does not show groundwater recharge, the volumetric share of precipitation undergoing preferential flow was set to zero.

B.5.3 Modelling erosion for different soil compartments

The proposed methodology distinguishes between compartments in the terrestrial environment as given in Table 5-1. One criterion for their distinction is water soil

Table B-8: Reported erosion rates in multimedia models

Erosion rate	Reference	Comment
0.03 mm/yr	Brandes et al. (1996)	for any soil
0.04 mm/yr	Hertwich et al. (1999)	Erosion of surface soil 0.0003 $kg/m^2/d$ divided by solid phase density of 2600 kg/m^3

erosion for which the erosion rate shall be derived in the following. It is noted here that only a differentiation of erosion rates according to compartments is implemented at present. A possible improvement of this situation is also described below.

Selection of a representative erosion rate for European conditions

There are only few reported values on erosion rates used in multimedia models (Table B-8). Their appropriateness shall be evaluated against assessed numbers of the measure 'sediment yield'. Sediment yield is defined as "(t)otal sediment outflow from a watershed ... in a specified period of time ... Usually expressed in weight per unit of time" (Deutsches Nationalkomitee für das internationale Hydrologische Programm (IHP) der UNESCO und das Operationelle Hydrologische Programm (OHP) der WMO, 1998, p. 134). It provides a rather reliable assessment of water soil erosion (Morgan, 1999). Although also containing eroded material originating from the rivers, these might serve as a rough estimate of what is transported from soil to water in a spatially-resolved way assuming that in-bed erosion equals the amount deposited within a catchment and no other long-term storage of suspended particulates within the catchment occurs.

The value of 0.04 mm/yr given in Table B-8 is used in CalTOX (Hertwich et al., 1999), a model developed for Californian conditions (McKone, 1993a). This value is substantially lower than the sediment yields given by Walling and Webb (1983) for California, ranging from 250 to more than 1000 $t/km^2/yr$ corresponding to 0.10 to above 0.38 mm/yr. This may be explained by the fact that the non-coastal areas in California are mountainous. CalTOX was designed in the first place to assist risk assessments of hazardous waste sites (in California, McKone, 1993a) which are most likely not located on steep slopes. For Europe, more than 50 % of the area show sediment yields below 50 $t/km^2/yr$ (= 0.02 mm/yr) whereas the rest ranges predominantly between 50 and 750 $t/km^2/yr$ (< 0.29 mm/yr) showing some peaks in the Mediterranean area with values above 1000 $t/km^2/yr$ (> 0.38 mm/yr). Thus, the erosion rate in SimpleBox 2.0 (Brandes et al., 1996) can be considered representative for rather large parts of Europe although heavily underestimating the more Mediterranean areas and overestimating erosion rates on about 50 % of the European area. This value which is also assumed by EUSES (European Commission, 1996a) is adopted here. It is also used when no further differentiation of the water soil erosion process in terms of compartments and/or zones is performed.

Distribution of the overall erosion rate to soil compartments

In order to allow for different erosion intensities on different soil compartments, the crop management factor (C-factor) of the Universal Soil Loss Equation (USLE; Wischmeier and Smith, 1978; Renard et al., 1997) is made use of according to what is presented in the main text (section 5.1.5). The resulting values are given in Table 5-7 on page 103.

Improvement of the water soil erosion process description

Due to the various factors influencing the soil erosion process (Wischmeier and Smith, 1978; Renard et al., 1997; Morgan, 1999), it is clear that erosion rates that only vary by compartment/land cover will fail to represent the real erosion rate occurring at a given site. On the other hand, there exist no quantitative models for the assessment of erosion rates at the regional scale to the knowledge of the author which is due to several problems as noted, for instance, by van der Knijff et al. (2000) and Wickenkamp et al. (2000). For a modelling approach that does not take into account temporally variable conditions in the environment (only 'quasi-dynamic', cf. section 2.3), there exists a possible improvement by making use of estimated sediment yields. Two groups have published global estimates on sediment yields (Milliman and Meade, 1983; Walling and Webb, 1983). The interaction of meteorological, soil-related and management-related parameters which are needed in order to model erosion (e.g., Wischmeier and Smith, 1978; Renard et al., 1997; Morgan, 1999) can be considered integrated in the sediment yield. Considering sediment yield would allow especially for differences between the south and the north of Europe in terms of rainfall erosivity factors (van der Knijff et al., 2000) and with respect to the grazing of different animals[45] which contribute to the explanation why soils of semi-arid and semi-humid areas to which the Mediterranean areas belong tend to have the highest observable erosion rates

[45] Small ruminants such as sheep and goats that are predominantly kept in Mediterranean areas bite off blades of grass closer to the soil surface than large ruminants leading to enhanced water soil erosion.

(Morgan, 1999). Estimated values for Europe range from below 50 to values around a few hundred (Milliman and Meade, 1983) to even above 1000 t/km^2/yr (Walling and Webb, 1983) corresponding to less than 0.02 and above 0.38 mm/yr assuming an average sediment density of 2600 kg/m^3.

In order to become even more sophisticated, a weighting scheme within the different catchments could allow for different land uses (variable C-factors as reported amongst other in Morgan, 1999 and Umweltbundesamt, 1999) similar to the compartment-specific erosion velocities as described above. Furthermore, it appears that former estimates have been either over- or underestimating sediment yields (Milliman and Syvitski, 1992) which should also be corrected accordingly. Additionally, there exist more advanced GIS-based techniques in order to describe for example the slope with respect to the USLE in a spatially-resolved context (e.g., Moore et al., 1993; Desmet and Govers, 1996). However, such attempts will not solve the general poor quantitative prediction of erosion in spatially-resolved applications (de Roo, 1993).

The use of the sediment yield is, however, left to future developments.

B.5.4 Components of the particle mass balance in surface freshwater bodies

Three processes are covered by the assessment methodology that are involved in the particle mass balance in the aquatic environment (cf. section 6.1.4):

- sediment deposition,
- resuspension, and
- sediment burial.

These will be presented in the following together with the derivation of values needed for their mathematical description (cf. sections A.3.11, A.3.12 and A.3.13) after exploring some general considerations.

Sediment particle inventory and general properties

Different sources of particles may be considered in the mass balance. Examples are soil erosion, sewer effluents and primary production in the water column (Brandes et al., 1996; Wania et al., 2000). All of the multimedia models reviewed provide constant values for the volume fraction of particles in the water column. These range from $2 \cdot 10^{-5}$ vol.-% (Mackay and Diamond, 1989; Wania et al., 2000) to $1 \cdot 10^{-3}$ vol.-% (Brandes et al., 1996, at the continental scale; Severinsen et al., 1996). The bulk of the reported values is in the order of 10^{-4} vol.-% (Mackay et al., 1992, 1996a; Wania and Mackay, 1995; Rantio and Paasivirta, 1996; Mackay and Hickie, 2000). One has to note, however, that suspended mat-

Table B-9: Characteristics of suspended matter as reported for some multimedia models and implications

Models	Stated values		Resulting values	
	Mass fraction of organic carbon	Density of suspended matter	Mass fraction of mineral matter[a]	Density of mineral matter[b]
	[weight-%]	[kg per m^3]	[weight-%]	[kg per m^3]
Mackay et al. (1992), Mackay et al. (1996a), Devillers et al. (1995)	20	1500	60	1575
Rantio and Paasivirta (1996)	22	1800	56	2321

a. Assuming that half of the organic matter mass consists of organic carbon (Schnitzer, 1978) and taking the complement as mineral matter.
b. Assuming an organic matter density of 1400 kg/m^3 (Scheffer and Schachtschabel, 1989).

ter contents in natural channels varies substantially with time and place due to factors such as magnitude of the flood, seasonal conditions, the source of the water and the sediment, and altitudinal location (Milliman and Syvitski, 1992; Shen and Julien, 1993).

As is argued in the main text (section 6.1.4), a simple mass balance for particles is followed which will only employ such constant inventories. As the present particle mass balance does not only cover organic suspended matter, the values on volume fractions of suspended particulates shall be compared to reported values. Before proceeding with this, the properties of suspended as well as sediment particles shall be defined.

The composition of the suspended matter as well as that of particles in the sediment varies considerably according to the information provided by several multimedia models (Tables B-9 and B-10). Assuming that the organic carbon mass makes up 50 % of the organic matter mass (Schnitzer, 1978) with an organic matter density of 1400 kg/m^3 (Scheffer and Schachtschabel, 1989) the respective mineral matter mass fractions as well as their densities are obtained. As can be seen from both Tables, the resulting mineral matter densities tend to be lower than

Table B-10: Characteristics of sediment solids as reported for some multimedia models and implications

Models	Stated values: Mass fraction of organic carbon [weight-%]	Stated values: Density of sediment solids [kg per m³]	Resulting values: Mass fraction of mineral matter[a] [weight-%]	Resulting values: Density of mineral matter[b] [kg per m³]
Mackay et al. (1992), Mackay et al. (1996a), Devillers et al. (1995)	4	2400	92	2559
Rantio and Paasivirta (1996)	20	2000	60	2800
Mackay (1991)	5	1500	90	1512
Mackay and Hickie (2000)	2.7 - 4.6	2000	94.6 - 90.8	2050 - 2091

a. Assuming that half of the organic matter mass consists of organic carbon (Schnitzer, 1978) and taking the complement as mineral matter.
b. Assuming an organic matter density of 1400 kg/m^3 (Scheffer and Schachtschabel, 1989).

that of clay minerals (2200 - 2900 kg/m^3) and of quartz (2650 kg/m^3, Scheffer and Schachtschabel, 1989) ranging from 1500 to 2800 kg/m^3. While the organic carbon content of the sediment particles as given in Table B-10 spans the value range found in other publications (from 3 to 20 vol.-%, Mackay and Diamond, 1989; Mackay and Southwood, 1992; Wania and Mackay, 1995; Brandes et al., 1996; Severinsen et al., 1996; Wania, 1996), the values for the organic carbon content of suspended matter as shown in Table B-9 are located at the higher end of the range from 0.04 (Wania et al., 2000) to 0.4 in the deep water zone of a lake (Wania, 1996) or in the tropic zone (Wania and Mackay, 1995). Like for other characteristics of the freshwater environment, a distinction of suspended solids in stream water and lakes is made. Generally, the organic matter content of suspended and deposited solids in streams is much smaller than that found in lakes. For this reason, the reported lower bound and upper bound values are used as an ori-

Table B-11: Characteristics of solids in the freshwater environment as used in the presented methodology

Property	Particle type	Stream	Lake
Mass fraction of organic carbon in ...	suspended matter	0.02[a]	0.4[b]
	sediment solids	0.005[c]	0.3[b]
Density of solids [kg per m^3][d] of ...	suspended matter	2469	1539
	sediment solids	2627	1726

a. Half the value as used in Wania et al. (2000) assumed for 'pure' stream conditions.
b. In the deep water zone of a lake (Wania, 1996).
c. Although the smallest value found is 0.02 for the northern-boreal and the polar zones in Wania and Mackay (1995) an even smaller value is adopted for 'pure' stream sediments which usually have an organic matter content below 1 % (Scheffer and Schachtschabel, 1989) due to water erosion and oxic conditions.
d. Assumptions: half of the organic matter mass consists of organic carbon (Schnitzer, 1978) and taking the complement as mineral matter; densities: 1400 kg_{OM}/m^3, 2550 $kg_{clay\ minerals}/m^3$ (for suspended solids) and 2650 kg_{MM}/m^3 (for sediment solids, Scheffer and Schachtschabel, 1989).

entation for the characterisation of stream and lake solids, respectively (Table B-11).

If no distinction was made, a value of 0.2 and 0.05 should be used for the mass fraction of organic carbon in suspended solids and sediment solids, respectively.

Based on the information on the respective organic carbon contents and the densities for organic and mineral matter, the respective densities of solids in the water column as well as in the sediment can be defined. The densities of suspended particles and sediment solids in streams and lakes are used as given in Table B-11 which were calculated according to:

$$\rho_{solids} = \frac{1}{\frac{fr\_w_{OM/solids}}{\rho_{OM}} + \frac{fr\_w_{MM/solids}}{\rho_{OM}}} \qquad \text{(B-11)}$$

where

ρ : density of bulk solids and their organic matter (OM) or mineral matter phases (MM) [kg per m^3]

fr_w : organic (OM) or mineral matter (MM) mass fraction of bulk solids [-].

Note that the mass fraction of organic carbon needs to be multiplied by a factor of two (Schnitzer, 1978) to arrive at the overall organic matter mass fraction. The remainder mass fraction consists of mineral matter. The assumed density of organic matter is 1400 kg/m^3 (Scheffer and Schachtschabel, 1989). Two different mineral matter densities are used for the computation of suspended solid and sediment solid densities. For suspended matter, the mineral phase's density is set to that of clay minerals, i.e., 2550 kg/m^3 (Scheffer and Schachtschabel, 1989), whereas for sediment solids it is set to that of quartz, i.e., 2650 kg/m^3 (Scheffer and Schachtschabel, 1989).

Comparing the densities in Tables B-9 and B-10 to those given in Table B-11, it is obvious that the reported values correspond more to the lake situation of the present study while the stream densities are higher than those given in the multimedia modelling literature.[46]

In Table B-12, the sediment delivered to the world's oceans and seas is given per river. The rivers are selected according to whether they are located in the geographical scope of WATSON and whether there is sufficient information available in Milliman and Syvitski (1992) for the derivation of a volume fraction of suspended matter in water. In order to arrive at volume fractions, the sediment discharge was divided by the product of the water discharge and the area. After unit adjustments and division by an assumed suspended particle density of 2469 kg/m^3 in streams (Table B-11), the respective volume fractions were obtained.

The derived volume fractions of suspended matter range from an exceptionally low value of $4 \cdot 10^{-5}$ vol.-% for a lowland river to $4 \cdot 10^{-2}$ vol.-% for mountainous rivers (Table B-12). These values, thus, tend to be larger than those adopted by the multimedia models cited above. Due to the fact that the values given in Table B-12 comprise fine particles active in chemical sorption as well as coarser ones, a value of $1 \cdot 10^{-3}$ vol.-% is adopted in the present study for stream waters which appears to be applicable to non-Alpine mountainous, upland and lowland European rivers. As a result, the concentration of suspended matter in freshwater streams is set to 0.02469 kg/m^3. In the absence of more specific data,

[46] In terms of its settling behaviour, the effective suspended particle density in water bodies is usually smaller due to water contained in the associations of the single particles (Shen and Julien, 1993). However, this is not taken account of by multimedia models. Rather, these only distinguish between phases (for values on volume fractions of suspended particles as assumed in multimedia models see above) and sub-phases such as organic carbon contents.

Table B-12: Water discharge, area, sediment discharge and volume fractions of transported sediment for several rivers in the geographical scope of WATSON as compiled in Milliman and Syvitski (1992)

River (country)	Water discharge [mm/yr]	Area [10^6 km^2]	Sediment discharge [10^6 t/yr]	Volume fraction[a] [vol.-%]
Mountain (1000-3000 m) - Alpine Europe				
Ebro (Italy, lower estimate)	220	0.085	1.5	0.003
Danube (Romania)	250	0.81	67	0.013
Po (Italy)	670	0.054	13	0.015
Rhone (France)	530	0.09	31	0.026
Arno (Italy)	400	0.0081	2.2	0.028
Tiber (Italy)	450	0.016	6.8	0.038
Ebro (Italy, higher estimate)	220	0.085	18	0.039
Mountain (1000-3000 m) - non-Alpine Europe				
Ardour (France)	670	0.016	0.24	0.001
Loire (France)	245	0.115	1.5	0.002
Garonne (France)	320	0.055	2.2	0.005
Upland (500-1000 m)				
Oder (Germany)	150	0.11	0.13	0.0003
Muonio Alv (Sweden)	500	0.024	0.36	0.001
Volga (Russia, Ukraine)	400	1.4	19	0.001
Elbe (Germany)	160	0.13	0.84	0.002
Pechora (former USSR)	425	0.25	6.1	0.002
Vistula (Poland)	165	0.2	2.5	0.003
Dnester (former USSR)	135	0.062	2.5	0.012

Table B-12: Water discharge, area, sediment discharge and volume fractions of transported sediment for several rivers in the geographical scope of WATSON as compiled in Milliman and Syvitski (1992)

River (country)	Water discharge [mm/yr]	Area [10^6 km^2]	Sediment discharge [10^6 t/yr]	Volume fraction[a] [vol.-%]
Lowland (100-500 m)				
Kalkkinen (Finland)	250	0.025	0.006	0.00004
Exe (UK)	860	0.0006	0.01	0.001
Weser (Germany)	230	0.038	0.33	0.002
Nene (UK)	160	0.0015	0.01	0.002
Kymijoki (Finland)	80	0.037	0.15	0.002
Dnieper (former USSR)	86	0.38	2.1	0.003
Wye (UK)	630	0.004	0.2	0.003
Creedy (UK)	500	0.00026	0.01	0.003
Bristol Avon (UK)	400	0.00067	0.02	0.003
Tyne (UK)	680	0.0022	0.13	0.004
Welland (UK)	200	0.00053	0.01	0.004
Seine (France)	130	0.065	1.1	0.005
Clyde (UK)	430	0.0019	0.11	0.005
Ystwyth (UK)	1100	0.00017	0.028[b]	0.006
Severn (UK)	380	0.0068	0.44	0.007

a. Volume fractions derived by assuming a suspended matter density of 2090 kg/m^3 which consists of 40 weight-% of organic matter with a density of 1400 kg/m^3 (Scheffer and Schachtschabel, 1989) and of 60 weight-% of mineral matter with a density of 2550 kg/m^3 which is the average of the range given for clay minerals by (Scheffer and Schachtschabel, 1989).

b. Value derived by multiplying the sediment yield of 164 t/km^2/year by the respective area.

a value for the volume fraction of suspended matter of $1 \cdot 10^{-4}$ vol.-% is assumed for lakes which complies with the bulk of the reported values in the multimedia literature (see above).

The corresponding value for the volume fraction of solids in sediments also needs to be specified. Reported values range from 0.1 (Mackay and Hickie, 2000) to 0.4 (Mackay, 1991; Rantio and Paasivirta, 1996).[47] Based on this information and using the respectively provided solid phase densities, the corresponding bulk densities range from about 1100 kg/m^3 (Rantio and Paasivirta, 1996; Mackay and Hickie, 2000) over 1185 kg/m^3 (Mackay, 1991) and 1280 kg/m^3 (Mackay et al., 1992, 1996a) to 1420 kg/m^3 (Devillers et al., 1995).

Shen and Julien (1993) report porosities or volume fractions of void spaces in sediments of between 44 and 17 % for fine sand to coarse gravel and boulder sediments, respectively. Thus, the pore volumes assumed by the multimedia models represent sediments which are made up of finer solids than fine sand which is most likely due to the fact that these represent lakes rather than streams. Additionally, the sediment compartments only comprise the active part of the overall sediments which is not as consolidated as the parts below. The median and the average of the reported volume fractions of sediments that consist of solids is 20 % which is adopted here.

Except for the sediment's volume fraction that consists of solids, a distinction between sediments and suspended matter in streams and in lakes has been made. Within WATSON, freshwater compartments may consist also of mixtures of lakes and streams. The respective property values, therefore, need to be determined taking into account both types of aquatic ecosystems. A weighting according to water and sediment volumes is, therefore, employed.

Sedimentation

Sedimentation is defined as the "(p)rocess of settling and depositing by gravity of suspended matter in water" (Deutsches Nationalkomitee für das internationale Hydrologische Programm (IHP) der UNESCO und das Operationelle Hydrologische Programm (OHP) der WMO, 1998, p. 133). It, thus, leads to a transfer of substances from the freshwater compartment to the sediment compartment. If sedimentation prevails over resuspension, this may lead to the ultimate removal of substances from the modelled system especially due to the 'sediment burial'

---

[47] Note that two values are used by Rantio and Paasivirta (1996): a value of 0.6 for sediment porosity corresponding to 40 vol.-% solids and a value of 0.05 for all segments concerning 'volume fraction of sediment solids'. It is unclear to the author how these match.

process assumed to occur (cf. section A.3.13) while degradation being usually largely reduced in sediments. Thus, modelling this process appropriately is rather important also in light of the availability of substances towards aquatic organisms (Håkanson, 1984).

Sedimentation together with erosion is an unresolved research area according to Shen and Julien (1993): "Despite extensive research effort, knowledge of erosion and sediment transport still remains incomplete, and there is no generally accepted formula to be used for an accurate solution of the sediment transport rate and watershed sediment yield" (p. 12.1). Sediment transport characteristics are determined by the size, shape, concentration, fall velocity, bulk density of sediment particles and properties such as coatings (Shen and Julien, 1993; Nicholas and Walling, 1996; Droppo et al., 1998; Aboul-Kassim and Simoneit, 2001a; Lick and McNeil, 2001). In the context of in-water chemical transport models, basically only those particles are of interest to which chemicals may be sorbed. These are mostly fine particles and colloids (although frequently measured as dissolved organic carbon) whose surfaces are especially efficient in sorbing metals and organic chemicals (Walling, 1983; McCutcheon et al., 1993; Aboul-Kassim and Simoneit, 2001a).

There have been only few attempts to represent still water areas unlike those with flowing waters in multimedia (-type) modelling exercises. This was done either by distinguishing different parts of lakes (Wania, 1996; Mackay and Hickie, 2000) or by explicitly accounting for stagnant water compartments (Beck et al., 2000; Scheringer et al., 2000a).

The first approach requires measured or estimated data on the different water bodies included in the assessment which is rather data-intensive and may be considered when further developing the model. At the same time it shall be noted that this will be a more process-based approach in agreement with the hydrological literature. The second approach would further extend the amount of compartments distinguished, leading to higher requirements in terms of resources (computation time, data storage). A more pragmatic approach has, therefore, been adopted.

Due to their small size and, thus, their fairly reduced settling velocity, those particles or suspended matter to which most of the assessed substances are attached are only allowed to settle in lakes and stagnant waters which is in line with Scheringer et al. (2000a) and Beck et al. (2000). In the absence of more specific information, it is assumed that sedimentation occurs in all lakes at a specified rate. In contrast, only 5 % of the in-stream water volumes are assumed to allow for sedimentation due to their low amount of stagnant waters. This volume fraction is substantially lower than the 25 % that were assumed by Scheringer et al. (2000a). However, these authors did not distinguish lakes explicitly. Also, their value appears to be rather high.

The overall volume fraction of stagnant waters in a given zone is calculated according to the following equation:

$$fr\_V_{\text{stagnant}}(w,z) = \frac{V_{\text{lake}}(w,z) + V_{\text{stream}}(w,z) \cdot 0.05}{V(w,z)} \qquad \text{(B-12)}$$

where

$$V_{\text{lake}}(w,z) = A_{\text{lake}}(w,z) \cdot d_{\text{lake}}(w) \qquad \text{(B-13)}$$

$$V_{\text{stream}}(w,z) = (A(w,z) - A_{\text{lake}}(w,z)) \cdot d_{\text{stream}}(w) \qquad \text{(B-14)}$$

$$V(w,z) = V_{\text{lake}}(w,z) + V_{\text{stream}}(w,z) \qquad \text{(B-15)}$$

where

A : area of the freshwater compartment as a whole or the lake present in zone z [m^2] (information available as described in sections B.2, B.3 and B.4)

d : depth of streams or lakes [m] (defined in section B.4)

fr_V : volume fraction of stagnant waters [-]

V : volume of the bulk freshwater compartment, its lake portion or its stream portion in zone z [m^3].

Another distinction is made in that sedimentation in freshwater bodies of zones that pour directly into the sea ('river mouth') is increased due to slower flow velocities, also called aggradation zone or "area of deposition" in an idealised fluvial system (Schumm, 1977). By default, $fr\_V_{\text{stagnant}}(w,z)$ is set to 21 % in these zones provided they are part of a larger drainage basin. This is guided by the idea that a smaller percentage of the deposition rate is resuspended in these areas than in other 'pure' stream zones (see footnote a. of Table B-13).

Reported values for sedimentation rates are given in Tables B-14 and B-15 for generic or evaluative and site-specific multimedia models, respectively. The values span six orders of magnitude when also considering the values in the order of $2 \cdot 10^{-5}$ metres per second (cf. Brandes et al., 1996; Scheringer et al., 2000a). Assuming that no inter-annual accumulation of suspended particulates occurs even in the large lakes which are assumed to are 74 metres deep (cf. section B.4.1), the net removal of these particles must be set accordingly. By 'net removal' from the water column the following three processes may principally be considered to be active for both organic and mineral particles: (a) sedimentation, (b) resuspension and (c) water advection out of the water body noting that organic particles may additionally undergo mineralization (see below). Due to the potentially long residence times of waters in large lakes, water advection is not further considered for this one year balance. Thus, the lower bound of the net sedimentation rate results by subtracting the resuspension velocity from the sediment deposition velocity:

$$v_{\text{net sedimentation}} = v_{\text{sedimentation}} - v_{\text{resuspension}} \quad \text{(B-16)}$$

where

v : velocity of particles while undergoing net sedimentation, sedimentation or resuspension [m^3 per m^2 per s] or [m per s].

In order for 74 metres to be cleared in a one year (balancing) period, a net sediment deposition rate of $2.35 \cdot 10^{-6}$ metres per second would be necessary. Following Stokes' law, this value is in the range of velocities obtained for temperatures between 5 and 10°C for a spheric particle with a radius of 1 μm (i.e., of the clay fraction) and a density of 1539 kg/m^3 (assumed for suspended particles in lakes, cf. Table B-11). The settling velocities range between $2.21 \cdot 10^{-6}$ and $2.56 \cdot 10^{-6}$ metres per second for a temperature of 5 and 10°C and a corresponding (absolute) water viscosity of $1.518 \cdot 10^{-3}$ and $1.307 \cdot 10^{-3}$ kg/m/s (McCutcheon et al., 1993), respectively. Thus, the value appears to be reasonable.

Within the presented methodology, it is not suggested to include the lumped process of net sedimentation but to rather address both sedimentation and resuspension separately. One, therefore, needs to set both of the single-process velocities on the right hand side of Eq. (B-16) accordingly. The ratios between the velocity of resuspension, burial and mineralization on the one hand and the sedimentation velocity on the other shall be used in order to derive the different velocities for large lakes and rivers separately. These are also provided in Tables B-14 and B-15. One can see that several authors do not take into account the mineralization of organic matter in the sediment while others consider them to amount between 5 % in lakes (Mackay and Hickie, 2000) to up to 30 % in rivers (Rantio and Paasivirta, 1996). In principle, one would need to distinguish between the mineral and organic phases of the respective sediment and suspended particles when taking account of mineralization. This is not done at present in WATSON. The relationships used in this study are given in Table B-13.

Table B-13: Relationships between the different process rates active in the particle mass balance for surface freshwater as assumed in this study

Relationships	Pure river	River mouth[a]	Pure lake
Ratio resuspension / sedimentation	95 %[b]	45 %	33 %
Ratio burial / sedimentation	5 %	55 %	67 %[c]
Ratio remainder / sedimentation	0 %[d]	0 %	0 %[e]

a. In order to obtain the ratios for river mouth situations while following the computations described below, a stagnant volume fraction of 21 % needs to be specified.
b. The highest reported value is 85 % for the shore line of a lake (Wania, 1996); due to the even higher flow rate in streams a higher value has been adopted; note that the 'effective' sedimentation is higher in lake and river mouth situations of larger rivers.
c. Value selection guided by the burial at the deep water zone of a lake (Wania, 1996).
d. In case mineralization was to be considered the value of 14 % as used in the POPCYCLING-Baltic model would be suggested to be used for organic matter in rivers (Wania et al., 2000).
e. In case mineralization was to be considered the value of 7 % as used for the southern segment of Lac Saint Louis would be suggested to be used for organic matter in lakes (Mackay and Hickie, 2000), owing to the smaller biological activity and lower temperatures throughout the course of a year.

The overall sedimentation rate in a freshwater compartment is calculated according to:

$$v_{\text{sedimentation, total}} = fr\_V_{\text{stagnant water}} \cdot v_{\text{sedimentation, lake}} + (1 - fr\_V_{\text{stagnant water}}) \cdot v_{\text{sedimentation, stream}} \quad \text{(B-17)}$$

where

v : velocity of particles while undergoing sedimentation or resuspension in pure streams, pure lakes or the mixture of the freshwater bodies present in a given zone ('total') [m^3 per m^2 per s] or [m per s]

fr_V : volume fraction of stagnant waters [-].

For a 'pure' lake situation, Eq. (B-17) reduces to:

$$v_{\text{sedimentation, total}} = 1 \cdot v_{\text{sedimentation, lake}} \quad \text{(B-18)}$$

so that the overall sedimentation rate is equal to that of a lake or still water body. Based on the relationships as given in Table B-13 and assuming a net sedimentation rate of $2.35 \cdot 10^{-6}$ metres per second for lakes, the respective sediment deposition velocity amounts to:

$$\begin{aligned} v_{\text{net sedimentation, lake}} &= v_{\text{sedimentation, lake}} - v_{\text{resuspension, lake}} \\ 2.35 \cdot 10^{-6} &= v_{\text{sedimentation, lake}} - 0.33 \cdot v_{\text{sedimentation, lake}} \\ \Rightarrow v_{\text{sedimentation, lake}} &= \frac{2.35 \cdot 10^{-6}}{1 - 0.33} = 3.50 \cdot 10^{-6} \end{aligned} \tag{B-19}$$

where

v : velocity of particles while undergoing net sedimentation, sedimentation or resuspension [m^3 per m^2 per s] or [m per s].

For still-water areas within streams, the same net sedimentation rate of $2.35 \cdot 10^{-6}$ metres per second as for lakes is adopted due to the compliance with Stokes' law. In contrast to lakes, streams only consist in parts of more or less still water portions. While in the present methodology the water flows are allowed to vary between zones (cf. section B.5.2), a more generic approach is taken for illustration purposes. Assuming a water flow velocity similar to that used by Scheringer et al. (2000a) which is 1 metre per second and which complies to the upper typical flow velocity as stated in Schwarzenbach et al. (1993) one can see that there is a difference of about five orders of magnitude between the net sedimentation rate and the flow velocity. Thus, sedimentation is negligible. In order to follow the computation of the overall sedimentation rate of a compartment as given in Eq. (B-17), however, an explicit value for the sedimentation rate under still-water conditions is needed.

Allowing the total resuspension rate to be 95 % of that of the total sedimentation rate (cf. Table B-13) and employing the formula for the overall sedimentation rate (Eq. (B-17)), one can derive the gross sedimentation rate according to:

$$\begin{aligned} 0.05 \cdot v_{\text{sedimentation, lake}} &= fr\_V_{\text{stagnant water}} \cdot v_{\text{sedimentation, lake}} + \\ &\quad (1 - fr\_V_{\text{stagnant water}}) \cdot v_{\text{sedimentation, stream}} \\ \Rightarrow v_{\text{sedimentation, stream}} &= 0 \end{aligned} \tag{B-20}$$

where

v : velocity of particles while undergoing sedimentation or resuspension in streams or lakes [m^3 per m^2 per s] or [m per s]

fr_V : volume fraction of stagnant waters [-].

As a result, the overall sediment deposition rates as computed according to Eq. (B-17) are $3.50 \cdot 10^{-6}$ and $1.75 \cdot 10^{-7}$ metres per second for lakes and streams, respectively. Both values for the (gross) sedimentation rate are in the range found in the literature although closer to the higher end (cf. Tables B-14 and B-15). Note that the net sedimentation rate in streams is significantly reduced due to the higher resuspension rate in streams.

Resuspension

Although different processes are involved in the resuspension and the sedimentation process, it is assumed here that when sedimentation is large resuspension is small mostly depending on the flow velocities of the water body. Resuspension affects the sediment compartment which is assumed to have a uniform depth (cf. section 6.1) irrespective of whether it is situated below waters of a stream or a lake. In order for resuspension to become active, first the so-called incipient motion needs to take place (Shen and Julien, 1993): "(s)ediment particles are moved by the flow whenever the magnitude of instantaneous fluid force acting on the sediment particle exceeds the resistance force for this particle to be moved" (p. 12.16). For turbulent flows which predominate in natural waters, this fluid force fluctuates rather substantially in time and may, therefore, require a similar approach as for intermittent rain in multimedia models (e.g., Hertwich et al., 2000; MacLeod et al., 2001; Hertwich, 2001) that are based on constant environmental conditions.

In any case, the degree of resuspension is considered to be a function of the magnitude of the water-sediment interface. Thus, a corresponding area fraction of sediments located below stagnant waters is defined:

$$fr\_A_{\text{stagnant}}(ws, z) = \frac{A_{\text{lake}}(ws, z) + A_{\text{stream}}(ws, z) \cdot 0.05}{A(ws, z)} . \qquad \text{(B-21)}$$

The respective terms are defined analogously to Eq. (B-12), replacing volumes by areas.

Reported values for resuspension rates are given in Tables B-14 and B-15 for generic or evaluative and site-specific multimedia models, respectively. Like for the sedimentation rate, the values span six orders of magnitude. For the site-specific models in Table B-15, resuspension rates in lake waters are in the order of 10^{-11} to 10^{-10} (Wania, 1996; Mackay and Hickie, 2000) whereas those for rivers are about 10^{-7} (Rantio and Paasivirta, 1996).

Table B-14: Reported invariant (organic) particle mass balances in surface freshwater bodies of non-site-specific multimedia models

Sedimentation rate [m/s]	Resuspension rate [m/s]	Sediment burial rate [m/s]	Ratio resuspension / sedimentation	Ratio burial / sedimentation	Ratio mineralization / sedimentation[a]	Reference and remarks
$1.27 \cdot 10^{-11}$	$3.17 \cdot 10^{-12}$	$9.51 \cdot 10^{-12}$	25 %	75 %	0 %	Devillers et al. (1995)
$1.39 \cdot 10^{-10}$	$5.56 \cdot 10^{-11}$	$5.56 \cdot 10^{-11}$	40 %	40 %	20 %	Mackay et al. (1992), Mackay et al. (1996a)
$1.39 \cdot 10^{-10}$	$5.56 \cdot 10^{-11}$	$5.56 \cdot 10^{-11}$	40 %	40 %	20 %	Wania and Mackay (1995); invariant for all non-polar zones
$2.09 \cdot 10^{-10}$	$1.46 \cdot 10^{-10}$	$6.34 \cdot 10^{-11}$	70 %	30 %	0 %	Severinsen et al. (1996); freshwater (burial termed 'netto sedimentation rate')
$6.11 \cdot 10^{-6}$	$3.42 \cdot 10^{-6}$	$1.83 \cdot 10^{-6}$	56 %	30 %	14 %	Wania et al. (2000); upper bound for freshwater
$8.73 \cdot 10^{-6}$	$4.89 \cdot 10^{-6}$	$2.61 \cdot 10^{-6}$	56 %	30 %	14 %	Wania et al. (2000); lower bound for freshwater

a. The remainder of 100 % minus what is resuspended and buried is considered to be the fraction which is mineralized.

Table B-15: Reported invariant (organic) particle mass balances in surface freshwater bodies of site-specific multimedia models

Sedimentation rate [m/s]	Resuspension rate [m/s]	Sediment burial rate [m/s]	Ratio resuspension / sedimentation	Ratio burial / sedimentation	Ratio mineralization / sedimentation[a]	Reference
$1.74 \cdot 10^{-11}$	$1.16 \cdot 10^{-11}$	$4.86 \cdot 10^{-12}$	67 %	28 %	5 %	Mackay and Hickie (2000); northern and eastern segment of Lac Saint Louis
$3.47 \cdot 10^{-11}$	$2.31 \cdot 10^{-11}$	$9.26 \cdot 10^{-12}$	67 %	27 %	7 %	Mackay and Hickie (2000); southern segment of Lac Saint Louis
$4.17 \cdot 10^{-10}$	$2.78 \cdot 10^{-10}$	$1.39 \cdot 10^{-10}$	67 %	33 %	0 %	Wania (1996); intermediate zone of a lake
$4.17 \cdot 10^{-10}$	$1.39 \cdot 10^{-10}$	$2.78 \cdot 10^{-10}$	33 %	67 %	0 %	Wania (1996); deep water zone of a lake
$5.56 \cdot 10^{-10}$	$4.72 \cdot 10^{-10}$	$8.33 \cdot 10^{-11}$	85 %	15 %	0 %	Wania (1996); shore line of a lake
$1.39 \cdot 10^{-9}$	$5.56 \cdot 10^{-10}$	$8.33 \cdot 10^{-10}$	40 %	60 %	0 %	Wania (1996); river delta in a lake
$3.17 \cdot 10^{-7}$	$1.90 \cdot 10^{-7}$	$3.17 \cdot 10^{-8}$	60 %	10 %	30 %	Rantio and Paasivirta (1996); River Kymijoki, invariant for all segments

a.The remainder of 100 % minus what is resuspended and buried is considered to be the fraction which is mineralized.

The overall resuspension rate in the present study is calculated according to the following equation taking into account one 'pure' resuspension rate for streams and one for lakes (or rather stagnant waters, cf. section A.3.12):

$$\begin{aligned} v_{\text{resuspension, total}} = {} & fr\_A_{\text{stagnant water}} \cdot v_{\text{resuspension, lake}} + \\ & (1 - fr\_A_{\text{stagnant water}}) \cdot v_{\text{resuspension, stream}} \end{aligned} . \qquad \text{(B-22)}$$

For a situation in which the freshwater body entirely consists of a lake, Eq. (B-22) reduces to:

$$v_{\text{resuspension, total}} = 1 \cdot v_{\text{resuspension, lake}} . \qquad \text{(B-23)}$$

According to the relationship between the resuspension rate and the sedimentation rate in lakes (cf. Table B-13), the overall resuspension rate for a 'pure' lake situation in the present study are, thus, given as:

$$\begin{aligned} v_{\text{resuspension, lake}} & = 0.33 \cdot v_{\text{sedimentation, lake}} \\ & = 0.33 \cdot 3.51 \cdot 10^{-6} = 1.156 \cdot 10^{-6} \end{aligned} . \qquad \text{(B-24)}$$

If the freshwater body consists purely of a river, Eq. (B-22) becomes:

$$\begin{aligned} v_{\text{resuspension, total}} & = fr\_A_{\text{stagnant water}} \cdot v_{\text{resuspension, lake}} + \\ & \quad (1 - fr\_A_{\text{stagnant water}}) \cdot v_{\text{resuspension, stream}} \\ & = 0, 05 \cdot v_{\text{resuspension, lake}} + (1 - 0, 05) \cdot v_{\text{resuspension, stream}} \end{aligned} . \qquad \text{(B-25)}$$

Substituting for the lake resuspension rate as calculated by Eq. (B-24) and allowing the overall in-stream resuspension rate to equal 95 % of the (actual) in-stream sedimentation rate (cf. Table B-13), one obtains Eq. (B-26).

The overall resuspension rate for lakes and streams as computed according to Eq. (B-22) using the values obtained by Eqs. (B-24) and (B-26) are $1.156 \cdot 10^{-6}$ and $1.66 \cdot 10^{-7}$ metres per second for lakes and streams, respectively. Both values for the (gross) resuspension rate are in the range found in the literature although closer to the higher end (cf. Tables B-14 and B-15).

$$
\begin{aligned}
v_{\text{resuspension, total}} &= 0.95 \cdot (0.05 \cdot v_{\text{sedimentation, lake}} + \\
&\quad (1 - 0.05) \cdot v_{\text{sedimentation, stream}}) \\
&= 0.05 \cdot v_{\text{resuspension, lake}} + (1 - 0, 05) \cdot v_{\text{resuspension, stream}} \\
\Rightarrow v_{\text{resuspension, stream}} &= \frac{[0.95 \cdot (0.05 \cdot 3.50 \cdot 10^{-6} + 0.95 \cdot 0)] - (0.05 \cdot 1.156 \cdot 10^{-6})}{1 - 0.05} \\
&= 1.143 \cdot 10^{-7}
\end{aligned}
\quad \text{(B-26)}
$$

Sediment burial

'Sediment burial' means a process that leads to the translocation of substances from the active layer to the inactive layer further down the sediment. It constitutes an ultimate loss process from the modelled system.

Several authors of multimedia fate models report rates or rather velocities for the sediment burial process which span six orders of magnitude (cf. Tables B-14 and B-15).

The overall burial rate in the present study is calculated analogously to Eq. (B-22) by taking into account one 'pure' burial rate for streams and one for lakes (or rather stagnant waters, cf. section A.3.13):

$$
v_{\text{burial, total}} = fr\_A_{\text{stagnant water}} \cdot v_{\text{burial, lake}} + (1 - fr\_A_{\text{stagnant water}}) \cdot v_{\text{burial, stream}} \,. \quad \text{(B-27)}
$$

For a situation in which the freshwater body entirely consists of a lake, Eq. (B-27) reduces to:

$$
v_{\text{burial, total}} = 1 \cdot v_{\text{burial, lake}} \,. \quad \text{(B-28)}
$$

According to the relationship between the burial rate and the sedimentation rate in lakes (cf. Table B-13), the overall burial rate for a 'pure' lake situation in the present study are, thus, given as:

$$
\begin{aligned}
v_{\text{burial, lake}} &= 0.67 \cdot v_{\text{sedimentation, lake}} \\
&= 0.67 \cdot 3.51 \cdot 10^{-6} = 2.35 \cdot 10^{-6}
\end{aligned}
\,. \quad \text{(B-29)}
$$

If the freshwater body consists purely of a river, Eq. (B-27) becomes:

$$
\begin{aligned}
v_{\text{burial, total}} &= fr\_A_{\text{stagnant water}} \cdot v_{\text{burial, lake}} + (1 - fr\_A_{\text{stagnant water}}) \cdot v_{\text{burial, stream}} \\
&= 0.05 \cdot v_{\text{burial, lake}} + (1 - 0.05) \cdot v_{\text{burial, stream}}
\end{aligned} \quad . \tag{B-30}
$$

Substituting for the lake burial rate as calculated by Eq. (B-29) and allowing the overall in-stream burial rate to equal 5 % of the (actual) in-stream sedimentation rate (cf. Table B-13), one obtains:

$$
\begin{aligned}
v_{\text{burial, total}} &= 0.05 \cdot (0.05 \cdot v_{\text{sedimentation, lake}} + \\
&\quad (1 - 0.05) \cdot v_{\text{sedimentation, stream}}) \\
&= 0.05 \cdot v_{\text{burial, lake}} + (1 - 0.05) \cdot v_{\text{burial, stream}} \\
\Rightarrow v_{\text{burial, stream}} &= \frac{[0.05 \cdot (0.05 \cdot 3.50 \cdot 10^{-6} + 0.95 \cdot 0)] - 0.05 \cdot 2.35 \cdot 10^{-6}}{1 - 0.05} \\
&= -1.143 \cdot 10^{-7}
\end{aligned} \quad . \tag{B-31}
$$

The overall sediment burial rate for lakes and streams as computed according to Eq. (B-27) using the values obtained by Eqs. (B-29) and (B-31) are $2.35 \cdot 10^{-6}$ and $8.76 \cdot 10^{-9}$ metres per second for lakes and streams, respectively. These correspond to the net sedimentation rates. Both values for the overall burial rate are in the range found in the multimedia modelling literature, the one for lakes being closer to the higher end (cf. Tables B-14 and B-15). The rather high sediment burial rate in lakes may also be due to the fact that in this study no mineralization of sediment particles is assumed to occur. In order to compare these values to values found in the literature, the burial velocities are converted into annual volumetric additions to sediments. The velocities are multiplied by the volume fractions of solids in the respective water column, i.e., $1 \cdot 10^{-4}$ and $1 \cdot 10^{-3}$ vol.-% for lakes and streams, respectively. The resulting values are 0.074 mm/yr, 0.003 mm/yr and 0.13 mm/yr for lakes, streams and river mouth locations, respectively. These are mostly within the range found for geologic aggradation rates (0.01 mm/yr to 3 mm/yr in the non-marine environment, Hohl, 1985) noting that under pure stream conditions a very small aggradation takes place. In particular the higher values found for deltas, i.e., 3 mm/yr, exceed those adopted for river mouths by one order of magnitude.

Note that the value obtained for the in-stream burial rate by Eq. (B-31) is negative. All of the velocities derived for streams (not only the velocity for burial, but also for sedimentation and resuspension (Eqs. (B-31), (B-20) and (B-26), respectively)) should, however, be regarded as hypothetical as these are not directly used in the process formulations (section A.3). These values are obtained in order to fulfil the following requirements:

- in order to provide a generally applicable computation of the overall process rates, the approach as given by Eq. (6-9) is followed which distinguishes between stagnant and non-stagnant domains within any freshwater compartment. Due to the heterogeneity of freshwater compartments ranging from pure streams over mixtures of streams and lakes to pure lakes, this methodological approach is adopted, and
- the overall in-stream net sedimentation rate, i.e., resulting sediment deposition rate minus resuspension rate, shall amount to 5 % of the lake net sedimentation rate (cf. Eq. (B-20)).

As a result, especially the negative value for the burial rate is hypothetical and is only used in order to yield a (non-negative) total process velocity. The hypothetic values for pure moving water conditions are, therefore, considered justified and scientifically defendable as long as they are consistently derived and used. As stated above, any water body is assumed to at least contain 5 % of still waters which assures that no negative end-values result.

B.5.5 Average surface temperature

The volatility of substances with non-negligible vapour pressures depends on the ambient temperature. Furthermore, exposure response functions may depend on temperature, such as for damages to materials (Tidblad et al. (1998) quoted in Friedrich and Bickel, 2001a). Therefore, the ambient temperature at the surface is needed.

Annual average temperature data for ground level air were taken from the EcoSense multi-source version for Europe on the EMEP 50 x 50 km grid. Although the heat contained in a volume of air consists of the sensitive as well as the latent heat, i.e., that is contained in the entrained humidity, the temperature was taken as the indicator for both components. This data processing, thus, assumes that the latent heat in air volumes of adjacent grid cells are so close that its influence on the total heat can be disregarded.

The temperature was distributed to the respective zones by area weighting. By doing so it was revealed that temperature data for the most southern EMEP 50 y row are missing (mostly Africa). This data gap was filled by assuming equal temperatures as in the next more northern EMEP 50 y row.

B.6 Spatial differentiation for the exposure and impact assessment

In contrast to the environmental fate model, the exposure and the impact assessments follow a spatial differentiation based on administrative units mostly according to the Nomenclature of Territorial Units for Statistics (Nomenclature des Unités Territoriales Statistiques, NUTS) used by the Statistical Office of the European Communities (EUROSTAT).[48] Thus, the information that is available in a spatially-resolved way is attributed to the different administrative levels distinguished. The highest resolution is available for the larger member states of the European Union for which NUTS level 3 is distinguished corresponding to municipalities (Fig. B-4). For countries that are not (yet) part of the European Union as of the beginning of 2004, usually only the countries themselves are distinguished. Exceptions which have one subdivision below country-level are Albania, Azerbaidjan, Bulgaria, the Czech Republic, Georgia, Hungary, Norway, Poland, Romania, Slovenia, Switzerland and the former Yugoslavia. Non-European Union countries with a threefold subdivision are Russia and the Ukraine (Fig. B-4).

B.6.1 Production-related data

There are presently two types of production-related data included in the assessment: the production and the yield.

Production data

In order to consider trade and to introduce a production-based human exposure assessment, one needs to know the actual amounts of food produced. These are taken from the EcoSense multi-source version database to the extent possible (e.g., wheat, barley, potatoes, rye, oats). Missing data on animal produce such as beef, pork, milk, poultry, eggs and pork as well as spinach are taken from the Food and Agriculture Organization of the United Nations' (FAO) statistical database (Food and Agriculture Organization of the United Nations - Statistics Division, 2002b, 2002a; Food and Agriculture Organization of the United Nations - Statistics Division, 2003) for the year 2000. Information on the production of cereals in Russia have been taken from the same source. The amounts of the respective food groups produced are shown in Table B-16.

The original data utilized are given for different levels of aggregation. Whereas the FAO data are given at country level (NUTS0 or equivalent), the in-

---

[48] Note that also the direct releases into water and soil are specified according to these administrative units.

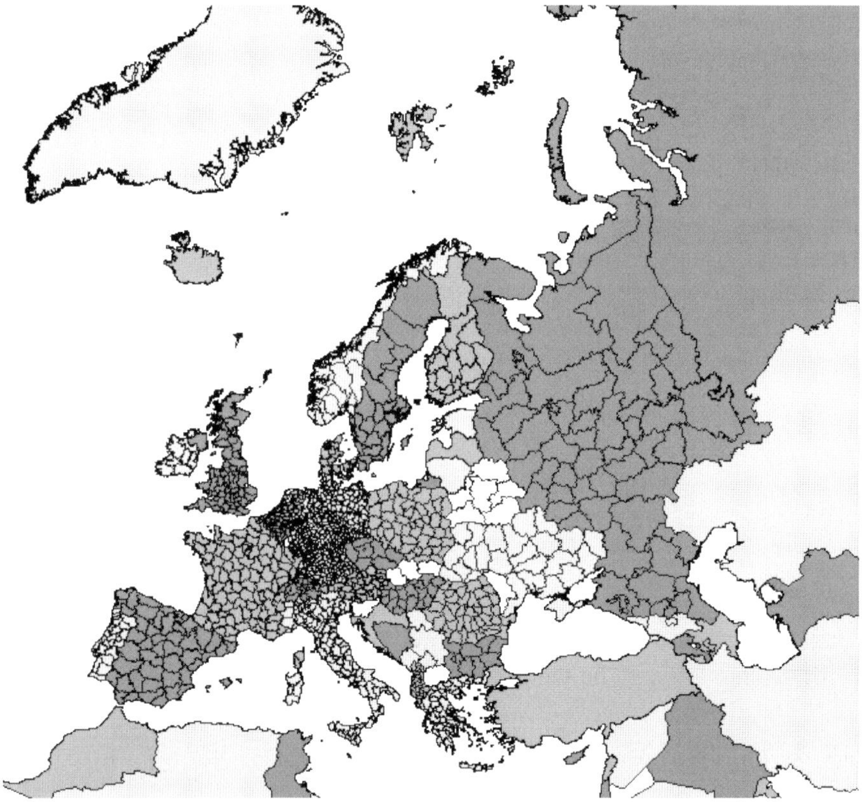

Fig. B-4: Subdivision of the geographical scope of the model into administrative units. Countries are distinguished by different shades of grey (see Fig. B-1 for the model's boundaries).

formation stored in the EcoSense database may be as detailed as at the municipality level. Apart from the FAO, information on agricultural production data contained in the EcoSense database were mostly extracted from the country-specific editions of the series by Statistisches Bundesamt (various volumes) which were issued in different years from 1991-1995 providing data at country level. Agricultural production data below the country level were to a large extent taken from the respective national statistical agencies (e.g., Statistisches Bundesamt in Germany, Istituto Nazionale di Statistica in Italy) or from the Statistical Office of the European Communities. All data are valid for the early nineties.

Table B-16: Annual national production of different produce [kt/yr]

Country	Beef and veal[a]	Cereals[b, c]	Cow milk, whole fresh[a]	Eggs[d]	Freshwater fish[d]	Spinach[e]	Pork[a]	Potatoes[b]	Poultry meat[d]
Albania	36	49	807	21	0.0008	0	6.8	65	4.0
Armenia	13	121	177	8.2	0.0002	0	2.4	163	0.46
Austria	203	2439	3340	86	0.0035	7.3	624	594	111
Azerbaijan, Republic of	10	170	196	5.8	0.0009	0	0.30	63	3.3
Belarus	269	3727	4490	182	0.0058	0	256	10000	76
Belgium	253	1908	3398	194	0.0013	75	981	1906	407
Bosnia and Herzegovina	13	1573	540	15	0.0025	0	5.0	0	8.4
Bulgaria	67	3762	1390	82	0.010	3.0	243	478	104
Croatia	27	1773	607	46	0.0037	0	114	507	33
Czech Republic	107	6631	2789	188	0.023	3.5	417	1460	215
Denmark	154	7669	4720	74	0.044	0	1624	1359	202
Estonia	15	462	629	16	0.0042	0	30	340	7.3
Faroe islands	0.077	0	0	0	0	0	0	0	0

Table B-16: Annual national production of different produce [kt/yr]

Country	Beef and veal[a]	Cereals[b, c]	Cow milk, whole fresh[a]	Eggs[d]	Freshwater fish[d]	Spinach[e]	Pork[a]	Potatoes[b]	Poultry meat[d]
Finland	91	3298	2450	59	0.072	0	173	798	64
France	1514	39318	24898	1038	0.064	109	2312	5464	2221
Georgia	48	168	619	20	0.0002	0	37	350	14
Germany	1301	36934	28300	901	0.060	60	3981	26170	801
Greece	66	2606	789	117	0.026	37	143	946	154
Hungary	49	3934	2145	176	0.019	7.0	622	1042	470
Iceland	3.6	0	107	0	0.0043	0	0	0	0
Ireland	577	1447	5160	32	0.024	0	226	584	123
Italy	1154	11739	11740	686	0.056	91	1478	2308	1089
Kazakhstan	63	2846	770	19	0.0056	0	28	289	6.9
Latvia	22	726	823	24	0.0017	0	32	701	7.2
Liechtenstein	0	0	12	0	0.0032	0	0	0	0
Lithuania	75	2706	1725	39	0.0036	0	84	1849	25
Luxembourg	22	107	291	0	0.0001	0	84	20	15
Macedonia	7.0	537	200	26	0.0018	0	9.0	180	4.8

Table B-16: Annual national production of different produce [kt/yr]

Country	Beef and veal[a]	Cereals[b, c]	Cow milk, whole fresh[a]	Eggs[d]	Freshwater fish[d]	Spinach[e]	Pork[a]	Potatoes[b]	Poultry meat[d]
Malta	1.6	9	48	6.0	0	0	9.1	13	5.3
Moldova, Republic of	21	926	555	32	0.0016	0	60	400	16
Netherlands	471	1338	11135	668	0.0071	49	1623	7699	754
Norway	91	1177	1699	48	0.466	0	103	455	43
Poland	349	19728	11889	424	0.052	0	1923	36270	626
Portugal	83	1749	1442	117	0.0012	14	317	1242	268
Romania	162	5692	4301	263	0.014	0	502	4143	259
Russian Federation	385	12163	6490	384	0.116	0	318	7671	153
Serbia and Montenegro	98	2821	1830	72	0.010	0	655	0	89
Slovakia	48	2378	1067	61	0.0023	1.1	164	483	104
Slovenia	42	221	649	23	0.0013	0.39	59	185	67
Spain	629	15536	5997	658	0.038	62	2904	5000	987
Sweden	150	3830	3297	102	0.0086	0	277	738	92

Table B-16: Annual national production of different produce [kt/yr]

Country	Beef and veal[a]	Cereals[b, c]	Cow milk, whole fresh[a]	Eggs[d]	Freshwater fish[d]	Spinach[e]	Pork[a]	Potatoes[b]	Poultry meat[d]
Switzerland	128	1064	3871	36	0.0030	17	225	908	49
Turkey	236	17158	5800	449	0.043	136	0.18	0	439
Ukraine	754	22300	12436	497	0.048	0	676	15000	193
United Kingdom	708	19841	14489	589	0.15	0	923	6445	1513

a. Year 2000 taken from Food and Agriculture Organization of the United Nations - Statistics Division (2002b).
b. Different years and sources.
c. Comprising wheat, barley, rye and oats.
d. Year 2000 taken from Food and Agriculture Organization of the United Nations - Statistics Division (2002a).
e. Year 2000 taken from Food and Agriculture Organization of the United Nations - Statistics Division (2003).

The exposure assessment is performed at the lowest administrative level distinguished (see Fig. B-4, 1355 administrative units in total) unless aggregation takes place. Different distribution schemes have been followed in order to distribute the food production and also population data from for instance the country level to the lowest administrative level distinguished. These schemes may be based on the total area (e.g., for human population), water volume (fish), or the land uses pastures (cattle) and arable land (all other agricultural produce). From the degree to which farm animals are kept outside (cf. section 7.1.1), it is clear that especially the distribution of farm animals other than cattle is difficult according to a particular land use. Rather than using a purely (total) area-weighted distribution scheme, the distribution scheme according to arable land is adopted in order to follow agricultural activity. Prior to distributing the animal produce eggs, poultry, beef and pork according to one of these schemes, however, the stock and production information available from the REGIO database (European Commission, 2003e) is used to distribute the FAO data to below country level to the extent possible.

Some countries shown in Fig. B-4 are not entirely covered by the models WATSON and EcoSense (cf. Fig. B-1). In case receptor data for example on production but also on population are only provided at the country level, this may lead to overestimates of the affected amounts of food produced and/or population living in the assessed area. For instance, Russia is only covered to 20 % in terms of space by both models. Adopting the country total for food production for instance is, therefore, misleading. Affected countries are Russia, Kazakhstan, Armenia, Azerbaijan, Turkey, Libya, Algeria and Morocco. The receptor data provided at the country level (NUTS0) are, therefore, corrected according to the area share of the respective countries in the geographical scope of the model. Total land areas were taken from Central Intelligence Agency (CIA) (2003) while the areas covered were derived from the WATSON database (Table B-17).

Data on yield

The second type of production-related data is the respective yield. This is needed for the assessment of the removal from the environmental fate model due to harvest of agricultural produce when exposed via atmospheric deposition (cf. section A.6.5). Note that in contrast to agricultural practice, this parameter needs to reflect the total mass produced on a given area over a one year period, accounting for potentially several harvests of the same crop. The values for spinach in the different countries were taken from Food and Agriculture Organization of the United Nations - Statistics Division (2003) for the year 2000.

Table B-17: Correction of country total receptor values according to area covered by WATSON

Country	Total area[a] [km^2]	Area covered [km^2]	Share [%]
Algeria	2381740	641750	27
Armenia	28400	10871	38
Azerbaijan	86100	16384	19
Kazakhstan	2669800	551390	21
Libya	1759540	517360	29
Morocco	2381740	21500	1
Russia	16995800	3449200	20
Turkey	770760	511960	66

a.Total land area taken from Central Intelligence Agency (CIA) (2003).

B.6.2 Human consumption data

According to the official report on nutrition for Germany (Deutsche Gesellschaft für Ernährung e.V., 2000), there are different types of data for the assessment of food uptake by a population. It is distinguished between use data ('Verbrauchsdaten') based on agricultural statistics and consumption data ('Verzehrsdaten') which are inquired at the end user level. The latter are not readily available for all countries covered by the present assessment (cf. the Euromonitor (1992) dataset discussed below). If consumption data are available, these are often only representative for a small sub-population of a country (e.g., a municipality; cf. consumption data for Catalans (Buckley-Golder et al., 1999) and the whole of Spain (Euromonitor, 1992 given in European Centre for Ecotoxicology and Toxicology of Chemicals, 1994)).

It was, therefore, explored to what degree the per capita food supply data of the FAO Food Balance Sheets (FBSs, Food and Agriculture Organization of the United Nations - Statistics Division, 2002a) which give the "quantities of food reaching the consumer" (ibid.) can be taken as a proxy for the real intake. The consumption data for several EU countries published by Euromonitor (1992) reproduced in European Centre for Ecotoxicology and Toxicology of Chemicals (1994) and European Commission (2003a) were compared to those provided by

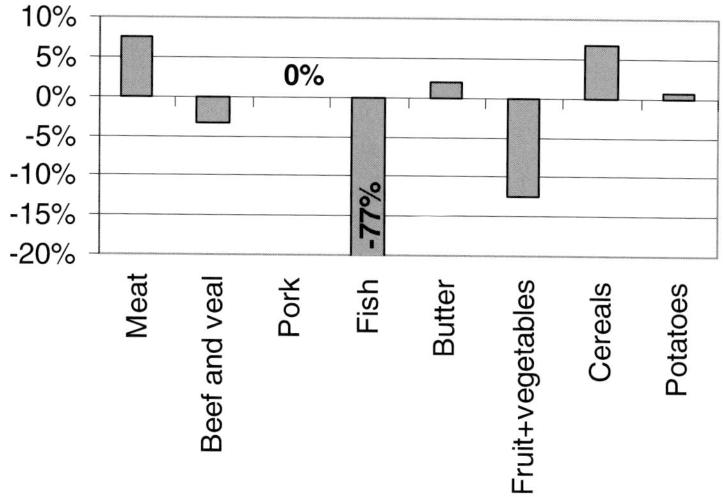

Fig. B-5: Example on the deviation of the food supply data (Food and Agriculture Organization of the United Nations - Statistics Division, 2002a) from the consumption data by Euromonitor (1992): EU15 countries in 1990

the FBSs. No reference year was stated which is why the comparison was done for the years 1990 through 1992. As an example, the result of the comparison for the European Union 15 (EU15) countries in 1990 is given in Fig. B-5. The following conclusions can be drawn:

- the most severe deviations occur for aggregated food items (e.g., meat, fish, fruit/vegetables),
- fish as well as fruit and vegetable supply as estimated by the FBS tend to overestimate the consumption given by Euromonitor (1992), and
- a simple derivation of a loss fraction of edible food in the households is not apparent.

However, one would expect that the supply is usually larger than the consumption. This can be explained by the fact that not all food that is assessed to be available for consumption is finally eaten (e.g., due to loss, plate-waste). Additionally, there are many gaps in deriving the FBSs particularly in the statistics of utilization for non-food purposes which might lead to a reduction of the estimated per capita food supply.[49] Within the assessment, use is made of the food supply data that are corrected by assuming that 5 % of the retailed food is lost in order to arrive at a more representative, country-dependent proxy of real consumption. In the equations, this is considered through the inclusion of the parameter $fr\_w_{\text{not consumed/food supply}}$.

It occurs that the agricultural production data for 'cow milk, whole, fresh' (Food and Agriculture Organization of the United Nations - Statistics Division, 2002b) are smaller than those given for 'milk - excluding butter' in the Food Balance Sheets (Food and Agriculture Organization of the United Nations - Statistics Division, 2002a) based on which the milk supply shall be determined. While both apparently exclude butter and cream, the difference is explicable by production of milk from animals other than cows (i.e., buffalos, goats and sheep). It is assumed that the per capita supply has the same milk composition as the domestic production. Based on this assumption, the 'milk - excl. butter' is converted into 'cow milk, whole, fresh' by a country-specific conversion factor ('share' in Table B-18) in order to yield the cow milk supply available for intake by humans.

The predicted substance concentrations in food are only valid for those food items that are produced within the geographical scope of the model. In order to know to what degree the European[50] food supply relies on imports or formulated inversely to what degree the European food production can sustain its food demand, the self-supply is derived from trade statistics at the border of Europe for the year 2000 (Food and Agriculture Organization of the United Nations - Statistics Division, 2002a; Food and Agriculture Organization of the United Nations - Statistics Division, 2003). In general, the amounts produced in Europe can at least sustain consumption as regards the food groups considered in the assessment (Table B-19). These self-supply figures only consider net trade effects. Import of food (and feed) produced outside the geographical area considered (also taking place to varying degrees), however, leads to a 'dilution' of the predicted pollutant concentrations due to the fact that the exposure assessment is confined to a certain portion of the world and all produce imported except for re-imports is, thus, considered unexposed. Nevertheless, it is assumed that people only take in food items produced within the area modelled. This applies to all food groups listed in Table B-19 except spinach. Although the case of spinach may be regarded is in-

---

49 See comment to the FBS data found at http://www.fao.org/waicent/faostat/agricult/fbs-e.htm.

50 By 'Europe', the following countries are meant: Albania, Austria, Belarus, Belgium, Bosnia and Herzegovina, Bulgaria, Croatia, Czech Republic, Denmark, Estonia, Finland, France, Germany, Greece, Hungary, Ireland, Italy, Latvia, Lithuania, Luxembourg, Macedonia, Malta, Republic of Moldova, Netherlands, Norway, Poland, Portugal, Romania, Russian Federation, Serbia and Montenegro, Slovakia, Slovenia, Spain, Sweden, Switzerland, Ukraine, United Kingdom.

Table B-18: Difference between cow milk production and overall milk production and assumed share of cow milk production with respect to the overall milk production

Country	Cow milk, whole, fresh production[a] [t/yr]	Milk - excluding butter (total inland production)[b] [t/yr]	Difference [t/yr]	Share [-]
Albania	807000	948007	141007	85%
Armenia	462000	473760	11760	98%
Austria	3340126	3364290	24164	99%
Azerbaijan, Republic of	1031110	1031110	0	100%
Belarus	4489600	4489600	0	100%
Belgium	3398296	3398296	0	100%
Bosnia and Herze-govina	540000	547100	7100	99%
Bulgaria	1389800	1706300	316500	81%
Croatia	2145000	2188740	43740	98%
Cyprus	146600	180200	33600	81%
Czech Republic	2789364	2805120	15756	99%
Denmark	4719800	4719800	0	100%
Estonia	628911	628911	0	100%
Finland	2450100	2450100	0	100%
France	24898000	25630100	732100	97%
Georgia	618900	618900	0	100%
Germany	28331216	28354410	23194	100%
Greece	789000	1958740	1169740	40%
Hungary	606816	615470	8654	99%

Table B-18: Difference between cow milk production and overall milk production and assumed share of cow milk production with respect to the overall milk production

Country	Cow milk, whole, fresh production[a] [t/yr]	Milk - excluding butter (total inland production)[b] [t/yr]	Difference [t/yr]	Share [-]
Iceland	107353	107353	0	100%
Ireland	5159788	5159790	2	100%
Italy	11741000	12891000	1150000	91%
Kazakhstan	3730200	3774690	44490	99%
Latvia	822983	824970	1987	100%
Liechten-stein	12000	12000	0	100%
Lithuania	1724700	1724700	0	100%
Luxem-bourg	290704	290704	0	100%
Macedonia	200000	240000	40000	83%
Malta	47969	49642	1673	97%
Moldova, Republic of	554800	571000	16200	97%
Netherlands	11135000	11135000	0	100%
Norway	1699000	1720500	21500	99%
Poland	11889300	11901860	12560	100%
Portugal	1994788	2132860	138072	94%
Romania	4301259	4622760	321501	93%
Russian Federation	31977000	32300000	323000	99%
Serbia and Montenegro	1830000	1862000	32000	98%

Table B-18: Difference between cow milk production and overall milk production and assumed share of cow milk production with respect to the overall milk production

Country	Cow milk, whole, fresh production[a] [t/yr]	Milk - excluding butter (total inland production)[b] [t/yr]	Difference [t/yr]	Share [-]
Slovakia	1067000	1123090	56090	95%
Slovenia	649300	649300	0	100%
Spain	6047000	6673000	626000	91%
Sweden	3297000	3300000	3000	100%
Switzerland	3871300	3887800	16500	100%
Turkey	8732041	9807500	1075459	89%
Ukraine	12436000	12710000	274000	98%
United Kingdom	14488000	14489000	1000	100%

a. According to Food and Agriculture Organization of the United Nations - Statistics Division (2002b).

b. According to Food and Agriculture Organization of the United Nations - Statistics Division (2002a).

significant, a correction factor is introduced in order for the exposure assessment to be applicable for any type of produce, regardless of the degree of self-supply. This correction factor is equal to the values given in Table B-19 ('degree of self-supply') setting values larger than 100 % to unity ('value adopted').

B.6.3 Further substance-independent data used in the exposure assessment

In the following, some of the variable parameter values are given that neither fall into the groups presented above nor are substance-dependent.

Farm animals take in different feed at varying rates. These are given for two exposure assessment frameworks separately (Tables B-21 and B-20).

Some of the bioconcentration factors are given as a ratio of dry weight concentrations in soil and produce, respectively (cf. section C.2). However, the food consumption information is given on a fresh weight basis. One, therefore, needs

Table B-19: Degree of self-supply in Europe[a] with respect to the food groups considered in the exposure assessment; derived based on (Food and Agriculture Organization of the United Nations - Statistics Division, 2002a; Food and Agriculture Organization of the United Nations - Statistics Division, 2003)

Food group	Degree of self-supply [%]	Value adopted [%]
Barley	112	100
Bovine Meat	100	100
Eggs	101	100
Freshwater Fish	101	100
Milk - Excluding Butter	108	100
Oats	106	100
Pork	103	100
Potatoes	102	100
Poultry Meat	101	100
Rye	104	100
Spinach	97	97
Wheat	107	100

a. See also footnote 50.

to perform a unit conversion correspondingly. The respective values used are given in Table B-22.

At present only wheat is considered as the main source of grains fed to farm animals. Its mass fraction of the total amount of grains eaten by farm animals as assumed in the assessment is given in Table B-23.

Table B-20: Ingestion of feed and soil particles by farm animals ($ING_{feed\ or\ soil}$) [kg DW/capita/s] according to United States - Environmental Protection Agency (1998)

Farm animal	Feed or soil	$ING_{feed\ or\ soil}$	Remark
Beef	Forage	$4.40 \cdot 10^{-5}$	forage consumption of typical beef cattle (Table in section 5.4.4.2, United States - Environmental Protection Agency, 1998)
	Grains	$4.40 \cdot 10^{-5}$	grain consumption of typical beef cattle (Table in section 5.4.4.2, United States - Environmental Protection Agency, 1998)
	Silage	$1.16 \cdot 10^{-5}$	silage consumption of typical beef cattle (Table in section 5.4.4.2, United States - Environmental Protection Agency, 1998)
	Soil particles	$3.47 \cdot 10^{-6}$	section 5.4.4.4 (United States - Environmental Protection Agency, 1998); the recommended value of 0.5 kg/day is for subsistence farmer beef cattle; thus, the quoted value by US-EPA 1990 of 0.3 kg/day which is representative for typical beef farmers' cattle is used
Cow milk and products	Forage	$7.18 \cdot 10^{-5}$	forage consumption of typical dairy farmer cattle (Table in section 5.4.5.2, United States - Environmental Protection Agency, 1998)
	Grains	$1.41 \cdot 10^{-4}$	grain consumption of typical dairy farmer cattle (Table in section 5.4.5.2, United States - Environmental Protection Agency, 1998)
	Silage	$2.20 \cdot 10^{-5}$	silage consumption of typical dairy farmer cattle (Table in section 5.4.5.2, United States - Environmental Protection Agency, 1998)

Table B-20: Ingestion of feed and soil particles by farm animals ($ING_{feed\ or\ soil}$) [kg DW/capita/s] according to United States - Environmental Protection Agency (1998)

Farm animal	Feed or soil	$ING_{feed\ or\ soil}$	Remark
Cow milk and products (continued)	Soil particles	$2.31 \cdot 10^{-6}$	section 5.4.5.4 (United States - Environmental Protection Agency, 1998); the recommended value of 0.4 kg/day is for subsistence farmer dairy cattle; thus, the quoted value by NC DEHNR of 0.2 kg/day is used which is representative for typical dairy farmers' cattle
Laying hens (eggs)	Grains	$2.31 \cdot 10^{-6}$	value for hens (section 5.6.1.2, United States - Environmental Protection Agency, 1998)
	Soil particles	$2.31 \cdot 10^{-6}$	value for hens (section 5.6.1.2, United States - Environmental Protection Agency, 1998)
Pork	Grains	$3.82 \cdot 10^{-5}$	section 5.5.1.2 (United States - Environmental Protection Agency, 1998)
	Soil particles	$4.28 \cdot 10^{-6}$	section 5.5.1.4 (United States - Environmental Protection Agency, 1998)
Poultry	Grains	$2.31 \cdot 10^{-6}$	section 5.6.1.2 (United States - Environmental Protection Agency, 1998)
	Soil particles	$2.31 \cdot 10^{-6}$	section 5.6.1.2 (United States - Environmental Protection Agency, 1998)

Table B-21: Ingestion of forage by farm animals (ING_{forage}) [kg DW/capita/s] according to International Atomic Energy Agency (2001)

Farm animal	ING_{forage}	Remark
Beef	$1.39 \cdot 10^{-4}$	Table XII (value for large animal, diet consists of fresh forage only, International Atomic Energy Agency, 2001)
Cow milk and products	$1.85 \cdot 10^{-4}$	Table XII (value for large animal, diet consists of fresh forage only, International Atomic Energy Agency, 2001)

Table B-22: Mass fraction of food dry matter ($fr\_w_{solid\ phase/bulk}$) [kg_{food} DW per kg_{food} FW]

Produce	$fr\_w_{solid\ phase/bulk}$	Remark
Cereals	0.9	on average 10 % moisture content for cereals assumed (Table 9-19, United States - Environmental Protection Agency, 1997a)
Fish	0.2468	average of carp, drum (fw), perch, pike and trout (all in raw status; Table 10-48, United States - Environmental Protection Agency, 1997a)
Meat	0.284	moisture content of beef (71.6%) taken as representative although varying from 68.3% for goose to 75.5% for wild duck (Table 11-21, United States - Environmental Protection Agency, 1997a)
Potatoes	0.1671	moisture content of 'potatoes (white) - whole' is 83.29% according to Table 9-19 in United States - Environmental Protection Agency (1997a)
Spinach	0.0842	moisture content of spinach is 91.58% according to Table 9-19 in United States - Environmental Protection Agency (1997a)

Table B-23: Mass fraction of grains fed to farm animals consisting of wheat ($fr\_w_{wheat/total\ grain}$) [-]

Farm animal	$fr\_w_{wheat/total\ grain}$	Remark
Beef and milk cattle	0.013	0.03 of cereals in fodder for cattle (rule of thumb), overall fodder consumption 11095100 t of which 4861700 t are cereals and 2153000 t are wheat in Germany from July 2003 through January 2004 (Menz, 2004)
Pork, poultry and laying hens	0.29	0.65 of cereals in fodder for non-cattle, overall fodder consumption 11095100 t of which 4861700 t are cereals and 2153000 t are wheat in Germany from July 2003 through January 2004 (Menz, 2004)

Appendix C Substance-dependent data

In this Appendix, substance-dependent data are compiled to the extent that these are not provided in the main text. Data presented are those needed for the environmental fate (section C.1) and exposure assessment (C.2). Additionally, monitoring data are given in section C.3. While substance-dependent data involved in the impact assessment step of the Impact Pathway Approach have been fully given in the main text (cf. section 7.3), it shall be noted that substance-dependent valuation is not foreseen to be performed. This is due to the circumstance that results at the impact level may be aggregated according to the health endpoint such as DALYs (cf. section 7.3). As a result, there is for instance no section on monetary valuation in this Appendix.

C.1 Substance properties influencing the environmental fate

In the context of multimedia models, it is assumed that there is thermodynamic equilibrium within compartments. This means that substances partition between different phases of a compartment according to their ideal partitioning coefficients. Partitioning can occur between the solid and aqueous phase ('solid-water partitioning coefficients'), the gas and solid phase ('air-solid partitioning coefficient') as well as the gas and aqueous phase ('air-water partitioning coefficient'). Although it is tried in this documentation to use 'air', 'soil' and 'water' only for the air, soil and water compartment(s), respectively and not for phases, these terms are used here nevertheless as the notions 'solid-water partitioning coefficient' as well as the 'air-water partitioning coefficient' are commonly used.

C.1.1 Solid-water partitioning coefficient

In order to determine the solid-water partitioning coefficient, there are different approaches for different substances.

Lipophilic, non-dissociating organic substances

For lipophilic, non-dissociating substances, it is most common to base the solid-water partition coefficient on the octanol-water partition coefficient (K_{ow}). Usually first an organic carbon-water partition coefficient (K_{oc}) is derived (e.g., Brandes et al., 1996; Seth et al., 1999; McKone and Bennett, 2003). However, there is evidence that the goodness of the correlation between these two parameters is to be questioned (e.g., Seth et al., 1999; Baker et al., 2000, 2001). Seth et al. (1999) have shown that the usually good correlation between these two coefficients basically stems from an autocorrelation of the activity coefficient of the dissolved chemical fraction. Due to differing activity coefficients in the octanol phase and the organic carbon phase, a single correlation for all organic chemical classes is likely to be less accurate than class-specific models. This is supported by the observation that lipophilic organic chemicals although showing similar K_{ow} values have significantly different K_{oc} values (Chiou et al., 1998). Thus, Seth et al. (1999) recommend to use the following relationship:

$$K_{oc} = 0.00035 \cdot K_{ow} \tag{C-1}$$

where

0.00035 : empirical factor, conversion of theoretical unit from l per kg to m^3 per kg performed

K_{oc} : organic carbon-water partitioning coefficient [kg/kg C_{org} per kg/m^3_{water}]

K_{ow} : n-octanol water partitioning coefficient [kg/$m^3_{octanol}$ per kg/m^3_{water}].

Note that this is the partitioning coefficient between the organic carbon and the aqueous phase. In order to arrive at the overall partitioning coefficient between the aqueous and the (total) solid phase and assuming that the amount of chemical in the non-organic-carbon solid phase is zero, the solid-water partitioning coefficient is calculated by multiplying the K_{oc} value by the organic carbon content of the compartment:

$$K_{sw} = fr\_w_{\text{organic carbon/solid phase}} \cdot K_{oc} = 0.00035 \cdot fr\_w_{\text{organic carbon/solid phase}} \cdot K_{ow} \tag{C-2}$$

where

0.00035 : empirical factor, conversion of theoretical unit from l per kg to m^3 per kg performed fr_w : mass fraction of organic carbon in solid phase [kg C_{org} per $kg_{solid\ phase}$] (defined as described in section B.5)

K_{oc} : organic carbon-water partitioning coefficient [kg/kg C_{org} per $kg/m^3{}_{water}$]

K_{ow} : n-octanol water partitioning coefficient [$kg/m^3{}_{octanol}$ per $kg/m^3{}_{water}$]

K_{sw} : solid-water partitioning coefficient [$kg/kg_{solid\ phase}$ per $kg/m^3{}_{water}$].

It needs to be stressed that the selection of a well predictive data estimation function for the solid-water partitioning coefficient is crucial as this is one of the most sensitive/important parameters in multimedia models when modelling semi-volatile organic substances (e.g., McKone, 1993b; Baker et al., 2001). As argued by Seth et al. (1999), class-specific regression models would be favourable. In particular, a separate relationship for Polycyclic Aromatic Hydrocarbons (PAHs) seems advisable (Chiou et al., 1998; Seth et al., 1999). A Quantitative Structure Activity Relationship (QSAR) that seems to be rather good in predicting K_{oc} values of (at least very hydrophobic) PAHs was presented by Baker et al. (2001). Although it is based on 'several easily calculable descriptors', the easiness comes with a profound knowledge of chemistry for deriving molecular connectivity indices which might not be available to all possible end users. Fairly recently, an entirely different approach has been proposed by Breivik and Wania (2003).

Trace elements

When acquiring data for heavy metals or trace elements, it is recommended to use solid-water partition coefficients (mostly referred to as K_d-values) of aged samples. 'Aged samples' means that the heavy metals applied to soil should be allowed some time to sorb to the soil matrix before the actual partitioning coefficient is determined.

Solid-water partition coefficients used

Within WATSON, the solid-water partition coefficients may be allowed to either depend on pH or on the organic carbon content, for trace elements or hydrophobic organic substances respectively. According to the prioritisation of substances (cf. section 3.2), the values used in this study are given in Table C-1.

Table C-1: pH-dependent solid-water partitioning coefficients (K_d) [$kg/kg_{solid\ phase}$ per $kg/m^3_{aqueous\ phase}$]

Trace element	pH range	K_d	Remarks
Arsenic	3.00 - 5.75	25.0	value for pH 4.9 adopted (United States - Environmental Protection Agency, 1998)
	5.75 - 6.25	26.9	geometric mean of value for pH 4.9 and 6.8 (United States - Environmental Protection Agency, 1998)
	6.25 - 7.25	29.0	value for pH 6.8 adopted (United States - Environmental Protection Agency, 1998)
	7.25 - 7.75	30.0	geometric mean of value for pH 6.8 and 8 (United States - Environmental Protection Agency, 1998)
	7.75 - 9.60	31.0	value for pH 8 adopted (United States - Environmental Protection Agency, 1998)
Cadmium	3.00 - 4.75	0.011	geometric mean of minimum and maximum value for pH 3-5 (Anonymous, 1999b)
	4.75 - 5.25	0.045	geometric mean of minimum and maximum values for pH 3-5 and 5-8 (Anonymous, 1999b)
	5.25 - 7.75	0.18	geometric mean of minimum and maximum value for pH 5-8 (Anonymous, 1999b)
	7.75 - 8.25	0.38	geometric mean of minimum and maximum values for pH 5-8 and 8-10 (Anonymous, 1999b)
	8.25 - 10.0	0.79	geometric mean of minimum and maximum value for pH 8-10 (Anonymous, 1999b)

Table C-1: pH-dependent solid-water partitioning coefficients (K_d) [$kg/kg_{solid\ phase}$ per $kg/m^3_{aqueous\ phase}$]

Trace element	pH range	K_d	Remarks
Chromium	3.00 - 5.75	1.20	value for pH 4.9 adopted, influence of competing anions and iron oxides not considered (United States - Environmental Protection Agency, 1998)
	5.75 - 6.25	46.5	geometric mean of value for pH 4.9 and 6.8, influence of competing anions and iron oxides not considered (United States - Environmental Protection Agency, 1998)
	6.25 - 7.25	1800	value for pH 6.8 adopted, influence of competing anions and iron oxides not considered (United States - Environmental Protection Agency, 1998)
	7.25 - 7.75	2782	geometric mean of value for pH 6.8 and 8, influence of competing anions and iron oxides not considered (United States - Environmental Protection Agency, 1998)
	7.75 - 9.60	4300	value for pH 8 adopted, influence of competing anions and iron oxides not considered (United States - Environmental Protection Agency, 1998)
Lead	3.75 - 6.75	0.88	geometric mean of minimum and maximum value for pH 4.0-6.3 and equilibrium lead concentrations of 1.0-99.9 µg/l (Anonymous, 1999b)
	6.75 - 8.75	3.11	geometric mean of minimum and maximum value for pH 6.4-8.7 and equilibrium lead concentrations of 1.0-99.9 µg/l (Anonymous, 1999b)
	8.75 - 11.0	7.01	geometric mean of minimum and maximum value for pH 8.7-11.0 and equilibrium lead concentrations of 1.0-99.9 µg/l (Anonymous, 1999b)

C.1.2 Air-water partitioning coefficient

The air-water partitioning coefficient is used when one has to deal with (semi-) volatile substances, i.e., those substances that have an appreciable vapour pressure at ambient temperatures. The (dimensionless) air-water partitioning coefficient can be derived from the Henry's law constant according to:

$$K_{\text{aw,p}} = \frac{H(p)}{R \cdot T(z)} \tag{C-3}$$

where

H : Henry's law constant of substance p [Pa $m^3{}_{water}$ per mol]

K_{aw} : air-water partitioning coefficient or dimensionless Henry's law constant of substance p [-]

R : universal gas constant [Pa $m^3{}_{gas}$ per K per mol]; 8.314510 (Lide, 2002)

T : absolute ambient temperature in zone z [K] (defined as described in section B.5.5).

The Henry's law constant of metals (except for mercury) and dissociated organic compounds are assumed to be negligible. These are set to zero.

C.1.3 Air-solid partitioning coefficient

Usually the partitioning between the aqueous phase on the one hand and the solid or gas phase on the other are known from which the air-solid partitioning coefficient can be derived. According to Gibbs' phase rule, the degree of freedom is the number of components (here: mole fractions) minus the number of phases (e.g., in aerated soils: three, in water bodies and sediments: two) plus a constant of two:

$$F = K - P + 2 \tag{C-4}$$

where:

F : Degrees of freedom

K : Number of components

P : Number of phases.

Assuming we have a system of three phases, i.e., the aqueous, the solid and the gas phase. A substance in the system may consequently have potentially three 'places' where it could stay. The three mole fractions are the components. If a substance partitions into each of these phases, the components equal the phases and the degree of freedom is always 2. This would be the case for a true multimedia substance, i.e., one that is volatile, soluble in water to some degree and that sorbs to solid phases. All three partitioning coefficients need to be known one of which is determined if the other two are known. If another substance avoids one of the phases the degree of freedom is always one as the number of components is smaller than the phases present in the system. The behaviour of such a substance is determined by the partitioning coefficient between the two phases in which it can be found. This is the case for example for non-volatile metals. If again another substance avoids two of the three phases then no partition coefficient needs to be known to determine the behaviour of the substance in the system.

Depending on the value of the air-water partitioning coefficient, the air-solid partitioning coefficient may also become zero for instance for metals (except for mercury) and dissociated organic substances.

C.2 Substance properties influencing the exposure

There are several substance-dependent parameters used in the exposure assessment. These may additionally depend on different exposure assessment frameworks. In the following, it is, therefore, distinguished whether the parameters for which the values will be given are used

- irrespective of the exposure assessment framework (section C.2.1),
- in relation to the Human Health Risk Assessment Protocol for Hazardous Waste Combustion Facilities (HHRAP, United States - Environmental Protection Agency, 1998, section C.2.2), or
- by generic models for use in assessing the impact of discharges of radioactive substances to the environment (International Atomic Energy Agency, 2001, section C.2.3).

Note that the latter exposure assessment is less detailed than the former.

C.2.1 Exposure-related data independent of the exposure assessment framework used

In order to assess the effective Intake Fraction, it is necessary to define the mass fraction of a substance contained in food or ambient air that has the potential to exert an adverse effect. The values assumed are given in Table C-2.

Table C-2: Mass fraction of a substance contained in food leading to an effect ($fr\_w_{effective/total}$) [-]

Trace element	Exposure route	$fr\_w_{effective/total}$	Remarks
Arsenic	Ingestion	0.03	upper bound (Baxter and Lewis, 2002)
	Inhalation	1	inorganic forms of arsenic dominate the releases from high-temperature processes (Pacyna, 1987) which still appears to be valid today (Agency for Toxic Substances and Disease Registry, 2000b)
Cadmium	Ingestion	1	
	Inhalation	1	
Chromium	Ingestion	0.1	upper bound (Anonymous, 2002)
	Inhalation	0.1	only about 10-18 % of total chromium being emitted to air by oil and coal fired power plants as the primary source of particle-bound chromium to air is in the hexavalent state (French et al., 1998)
Lead	Ingestion	1	
	Inhalation	1	

C.2.2 Data related to the exposure assessment framework according to United States - Environmental Protection Agency (1998)

In the exposure assessment according to United States - Environmental Protection Agency (1998) several parameters are used which depend on the substance and sometimes also on the animal or plant through which humans are exposed (cf. section A.7). The values used are given in the following.

At equilibrium, the passive uptake of substances by an organism from its environment can be described with the help of the bioconcentration factor (BCF).

Table C-3: Bioconcentration factors (BCF) aqueous phase-freshwater fish [m^3/kg FW] (source: United States - Environmental Protection Agency, 1998)

Trace element	BCF	Remarks
Arsenic	0.02	Table A-3-14 (ibid.), BCF_{fish}, units adjusted
Cadmium	0.25	Table A-3-35 (ibid.), BCF_{fish}, units adjusted
Chromium	0.28	Table A-3-52 (ibid.), BCF_{fish}, units adjusted
Lead	0.008	Table A-3-128 (ibid.), BCF_{fish}, units adjusted, use of BAF instead of BCF

Depending on the medium from which the substances are taken up, one can distinguish BCFs for aquatic organisms from those for terrestrial organisms. Accordingly, the BCFs for fish and for vegetal produce are given separately in Tables C-3 and C-4, respectively.

Unlike passive uptake by plants and fish, farm animals actively take up feed and drinking water. In order to assess the concentration in animal products from daily pollutant intake at equilibrium, use is made of biotransfer factors (BTFs, Table C-5). Note the limited availability of BTFs for eggs, pork and poultry.

According to United States - Environmental Protection Agency (1998), uptake by root crops from soil is formulated in a K_{ow}-dependent way for any substance by introducing an empirical correction factor. Its value is 0.01 if the logarithm of the K_{ow} value is greater than 4 and 1 else. This is in line with the findings of Trapp (2002) for the dynamic case, however, at a different threshold. One may, therefore, consider to introduce a two-threshold approach where a correction factor of 0.1 could be used for instance at a log K_{ow} in the range of 2 to 4. Note that in the range between log K_{ow} from 1 or 2 to 4 the distribution behaviour of substances between aqueous phase and lipid phase of plants is in transition (cf. Figure 2 in Riederer, 1995).

As all trace elements considered in the present study have rather low values for K_{ow}, their correction factors are all set to unity (Table C-6).

Table C-4: Bioconcentration factors (BCF) for different vegetal produce [mol/kg plant DW per mol/kg soil DW] (source: United States - Environmental Protection Agency, 1998)

Trace element	Produce	BCF	Remarks
Arsenic	Aboveground exposed produce	0.013	Table A-3-14, Br_{ag}, adapted to 30 cm soil depth (see comment on page A-3-21, ibid.)
	Belowground produce	0.016	Table A-3-14, $Br_{rootveg}$, adapted to 30 cm soil depth (see comment on page A-3-19, ibid.)
	Cereals	0.008	Table A-3-14, Br_{grain}, adapted to 30 cm soil depth (see comment on page A-3-21, ibid.)
	Grass, forage	0.072	Table A-3-14, Br_{forage}, adapted to 30 cm soil depth (see comment on page A-3-2, ibid.1)
	Silage	0.072	Table A-3-14, Br_{forage}, adapted to 30 cm soil depth (see comment on page A-3-21, ibid.), value also applies to silage
Cadmium	Aboveground exposed produce	0.25	Table A-3-35, Br_{ag}, adapted to 30 cm soil depth (see comment on page A-3-21, ibid.)
	Belowground produce	0.13	Table A-3-35, $Br_{rootveg}$, adapted to 30 cm soil depth (see comment on page A-3-19, ibid.)
	Cereals	0.12	Table A-3-35, Br_{grain}, adapted to 30 cm soil depth (see comment on page A-3-21, ibid.)
	Grass, forage	0.73	Table A-3-35, Br_{forage}, adapted to 30 cm soil depth (see comment on page A-3-21, ibid.)
	Silage	0.73	Table A-3-35, Br_{forage}, adapted to 30 cm soil depth (see comment on page A-3-21, ibid.), value also applies to silage

Table C-4: Bioconcentration factors (BCF) for different vegetal produce [mol/kg plant DW per mol/kg soil DW] (source: United States - Environmental Protection Agency, 1998)

Trace element	Produce	BCF	Remarks
Chromium	Aboveground exposed produce	0.0049	Table A-3-52, Br_{ag}
	Belowground produce	0.0045	Table A-3-52, $Br_{rootveg}$
	Cereals	0.0045	Table A-3-52, Br_{grain}
	Grass, forage	0.0075	Table A-3-52, Br_{forage}
	Silage	0.0075	Table A-3-52, Br_{forage}, value also applies to silage
Lead	Aboveground exposed produce	0.014	Table A-3-128, Br_{ag}
	Belowground produce	0.009	Table A-3-128, $Br_{rootveg}$
	Cereals	0.009	Table A-3-128, Br_{grain}
	Grass, forage	0.045	Table A-3-128, Br_{forage}
	Silage	0.045	Table A-3-128, Br_{forage}, value also applies to silage

Table C-5: Biotransfer factors (BTF) relating daily pollutant intake to contents in animal produce [s·capita/kg FW] (source: United States - Environmental Protection Agency, 1998)

Trace element	Produce	BTF	Remarks
Arsenic	Beef and veal	173	Table A-3-14, Ba_{beef}, units adjusted
	Cow milk and products	518	Table A-3-14, Ba_{milk}, units adjusted
	Eggs	n/a	Table A-3-14, Ba_{egg}, not defined
	Pork	n/a	Table A-3-14, Ba_{pork}, not defined
	Poultry	n/a	Table A-3-14, $Ba_{chicken}$, not defined
Cadmium	Beef and veal	10.4	Table A-3-35, Ba_{beef}, units adjusted
	Cow milk and products	0.56	Table A-3-35, Ba_{milk}, units adjusted
	Eggs	216	Table A-3-35, Ba_{egg}, units adjusted
	Pork	16.5	Table A-3-35, Ba_{pork}, units adjusted
	Poultry	9158	Table A-3-35, $Ba_{chicken}$, units adjusted
Chromium	Beef and veal	475	Table A-3-52, Ba_{beef}, units adjusted
	Cow milk and products	130	Table A-3-52, Ba_{milk}, units adjusted
	Eggs	n/a	Table A-3-52, Ba_{egg}, not defined
	Pork	n/a	Table A-3-52, Ba_{pork}, not defined
	Poultry	n/a	Table A-3-52, $Ba_{chicken}$, not defined
Lead	Beef and veal	25.9	Table A-3-128, Ba_{beef}, units adjusted
	Cow milk and products	21.6	Table A-3-128, Ba_{milk}, units adjusted

Table C-5: Biotransfer factors (BTF) relating daily pollutant intake to contents in animal produce [s·capita/kg FW] (source: United States - Environmental Protection Agency, 1998)

Trace element	Produce	BTF	Remarks
Lead (continued)	Eggs	n/a	Table A-3-128, Ba_{egg}, not defined
	Pork	n/a	Table A-3-128, Ba_{pork}, not defined
	Poultry	n/a	Table A-3-128, $Ba_{chicken}$, not defined

Table C-6: Empirical correction factor ($emp_{BCF,\ root\ crop}$) for equilibrium uptake by belowground produce depending on the substance's octanol-water partitioning coefficient (K_{ow}) [-] (source: United States - Environmental Protection Agency, 1998, p. 5-35)

Trace element	$emp_{BCF,\ root\ crop}$
Arsenic	1
Cadmium	1
Chromium	1
Lead	1

Table C-7: Mass fraction adhering to aboveground exposed produce during wet deposition ($fr\_w_{adhere/wet\ deposition}$) [-] (source: United States - Environmental Protection Agency, 1998, Table B-2-7, p. B-78; value for cations and insoluble particles)

Trace element	$fr\_w_{adhere/wet\ deposition}$
Arsenic	0.6
Cadmium	0.6
Chromium	0.6
Lead	0.6

The exposure assessment by United States - Environmental Protection Agency (1998), furthermore, distinguishes between cations and anions in terms of their adhesion to vegetal surfaces upon intercepted wet deposition (Table C-7).

C.2.3 Data related to the exposure assessment framework according to International Atomic Energy Agency (2001)

During model evaluation, a second exposure assessment framework has been employed (cf. Table 9-4). Table C-8 provides the corresponding values used.

Table C-8: Parameter values used for the exposure assessment according to International Atomic Energy Agency (2001)

Trace element	Parameter	Unit	Receptors	Value[a]
Cadmium	bioconcentration factor for aboveground produce	mol/kg plant DW per mol/kg soil DW	Grass, forage	5
	bioconcentration factor soil-plant	mol/kg plant FW per mol/kg soil DW	All crops considered	0.5
	biotransfer factor daily pollutant intake to milk	s/m^3	Cow milk and products	1728000
	biotransfer factor relating daily pollutant intake to meat	s·capita/kg FW	Beef and veal	86.4
Lead	bioconcentration factor for aboveground produce	mol/kg plant DW per mol/kg soil DW	Grass, forage	0.1
	bioconcentration factor soil-plant	mol/kg plant FW per mol/kg soil DW	All crops considered	0.02
	biotransfer factor daily pollutant intake to milk	s/m^3	Cow milk and products	25920
	biotransfer factor relating daily pollutant intake to meat	s·capita/kg FW	Beef and veal	60.48

a. Found in Table XI, adherent soil particles are included.

C.3 Monitoring data on media and food concentrations

In Chapter 9, a comparison of the model results in terms of concentrations in different media and foodstuff with measured data has been carried out. The monitoring data as used in the Figures 9-3 through 9-6 are taken from the data compiled in Tables C-9 through C-12 for arsenic, cadmium, chromium and lead, respectively. The values used are highlighted in bold. If the lower limit was reported to be below the detection limit (indicated by a ’<’ before the numbers), half of that value was taken.

Table C-9: Reported arsenic concentrations in environmental media and foodstuff

Medium or food item	Type of value	Value	Unit	Remarks
Upper continental crust	expectation value/range	**2.0**	[mg/kg]	Table 1 (Wedepohl, 1995); natural background value
Any soil	total range	**0.07-95**	[mg/kg DW]	Table 120 (Kabata-Pendias and Pendias, 2001); minimum and maximum values in Fig. 9-3
		<0.2-83	[mg/kg DW]	only top soils and particles smaller than 2 mm considered (Reimann and de Caritat, 1998)
	expectation value/range	0.1-20	[mg/kg]	Gebel (1999)
		0.5-**6.6**	[mg/kg DW]	median range; only top soils and particles smaller than 2 mm considered (Reimann and de Caritat, 1998); median value in Fig. 9-3
		0.2-41	[mg/kg DW]	arithmetic mean, Table 120 (Kabata-Pendias and Pendias, 2001)
	maximum value due to local contamination	100-2500	[mg/kg]	copper processing (Gebel, 1999)
		2500	[mg/kg DW]	metal processing, Table 121 (Kabata-Pendias and Pendias, 2001)
		2000	[mg/kg DW]	chemical works, Table 121 (Kabata-Pendias and Pendias, 2001)
Agricultural soil	total range	**<0.2-19**	[mg/kg DW]	only top soils and particles smaller than 2 mm considered (Reimann and de Caritat, 1998); minimum and maximum values in Fig. 9-3

Table C-9: Reported arsenic concentrations in environmental media and foodstuff

Medium or food item	Type of value	Value	Unit	Remarks
Agricultural soil (continued)	expectation value/range	**1.55-6.6**	[mg/kg DW]	median range; only top soils and particles smaller than 2 mm considered (Reimann and de Caritat, 1998); median value in Fig. 9-3 obtained by averaging
	maximum value due to local contamination	700	[mg/kg]	arsenic-containing herbicide application (Gebel, 1999)
		625	[mg/kg DW]	application of arsenical pesticides, Table 121 (Kabata-Pendias and Pendias, 2001)
Surface water	total range	**$<1 \cdot 10^{-5}$ - $2.5 \cdot 10^{-2}$**	[mg/l]	unfiltered samples (Reimann and de Caritat, 1998); minimum and maximum values in Fig. 9-3
	expectation value/range	**$2 \cdot 10^{-4}$ - $1.4 \cdot 10^{-3}$**	[mg/l]	median range, unfiltered samples (Reimann and de Caritat, 1998); median value in Fig. 9-3 obtained by averaging
Sediments	total range	**<2-1305**	[mg/kg DW]	only particles smaller than 0.18 mm considered (Reimann and de Caritat, 1998); minimum and maximum values in Fig. 9-3
	expectation value/range	**2-12**	[mg/kg DW]	median range, only particles smaller than 0.18 mm considered (Reimann and de Caritat, 1998); median value in Fig. 9-3 obtained by averaging
Cereals	total range	**<0.1-365**	[µg/kg FW]	range for baking goods and cereals, Table 1 (Gebel, 1999); minimum and maximum values in Fig. 9-3

Table C-9: Reported arsenic concentrations in environmental media and foodstuff

Medium or food item	Type of value	Value	Unit	Remarks
Cereals (continued)	expectation value/range	**24.5**	[µg/kg FW]	arithmetic mean for baking goods and cereals, Table 1 (Gebel, 1999); 'median' value in Fig. 9-3
		0.3-40	[µg/kg FW]	Table 122 (Kabata-Pendias and Pendias, 2001) [a]
Potatoes	expectation value/range	**14.2**	[µg/kg FW]	arithmetic mean, baked potatoes, Table 1 (Gebel, 1999); 'median' value in Fig. 9-3
		5.0-33.4	[µg/kg FW]	Table 122 (Kabata-Pendias and Pendias, 2001); minimum and maximum values in Fig. 9-3 [a]
	maximum value	183	[µg/kg FW]	tuber peels after application of arsenical pesticides, Table 123 (Kabata-Pendias and Pendias, 2001) [a]
Vegetables	total range	<0.1-84	[µg/kg FW]	range, Table 1 (Gebel, 1999)
	expectation value/range	7.0	[µg/kg FW]	arithmetic mean, Table 1 (Gebel, 1999)
Spinach	expectation value/range	**16.8-126**	[µg/kg FW]	Table 122 (Kabata-Pendias and Pendias, 2001) [a]; minimum and maximum values in Fig. 9-3; 'median' value in Fig. 9-3 obtained by averaging

Table C-9: Reported arsenic concentrations in environmental media and foodstuff

Medium or food item	Type of value	Value	Unit	Remarks
Freshwater fish	total range	**29-555**	[µg/kg FW]	range, Table 1 (Gebel, 1999); minimum and maximum values in Fig. 9-3
	expectation value/range	**160**	[µg/kg FW]	arithmetic mean, Table 1 (Gebel, 1999); 'median' value in Fig. 9-3
Milk and dairy products	total range	**<0.4-26.0**	[µg/kg FW]	range, Table 1 (Gebel, 1999); minimum and maximum values in Fig. 9-3
	expectation value/range	**33.8**	[µg/kg FW]	arithmetic mean, Table 1 (Gebel, 1999); 'median' value in Fig. 9-3
Meat	expectation value/range	**6**	[µg/kg FW]	arithmetic mean, Table 1 (Gebel, 1999); 'median' value in Fig. 9-3
Poultry	expectation value/range	35.9	[µg/kg FW]	arithmetic mean, Table 1 (Gebel, 1999)

a. Converted from mg/kg DW into mg/kg FW according to mass fractions of food dry matter (cf. Table B-22).

Table C-10: Reported cadmium concentrations in environmental media and foodstuff

Medium or food item	Type of value	Value	Unit	Remarks
Upper continental crust	expectation value/range	**0.102**	[mg/kg]	Table 1 (Wedepohl, 1995); natural background value
Any soil	total range	**<0.01-40.9**	[mg/kg DW]	only top soils and particles smaller than 2 mm considered (Reimann and de Caritat, 1998); minimum and maximum values in Fig. 9-4
		0.01-4	[mg/kg DW]	Table 71 (Kabata-Pendias and Pendias, 2001)
	expectation value/range	0.117-**0.7**	[mg/kg DW]	median range; only top soils and particles smaller than 2 mm considered (Reimann and de Caritat, 1998); median value in Fig. 9-4
		0.06-1.1	[mg/kg DW]	arithmetic mean, Table 71 (Kabata-Pendias and Pendias, 2001)
		<0.01-0.5	[mg/kg DW]	Table 8.1 (Stoeppler, 1992)
	maximum value due to local contamination	1781	[mg/kg DW]	metal processing, Table 72 (Kabata-Pendias and Pendias, 2001)
		10	[mg/kg DW]	roadside, Table 72 (Kabata-Pendias and Pendias, 2001)
		<0.2- >50	[mg/kg DW]	typical polluted value, Table 8.1 (Stoeppler, 1992)
Agricultural soil	total range	**<0.01-3.8**	[mg/kg DW]	only top soils and particles smaller than 2 mm considered (Reimann and de Caritat, 1998); minimum and maximum values in Fig. 9-4
		0.037-0.908	[mg/kg DW]	Table 2.8 (Traina, 1999)

Table C-10: Reported cadmium concentrations in environmental media and foodstuff

Medium or food item	Type of value	Value	Unit	Remarks
Agricultural soil (continued)	expectation value/range	0.117-**0.3**	[mg/kg DW]	median range; only top soils and particles smaller than 2 mm considered (Reimann and de Caritat, 1998); median value in Fig. 9-4
		0.2-1.0	[mg/kg]	rural areas, Table 1 (Ewers and Wilhelm, 1995)
		0.5-1.5	[mg/kg]	urban areas, Table 1 (Ewers and Wilhelm, 1995)
	maximum value due to local contamination	167	[mg/kg DW]	sludged, irrigated, or fertilized farmland, Table 72 (Kabata-Pendias and Pendias, 2001)
Surface water	total range	**$<2 \cdot 10^{-6}$- $9.6 \cdot 10^{-3}$**	[mg/l]	unfiltered samples (Reimann and de Caritat, 1998); minimum and maximum values in Fig. 9-4
	expectation value/range	**$<2 \cdot 10^{-5}$- $2.9 \cdot 10^{-4}$**	[mg/l]	median range, unfiltered samples (Reimann and de Caritat, 1998); median value in Fig. 9-4 obtained by averaging
		$<5 \cdot 10^{-5}$- $2 \cdot 10^{-4}$	[mg/l]	dissolved and particulate bound, Table 8.1 (Stoeppler, 1992)
		$1 \cdot 10^{-5}$- $4 \cdot 10^{-5}$	[mg/l]	Table 1 (Ewers and Wilhelm, 1995)
River sediments	expectation value/range	**0.04-0.8**	[mg/kg DW]	Table 8.1 (Stoeppler, 1992); minimum and maximum values in Fig. 9-4; median value in Fig. 9-4 obtained by averaging

Table C-10: Reported cadmium concentrations in environmental media and foodstuff

Medium or food item	Type of value	Value	Unit	Remarks
River sediments (continued)	maximum value due to local contamination	30-800	[mg/kg DW]	typical polluted value, Table 8.1 (Stoeppler, 1992)
Cereals	total range	**<0.0011-1.44**	[mg/kg FW]	Table 75 (Kabata-Pendias and Pendias, 2001); minimum and maximum values in Fig. 9-4 [a]
	expectation value/range	**0.012-0.244**	[mg/kg FW]	median range, Table 75 (Kabata-Pendias and Pendias, 2001); median value in Fig. 9-4 obtained by averaging [a]
		≤0.04	[mg/kg FW]	wheat flour, wheat bread, bran, potatoes root and foliage vegetables, rice, Table 8.1 (Stoeppler, 1992)
Potatoes	total range	**0.0003-0.435**	[mg/kg FW]	Table 2 (Ewers and Wilhelm, 1995); minimum and maximum values in Fig. 9-4
	expectation value/range	**0.001-0.09**	[mg/kg FW]	median range, Table 73 (Kabata-Pendias and Pendias, 2001); median value in Fig. 9-4 obtained by averaging
		≤0.04	[mg/kg FW]	wheat flour, wheat bread, bran, potatoes root and foliage vegetables, rice, Table 8.1 (Stoeppler, 1992)
		0.016	[mg/kg FW]	median, Table 2 (Ewers and Wilhelm, 1995)

Table C-10: Reported cadmium concentrations in environmental media and foodstuff

Medium or food item	Type of value	Value	Unit	Remarks
Spinach leaves	maximum value due to local contamination	**0.33** - 0.54	[mg/kg FW]	Table 74 (Kabata-Pendias and Pendias, 2001); 'median' value in Fig. 9-4 [a]
Fish	expectation value/range	**<0.0025**	[mg/kg FW]	fish muscle, Table 8.1 (Stoeppler, 1992); median value in Fig. 9-4 [a]
Meat	expectation value/range	**≤0.005**	[mg/kg FW]	meat from various animals, Table 8.1 (Stoeppler, 1992); median value in Fig. 9-4
		<0.05	[mg/kg FW]	Ewers and Wilhelm (1995)
Eggs	expectation value/range	**<0.05**	[mg/kg FW]	Ewers and Wilhelm (1995); median value in Fig. 9-4
Milk and dairy products	expectation value/range	**≤0.001**	[mg/kg FW]	Table 8.1 (Stoeppler, 1992); median value in Fig. 9-4
		<0.05	[mg/kg FW]	Ewers and Wilhelm (1995)

a. Converted from mg/kg DW into mg/kg FW according to mass fractions of food dry matter (cf. Table B-22).

Table C-11: Reported chromium concentrations in environmental media and foodstuff

Medium or food item	Type of value	Value	Unit	Remarks
Upper continental crust	expectation value/range	**35**	[mg/kg]	Table 1 (Wedepohl, 1995); natural background value
Any soil	total range	1-**1500**	[mg/kg DW]	Table 137 (Kabata-Pendias and Pendias, 2001); maximum value in Fig. 9-5
		0.2-838	[mg/kg DW]	only top soils and particles smaller than 2 mm considered (Reimann and de Caritat, 1998); minimum value in Fig. 9-5
	expectation value/range	19.1-**80**	[mg/kg DW]	median range; only top soils and particles smaller than 2 mm considered (Reimann and de Caritat, 1998); median value in Fig. 9-5
		10-90	[mg/kg]	Table 1 on environmental loads (Hertl and Merk, 1999); values may, therefore, represent expectation values of non-pristine soils
		7-221	[mg/kg DW]	arithmetic mean, Table 137 (Kabata-Pendias and Pendias, 2001)
Agricultural soil	total range	**<5-510**	[mg/kg DW]	only top soils and particles smaller than 2 mm considered (Reimann and de Caritat, 1998); minimum and maximum values in Fig. 9-5
	expectation value/range	**19.1-57**	[mg/kg DW]	median range; only top soils and particles smaller than 2 mm considered (Reimann and de Caritat, 1998); median value in Fig. 9-5 obtained by averaging
Surface water	total range	**$<1 \cdot 10^{-4}$ - 0.179**	[mg/l]	unfiltered samples (Reimann and de Caritat, 1998); minimum and maximum values in Fig. 9-5

Table C-11: Reported chromium concentrations in environmental media and foodstuff

Medium or food item	Type of value	Value	Unit	Remarks
Surface water (continued)	expectation value/range	0.001-0.01	[mg/l]	Table 1 on environmental loads (Hertl and Merk, 1999); values may, therefore, represent expectation values of non-pristine freshwater
		$<1 \cdot 10^{-4}$ - $9.7 \cdot 10^{-3}$	[mg/l]	median range, unfiltered samples (Reimann and de Caritat, 1998); median value in Fig. 9-5 obtained by averaging
Sediments	total range	**<5-3176**	[mg/kg DW]	only particles smaller than 0.18 mm considered (Reimann and de Caritat, 1998); minimum and maximum values in Fig. 9-5
	expectation value/range	**64-161**	[mg/kg DW]	median range, only particles smaller than 0.18 mm considered (Reimann and de Caritat, 1998); 'median' value in Fig. 9-5 obtained by averaging
Cereals	expectation value/range	4	[µg/kg]	Hertl and Merk (1999) [a,b]
		1.4-55	[µg/kg FW]	Table 138 (Kabata-Pendias and Pendias, 2001) [b]; minimum and maximum values in Fig. 9-5; 'median' value in Fig. 9-5 obtained by averaging
Potatoes	expectation value/range	**3.5**	[µg/kg FW]	Table 138 (Kabata-Pendias and Pendias, 2001) [b]; median value in Fig. 9-5
Vegetables	expectation value/range	**2.5**	[µg/kg]	Hertl and Merk (1999) [a,b]; median value in Fig. 9-5

Table C-11: Reported chromium concentrations in environmental media and foodstuff

Medium or food item	Type of value	Value	Unit	Remarks
Freshwater fish	expectation value/range	**27.2**	[μg/kg]	Hertl and Merk (1999) [a,b]; median value in Fig. 9-5
Milk and dairy products	expectation value/range	**100**	[μg/kg]	Hertl and Merk (1999) [a]; median value in Fig. 9-5
Meat	expectation value/range	**78.8**	[μg/kg]	Hertl and Merk (1999) [a,b]; median value in Fig. 9-5

a. There is neither an indication of whether the concentration is given for fresh or dry weight nor whether the values are representative for 'pristine' or contaminated situations; it is assumed that the concentrations provided for foodstuff other than milk and dairy products is on a dry weight-basis.
b. Converted from mg/kg DW into mg/kg FW according to mass fractions of food dry matter (cf. Table B-22).

Table C-12: Reported lead concentrations in environmental media and foodstuff

Medium or food item	Type of value	Value	Unit	Remarks
Upper continental crust	expectation value/range	**17**	[mg/kg]	Table 1 (Wedepohl, 1995); natural background value
Any soil	total range	3-16338	[mg/kg DW]	only top soils and particles smaller than 2 mm considered (Reimann and de Caritat, 1998)
		1.5-286	[mg/kg DW]	Table 110 (Kabata-Pendias and Pendias, 2001)
		1.5-888	[mg/kg DW]	Table 2.21 (Nriagu, 1978); minimum and maximum values in Fig. 9-6
	expectation value/range	7.45-40	[mg/kg DW]	median range; only top soils and particles smaller than 2 mm considered (Reimann and de Caritat, 1998)
		7.9-84	[mg/kg DW]	arithmetic mean, Table 110 (Kabata-Pendias and Pendias, 2001); 'median' value in Fig. 9-6 obtained by averaging
	maximum value due to local contamination	18500	[mg/kg DW]	metal processing, Table 111 (Kabata-Pendias and Pendias, 2001)
		30000	[mg/kg DW]	'geologically polluted' soils, Table 2.11 (Nriagu, 1978)
		7000	[mg/kg DW]	roadside, Table 111 (Kabata-Pendias and Pendias, 2001)
Agricultural soil	total range	3-192	[mg/kg DW]	only top soils and particles smaller than 2 mm considered (Reimann and de Caritat, 1998)

Table C-12: Reported lead concentrations in environmental media and foodstuff

Medium or food item	Type of value	Value	Unit	Remarks
Agricultural soil (continued)	total range (continued)	**1.5-888**	[mg/kg DW]	Table 2.21 (Nriagu, 1978); minimum and maximum values in Fig. 9-6
	expectation value/range	7.45-14	[mg/kg DW]	median range; only top soils and particles smaller than 2 mm considered (Reimann and de Caritat, 1998)
		10-247	[mg/kg DW]	Table 2.21 (Nriagu, 1978); 'median' value in Fig. 9-6 obtained by averaging
	maximum value due to local contamination	3916	[mg/kg DW]	sludged farmland, Table 111 (Kabata-Pendias and Pendias, 2001)
Surface water	total range	**$<10^{-5}$-0.58**	[mg/l]	unfiltered samples (Reimann and de Caritat, 1998); minimum and maximum values in Fig. 9-6
	expectation value/range	**$2.1 \cdot 10^{-4}$-$3.4 \cdot 10^{-3}$**	[mg/l]	median range, unfiltered samples (Reimann and de Caritat, 1998); 'median' value in Fig. 9-6 obtained by averaging
Lake sediments	total range	**<0.1-5000**	[mg/kg DW]	Nriagu (1978); minimum and maximum values in Fig. 9-6

Table C-12: Reported lead concentrations in environmental media and foodstuff

Medium or food item	Type of value	Value	Unit	Remarks
Lake sediments (continued)	expectation value/range	**16**	[mg/kg DW]	Nriagu (1978); 'median' value in Fig. 9-6 obtained by averaging the lake value with the river value
		95	[mg/kg DW]	average lake sediment concentration with evidence of pollution (Nriagu, 1978)
River sediments	total range	3.9-3700	[mg/kg DW]	Table 2.29 (Nriagu, 1978)
	expectation value/range	**23**	[mg/kg DW]	Nriagu (1978); 'median' value in Fig. 9-6 obtained by averaging the lake value with the river value
		98	[mg/kg DW]	average riverine sediment concentration with evidence of pollution (Nriagu, 1978)
Cereals	total range	**<0.01-40**	[mg/kg FW]	Table 113 (Kabata-Pendias and Pendias, 2001) [a]; minimum and maximum values in Fig. 9-6
	expectation value/range	0.01-0.71	[mg/kg FW]	arithmetic mean range, Table 113 (Kabata-Pendias and Pendias, 2001) [a]
		0.05-**0.06**	[mg/kg FW]	median, Table 2b (Wilhelm and Ewers, 1999); median value in Fig. 9-6
	maximum value	0.45	[mg/kg FW]	98th percentile, Table 2b (Wilhelm and Ewers, 1999)
		40	[mg/kg FW]	Table 113 (Kabata-Pendias and Pendias, 2001) [a]

Table C-12: Reported lead concentrations in environmental media and foodstuff

Medium or food item	Type of value	Value	Unit	Remarks
Potatoes	expectation value/range	**0.08-0.50**	[mg/kg FW]	arithmetic mean range, Table 112 (Kabata-Pendias and Pendias, 2001) [a]; maximum and 'median' values in Fig. 9-6
		0.03	[mg/kg FW]	median, Table 2b (Wilhelm and Ewers, 1999); minimum value in Fig. 9-6
	maximum value	0.19	[mg/kg FW]	98th percentile, Table 2b (Wilhelm and Ewers, 1999)
		425	[mg/kg AW]	metal processing, ash weight basis, Table 115 (Kabata-Pendias and Pendias, 2001)
Leafy vegetables	expectation value/range	**0.04**	[mg/kg FW]	median, Table 2b (Wilhelm and Ewers, 1999); median value in Fig. 9-6
	maximum value	0.81	[mg/kg FW]	98th percentile, Table 2b (Wilhelm and Ewers, 1999)
		27.1	[mg/kg FW]	metal processing, Table 115 (Kabata-Pendias and Pendias, 2001) [a]
Fish	expectation value/range	**0.03**	[mg/kg FW]	median, Table 2a (Wilhelm and Ewers, 1999); median value in Fig. 9-6
	maximum value	0.37	[mg/kg FW]	98th percentile, Table 2a (Wilhelm and Ewers, 1999)
Eggs	expectation value/range	0.02	[mg/kg FW]	median, Table 2a (Wilhelm and Ewers, 1999)

Table C-12: Reported lead concentrations in environmental media and foodstuff

Medium or food item	Type of value	Value	Unit	Remarks
Eggs (continued)	maximum value	0.46	[mg/kg FW]	98th percentile, Table 2a (Wilhelm and Ewers, 1999)
Milk and dairy products	expectation value/range	0.01	[mg/l]	median for milk, Table 2a (Wilhelm and Ewers, 1999)
		0.07	[mg/kg FW]	median for cheese, Table 2a (Wilhelm and Ewers, 1999); median value in Fig. 9-6
	maximum value	0.04	[mg/l]	98th percentile for milk, Table 2a (Wilhelm and Ewers, 1999)
		1.17	[mg/kg FW]	98th percentile for cheese, Table 2a (Wilhelm and Ewers, 1999)
Pork	expectation value/range	**0.08**	[mg/kg FW]	median, Table 2a (Wilhelm and Ewers, 1999); median value for beef in Fig. 9-6
	maximum value	0.53	[mg/kg FW]	98th percentile, Table 2a (Wilhelm and Ewers, 1999)

a.Converted from mg/kg DW into mg/kg FW according to mass fractions of food dry matter (cf. Table B-22).

Appendix D Symbols, indices and compartment acronyms used for parameter and process description

In this Appendix, the symbols used in documenting equations are defined and described. Note that the symbols found in this part of the Appendix have not been used in section A.1 which is on the description of the overall matrix computations.

Table D-1 describes the symbols following the rule that for each symbol there is only one unit permitted. Table D-2 lists the dependencies as given in parentheses. These depend on the table (i.e., the necessary fields to be specified in order to define a value, 'degrees of freedom') in which the respective parameter is stored. Table D-3 shows the acronyms used for the compartments.

When defining the parameters in the database indices in parameter symbols are denoted by square brackets. These indices specify the context of a parameter more clearly when necessary.

In case the parameter is a value relating two values of the same unit (fractional value) the declaration in square brackets first states the numerator followed by a slash ('/') and then the denominator term.

Table D-1: Symbols and corresponding unique units used

Symbol	Name	Unit
aux	auxiliary parameter (e.g., for intermediate calculations)	variable
A	area	m^2
ATMDEP	atmospheric deposition	$kg/m^2/s$
BCF_dw/dw	bioconcentration factor in dry weight per dry weight	kg dry weight per kg dry weight
BCF_dw/fw	bioconcentration factor in dry weight per fresh weight	kg dry weight per kg fresh weight
BCF_V/fw	bioconcentration factor in volume per fresh weight	m^3/kg fresh weight
BW	body weight	kg per person
β_{ED10}	slope factor based on effective dose affecting 10 % of a population over background	individual lifetime risk per mg/kg Body Weight/day
C_w/v	concentration in weight per volume	kg/m^3
C_w/fw	concentration in weight per fresh weight	kg/kg FW of medium
C_w/dw	concentration in weight per dry weight	kg/kg DW of medium
C_w/w$_{phase\ x}$	concentration in weight per weight of phase x	kg/kg of phase x
d	depth	m
DALY	Disability Adjusted Life Years	years lost-equivalents (per incidence)
ED	equilibrium distribution relating bulk concentration to single phase concentration	kg/m^3 bulk per kg/m^3 phase

Table D-1: Symbols and corresponding unique units used

Symbol	Name	Unit
emp	empirical factor	(variable, only theoretical)
FCTF_t/v	food chain transfer factor in time per volume	s/m^3
FCTF_t/w	food chain transfer factor in time per weight	s/kg
fr_A	area fraction	-
fr_Q	discharge fraction	-
fr_r	fraction of a receptor belonging to a subgroup (e.g., risk groups within a population)	-
fr_v	'velocity' fraction, i.e., $m^3/m^2/s$ affected volume per $m^3/m^2/s$ bulk	-
fr_V	volume fraction	-
fr_w	mass fraction	-
H	Henry's law constant	$Pa{\cdot}m^3/mol$
IF	Intake Fraction	-
ING	intake rate (or ingestion) of, e.g., food and feed, but also soil per head (= caput)	kg fresh weight/ capita/s
INH	inhalation rate per head (= caput)	m^3/capita/s
IR	intake rate of, e.g., food and feed, but also soil (overall, aggregated)	kg/s
IR_p	personal intake rate	kg/capita/s
k	process rate in the environmental fate matrix	m^3/s
K_{ow}	n-octanol water partition coefficient	-
K_{sw} (or K_d)	solid-water partition coefficient	m^3/kg
ln(2)	natural logarithm of 2	-
M	mass	kg
MW	molecular weight	kg/mol

Table D-1: Symbols and corresponding unique units used

Symbol	Name	Unit
P	production, e.g., of food	kg fresh weight/s
pH	negative common logarithm of the hydronium ion activity	-
Q	discharge	m^3/s
R	universal or molar gas constant	$Pa{\cdot}m^3/mol/K$
r	rate	1/s
rho or ρ	density	kg/m^3
S	source strength, emission rate	kg/s[a]
SOL	solubility	kg/l
T	temperature	K
t	time	s[a]
V	volume	m^3
v	velocity	m/s
Y_dw	Yield based on dry weight	kg dry weight per m^2
Y_fw	Yield based on fresh weight	kg fresh weight per m^2
YLD	Years of Life lived with a Disability	years lost-equivalents (per incidence)
YOLL	Years of Life Lost	years lost (per incidence)

a. There are instances in this document where the time is given in years and not in seconds.

Table D-2: Symbols used to show degrees of freedom. Symbols occur in parentheses or as indices

Symbol	Meaning
c	compartment or compartment group
d	dependency on other parameters (e.g., pH)
e	exposure framework
i	impact or effect (type)
n	nation or other administrative unit
p	pollutant, substance
r	receptor
s	scenario
t	time
z	zone or (base) region

Table D-3: Compartment acronyms employed

Compartment	Acronym
air	a
fresh**w**ater body	w
fresh**w**ater **s**ediment	ws
ground**w**ater	gw
glacier	gl
impervious surface (**u**rban/built-up area)	u
(**b**are or) non-vegetated land	b
(semi-) **n**atural ecosystems	n
pasture/grassland	p
arable (or **ag**ricultural) land	ag

Index

F

H

I

L